S0-ASF-800

DIAGNOSTIC
IMAGING
REVIEW

DIAGNOSTIC IMAGING REVIEW

Gordon Gamsu, M.D.
Professor of Radiology and Vice Chairman
Cornell University Medical Center
New York, New York

Maitray D. Patel, M.D.
Chief of Ultrasound
San Francisco General Hospital

Assistant Professor of Radiology
University of California, San Francisco, School of Medicine
San Francisco, California

Senior Associate Consultant
Mayo Clinic Arizona
Scottsdale, Arizona

W.B. SAUNDERS COMPANY
A Division of Harcourt Brace & Company
Philadelphia • London • Toronto • Montreal • Sydney • Tokyo

W.B. SAUNDERS COMPANY
A Division of Harcourt Brace & Company

The Curtis Center
Independence Square West
Philadelphia, Pennsylvania 19106

Library of Congress Cataloging-in-Publication Data

Diagnostic imaging review / [edited by] Gordon Gamsu, Maitray Patel.

p.   cm.

ISBN 0–7216–3801–5

1. Diagnostic imaging.   I. Gamsu, Gordon.   II. Patel, Maitray.
   [DNLM: 1. Diagnostic Imaging.   WN 180 D5365 1998]

RC78.7.D53D5284 1998   616.07′54—dc21

DNLM/DLC   97–41325

DIAGNOSTIC IMAGING REVIEW   ISBN 0–7216–3801–5

Copyright © 1998 by W.B. Saunders Company

All rights reserved. No part of this publication may be reproduced or transmitted in any form or by any means, electronic or mechanical, including photocopy, recording, or any information storage and retrieval system, without permission in writing from the publisher.

Printed in the United States of America

Last digit is the print number: 9   8   7   6   5   4   3   2   1

To my wife, Indu,
and my parents, Kailas and Dasharath (MDP)

To Gay Morris-Gamsu and Jessica Gamsu,
who make it all worthwhile (GG)

Contributors

Barbara Binkert, M.D.
Associate Professor of Clinical
  Radiology,
  Cornell University Medical College;
  Associate Attending Radiology,
  New York Hospital-Cornell
  Medical Center,
  New York, New York
Nuclear Medicine

Calvin J. Cruz, Jr., M.D., Ph.D.
Minneapolis Radiology Associates,
  Minneapolis, Minnesota
Neuroimaging

Steven D. Frankel, M.D.
Assistant Clinical Professor of
  Radiology,
  University of California, San
  Francisco,
  School of Medicine, San Francisco,
  California
*Genitourinary Tract Imaging,
  Breast Imaging*

Gordon Gamsu, M.D.
Professor of Radiology and Vice
  Chairman, Cornell University
  Medical Center, New York, New
  York
*Thoracic Imaging,
  Heart and Great Vessel Imaging*

Stanley J. Goldsmith, M.D.
Professor of Radiology and Professor of
  Medicine,
  Cornell University Medical College;
  Director, Nuclear Medicine,
  Attending Radiology, and
  Co-Director, Nuclear Cardiology,

New York Hospital-Cornell Medical
  Center,
  New York, New York
Nuclear Medicine

James Hurley, M.D.
Associate Professor of Radiology and
  Associate Professor of Medicine,
  Cornell University Medical College;
  Associate Director, Department of
  Nuclear Medicine, New York
  Hospital-Cornell Medical Center,
  New York, New York
Nuclear Medicine

Carl L. Kalbhen, M.D.
Assistant Professor of Radiology,
  Loyola University of Chicago Stritch
  School of Medicine,
  Maywood, Illinois
Genitourinary Tract Imaging

Alan Laorr, M.D.
Radiologist, Fairview-University
  Medical Center;
  Musculoskeletal Radiologist;
  Suburban Radiologic Consultants,
  Ltd.,
  Minneapolis, Minnesota
Musculoskeletal Imaging

Maitray D. Patel, M.D.
Chief of Ultrasound, San Francisco
  General Hospital, Assistant Professor
  of Radiology, University of
  California, San Francisco, School of
  Medicine, San Francisco, California
*Alimentary Tract Imaging,
  Abdominal Viscera Imaging,
  Ultrasound*

Charles G. Peterfy, M.D., Ph.D.
Assistant Professor of Radiology,
   Medical Director of MRI Research,
   and Osteoporosis and
   Arthritis Research Group,
   Department of Radiology, University
   of California, San Francisco, School
   of Medicine, San Francisco,
   California
Musculoskeletal Imaging

Tracy Samples, M.D.
Chief, Pediatric Radiology,
   60th Medical Group David Grant
   Medical Center,
   Travis AFB, California
Pediatric Imaging

Scott Schultz, M.D.
Chief, Interventional Radiology,
   North Memorial Medical Center,
   Minneapolis, Minnesota
Interventional Radiology

Douglas Sides, M.D.
Raritan Radiology Associates,
   Perth Amboy, New Jersey
Ultrasound

Preface

As they approach their senior year, radiology residents begin to contemplate seriously one of the last challenges to their training years—board examinations. These residents are often perplexed as to the best way to prepare for these examinations. After all, most have been diligently reading textbooks, reviewing teaching files, and attending conferences during the preceding 3½ years; how does one begin to review this information and fill the gaps in one's knowledge? The dilemma is not unique to residents. Radiologists in practice often need to review periodically the fundamentals of radiology, especially the subspecialty areas in which they do not practice daily.

The difficulties faced by these individuals include the facts that (1) radiology textbooks are usually designed to impart information by describing diseases and demonstrating their imaging manifestations, whereas radiologists are required to recognize imaging manifestations and generate reasonable differential diagnoses; (2) residents and practicing radiologists have not usually organized their notes in a central place and in ways that make these notes accessible; and (3) while reviewing material many have difficulty in assessing which facts and concepts they have truly mastered and which they have momentarily memorized or merely glossed over.

Diagnostic Imaging Review was created to help radiologists overcome these obstacles. The book is of greatest value if used as a study companion and workbook. This text does not represent a review of all of radiology, and it should not be considered an all-inclusive compendium. It assists in the organization of material learned while participating in conferences, reviewing teaching files, studying reference works, and practicing radiology.

The book is organized into 12 chapters, each of which covers material relevant to one of the recognized sections of diagnostic imaging. Gastrointestinal imaging is subdivided into Alimentary Tract Imaging and Abdominal Viscera Imaging. Most chapters comprise three sections: an introductory overview, relevant differential diagnoses with discussion of features, and a list of disease entities considered to be the most important in that subspecialty area.

The introductory overview outlines an approach to imaging within the subspecialty.

The second section lists basic differential diagnoses for particular findings and discusses pertinent features of each diagnostic possibility as relates to that finding. This section is organized in a two-column format. On the right are differential diagnosis lists and the information regarding these entities. Included are figure references from important texts, listed by page number so that the reader can quickly review the appearances of various states and compare them with the images of other entities for their differentiation. We hope that the reader will note additional figure references from books and journals when encountered in daily reading.

Questions that test the reader's understanding of the material are presented on the left-hand column in the differential diagnosis section. These allow periodic self-evaluation. When possible, we have focused the questions on issues that help to distinguish one entity from another. The questions are not all inclusive. Once the reader has gained experience with a particular differential diagnosis and understands the concepts underlying these differences, additional questions or comments can be added. The best time to write questions is after the initial reading of the subject. For instance, a senior resident might spend time contemplating and recording important additional questions on the material. The act of writing questions is an important learning exercise, and the existing questions can serve as templates for this process.

The third section of most chapters is an alphabetical listing of entities relevant to the subspecialty field with important clinical and imaging data. The information is essential to the understanding of the important entities in each area of imaging. This section may be amended with the reader's own notes. When reviewing the differential diagnosis lists in section two, the reader can refer to section three to review basic information regarding any particular disease. This material represents the core information that an individual should be ready to proffer when discussing a particular diagnosis or disease.

This volume is the product of the collaborative efforts of a number of radiologists. We wish to thank the authors of each chapter for their efforts in conforming to a novel style. The book would not have been possible without the extensive editorial assistance of Ms. Barbara Cohen-Kligerman, who developed each chapter and was instrumental in ensuring that the authors completed their manuscripts. We also extend our gratitude to Lisette Bralow and the staff at W.B. Saunders Company for their assistance in compiling this text. Even though every attempt has been made to be as accurate as possible, factual oversights do occur. Both editors welcome comments and corrections.

We envision a text that provides the structure for referencing images and recording short notes that radiologists, in training and in practice, may encounter over the years, and a tool that provides the means for periodic rapid memory refreshment. Used this way, we hope that *Diagnostic Imaging Review* proves valuable to all students of radiology.

GORDON GAMSU, M.D.
MAITRAY D. PATEL, M.D.

Contents

Thoracic Imaging

■ Gordon Gamsu, M.D.

OVERVIEW

Thoracic imaging has a vocabulary of its own. Many of these terms are confusing and must be understood. A selected list of important thoracic imaging terms can be found in the Appendix.

ANATOMY AND PHYSIOLOGY

A few important facts need to be known about the anatomy and physiology of the lungs.

Lung Anatomy

The Airways. The airways are branching tubular structures, starting with the trachea, which is 10 to 12 cm long and 15 to 25 mm in diameter. The "conducting airways" are those without alveoli; they divide dichotomously for 12 to 27 generations, reaching the terminal bronchioles. The terminal bronchiole is the last nonalveolated airway. Bronchi have cartilage in their walls; bronchioles do not. Bronchioles have an internal diameter of about 1 mm or less. There are about 30,000 terminal bronchioles and thus 30,000 acini.

Beyond the terminal bronchioles are five to nine generations of respiratory bronchioles (partially alveolated) and alveolar ducts (all alveoli), terminating in alveolar sacs. There are approximately 300,000,000 alveoli, which are present by 8 to 10 years of age and increase in size until maturity. The regions beyond the terminal bronchioles are called the *exchange* portion of the respiratory system, because alveoli are present along the walls of all of these structures where gas exchange occurs. The general term for the lung beyond the conducting airways is the *lung parenchyma*, including the airways, small blood vessels, and support structures of the lung.

Pulmonary Arteries and Veins. The pulmonary arteries divide in a manner similar to that of the bronchi ("oak tree" branching pattern) and accompany the bronchi from the hila to the respiratory bronchioles. The pulmonary veins ("pine tree" branching pattern) are separate from the arteries and bronchi and have their own investing interstitial space in the interlobular septa. The smaller pulmonary venules lie in the interlobular septa, between the lobules. The pulmonary circulation is low pressure and capable of marked recruitment when cardiac output increases.

Bronchial Arteries and Veins. About 1% of the cardiac output goes through the bronchial arteries, which arise from the aorta near the tracheal bifurcation. There are usually two or three bronchial arteries that supply blood to the larger airways. Approximately half of the bronchial blood flow returns via systemic veins to the right heart and the other half via the pulmonary veins to the left side of the heart, having bypassed the pulmonary capillary bed.

Pulmonary Lymphatics. Lymphatics are present in the pleura, around veins, and around the bronchoarterial axis. Lymph from interstitial lung fluid flows to the hilar and mediastinal lymph nodes.

Pleura. The pleura consists of a mesothelial layer, a subepithelial layer, and a fibrovascular layer. The subepithelial layer is in direct contact with the interstitial space of the lung.

Pulmonary Physiology

The lung has both respiratory and metabolic functions. Although the latter are extremely important, the radiologist does not need to know much more than that the lung is capable of metabolic activity and does such things as convert angiotensin-1 to angiotensin-2 and extract serotonin.

The respiratory functions of the lungs are evaluated by pulmonary function studies. A radiologist needs to know the normal divisions of lung volumes (Table 1–1); the different measurements of flow rates, including the forced expiratory volume in 1 second (FEV_1) (usually recorded as a percentage of forced vital capacity [FVC]); what a flow:volume loop is; and FEF 25 to 75% (the flow rate expired between 25 and 75% of vital capacity).

Diffusing capacity is an important concept. It is measured by determining the diffusion of the highly soluble and diffusible gas carbon monoxide. It reflects the alveolar surface area in contact with the air on one side and thin-walled blood vessels on the other side. Disturbances in the diffusing capacity can be seen with any cause of decrease in the size of this membrane. Obstructive lung diseases such as emphysema and interstitial lung diseases can diminish the lung's diffusing capacity. In most circumstances, the disruption in diffusing capacity is from a mismatch of ventilation and perfusion. In only a few situations is the alveolar:capillary wall thickening sufficient to disturb diffusion of oxygen or carbon monoxide.

The pulmonary circulation is a low-pressure system with mean pressure of less than 22 torr, systolic pressure of less than 30, and diastolic pressure of approximately 14. The flow through the system can increase by 10-fold with virtually no increase in pressure, because of massive recruitment of parallel pathways. Diffusing capacity increases slightly with exercise, and the alveolar-arterial oxygen difference decreases with exercise. Diffusing capacity increases with left heart failure.

Table 1–1. Static Lung Volumes

TLC	Total lung capacity
VC	Vital capacity
RV	Residual volume
FRC	Functional residual capacity
TV	Tidal volume
IRV	Inspiratory reserve volume
ERV	Expiratory reserve volume
IC	Inspiratory capacity

INTERPRETATION OF CHEST IMAGES
Modalities

Chest Radiograph. In the patient with suspected intrathoracic disease, the chest radiograph is indivisible from the clinical examination. In many instances, it is obtained before the physical examination. This is not only expedient but also emphasizes the importance of using the chest radiograph and physical examination in combination.

Computed Tomography (CT) Scans. CT scans most often are used to give better information about the structure and density of a lesion first detected from a chest radiograph.

In an increasing number of situations (listed below), thoracic CT or high-resolution CT (HRCT) is used for the following:

Detection of lesions
> In high-risk situations, e.g., interstitial disease, bronchiectasis, emphysema
> In symptomatic patients with a normal chest radiograph
> In patients with unexplained abnormalities of pulmonary function

Localization for invasive procedures
> Aspiration biopsies
> Bronchoscopy (airway lesions and mediastinal nodes)
> Choosing the optimal site for open-lung biopsy or video-assisted thoracic surgery (VATS)
> Pleural drainage procedures

Appropriateness of mediastinoscopy
Staging of lung cancer
Volume reduction surgery
Detection of thoracic metastases or extent of lymphoma
Evaluate complex pleuropulmonary problems
Detect pulmonary emboli (spinal CT)

Magnetic Resonance Imaging (MRI). MRI has a limited clinical role in the thorax at this time, outside of the heart. The few indications are for the relationship of masses to vascular structures such as the pulmonary arteries and superior vena cava (SVC). It does not detect mediastinal/lung lesions better than CT does. MRI characterization of lesions for malignancy/tissue composition has been disappointing. Angiography with spiral CT is going to challenge MRI, even for vascular thoracic abnormalities such as dissections.

Other Modalities. Other modalities such as bronchography, pulmonary arteriography, and fluoroscopy of the thorax are being used with decreasing frequency or have been abandoned.

Interpretation

Chest Radiographs. Interpretation of chest radiographs (as well as CT and MRI images) requires experience that can be obtained only by reviewing a large number of studies. Sophisticated interpretation is mostly a learned skill. Each interpreter should develop a search pattern when viewing images, incorporating certain basic features. *One should have a routine that becomes second nature;* one's interpretations then will be more thorough and rewarding.

The most common errors in thoracic imaging occur when:

> The search process is halted after the first abnormal observation is made
> The interpreter's attention is captured by an obvious abnormality and less apparent findings go undetected
> The importance of a perceived abnormality is rejected (70% of "misses")

Most abnormalities that are missed can be detected with a methodical viewing of the radiographs (it sounds pedantic, but is true). Outlined as follows is a 10-point plan for reading the chest radiograph.

1

Before starting:

1. Review the **patient's name, age, sex**, and **clinical information** from the request form (if no clinical information is provided, state so in your report). This will give you a reasonable idea that you are dealing with the correct patient.
2. Make an overall assessment of the **quality of the examination**, noting the following:

    Exposure (with the presently suggested techniques, the intervertebral disc spaces in the lower thoracic spine should be visible)

    Rotation (use the relationship of the upper spinous processes to the medial ends of the clavicles)

    Whether any significant areas have been *coned off* of the radiograph

    Any *artifacts*
3. Compare one side of the thorax to the other for **symmetry,** noting:

    Relative height of the hemidiaphragms (at the same time check that the depth of inspiration is adequate: anterior right ribs to the top of the right hemidiaphragm on the posteroanterior [PA] view; 4th to 6th)

    Equal lucency of the lungs; symmetric distribution of the size and number of the pulmonary vessels; equal overall density of the lungs; equal position of the scapulae, ensuring that they do not obscure the lungs
4. Look at the whole radiograph as an entity for **any obvious abnormalities**, e.g., missing scapula; forequarter/arm missing; destroyed rib/vertebra; large mediastinal/lung mass. Most abnormalities have been detected by this time (about 10 seconds, and the systematic search has not started yet!).

The search now begins. There are many ways to read a chest radiograph. We start the search process with:

5. The **heart** (cardiac silhouette) and **aorta**.

    These should be studied as a unit, as they often reflect concomitant disease

    Use both the PA and lateral views together; they are one examination
6. Move to the remainder of the **mediastinum**, paying special attention to the

    Right paratracheal stripe

    Azygoesophageal recess

    Tracheal air column

    and, if present,

    Esophageal air columns

    Mediastinal stripes

    Silhouetting of any of the interfaces between lung and mediastinum

    Any mediastinal masses or bulges
7. While you are up at the top of the radiograph, look at the:

    Trachea

    Soft tissues of the neck

    Apices of the lungs for any concavity or masses

    Rib destruction in association with a superior sulcus tumor is one of the most common misses
8. Now start down the **lungs**, going from side to side

    It is unlikely that one will miss something in the middle of a lung with a systematic search, so concentrate on the more difficult areas, i.e.,

    Behind the first rib and clavicle

    Behind the heart to the left and right sides of the spine

    Behind the hemidiaphragms

    Identify all fissures and their positions
9. Go to the **hila**, again using the PA and lateral views together

    The hila are complex, so use the "bare" areas, such as the posterior wall of the intermediate bronchus, the left anterior hilar window, and the relative position of the arteries, veins, and bronchi
10. Finally, glance at the **soft tissues of the chest wall** and **ribs**

Even though it sounds sacrilegious, you don't have time to look at each rib completely; moreover, if your search up to now has been unrevealing, it is unlikely that an asymptomatic chest wall lesion will be found (this is obviously modified if the patient, for instance, has a history of prior breast carcinoma).

The normal chest radiograph should be read in 45 to 90 seconds. In any less time, things will be missed; in any more time, the false-positive rate will increase.

CT/MRI Studies. Below is an 11-point plan for reading CT and MRI studies.

1. Start with the identification of the **patient**, including **age** and **sex**.
   Clinical information is even more important; it is essential to know why the examination was undertaken (in most circumstances, the person reading the study also monitored it, and these facts will already have been established).

2. Make an overall assessment of the quality of the examination and whether it can be interpreted. The major problems are:
   Missing slices
   Inappropriate window settings
   Motion degradation of the lung images
   An incomplete study
   A percentage of studies have to be repeated. For CT, it is most important to know whether IV contrast was administered; for MRI, the exact sequences and modifiers, e.g., fat-suppression, should be known.
   The systematic search now starts.

3. Start with the **mediastinal images**, at the **aortic** arch; it is easier to identify the vessels of the mediastinum (arteries and veins).

4. Work upward, identifying normal:
   Vessels and **structures**
   Trachea and **esophagus**
   Any nodes
   Go back and forth if necessary. Make sure you have identified the extra-thoracic **trachea** and **larynx,** if they are included.

5. Then go caudad (toward the feet), identifying:
   Systemic and **pulmonary vessels** in their mediastinal courses
   AP window and **subcarinal space** are the difficult areas to see. Both of these sites have compound appearances and are subject to partial volume averaging.

6. This is a good time to survey the **hila**.
   After intravenous (IV) contrast, the hila are easy to see; without it, they can be difficult. The most difficult area is where the right pulmonary artery curves inferiorly after giving off the anterior trunk (upper division); at this site there is a collection of fat and the area is subject to partial volume effects.

7. Move farther down and observe the
   Heart, pericardium and **paracardiac areas**, paying special attention to the circumcardiac nodes
   A lot of information can be gleaned about the heart's size and the presence of coronary artery calcification (findings that are often neglected on thoracic CT)

8. This is a good time to study the **upper abdomen**, especially the liver and adrenal glands.

9. Now proceed to the **lungs**:
   Search these systematically from apex to base, ensuring that each level and side is viewed.
   It is a good idea to mark any sites of abnormality, so they are not forgotten during dictation, and they will be evident to colleagues on follow-up studies.

10. Consider whether it is important to go to the console to do the following:
    Review any slices at other window settings
    Display the pixel density map of a region or obtain a region-of-interest measurement.
    Objectively measure the size of a lesion

11. Finally, before dictating your report, think about whether any additional scans are warranted, e.g.:
    Thin-section nodule densitometry
    Repeat hilar images with contrast

Details of the interpretation of the images, although very important, are beyond the scope of this section.

CONGENITAL LUNG LESIONS

An understanding of congenital abnormalities of the lung is based on knowledge of a few rudimentary facts about how the lung develops:

> The lungs arise from the foregut as two connected buds
> The intraparenchymal pulmonary vessels develop with the lung buds
> The extraparenchymal pulmonary arteries are from the primitive dorsal and ventral arterial arches
> The fetal lung has extensive systemic arterial connections that regress before birth

The major lung anomalies are from:

> Abnormal bronchial development, which can be classified as:
>> Lack of branching
>> Abnormal occlusions
>> Abnormal buds
>> Lack of differentiation
> Abnormal development of the lung vessels, including:
>> Fistulas
>> Obstructions
>> Lack of regression

Specific lung anomalies are outlined in Table 1–2.

MEDIASTINUM AND HILA

Several classifications divide the mediastinum into different compartments. For chest radiographs, the easiest and best system is as follows:

> Anterior: sternum to a line following the anterior wall of the trachea and posterior border of the heart (tracheocardiac line); contents are the heart,

Table 1–2. Specific Anomalies of the Lung

Developmental absence of lung tissue
  Agenesis
  Aplasia
  Hypoplasia
Bronchial anomalies
  Tracheal bronchus
  Pig bronchus
  Bridging bronchus
  Bronchial isomerism
Foregut: Bronchial (bronchogenic) and esophageal cysts
  Congenital bronchial cysts
  Congenital esophageal cysts
Bronchial atresia
Congenital lobar emphysema
Cystic adenomatoid malformation
Pulmonary arteriovenous malformation (fistula)
Congenital proximal pulmonary artery interruption
Congenital unilateral pulmonary vein atresia
Systemic vascular anomalies
  Hypogenetic lung (scimitar syndrome)
  Pulmonary sequestration
    Intralobar sequestration
    Extralobar sequestration
  Systemic arterial supply to the lung

1

ascending aorta and great vessels, SVC and bracheocephalic veins, thymus, anterior lymph nodes, and ectopic parathyroids (2%)

Middle: tracheocardiac line to a line parallel to and 1 cm behind the anterior border of the vertebral bodies; contents are the trachea, esophagus, many lymph nodes, thoracic duct, vagus nerves, sympathetic nerve chains, and azygos veins

Posterior: behind the middle compartment to the posterior chest wall; contents are the spinal nerves, spine and paraspinous soft tissues, lymph nodes, and descending aorta

The aorta is in all three mediastinal compartments.

A variation of the foregoing classification divides the mediastinum into superior and inferior compartments. The superior compartment is above a line joining the sternomanubrial junction to the fourth intervertebral disc space. The inferior is below this line and is divided into the three previous anterior, middle, and posterior compartments.

On CT, the mediastinum is classified differently. From front to back, the mediastinal spaces (compartments) are as follows:

Pre(cardio)vascular including the retrosternal
Paracardiac
Pretracheal
Paratracheal
Paraesophageal
Subcarinal
Paraspinal

PULMONARY NEOPLASMS

The lungs are the most common site for both primary and secondary neoplasms. A detailed understanding of their presentation is essential. This section presents specific topics of importance, but is not a comprehensive review.

The Solitary Pulmonary Nodule (SPN). A solitary pulmonary nodule occurs in approximately two of every 1000 chest radiographs. In most patients, it is small (less than 2 cm), overtly calcified, and can be reported as being of no consequence.

The differential diagnosis (DD) is extensive (Table 1–3), but conceptually SPNs are classified into three groups: definitely benign, definitely malignant, and indeterminate.

Management of the patient with a SPN is directed towards determining whether the nodule is benign or not, deciding on the sequence of studies required to make this determination, and deciding on any interventions for confirmation and treatment. The factors involved in these decisions are both clinical and the results of imaging studies. The eight most important factors are:

Age
Patients under 30 years old are unlikely to have a pulmonary malignancy
Those over 40 years old are more likely (less important factor)
Symptoms (e.g., hemoptysis)
Any patient with symptoms that could be attributed to the SPN must be investigated until a definite diagnosis is reached (important factor)
Site
Lesions have a predilection for certain sites (e.g., arteriovenous malformations [AVM], lower lobes; sequestration, posterior basal segments of the lower lobes; adenocarcinoma, upper lobes, more often right than left) (less important factor)
Geography
Helps determine the frequency and type of granulomas that may be present (less important factor)
Prior malignancy
The site of origin and latency can suggest the likelihood of an SPN being a metastasis (less important factor)

Table 1–3. Differential Diagnosis of Single Pulmonary Nodule

Inflammatory
  Granuloma (tuberculosis, histoplasmosis, coccidioidomycosis)
  Hydatid (rare)
Neoplastic
  Primary lung carcinoma
  Solitary metastasis
  Adenoma (carcinoid less common than cylindroma)
  Hamartoma
Vascular
  Infarct
  Arteriovenous malformation
  Pulmonary artery aneurysm
Congenital
  Bronchogenic cyst
  Sequestration
Collagen vascular disease
  Rheumatoid arthritis (rare)
  Caplan's syndrome (rare)
  Plasma cell granuloma (rare)
Miscellaneous
  Artifact
  Pleural plaque
  Pseudotumor
  Chest wall/breast mass
  Skin lesion

Stability
  Lesions stable for 2 years are most likely benign; beware of the occasional alveolar cell carcinoma
  Most primary lung carcinomas double in volume (increase in diameter by 1.2-fold) in 30 to 450 days (important factor)
Calcification
  Must be central, diffuse, popcorn, or laminated (bulls-eye) to be significant
  Up to 10% of carcinomas contain calcium that can be detected on CT (important factor)
Imaging features
  Certain features seen on radiographs or CT can be highly suggestive of whether a nodule is malignant or not (Table 1–4) (important factor)

The imaging studies used for evaluation of the SPN are chest radiographs and CT scans (with thin sections). Chest radiographs can demonstrate many of the findings in Table 1–4, especially stability. CT is more accurate for showing contour, edge, calcification, cavitation, adenopathy, and satellites. MRI at present has no part in evaluation of the SPN, unless a vascular structure is suspected.

Table 1–4. Discriminatory Imaging Features in a Solitary Pulmonary Nodule

Feature	Malignant	Benign
Contour	Spiculated/smooth	Smooth
Size	>2 cm	<2 cm
Stability	Doubles 30–450 days	>2 years
Calcification	Eccentric/absent	Central/diffuse
Edge	Ill defined	Well defined
Cavitation	Highly suggestive	Absent unless active
Shape	Irregular	Round/ovoid
Adenopathy	Highly suggestive	Absent
Satellites	Present/absent	Absent
Air-bronchograms	Present/absent	Absent

The SPN is classified as benign, malignant, or indeterminate based on all of the clinical and imaging information. In most circumstances, the patient is asymptomatic and the nodule is detected from a chest radiograph obtained for other reasons. If the chest radiograph does not clearly show that the nodule is benign, CT is obtained (initially, thin sections through the nodule without contrast; then a complete CT with contrast, if the nodule is suggestive of a primary carcinoma). Recent studies indicate that nodules that do not enhance with IV contrast by more than 10 H (on CT) are benign.

Benign SPN. To be considered benign, an SPN should fulfill most of the criteria in Table 1–4; it should occur in a young patient and be calcified, solid, small (less than 2 cm), stable, smooth, round or ovoid, and have a well-defined edge. Some "nodules," in which CT may be definitive for diagnosis, include mucous plugs, rounded atelectasis, fungus ball, pleural plaque, focal consolidation, AVM, and hamartoma.

Malignant SPN. A malignant SPN should fulfill most of the following criteria: occur in an older patient; occur in a smoker; cause symptoms; be large or small, ill defined, growing, and spiculated; and have cavitation, absent or peripheral calcification, and adenopathy.

Indeterminate SPN. Indeterminate SPN are small (less than 2 cm), solid, smooth, and well defined; the stability is unknown, adenopathy is absent, and the nodule is asymptomatic.

The approach to an SPN is as follows:

Benign
  Follow-up radiograph in 6 to 12 weeks, or nothing, if absolutely certain of benignity
Malignant
  CT for staging
  Needle biopsy for confirmation in some cases
  Mediastinoscopy and/or resection depending on patient's clinical status
Indeterminate
  Must be investigated as soon as possible
  A nodule should remain in this category for as short a time as possible

If there is some suspicion that the SPN could be a benign reversible process (e.g., recent infection; possible infarct), a follow-up radiograph is obtained in 2 to 4 weeks. If the SPN has not become significantly smaller, evaluation is necessary. The evaluation procedures can include CT, CT densitometry, biopsy, repeat biopsy, and thoracotomy.

CT is more sensitive for detecting calcium than radiographs and can reasonably quantify the calcium content of pulmonary nodules. In approximately half of the cases, the calcium is visible as a dense nodule (looks white). In the other half with a positive CT, the calcium is detected by high CT (Hounsfield) numbers. The high numbers (15% of the surface area of the nodule embracing contiguous pixels through the nodule) must be above 150 to 200 H. Calcium should be diffuse or central. Some radiologists favor a commercially available, standardized phantom to which the density of the nodule can be compared. In some cases, CT can also demonstrate areas of fat in the nodule (negative H values inside the nodule), indicating that it is probably a hamartoma. *Beware of partial volume averaging causing false-negative numbers near the edge of the nodule.* Approaches to the SPN vary among institutions; have a considered approach, but be accepting of others.

Bronchogenic Carcinoma. Bronchogenic carcinoma is the most common fatal malignancy in men and women (breast cancer is more common in women but has a better prognosis). Overall 5-year survival is 10 to 15%. Survival varies greatly by the following factors:

Cell type, e.g., small cell bronchogenic carcinoma has an especially poor prognosis and is not generally considered resectable; an occasional small cell bronchogenic carcinoma (SCBC) presenting as an SPN is resected, although these are probably poorly differentiated carcinoids, i.e., amino precursor up-take decarboxylation (APUD) type II tumors

Extent of tumor at the time of detection (most important). An SPN of less than 2 cm in diameter and without adenopathy has a 5-year survival of 40 to 60%. The prognosis is progressively worse the larger and more extensive the tumor.

Histologic Types of Lung Cancer. All but a small percent of lung cancers are composed of four main histologic types and their variants and dedifferentiated forms (Table 1–5), as follows:

Epidermoid carcinoma
    No longer the most common type
    Tends to arise centrally in the segmental and more proximal bronchi
    Causes "early" symptoms
    Most common type to produce atelectasis
Adenocarcinoma
    Most common type
    Tends to arise in the periphery of the lung
    Said not to have a strong statistical relationship to smoking (the evidence for this statement is weak)
Small cell undifferentiated carcinoma (oat cell carcinoma is a subgroup of SCBC)
    Tends to occur centrally
    Frequently has marked mediastinal adenopathy
    May present as a mediastinal mass
    Tumor arises from neuroectodermal tissue
    Has a strong resemblance clinically and histologically to malignant lymphoma
    Is relatively radiosensitive but recurs and has a terrible prognosis
Large cell undifferentiated carcinoma
    Similar to adenocarcinoma in its radiologic and histologic characteristics and survival statistics
    Frequently presents as a large mass

Other less common varieties include the following:

Bronchoalveolar cell carcinoma
    Variant of adenocarcinoma
    Tends to occur in the lung periphery and in the vicinity of a scar
    Presents as
        1. An SPN that can be very slow growing (doubling time, more than 2 years)
        2. Lung consolidation
        3. Diffuse nodules
    Biologically has two forms
        1. Focal, usually an ill-defined SPN or region of opacity (by definition limited to one lobe); CT is the best way to make this determination, and thus resectability

Table 1–5. Radiologic Findings in Lung Cancer (%)

Findings	Epidermoid	Adenocarcinoma	Small Cell	Large Cell
Peripheral lesion (nodule or mass)	31	74	32	65
Atelectasis	37	10	18	13
Consolidation	20	15	24	25
Hilar enlargement	40	18	78	32
Mediastinal enlargement	2	3	13	10
Pleural effusions	4	5	5	2
No abnormalities	3	1	0	0
Multiple abnormalities	37	30	62	43

2. Diffuse (more than one lobe involved) and not resectable

Alveolar cell carcinoma is in the differential diagnosis of a focal area of consolidation with multiple pulmonary nodules and in the differential diagnosis of chronic consolidation

Giant cell carcinoma

Unusual, highly malignant variant of adenocarcinoma with bizarre giant cells

Large

Often peripheral and involving the chest wall

Bronchial carcinoid

Formerly considered a "bronchial adenoma"; accounts for approximately 1 to 2% of primary lung malignancies; most often in the central bronchi and uncommonly in the trachea

Presentations of Bronchogenic Carcinoma. There are five major and eight minor presentations of bronchogenic carcinoma. The major presentations are as follows:

1. SPN

Approximately one third of lung carcinoma presents as:

A nodule (less than 3 or 4 or 5 cm in diameter, depending on the definition used) or

A mass; most are adenocarcinoma or large cell undifferentiated carcinoma

2. Atelectasis/consolidation

Approximately half of all lung carcinoma demonstrates atelectasis or consolidation, or both

Central obstructing tumors cause one of the following:

Obstructive atelectasis

A drowned lobe (obstructed and fluid filled, sometimes with mucus bronchograms)

Hyperinflation (rarely) from a ball-valve effect

Consolidation with preservation of bronchial patency and air bronchograms is found with alveolar cell carcinoma and on HRCT with adenocarcinoma manifesting as a small nodule

Endobronchial tumors that arise distal to segmental bronchi often do not cause atelectasis because collateral ventilation maintains normal lung expansion

3. Hilar/mediastinal enlargement

Hilar and/or mediastinal masses caused by nodal metastasis are present in 20 to 60% of lung cancers at the time of presentation (incidence varies widely among studies and is the reason why the results of many investigations are so different) (for practical purposes use 20 to 25%)

Nodal metastases are the most important part of lung cancer staging and are discussed later

4. Pleural abnormalities

Not uncommon (5%)

Small effusions and direct tumor extension to the pleural surface are the most common ways cancer involves the pleura

Lung cancer tends to respect the visceral pleural surface but can infiltrate the pleura and cross fissures

Pleural effusion that does not contain malignant cells can result from lymphatic obstruction and does not by itself indicate that the tumor is unresectable

CT after IV contrast, MRI, and pleuroscopy are the best methods for detecting pleural metastases

5. Chest wall abnormalities

1 to 5% of cases of lung carcinoma involve the pleura

Chest wall involvement is very likely if the patient presents with chest pain

Most common with superior sulcus tumors and peripheral undifferentiated tumors

Best methods of detection are rib detail radiographs, CT, bone scans, and MRI for the superior sulcus and paravertebral regions

1

Less common findings with lung carcinoma include the following:

6. Normal chest radiograph

   In 1 to 3% of lung carcinomas the chest radiograph is normal and cytologic study of sputum or bronchoscopy is abnormal

   The tumor may be very small or superficial and endobronchial

   In about half of these cases the tumor can be shown with CT

7. Mediastinal mass

   1 to 5% of bronchogenic carcinoma presents as a mediastinal (usually anterior) mass

   It may not be the result of nodal metastases and there is no visible lung mass

   SCBC can arise in the mediastinum from rests of neural cells

   Epidermoid/undifferentiated carcinoma can also present in this way; the primary tumor becomes visible later or the tumor arises from mediastinal rests of cells

8. SVC syndrome

   Usually from direct mediastinal invasion by a paramediastinal primary

   Can also be from extranodal spread of metastases

   Confirmation is with CT or MRI

   The tumor is invariably unresectable

   75% of SVC syndromes are from lung carcinoma; reverse ("down-hill") varices may be found

9. "Double-lesion" sign; atelectasis of more than one lobe on the right side (specifically the right upper lobe [RUL] and right middle lobe [RML]) can be seen with:

   Two endobronchial lesions

   One endobronchial lesion and obstruction from hilar nodal metastasis or infiltrating mass

   Two independent causes, e.g., tumor and a foreign body

   A lesion involving the main bronchus: with progressive stenosis of the right main bronchus, the order of collapse of the lobes is RML, followed by RUL then right lower lobe (RLL)

10. Calcification

    Calcified lung tumors result from the following causes:

      Engulfed granuloma, usually eccentric

      Calcified bronchogenic carcinoma; rare on radiographs, uncommon on CT or specimen radiographs (perhaps 10%)

      Calcium-accumulating metastasis, e.g., osteogenic sarcoma

    For visible calcium in nodules to be considered benign on CT, it should be central, popcorn, diffuse, or bulls-eye.

11. Shrinking carcinoma

    A nodule being followed for presumed benignity sometimes appears to become smaller but still turns out to be bronchogenic carcinoma

    The presumed reason is that inflammatory reaction around the nodule can decrease its conspicuousness, leading to the mistaken conclusion of a decrease in size

    Technical factors, e.g., penetration of the radiograph, can make a nodule appear smaller

    Always confirm that a nodule is smaller with serial radiographs at 3- to 6-week intervals for two or three cycles

12. Malignant bulla

    Bronchogenic carcinoma has some propensity to arise in the walls of bullae

    Progressive thickening of the wall of a bulla suggests infection or neoplasm

    Fluid in a bulla is by far most commonly benign and should not be considered significant unless other findings are present, e.g., focal wall thickening

13. Two primary bronchogenic carcinomas

    Two synchronous or metachronous primary bronchogenic carcinomas is not a rare finding

They have to be of different histologic types not to be considered a
primary and metastasis
Approximately 10% of patients surviving one lung carcinoma develop a
second primary tumor sometime later
With two indeterminate lung nodules:
Biopsy the newer, if one has been stable or shows features of benignity
Biopsy both
Median sternotomy and bilateral resection

Lung Cancer Staging. Only two imaging modalities are routinely used for the staging of lung carcinoma, namely, chest radiographs and CT scans (to include the adrenals, liver, and spleen). Most often these are the only two imaging procedures. Others have been tried (e.g., MRI of the brain or bone scans and various angiographic studies). Brain/bone imaging should be reserved for situations in which symptoms or laboratory tests suggest metastases are present. In patients with adenocarcinomas and mediastinal metastases, MRI of the head should be obtained. If any systemic symptoms are present, all sites of potential metastases should be evaluated, not only the symptomatic organ system. At times the chest radiograph is the only imaging study required. The patient can go straight to a definitive staging procedure (e.g., bronchoscopy or mediastinoscopy). For example, if mediastinal adenopathy is visible, CT of the thorax is unlikely to give additional information that will change the staging and resectability of the tumor. The patient can go directly to a staging mediastinoscopy to confirm nonresectability. In most circumstances, the diagnosis of an unresectable tumor is confirmed.

The role of CT in evaluating suspected bronchogenic carcinoma is to:

1. Determine whether invasive staging procedures are indicated for diagnosis, and which would be most successful (e.g., aspiration biopsy, bronchoscopy with or without transbronchial biopsy, mediastinoscopy, paramedian mini-thoracotomy, thoracotomy, thoracoscopy, adrenal/liver biopsy)
2. Demonstrate the site(s) most likely to provide a histologic diagnosis for staging
3. Show that the tumor is not resectable, beyond a reasonable doubt
4. Demonstrate the absence of visible spread and that the patient should go directly to thoracotomy
5. Show unsuspected significant concomitant disease

Additional uses include the following:

6. Localization for CT-guided biopsies
7. Planning radiotherapy
8. Detect endobronchial disease to direct bronchoscopy
9. Appearances and calcium content of an SPN

In patients with lung carcinoma, the anatomic extent of the tumor at the time of detection is the major determinant of prognosis and also determines the therapeutic approach.

The cell type and degree of differentiation have a lesser influence on outcome (excluding SCBC). This has led to the adoption of a precise anatomic staging system that is rigorously applied in most cases. The most widely used staging classification is the TNM classification of the American Joint Committee on Cancer Staging. This system was modified in 1986 to reflect the more aggressive surgical approach to lung carcinoma. The classification is based on the extent of tumor, as determined using all available clinical and imaging studies. The system defines the following:

The size, extent, and morphology of the primary tumor (T)
The presence of hilar and mediastinal nodal involvement (N)
The presence of distant metastases (M)

The stages in the TNM system are delineated in Table 1–6. Excellent correlation is found between tumor stage and survival after treatment.

Imaging studies are obtained for two reasons, staging of the lung cancer and defining the precise relationship of the tumor to important thoracic structures, *which may affect resectability and operative approach, but not staging.*

Table 1–6. Lung Cancer Staging

	Tumor	Node	Metastases
Occult carcinoma	Tx	N0	M0
Stage 0	Tis	N0	M0
Stage I	T1	N0	M0
	T2	N0	M0
Stage II	T1	N1	M0
	T2	N1	M0
Stage IIIa	T3	N0	M0
	T3	N1	M0
	T1–3	N2	M0
Stage IIIb	Any T	N3	M0
	T4	Any N	M0
Stage IV	Any T	Any N	M1

In general, non-small cell bronchogenic carcinomas (NSCBC) are resectable when the following conditions are met:

> They are confined to one hemithorax
> Invasion of the chest wall, mediastinum, or diaphragm is limited, permitting removal
> Nodal metastases are intracapsular and ipsilateral and do not extend above the level of the top of the aortic arch
> No distant metastases are present

These features define stages I, II, and IIIa (T0–3, N0–2, and M0). Exceptions exist depending on the aggressiveness of the surgeon; for instance, some surgeons resect a solitary brain metastasis with an otherwise resectable lung carcinoma.

Nonresectable tumors (NSCBC) have done the following:

> Invaded or encased cardiovascular or aerodigestive tract organs
> Invaded the spine or sternum
> Involved contralateral nodes
> Spread beyond the nodes within the mediastinum
> Metastasized distantly

These features define stages IIIb and IV (T4 or N3 or M1).

Accuracy of CT in Staging Bronchogenic Carcinoma. Understanding the strengths and limitations of imaging modalities in various situations is important. Extensive studies have looked at most aspects of the sensitivity (how good the technique is in not missing disease when it is present) and specificity (how good the technique is in excluding disease when it is absent) of CT and MRI.

MEDIASTINAL LYMPHADENOPATHY. Mediastinal lymph node is by far the most common site for metastases for spread of metastis bronchogenic carcinoma. The reported incidence varies widely, but should be about 20 to 25%. It is necessary to distinguish between *ipsilateral* (use the midpoint of the trachea) enlarged nodes (N2), which are considered resectable by many surgeons, and *contralateral* (N3) nodes, which are not considered resectable. For "enlarged" use 1 cm, even though some (approximately 5%) normal mediastinal nodes can be up to 1.5 cm in the short axis (the diameter measured on normal transverse CT scans).

The sensitivity of CT for detecting tumor-containing mediastinal nodes is about 65%; somewhat better than guessing, but not much! MRI has the same sensitivity. The low figure is the result of missed enlarged nodes containing tumor (perhaps spiral CT will improve this) and tumor in normal-sized nodes.

The specificity is only about 80%, limited by reactive enlarged nodes. The accuracy of CT is thus only about 70%, limited by its sensitivity and specificity. That of MRI is about the same.

Important caveats are as follows:

1. When CT is used in combination with good clinical judgment, it is unusual

for a patient to be denied surgery when the lung carcinoma would have been resectable

2. A bulky mediastinal mass is invariably nonresectable, even without organ invasion
3. Patients should not be denied surgery when the only finding is enlarged, well-defined mediastinal (N2 or 3) nodes; tumor in these nodes must be confirmed histologically and cytologically

DIRECT INVASION BY BRONCHOGENIC CARCINOMA. The frequency of invasion of the mediastinum or thoracic cage by lung carcinoma is approximately 5 to 10%, which makes it less common than nodal metastases. Limited invasion is resectable except when it involves the spine; sternum; AP window and recurrent laryngeal nerve; back of the left atrium; and central pulmonary veins, aorta, and great arteries. Most paramediastinal or peripheral lung carcinomas that abut the mediastinum or chest wall have not invaded these structures or, if they have, they are still resectable. Nonresectable mediastinal invasion is almost always obvious on CT as a bulky mass or encasement of organs. CT is poor for detecting subtle mediastinal or chest wall invasion by lung carcinoma (accuracy only 40 to 70%); thus, the tumor should be called "potentially resectable" unless it is obviously not.

CT findings that may indicate transpleural (mediastinal/chest wall) invasion are as follows:

1. A large, flat mass with more than 3 cm contact with the costal/mediastinal pleura
2. Pleural thickening adjacent to the mass
3. A mass in the soft tissues of the chest wall/mediastinum
4. Rib destruction (found only 5% of the time)
5. Increased density of the extrapleural fat
6. Organ encasement

Superior sulcus (Pancoast's) tumors are a subgroup of bronchogenic carcinomas with the same histologic types as the other NSCBC, but they have different biologic activity. They tend to invade superiorly, medially, and posteriorly.

MRI (which is better) and CT are used to detect extension into the following areas:

1. Spine and spinal canal
2. Superior mediastinum
3. Subclavian vessels
4. Brachial plexus

These modalities are also used to define the extent of the tumor before and after radiation therapy, which may be given before or after surgery.

PLEURAL INVOLVEMENT. Bronchogenic carcinoma can respect the pleura, cross the pleura, involve the pleura diffusely, or cause pleural effusion without direct involvement. *All pleural effusions in a patient with suspected lung carcinoma are significant and must be evaluated.* Evaluation is initially with thoracentesis/thoracoscopy with or without biopsy. The presence of malignant cells indicates nonresectability. Patients without malignant cells should undergo HRCT to look for lymphangitic spread.

DISTANT METASTASES. Metastases beyond the confines of the involved hemithorax are considered distant and preclude resection. Common sites are supraclavicular nodes, liver, adrenal glands, bone (lytic metastases distal to the wrist and ankle are almost always from the lung), brain, and contralateral lung.

Caveats include the following:

1. If any symptoms suggest metastases, all sites should be investigated
2. The adrenals and entire liver should be included in any CT study of the thorax for lung carcinoma

The incidence of adrenal and liver metastases is probably about 10 to 12% for each (figures vary) at initial presentation. CT has been shown to be unable to distinguish between smaller benign and malignant adrenal masses, unless the mass has a CT density below 10 H (on unenhanced scans). New, opposing-phase MRI shows some promise in distinguishing between an adenoma and metastasis. A biopsy sample should be taken from any indeterminate adrenal mass that is more

1

than 1 or 2 cm in diameter. Some radiologists start their CT examination for lung carcinoma with a large contrast bolus through the liver (not necessary with spiral CT).

CENTRAL EXTENT OF THE TUMOR. Carcinomas that arise centrally in and around the hila most frequently spread centrally. Their relationship to the bronchi and other hilar and mediastinal structures defines resectability and determines additional evaluation. Tumors arising in proximal bronchi often cause atelectasis of the distal lung segments, the lobes, or the whole lung. Once the lung has collapsed, imaging studies have difficulty separating the tumor from the surrounding collapsed lung. Contrast-enhanced CT or T2-weighted MRI images have been tried without much success. More important is the proximal extent of the tumor and its relationship to the following structures:

1. Bronchi
   Thin (5 mm) CT sections can sometimes show tumor within the lumen of a bronchus or a bronchus abruptly terminating in the mass with an amputated appearance; in these instances, bronchoscopy usually demonstrates endobronchial tumor
   If the bronchus terminates in the mass with a tapered appearance, CT cannot distinguish between extrinsic compression and an endobronchial tumor involving the airway mucosa
   CT also cannot show proximal submucosal extension of tumor, which is common and important
   Tumor within 2 cm of the tracheal carina is often resectable (newer surgical techniques allow resection of the distal trachea)
2. Vessels
   Tumors surrounding the SVC (medial to it), occluding the SVC, or causing an SVC syndrome are not resectable
   Tumor contacting more than half the circumference of the aorta is very likely to be nonresectable
   Tumor mass narrowing the pulmonary arteries within the mediastinum is nonresectable
3. Mediastinum
   Tumor extending into the mediastinum and crossing the midline is nonresectable
   In all of these situations good contrast between vessels and mass is required. This is obtained with contrast-enhanced CT.
4. Fissures
   Conventional CT cannot show a central tumor's relationship to the central interlobar fissures. When a pneumonectomy is not clinically possible, HRCT should be obtained through the tumor

Bronchial "Adenomas" and Benign Tumors. Primary lung tumors, with the exception of bronchogenic carcinoma, are uncommon. The most frequent benign tumors are:

Hamartomas
Lipomas
Fibromas

All of these tend to arise in the walls of bronchi. Less common are:

Granular cell myoblastomas
Chondromas
Leiomyomas
Neurogenic tumors
Papillomas

All of these tend to cause bronchial obstruction and may contain calcifications; usually they cannot be distinguished from each other.

Bronchial adenomas are often considered benign because they are slow growing. This is totally wrong, because all of them are malignant.

Chondrohamartoma.   The third most common cause of an SPN is chondrohamartoma. These tumors originate from the stroma of the bronchial wall and consist of normal embryologic components in a disorganized mass. Cartilaginous elements are always present.

Rounded (Round) Atelectasis.   Although this entity is not a neoplasm, it is important to consider. It is a form of pulmonary pseudotumor found in conjunction with a fibrothorax (diffuse pleural thickening). It was originally described with tuberculosis, but is now mostly seen with asbestos-related diffuse pleural disease.

PULMONARY INFECTIONS

Pneumonia.   Pneumonia is the sixth leading cause of death in the United States. It is the most common cause of death from hospital-acquired infection. Pneumonia can be divided into three groups, caused by different organisms and with different significances, as follows:

1. Community-acquired: any pneumonia contracted away from a hospital setting
2. Nosocomial: any pneumonia contracted in a hospital setting
3. Immunocompromised: any pneumonia in an immunocompromised patient; the prevalence of different organisms varies according to the cause of the immunodeficiency

Predisposing factors and common organisms for the various types of pneumonia are shown in Table 1–7.

Pulmonary Findings in Human Immunodeficiency Virus (HIV) Infection.   HIV is a retrovirus. There have been approximately 1.0 to 1.5 million cases in the United States. The prevalence of acquired immune deficiency syndrome (AIDS) in the United States is about 250,000 cases with the older definition (500,000 with the newer definition using a low CD4 count); about 250,000 deaths (1995). The thorax is the most common site for abnormalities in HIV-positive individuals. *Pneumocystis carinii* pneumonia is the most common cause of pneumonia in AIDS patients, affecting 60 to 80% of patients.

Mycobacterial Infection.   HIV infection has caused a marked increase in the previously declining incidence of TB. It is estimated that up to 8% of patients with AIDS will be infected with TB; the incidence is much higher in Africa.

Fungal Infections.   Fungal infections are much less common than mycobacterial infections as a cause of pneumonia; they account for less than 5% of pneumonias. Cryptococcus is the most common organism. It causes central nervous system (CNS) disease in more than 90% of infected patients. Histoplasmosis, coccidioidomycosis, candidiasis, and aspergillosis have all been described but are not particularly common.

Bacterial Infections.   Pyogenic bacterial infections are seen with increased frequency in patients with AIDS. Bacteria account for 3 to 10% of pneumonias. The use of radiographic findings to suggest the organism in AIDS is fraught with danger and is attempted with caution.

Neoplasms.   From the beginning, the association between AIDS and certain neoplasms was obvious, but for other cancers the association is still inconclusive (Table 1–8).

Miscellaneous HIV-Related Diseases.   Miscellaneous HIV-related diseases include nonspecific interstitial pneumonitis (a poorly documented noninfectious interstitial inflammation with a benign course), lymphocytic interstitial pneumonitis (an indicator disease in children), and bronchiectasis, which is being seen with increasing frequency in HIV-positive individuals.

Table 1–7. Predisposing Factors and Common Organisms in Pneumonia

Type	Predisposing Factors	Organisms
Community acquired	None	*Streptococcus pneumoniae* *Mycoplasma pneumoniae, Chlamydia pneumoniae, Legionella* spp, viruses
	Alcoholism	*S. pneumoniae,* gram-negative bacilli (e.g., *Klebsiella*)
	Chronic bronchitis	*S. pneumoniae, Haemophilus influenzae*
	Advanced age	*S. pneumoniae, Staphylococcus aureus*
	Recent viral pneumonia	*S. aureus, S. pneumoniae, H. influenzae*
	Recurrent aspiration	Anaerobes, especially microaerophilic streptococci and peptococci
	Cystic fibrosis	*Pseudomonas* spp, *S. aureus*
	Hyposplenism	*S. pneumoniae*
Nosocomial pneumonia	Intensive care unit (ICU) occupancy, thoracic/upper abdominal surgery, age, intubation, impaired mentation, use of antibiotics to which the organism is insensitive	Gram-negative bacilli, especially *Pseudomonas* and *Klebsiella* spp; *Escherichia coli; Proteus mirabilis; Enterobacter* and *Serratia* spp; *S. aureus; S. pneumoniae;* anaerobes
Immunocompromised pneumonia	Human immunodeficiency virus (HIV) infection	*Pneumocystis carinii, S. pneumoniae,* tuberculosis, *Nocardia asteroides,* atypical mycobacteria, cryptococci, other opportunistic organisms
	Transplantation	Cytomegalovirus (CMV), *Aspergillus fumigatus;* herpes simplex; *P. carinii; S. aureus*
	Cancer (especially hematopoietic)	*Candida* spp, *Aspergillus* spp, CMV, herpes simplex, gram-positive cocci, others
	Chemotherapy, debility, steroids, age?, radiation?	

Diffuse Lung Disease

Diseases that involve the lungs diffusely (or multifocally) can be categorized into the following four major groups based on radiographic and/or CT features:

Alveolar diseases
Interstitial diseases
Vascular diseases
Airway diseases

Table 1–8. AIDS-Related Neoplasms

Definite
  Kaposi's sarcoma
  B-cell lymphoma
  Hodgkin's disease
Likely
  Non-Hodgkin's lymphoma
  Cervical cancer
  Myosarcoma (in children)
  Bronchogenic carcinoma

Table 1–9. Principal Causes of Diffuse Alveolar Consolidations

Cardiogenic pulmonary edema
Noncardiogenic pulmonary edema
Renal failure and fluid overload
Adult respiratory distress syndrome (ARDS)
Diffuse lung injuries
Infectious pneumonias
Drug-induced pneumonitis
Eosinophilic pneumonias
Alveolar hemorrhage
Pulmonary alveolar proteinosis
Alveolar cell carcinoma

Each group has its own diagnostic significance and specific appearance. The different groups can coexist, and frequently only the dominant features are visible. Although the groups are described in anatomic terms, there may not be a precise pathologic correlation with any one pattern.

Alveolar Disease. Synonyms for alveolar disease are *alveolar-filling, consolidation, air space,* and *air-space filling.* The components that characterize these diseases are:

1. Acinar nodules
2. Multiple soft, fluffy, confluent opacities
3. Air-bronchograms
4. Obscuration of the lung vessels
5. Opacity marginated by pleural surfaces
6. Ground-glass opacities (an early manifestation of alveolar disease)

The causes of diffuse alveolar consolidations are listed in Table 1–9.

Interstitial Disease. Diseases that predominantly involve the interstitium of the lung show various diffuse findings on chest radiographs and CT scans, which indicate the site of abnormality. The radiologic term *interstitial disease* is descriptive and is not synonymous with the pathologic definition of interstitial disease. Caveats are as follows:

Although patients with an interstitial radiographic appearance show pathologic interstitial disease, the alveoli may also be involved, and this involvement may dominate
Diffuse interstitial disease can be present with a normal chest radiograph (10 to 25%)
Diffuse interstitial disease can manifest as a pure alveolar "pattern" on radiographs

The principal interstitial patterns are presented in Table 1–10 and the causes of a diffuse interstitial pattern in Table 1–11.

Vascular Disease. Diffuse vascular disease is characterized by abnormal vascular caliber, abnormal vascular clarity, and several of the findings that can be ascribed to interstitial and alveolar disease. Abnormal vascular caliber and its distribution comprise a distinct subset of diffuse lung disease. The diseases can be the following:

Pulmonary arterial
Pulmonary hypertension
Left-to-right shunts
Pulmonary vascular occlusive diseases

Findings involve changes in arterial caliber and number.

Pulmonary venous
Venous hypertension/left heart failure
Veno-occlusive disease

Table 1–10.   Diffuse Interstitial Patterns*

Pattern	Characteristics
Micronodular	Profusion of 1.5–2 mm nodules, granular appearance
Miliary	Profusion of 2–10 mm nodules (usually 2–5)
Nodular	Profusion of 5–20 mm nodules
Reticular	Linear pattern with fishnet or mosaic appearance; also with horizontal lines (e.g., Kerley's)
Honeycomb	Cystic structures (3–10 mm in diameter) that share common space
Reticulonodular	Mixed miliary and reticular
Cystic	Thin-walled, air-containing spaces larger than 1 cm in diameter with visible walls

*More than one finding is frequently present; the dominant finding should be considered.

Findings can be acute or chronic and can show caliber changes, interstitial fluid accumulation, alveolar flooding, and obscuration of vessels
Pulmonary capillary
Changes in capillary permeability can allow fluid accumulation in the interstitium of the lungs and the alveolar spaces

Airways Disease.   It is extremely useful to recognize that diseases of the airways can result in distinctive findings. Diffuse airways disease has features that can be mistaken for interstitial disease. The diseases include chronic bronchitis, asthma, bronchiectasis, and emphysema. The characteristic findings are:

1. Visible dilated bronchi (parallel lines, "tram-tracks")
2. Irregularity of the pulmonary vessels
3. Diffuse increased opacity to the lungs ("dirty chest")
4. Preserved/increased lung volumes
5. Often pulmonary hypertension

Conclusions.   The initial interpretation of a chest radiograph that is diffusely abnormal can be unnerving. HRCT provides much more information than chest radiographs and is obtained in almost all cases in which a diagnosis is not known (and often when it is). An open biopsy is required for a definitive diagnosis in more than 50% of cases of chronic diffuse lung disease. Associated clinical and radiological findings give clues to the diagnosis in many cases. A diffusely abnormal chest radiograph should be approached logically, along the following lines:

1. Decide if the radiograph is truly abnormal (sometimes difficult)
2. Decide on the dominant feature by focusing on a small representative area of lung (the diamond-shaped area between four ribs is good)

Table 1–11.   Causes of a Diffuse Interstitial Pattern

Fibrosing alveolitis (idiopathic pulmonary fibrosis, IPF)
Inhalation disorders (inorganic or organic)
Drug-induced lung disorders
Histiocytosis X (Langerhans' giant cell disease)
Desquamative interstitial pneumonitis (DIP)
Malignant neoplasms (lymphangitic carcinomatosis)
Lymphoproliferative disorders
Infectious processes
Hypersensitivity pneumonitides
Edema
Sarcoidosis
Pulmonary hemosiderosis
Collagen vascular diseases

3. Look for clues such as pleural disease, adenopathy, calcification, bony abnormalities, pulmonary hypertension
4. Decide on the distribution of disease
5. Obtain old radiographs for comparison
6. Use all available clinical information
7. Suggest additional tests, especially HRCT
8. Give a differential diagnosis
9. Suggest a site for the biopsy sample (usually based on the HRCT)
10. Be supportive of your clinician. He or she often knows less about what's going on than you do!

APPENDIX

Anatomic and Physiologic Definitions

Several anatomic concepts are specific to the lung and should be known. The terms for these concepts relate to specific anatomic features that may or may not be visible on radiographs or CT scans.

Acinus: The portion of lung subtended by a single terminal bronchiole. Consists of respiratory bronchioles, alveolar ducts, and alveolar sacs together with their support and vascular structures. The acinus is not anatomically separated from the surrounding lung and not visible on radiographs or CT scans.

Alveolar pores (pores of Kohn): Microscopic communications between alveolar spaces through alveolar walls. One of the three pathways for collateral ventilation. The other two are the canals of Lampert and the channels of Martin.

Anterior junction line: Region in the anterior mediastinum where the two lungs approximate behind the sternum. Appears radiographically as a vertical opacity below the manubrium overlying the trachea and often projecting slightly toward the left inferiorly. If more than pencil-line thick, becomes invisible.

Aortopulmonary window: The region of the mediastinum beneath the aortic arch and above the left pulmonary artery. Lung penetrates the mediastinum to a variable extent at this site. The window contains the ductal ligament, the left recurrent laryngeal nerve, and lymph nodes. The base of the aortopulmonary window is formed by the left wall of the trachea, the left main bronchus, and the esophagus. On frontal radiographs the aortopulmonary window should be concave or straight.

Azygoesophageal recess: A region on the inferior posterior right side of the mediastinum where the right lower lobe contacts the mediastinal structures between the heart anteriorly and the spine posteriorly. The medial boundaries are formed variably by the aorta, esophagus, azygos vein, and left lung.

Hilum: Anatomically defined as a depression on the medial side of the lung where the vessels, bronchi, and associated structures enter. Radiologically, it is defined as the region where the vessels and bronchi exit the mediastinum and become visible by their contact with the air-containing lungs. The peripheral extent is usually considered to be as far as segmental or subsegmental bronchi.

Lobule: A unit of lung structure. The commonly used division is the "secondary pulmonary lobule," marginated by interlobular septa. The lobule can contain from two to more than 20 acini and can be from 1 to more than 4 cm on a side.

Paraspinous lines: The interface between the lung and the soft tissues surrounding the thoracic vertebral column. On chest radiographs, on the left side, the paraspinous line may be from several millimeters to 1 cm or more lateral to the vertebral column, depending on the position of the aorta. On the right side, the paraspinous line should be no more than a few millimeters from the vertebral column. The paraspinous lines can be displaced laterally by numerous causes, such as bleeding, infection, adenopathy, or tumor. Close inspection often shows that the paraspinous line is not an interface but a linear opacity marginated medially by fat density and laterally by the lung.

Posterior superior junction line: A vertically oriented linear or curvilinear opacity produced by the pleural surfaces contacting each other behind the esophagus. It is variably visible projecting above the manubrium through the tracheal air column on frontal radiographs. Thickening, distortion, or displacement of this line is almost never of any diagnostic value.

Posterior tracheal stripe: A vertical linear opacity 2 to 5 mm in width visible on lateral chest radiographs, representing the soft tissues between air in the trachea in front and air in the right lung or esophagus behind. Thickening of this stripe may reflect esophageal pathology but is often deceptive.

Right paratracheal stripe: A vertically oriented linear opacity 2 to 4 mm in width comprising the soft tissues between air in the trachea and the air in the right lung. Thickening of this stripe is invariably abnormal and needs to be explained. It is a useful radiographic sign.

Radiographic Definitions (Abnormal Findings)

Acinar nodules: Round, poorly defined, discrete or confluent nodular opacities, each about 4 to 8 mm in diameter. When confluent, they produce an inhomogeneous opacification of the lungs. (Also used in CT.)

Air bronchogram: Air within bronchi, visible because of consolidation of the surrounding lung parenchyma. (Also used in CT.)

ARDS (Adult respiratory distress syndrome, high-protein pulmonary edema): A physiologic-radiologic-pathologic combination defining a condition in which a patient with normal or near-normal lung function experiences respiratory failure, including hypoxemia, partially reversible by positive end-expiratory pressure (PEEP); diffusely increased lung opacity on radiographs; and abnormal capillary permeability. Noncardiogenic pulmonary edema is a form of ARDS, but it is usually more rapidly reversible. More recent definitions include an increase in the alveolar-arterial oxygen gradient. The pathology is referred to as *DAD*, diffuse alveolar damage.

Atelectasis: Reduced volume of all or part of a lung (not as a result of surgical resection). Most commonly considered obstructive or nonobstructive. Atelectasis should always be qualified in terms of anatomic region (e.g., subsegmental, segmental, lobar), or in terms of being nonanatomic (e.g., platelike, linear, discoid).

Rounded atelectasis: A region of lung usually about the size of a segment or less, which is pleural based and collapsed to form a lentiform or rounded structure. The vessels and bronchi entering the area of atelectatic lung have a comet-shaped configuration. Key diagnostic features are direct contact with a region of diffuse pleural thickening along the costal or diaphragmatic pleura, decreased volume in the containing lobe, and a lentiform shape. It can contain calcifications or air-bronchograms and is usually stable over many years. The term *trapped lung* has been used synonymously with rounded atelectasis, but is poor.

Bleb: A gas-containing space within the layers of the visceral pleura. Radiographically must be pleural based and have a pencil-line thin wall. A bleb is one of the causes of thin-walled cystic spaces.

Bulla: Region of lung destruction 1 cm or more in diameter. If not infected, the wall must be pencil-line thin. It may or may not be associated with other features of emphysema.

Cavity: A hole within a pulmonary mass, nodule, or region of consolidation. The wall must be thicker than a pencil line. It can be malignant or benign.

Coin lesion: A well-circumscribed spherical opacity within the lung, usually defined as less than 3 cm in diameter.

1

Cyst (synonym: *thin-walled cystic space*): Includes all gas-containing, thin-walled spaces within the lung. An especially useful term because it does not mislead by ascribing a single cause to the space. (Also used in CT.)

Density: A region of increased tissue within the lung from multiple causes and with multiple appearances. The term *opacity* is now more commonly used. (Also used in CT.)

Dirty chest: A chest radiographic appearance of a diffuse increase in parenchymal opacity without specific features of interstitial lung disease. The small vessels are often poorly marginated and appear discontinuous. It is seen in association with smoking or chronic bronchitis. It is a subjective and not very specific appearance.

Doubling time: The time in days for a nodule to double in volume (i.e., increase in diameter by 1.2). Is a measure of the rate of growth of a spherical lung lesion. Most malignant lung lesions have a doubling time of between 30 and 450 days.

Egg-shell calcification: Peripheral circumferential calcification usually found in lymph nodes. It is seen most commonly with silicosis and sarcoidosis.

Emphysema: Irreversible enlargement of air spaces distal to terminal bronchioles, with destruction of alveolar walls. The CT appearance is of gas-containing holes within the lung, usually sublobular in size. It is often divided into centrilobular and panlobular, although the distinction between the two is not clear cut. Paraseptal (cicatricial) emphysema consists of enlarged air spaces around regions of lung scarring. Areas of emphysema are not marginated by walls unless completely replacing an entire lobule.

Fibronodular opacities: Refers to round and linear opacities, usually in the upper lobes of the lungs and usually implying inactive granulomatous disease. Unless stable on serial radiographs, activity is indeterminate.

Ground-glass: A fine increase in opacity focally or diffusely in the lungs, sometimes with a slightly granular texture. It implies increased soft tissue (e.g., water, blood, cells, phospholipid) and decreased air within the involved region. It is not specific for either alveolar or interstitial lung diseases, because swelling of alveolar walls can produce the same finding. (Also used in CT.)

Honeycombing: A radiographic appearance of small (less than 1 cm in diameter) air-containing spaces with relatively thick walls, and walls that are common to adjacent spaces. It represents a combination of destruction of lung parenchyma with fibrosis and coalescence of the residual alveolar walls. The term should be used specifically and, when accurate, implies destructive, fibrotic lung disease. (Also used in CT.)

Hypertension (pulmonary): Sustained elevation of the pulmonary artery pressure above a mean pressure of 22 or a systolic pressure of 30 mm Hg.

Infarct (pulmonary): A region of damaged tissue caused by interruption of the pulmonary arterial blood supply, most commonly from an embolus. The region of infarction may contain edema fluid, blood, or frankly necrotic material. Usually hump-shaped and pleura-based (may be against a fissure). Does not necessarily indicate necrosis, so it can clear rapidly.

Infiltrate: A region of increased opacity within the lung, not having the appearance of a mass and usually ill defined. *Infiltrate* is a poor term that is frequently misunderstood by clinicians to imply pneumonia.

Interstitium: A space in the lung surrounding vessels and bronchi and containing the support elements of the lung. Fluid and cells can accumulate in the interstitium. Consists of three interconnecting compartments: *central interstitium*, surrounding the pulmonary artery, bronchi, and veins, as far as the level of the terminal bronchiole; *interlobular interstitium*, surrounding the secondary pulmonary lobule and connecting with the subpleural interstitium; and *alveolar wall interstitium*, containing the small branches of the pulmonary vessels and the lymphatics. (Also used in CT.)

Kerley lines: See *septal lines.*

Markings: A vague, meaningless, descriptive term often used in a phrase such as "diffuse increased lung markings." It is used when hedging on deciding whether the lungs are diffusely abnormal or not. (The national plant of the radiologist is the hedge!)

Mass: A solid region within the lung, more than 3 to 5 cm in diameter (depending on definition). Usually nearly spherical and usually does not contain air bronchograms. (Also used in CT.)

Miliary pattern: Innumerable small nodular opacities throughout the lung, by definition 2 to 10 mm in diameter (usually less than 5 mm). Often indicates a diffuse granulomatous disease but may be seen with pulmonary metastases. (Also used in CT.)

Mucoid impaction: Dilated, mucus-filled bronchi producing tubular branching opacities within the lung ("finger-in-glove" when referring to large bronchi; "tree-in-bud" for small airways).

Nodule: A focal opacity less than 3 cm with a near-spherical shape and uniform density. It may be calcified or contain a cavity.

Opacity: A descriptive term indicating a region of abnormal attenuation within the lung. To a large extent, this term has replaced *density* when referring to abnormal lung regions. Can be quantified as "focal," "diffuse," "nodular," or "confluent."

Platelike atelectasis (discoid atelectasis, Fleischner's lines): Linear opacities 2 to 10 cm or more in length, often parallel to the diaphragm.

Pneumatocele: Another one of the thin-walled cystic spaces in the lung. It used to be limited to a thin-walled space occurring as the result of staphylococci or other pyrogenic pneumonia and not cavitation. It also had to be very large. Now the term is used in conjunction with any thin-walled space occurring after infection. Pneumatoceles are often unstable, disappearing in weeks to months. "Pneumatoceles" seen with *Pneumocystis carinii* pneumonia in patients with AIDS most frequently do not resolve.

Pneumothorax: Air (which soon becomes nitrogen) in the pleural space.

Primary complex: Granuloma plus hilar or mediastinal lymph node enlargement. Also refers to a lung granuloma (with or without calcification) and calcified hilar or mediastinal lymph nodes. The term *Ranke focus* or *Ghon complex* describes the same thing. These last two terms should be abandoned.

Profusion: A qualitative expression of the relative involvement of the lung by a diffuse process. Often used in pneumoconiosis to indicate the number of small round or linear (irregular) opacities with reference to standard radiographs.

Reticular pattern: Innumerable linear opacities form a summation to cause a network appearance to the lungs. It may also be caused by lines and nodules.

Reticulonodular pattern: The same as reticular pattern, but the linear opacities form a summation to produce a network plus a nodular appearance.

Septal lines: Linear opacities resulting from abnormal material in interlobular or other interstitial spaces of the lung. (Also used in CT.)
   Kerley A lines: Large lines 3 to 4 cm long connecting the peripheral with the central interstitium.
   Kerley B lines: Interlobular lines less than 2 cm in length and extending to or near the pleural surface.
Kerley A lines can branch, but Kerley B lines cannot.

Silhouette sign: Obliteration of a normal anatomic interface between the lung and the mediastinum caused by accumulation of soft-tissue equivalent material in the lung parenchyma.

CT Definitions (Abnormal Findings)

CT and high resolution CT (HRCT) have certain terms that are specific to findings on these studies. Some of the important ones follow.

Acinar nodule: The same as an air-space nodule. The two terms are used interchangeably.

Air space consolidation: An increase in lung opacity that results from replacement of alveolar gas by some other material, which obscures the underlying lung structure.

Air-space nodule: A small nodule, usually ill-defined, ranging from 5 mm to 1 cm in diameter, frequently associated with a small airway.

Architectural distortion: An appearance to the lung in which the normal vascular and bronchial arrangements are disturbed. It implies fibrosis. The appearance may vary from subpleural nodules reflecting collapsed secondary lobules, to a more global disturbance in the normal branching appearance of the lungs' architecture.

Bronchocentric: Describes the locus of a disease process surrounding small peripheral bronchi/bronchioles and usually having a nodular appearance.

Centrilobular: Defines a process in proximity to the center of the secondary lobule, at which site a small bronchus and pulmonary artery are found. Each pulmonary lobule can have several centrilobular structures. (Sometimes used synonymously with bronchocentric.)

Dependent lung opacity (density): Subpleural density or opacity in the most dependent portion of the lung, resulting from the relative airlessness of this area. It can be seen in normal or abnormal situations.

Interlobular septal thickening: Several terms have been used to describe thickening of interlobular septa, including *short lines, large reticular pattern, peripheral arcades, polygonal arcades, polygons, exagones, parenchymal bands*, and *long lines*. Lines are from 1 to 5 or 6 cm in length.

Intralobular interstitial thickening: Describes a fine linear pattern of thickening of the support structures within the secondary pulmonary lobule, especially well seen in alveolar proteinosis and sometimes interstitial lung fibrosis ("small" or "fine" reticular pattern).

Mosaic perfusion: Regional differences in lung opacity (and often in vascular caliber) caused by vascular obstructive disease. The same term has been used to describe the decreased lung attenuation resulting from parenchymal changes associated with airway disease. Distinction should be made between the two situations.

Regional inhomogeneity: An abnormal situation of regional differences in lung parenchymal attenuation in which the underlying lung architecture can be seen to be preserved. Regional inhomogeneity may be caused by increased attenuation, i.e., ground-glass opacities, decrease in attenuation associated with abnormal airways, or decreased attenuation associated with vascular obstructive disease.

Signet-ring sign: A dilated bronchus (indicates bronchiectasis) and its associated pulmonary artery, producing the appearance of a stone on a ring.

Subpleural line: A pencil-line, or slightly thicker, linear opacity varying from less than 1 to several cm in length that is parallel to and within about 1 cm of the costal pleural surface. When visible only in a "dependent" lung, it can reflect transient atelectasis; its presence in a nondependent lung may reflect interstitial fibrosis.

Traction bronchiectasis: Dilated, beaded bronchi found in areas of interstitial fibrosis, especially with honeycombing.

THORACIC IMAGING DIFFERENTIAL DIAGNOSES

Mediastinum
  Anterior mediastinal masses
  Middle mediastinal masses
  Posterior mediastinal masses
  Fatty mediastinal lesions
  Cystic mediastinal masses
  Diffuse mediastinal widening:
  Pneumomediastinum
  Bilateral hilar or mediastinal lymphadenopathy
  Hilar/mediastinal lymphadenopathy in AIDS
  Calcification
  Unilateral hilar enlargement
Airways
  Trachea
  Bronchi
Lungs
  Focal Lung Disease
  Diffuse/Multifocal Lung Disease
Pleura
  Pneumothorax
  Unilateral pleural effusion with otherwise normal chest radiograph
  Predominantly left-sided pleural effusion
  Predominantly right-sided pleural effusion
  Pleural effusion associated with lung consolidation or mass
  Pleural mass
  Pleural calcification
  Smooth pleural thickening
Chest Wall
  Unilateral elevated hemidiaphragm
  Bilateral elevated hemidiaphragms
  Chest wall mass
  Rib lesion with surrounding soft tissue mass
  Malignant chest wall tumors in children

MEDIASTINUM

ANTERIOR MEDIASTINAL MASSES

Name three anterior mediastinal masses that also can be masses in the middle mediastinum. Which anterior mediastinal masses can contain calcified foci?

Retrosternal goiter
Elongated/aneurysmal dilatation of innominate artery
Thymic masses
Germ cell neoplasms
Lymphoma
Ascending aortic aneurysm
Rarer tumors/masses

Retrosternal Goiter

- 1 to 3% of goiters enter thorax
- Sharply defined, smooth mass above aortic arch
- May contain calcification and may compress the trachea
- Most common cause of cervical tracheal displacement (usually laterally, posteriorly)
- Rarely situated between trachea and esophagus (anterior tracheal displacement)

FIGURES F.P.: 16–2; A.W.: 19–18

Elongated/Aneurysmal Dilatation of Innominate Artery

- Usually does not displace trachea
- Above aortic arch and on right side

Thymic Masses

- Thymoma
    - ¶ 15% of patients with myasthenia gravis have thymoma
    - ¶ 30 to 50% of thymomas in adults are malignant
    - ¶ 50% of patients with thymoma have myasthenia
    - ¶ Malignancy (extracapsular invasion) suggested by large size, mediastinal invasion, transpleural spread (15%)

FIGURES F.P.: 16–8/9/10/11; A.W.: 19–14

- Nodular thymic hyperplasia
- Lymphoma and leukemia
- Thymic carcinoma
- Thymic carcinoid
- Thymolipoma
    - ¶ Does not have appearance of focal thymic mass
    - ¶ Large, predominately fat-containing, benign anterior mediastinal tumors

FIGURES F.P.: 16–14; A.W.: 19–9

Germ Cell Neoplasms

- Benign teratoma
    - ¶ 50% of germ cell tumors in adults
    - ¶ More than one germ layer
    - ¶ Most arise in thymus
    - ¶ Most cystic and contain ectodermal elements
    - ¶ Fluid, fat, calcium
    - ¶ Large anterior mediastinal cyst

FIGURES F.P.: 19–17; A.W.: 16–19

- Teratocarcinoma

1

- Dermoid
- Seminoma
- Choriocarcinoma
- Embryonal cell carcinoma
- Endodermal sinus tumors
    ¶ 80% benign, 20% malignant; can be large
    ¶ On CT may contain calcium, fat, fluid levels, bone
    ¶ Malignancy suggested by mediastinal infiltration, large size, and extension to pleura

FIGURES   A.W.: 19–17

Lymphoma

- May arise from the thymus or lymph nodes
- Bulky anterior mediastinal adenopathy the most common radiographic finding with Hodgkin's lymphoma (sarcoid rarely involves anterior mediastinal nodes)

Ascending Aortic Aneurysm

- May be indistinguishable on chest radiographs from other anterior mediastinal masses
- Curvilinear calcifications are suggestive
- Must not be confused with sinus of Valsalva aneurysm

Rarer Tumors/Masses

- Lymphangioma
    ¶ Upper anterior mediastinum with or without cervical mass
    ¶ Often has associated venous malformations
- Mesenchymal tumors
- Parathyroid tumors
    ¶ Approximately 5% of parathyroid adenomas arise in the mediastinum, most commonly in front of ascending aorta but may be in middle or posterior mediastinum
- Morgagni's hernia
    ¶ Cardiophrenic angle mass
- Benign lymphoid hyperplasia (Castleman's disease, angiofollicular lymphoid hyperplasia)
    ¶ More common in middle or posterior mediastinum; chronic, lobulated, highly vascular masses

MIDDLE MEDIASTINAL MASSES

Name three malignant and three benign causes of a middle mediastinal mass. Which are the two most common neoplasms?

Lymph node enlargement
Bronchogenic cyst
Bronchogenic carcinoma
Aortic aneurysm
Reduplication cyst of esophagus (foregut cyst)
Chronic mediastinitis
Tracheal neoplasms
Castleman's disease (angiofollicular lymphoid hyperplasia)

Middle Mediastinum Location

- Between anterior wall of trachea/posterior border of heart and 1 cm behind anterior margins of vertebral bodies

1

Lymph Node Enlargement

- Most common cause metastases from bronchogenic carcinoma or extrathoracic malignancies
- Lymphoma

FIGURES   A.W.: 16–42/44

- Granulomatous infections
- Sarcoidosis

Bronchogenic Cyst

- Well defined round or oval mass 1 to 10 cm in diameter
- Most common round mass within 5 cm of tracheal carina

Bronchogenic Carcinoma

- May arise in central bronchi or within mediastinum
- Most commonly squamous cell or small cell carcinoma
- Occasionally metastatic from lung primary in which primary not apparent on chest radiographs

Aortic Aneurysm

- Rim calcification useful
- May be traumatic (pseudoaneurysm) or atherosclerotic
- Rarer causes include dissection, mycotic aneurysm

FIGURES   F.P.: 19–28

Reduplication Cyst of Esophagus (Foregut Cyst)

- Often indistinguishable from a bronchogenic cyst (thus, better to refer to both as *foregut cysts*)

Chronic Mediastinitis

- Granulomatous mediastinitis most commonly presents as focal mediastinal mass
- Contains multiple sites of calcification
- May encase and narrow vascular structures and/or airways

FIGURES   F.P.: 19–3/4/5

Tracheal Neoplasms

- Mixed salivary gland tumors (cylindroma); most common: adenoid cystic carcinomas
- Carcinoid tumors
- Squamous/adenocarcinomas
- May have large extratracheal components
- Any soft tissue mass within tracheal cartilages as seen on CT is abnormal and requires investigation

FIGURES   F.P.: 11–6

Castleman's Disease (Angiofollicular Lymphoid Hyperplasia)

- Chronic, slow growing, low grade "malignancy"
- Hyaline vascular subtype (80%) enhances markedly with intravascular contrast material

Name two neurogenic tumors that arise in the posterior mediastinum. What organ systems can give rise to masses in the anterior, middle, and posterior mediastinum?

POSTERIOR MEDIASTINAL MASSES

Neurogenic neoplasm
Vertebral neoplasm
Abscess
Descending aortic aneurysm
Extramedullary hematopoiesis
Thoracic meningocele

Posterior Mediastinum Location

• Behind 1 cm from anterior margin of vertebral bodies

Neurogenic Neoplasm

• Neurofibromas and neurilemmomas in adults
• Ganglion neuromas and neuroblastomas in children
• Arise from spinal nerves or sympathetic nerve chain
• Calcification rare but may signify malignancy

FIGURES   F.P.: 19–32; A.W.: 16–60/61/62/63

Vertebral Neoplasm

• Osteochondroma, aneurysmal bone cyst, chondrosarcoma, osteogenic sarcoma, Ewing's sarcoma, myeloma, and metastases
• Soft tissue masses uncommon

Abscess

• Disk space and adjacent vertebral bodies involved

Descending Aortic Aneurysm

• Features are typical

Extramedullary Hematopoiesis

• More common in the lower half of the dorsal vertebral column
• Often bilateral, lobulated or smooth masses
• Bony changes of associated hemolytic anemia usually present
• Splenomegaly

Thoracic Meningocele

• Usually with neurofibromatosis
• Associated vertebral body anomalies

FATTY MEDIASTINAL LESIONS

Mediastinal lipomatosis
Mediastinal lipoma/liposarcoma
Thymolipoma
Morgagni's hernia containing omentum
Epicardial fat pad
Paraesophageal hernia containing fat
Extramedullary hematopoiesis (rarely fatty)
Chylolymphatic cyst
Teratoma, fat containing

FIGURES   F.P.: 19–20/21/22

Mediastinal Lipoma/Liposarcoma

• Most commonly adjacent to diaphragm

CYSTIC MEDIASTINAL MASSES

Name five cystic mediastinal masses.

Thymic cysts
Cystic degeneration in thymic Hodgkin's disease
Germ cell tumors
Foregut cyst, bronchogenic cyst, or reduplication cyst of esophagus
Neuroenteric cyst
Meningocele
Pancreatic pseudocyst
Lymphangioma/cystic hygroma
Mediastinal abscess
Hematoma
Goiter, cystic elements

Thymic Cysts

• Usually degenerative cysts in thymoma or germ cell tumor
• Congenital thymic cysts rare

Pancreatic Pseudocyst

• Presents through aortic hiatus

DIFFUSE MEDIASTINAL WIDENING

Lipomatosis
Diffuse lymphoma
Small cell bronchogenic carcinoma
Diffuse mediastinitis
Anaplastic/poorly differentiated squamous cell carcinoma
Hematoma

PNEUMOMEDIASTINUM

Name four causes of a pneumomediastinum that are unrelated to instrumentation or artificial ventilation.

Spontaneous
Barotrauma
Injury
Vomiting
Extension of retroperitoneal gas
Extension of cervical gas
Postoperative

Spontaneous

• Asthma
• Coughing or exercise
• Decompression (during diving)

1

Barotrauma

• With high peak inspiratory ventilatory pressures

Injury

• To esophagus, larynx, trachea, or bronchi during instrumentation
• Traumatic perforation of esophagus, trachea, or major bronchi

Vomiting

• With Boerhaave's syndrome

FIGURES   F.P: 19–7/8

BILATERAL HILAR OR MEDIASTINAL LYMPHADENOPATHY

Name four causes of bilateral hiIaradenopathy.

Sarcoidosis
Bronchogenic carcinoma (usually unilateral)
Lymphoma
Tuberculosis (usually unilateral)
Histoplasmosis
Coccidioidomycosis (usually unilateral)
Mycoplasma pneumonia
Viral disease
Bacterial infections (usually unilateral)
Leukemia
Metastases from extrathoracic primaries
Silicosis
Cystic fibrosis
Langerhans' giant cell disease

Sarcoidosis

• Bilateral hilar and right paratracheal adenopathy most common on chest radiographs (1, 2, 3 sign)
• Bilateral hilar and bilateral mediastinal adenopathy most common on CT
• Prevascular adenopathy uncommon
• Enlargement tends to decrease as parenchymal disease increases
• Except for withdrawal of treatment, adenopathy rarely increases once present
• Peripheral hilar (tracheobronchial) adenopathy has a good prognosis

Bronchogenic Carcinoma

• Adenopathy almost always ipsilateral
• Bilateral mediastinal adenopathy can occur
• Upper lobe tumors rarely extend to inferior hilar nodes
• Distribution of mediastinal adenopathy not predictive of side of primary tumor

Lymphoma

- Anterior mediastinal adenopathy most common presentation of Hodgkin's disease
- Non-Hodgkin's lymphomas more likely to involve multiple nodal sites
- Massive adenopathy in HIV-positive patient suggests B-cell lymphoma
- Lymph nodes calcify after radiation therapy but rarely after chemotherapy
- Detection of hilar nodes important for therapy in Hodgkin's disease

Tuberculosis

- Usually primary tuberculosis
- Usually unilateral and on side of lung disease

Histoplasmosis

- Unpredictable distribution of nodal involvement
- Calcification of nodes common

Coccidioidomycosis

- Unilateral and on same side as parenchymal disease
- Contralateral mediastinal nodal enlargement indicative of possible dissemination

Mycoplasma Pneumonia

- Unilateral/bilateral hilar and mediastinal adenopathy
- Common in children

Viral Disease

- Many viral infections can produce hilar adenopathy

Bacterial Infections

- Rare; most bacterial infections do not cause adenopathy, except lung abscesses

Leukemia

- Nodal enlargement in up to 20% of cases

Metastases From Extrathoracic Primaries

- Midline tumors including head and neck squamous cell carcinoma; medullary carcinoma of the thyroid, breast, kidney, genitourinary tract, and testis; melanoma
- May be unilateral or bilateral

Silicosis

- Bilateral hilar enlargement
- Eggshell calcifications

Cystic Fibrosis

· Unilateral or bilateral hilar enlargement common (adenopathy and later pulmonary hypertension)
· Findings suggesting airway disease (atelectasis, tram-tracks, mucus plugs, abscesses, hyperinflation, hemoptysis)

Langerhans' Giant Cell Granulomatosis

· Histiocytosis X

Rare Causes

· Drug induced: dilantin/trimethadione

HILAR/MEDIASTINAL ADENOPATHY IN AIDS

List the four most common causes of mediastinal adenopathy in patients with AIDS.

Kaposi's sarcoma
TB
Lymphoma
Cryptococcosis

UNILATERAL HILAR ENLARGEMENT

List five causes of unilateral hilar enlargment.

Granulomatous disease
    TB
    Coccidioidomycosis
    Histoplasmosis
Bronchogenic carcinoma
Lymphoma
Surgical shunt
Post stenotic from pulmonary valvular stenosis
Pulmonary artery coarctation
Pulmonary embolism
Partial absence of left pericardium
Pulmonary arteriovenous fistula

FIGURES A.W.: 16–46/50

Surgical Shunt

· Corrective surgery for right heart outflow obstruction

Post Stenotic

· Pulmonic valvular or supravalvular stenosis

Pulmonary Artery Coarctation

· Especially after congenital rubella

MEDIASTINAL CALCIFICATION

Lymph node
Granulomatous infections (especially histoplasmosis)
Silicosis
Contrast material ("pseudo" calcification)
Sarcoidosis

EGGSHELL CALCIFICATION

Name two causes of eggshell calicification.

Silicosis
Pneumoconiosis of coal workers (rare)
Sarcoidosis
Lymphoma after radiation (rare)

CARDIAC CALCIFICATION

Aortic/mitral valves
Coronary arteries
Annulus of aortic/mitral valves
Pericardium
Myocardium
Endocardium (i.e., thrombus)
Tumors (e.g., myxoma)

AIRWAYS

TRACHEA

FOCAL MASS

Name five causes of a focal tracheal mass.

Inflammatory polyp/papilloma
Adenoma (mixed salivary gland tumor/cylindroma)
Tracheal carcinoma
Invasion
Metastases
Lymphoma
Other tumors
Hematoma
Papillomatosis
Rare causes
    Rheumatoid
    Sarcoidosis
    Coccidioidomycosis
    Scleroma
    Wegener's granulomatosis
    Foreign body

Inflammatory Polyp/Papilloma

- Occurs after instrumentation or tracheotomy
- Presents as pedunculated or sessile mass
- Not neoplastic

Adenoma (Mixed Salivary Gland Tumor/Cylindroma)

- All low grade malignancies
- Represents 40% of tracheal neoplasms
- Metastasizes late
- Most common: adenoid cystic carcinomas; second most common: mucoepidermoid carcinomas
- Carcinoids constitute less than 10% of tracheal "adenomas"

FIGURES   A.W.: 8–60/61

1

Tracheal Carcinoma

- Irregular or annular can extensively invade through tracheal wall
- Can also spread regionally to nodes and invade adjacent structures
- CT to determine overall length of tumor and size of the extratracheal mass
- Up to 6 cm of trachea can be resected
- Most common: squamous cell carcinoma, adenocarcinoma, small cell carcinoma

Invasion

- From neoplasms near trachea
- Most common neoplasms invading trachea arise from lung, larynx, thyroid, and esophagus
- Difficult to distinguish from primary tracheal neoplasm
- Any soft tissue within cartilaginous tracheal rings on CT is abnormal

FIGURES F.P.: 11–6

Metastases

- Tumors that metastasize directly to tracheal wall: renal cell carcinoma, melanoma, breast carcinoma, and colon carcinoma

Lymphoma

- May involve tracheal wall

Other Tumors

- Unusual tumors arising from wall of trachea include neurogenic tumors, smooth muscle tumors, fibromas, hemangiomas, and chondromas

Papillomatosis

- Laryngeal papillomatosis spreads to trachea and bronchi in ± 4% of cases
- Usually only after tracheal instrumentation/tracheotomy
- More common in adolescence and young adulthood

DIFFUSE NARROWING

Which cause of diffuse tracheal narrowing is only in the lateral dimension?

Saber-sheath trachea
Relapsing polychondritis
Osteochondroplastica
Amyloidosis

Saber-Sheath Trachea

- Narrowing only in lateral dimension and intrathoracic trachea
- By definition AP diameter more than twice the lateral diameter
- Associated with chronic obstructive pulmonary disease (COPD)

Relapsing Polychondritis

- Smooth uniform narrowing of trachea
- Tracheal cartilages thickened and wall thickened on CT

Osteochondroplastica

- Irregular nodular narrowing with osteoid and chondroid elements

Amyloid

- Can occasionally have diffuse tracheal narrowing, as can rheumatoid, sclerodema and Wegener's granulomatosis

FIGURES   F.P.: 11–7/8; A.W.: 17–2/3/4

FOCAL NARROWING

Traumatic stricture
Neoplasms
Inflammatory masses
Extrinsic compression
Vascular ring
Congenital complete tracheal ring (rare)

Traumatic Stricture

- After intubation
- After tracheotomy
- Circumferential after injury from tracheotomy balloon

Extrinsic Compression

- Caused by vascular malformation, neoplasms, or goiter

Vascular Ring

- Posterior impression from anomalous subclavian in middle to upper third
- Posterior impression immediately above carina with anomalous origin of left pulmonary artery from right

BRONCHI

LOBAR/SEGMENTAL ATELECTASIS

What is the most common cause of lobar atelectasis in hospitalized patients?

Name four causes of benign bronchial strictures.

Intraluminal
    Foreign body
    Mucus plugs
    Bronchial metastases
In the wall
    Non-small cell carcinoma of bronchus
    Bronchial adenoma
    Carcinoids
    Chondrohamartoma
    Noninfectious granulomatous disease
    Sarcoidosis
    Wegener's granulomatosis

Infectious granulomatous disease
Tuberculosis
Collagen vascular disease
Congenital bronchial atresia
Bronchiectasis
Trauma
Middle lobe syndrome
Lymphadenopathy

FIGURES   F.P.: 4–19 to 37; F.P.: 4–42 to 69

Foreign Body

- Most common: peanut: next a tooth
- History may not be revealing
- CT usually shows intraluminal mass

Mucus Plugs

- Especially cystic fibrosis and complicated asthma with allergic bronchopulmonary aspergillosis
- Postoperative multiple mucus plugs the most common cause of atelectasis in hospitalized patients

Bronchial Metastases

- Renal cell, breast, melanoma, and colon (all rare)

Non-Small Cell Carcinoma of Bronchus

- Most commonly arises in third to fifth generation bronchi
- Atelectasis the presenting finding in approximately 20% of non-small cell bronchogenic carcinoma

Bronchial Adenoma

- Carcinoids constitute 80% of bronchial adenomas

Chondrohamartoma

- Rarely presents as endobronchial mass

Noninfectious Granulomatous Disease

- Especially sarcoidosis, Wegener's granulomatosis

Infectious Granulomatous Disease

- Tuberculosis and fungal infections
- May not show other features of infection
- Narrowing can result from granulomas in wall or mucosal strictures

Collagen Vascular Disease

- Rheumatoid rarely presents as bronchostenosis

Congenital Bronchial Atresia

- Most common site: left upper lobe
- Proximal mass represents dilated poststenotic, mucus filled airway

1

- Distal lung hyperlucency invariably present
- Right middle lobe second most common site

Bronchiectasis

- Lobar or segmental collapse from combination of mucus impaction and abnormal lung compliance

Trauma

- Fractured bronchus or bronchial tear
- Associated with mucosal or submucosal hematoma and bronchial obstruction
- Cardinal features: pneumothorax/pneumomediastinum and non-collapsing, non-reexpanding opacified lung

Middle Lobe Syndrome

- Represents nonobstructive atelectasis of middle lobe
- Originally described with prior compression resulting from TB lymphadenopathy causing lobar collapse followed by resolution of adenopathy
- Middle lobe because it is small and has difficulty reexpanding once collapsed
- Now in most cases postinfectious with scarring

Infectious Lymphadenopathy

- Was once common cause of atelectasis in children, especially those with tuberculosis
- Now rare

LUNGS

FOCAL LUNG DISEASE

SOLITARY NODULE (DIAMETER < 3 CM)

List six causes of a solitary pulmonary nodule that will not double in size in 2 years.

Malignant neoplasm
Inflammation/infection
Benign neoplasm
Splenosis and endometrial tissue deposits
AVM
Infarct
Bronchogenic cyst
Caplan's syndrome
Pseudo masses

General

- Seen on 2 of 1,000 chest radiographs
- Of resected lesions about 50% malignant
- May be neoplastic or benign

FIGURES   F.P.: 8–18 to 20; A.W.: 4–14 to 82

Malignant Neoplasm

- See Table 1–4 in *Overview* for features distinguishing benign from malignant SPN

- Bronchogenic carcinoma (20 to 60%)
- Lymphoma (rare)
- Sarcoma (rare)
- Adenoma (carcinoid, less than 5%)
- Solitary metastases (4 to 6%)
    ¶ 60% of solitary metastases from colon; others include kidney, ovary, testes, melanoma, and sarcoma
- Pleural fibroma

Inflammation/Infection

- Granuloma (20 to 60%); includes tuberculoma, histoplasmoma, coccidioidoma, and cryptococcoma
- Hydatid cyst (rare)
- Rounded atelectasis (usually more than 3 cm)
- Plasma cell granuloma
- Infectious/inflammatory: rheumatoid (necrobiotic) nodules

Benign Neoplasm

- Hamartoma (chondrohamartoma)(6 to 8%)
- Lipoma, fibroma, neurogenic tumor (all less than 5%)
- Intraparenchymal lymph nodes; common but small (usually less than 5 mm in diameter) and subpleural

Splenosis and Endometrial Tissue Deposits

- Rare benign lesions

Vascular

- Arteriovenous malformation (less than 5%)
- Hemangioma
- Infarct
- Pulmonary vein varix

Congenital

- Intraparenchymal bronchogenic cyst (less than 5%)
- Pulmonary sequestration

Inhalational

- Progressive massive fibrosis (PMF)
- Affects upper lobes, with marked hilar elevation
- Occupational history invaluable
- Less obvious grades of PMF can be seen on CT, caused by coalescence of silicotic nodules

FIGURES F.P.: 12–5/6; A.W.: 4–88

Pseudo Masses

- Nipple, mole, skin lesion
- Artifact
- Encapsulated fissural fluid
- Pleural plaque
- Callus/rib lesion

SOLITARY MASS (DIAMETER > 3 CM)

Bronchogenic carcinoma
Tuberculoma, histoplasmoma
Hydatid cyst (uncommon)
Chondrohamartoma
Lung abscess
Bronchoalveolar cell carcinoma
Solitary metastases
Rheumatoid (necrobiotic) nodule
Bronchogenic cyst
PMF

MULTIPLE NODULES/MASSES (ANY SIZE)

List five sites of neoplasms that tend to metastasize to the lungs as multiple pulmonary nodules.

Metastases
Lymphoma
Granulomatous infection
    MTB
    Coccidioidomycosis
    Histoplasmosis
Multifocal bronchoalveolar cell carcinoma
Multiple chondrohamartomas
Multiple AVMs
Laryngeal papillomatosis spread
Collagen vascular disease
    Wegener's granulomatosis
    Rheumatoid necrobiotic nodules
    Caplan's syndrome
Noninfectious granulomatous disease
    Sarcoid
    Bronchocentric granulomatosis
    Foreign body granulomas
    Langerhans' giant cell granulomatosis
Mucoid impaction
Trauma
Viral infection
    CMV
    Respiratory syncytial virus
    Measles
Nodular *P. carinii* pneumonia

FIGURES   F.P.: 6–31 to 56; A.W.: 4–85/86

Metastases

• Especially melanoma, sarcomas, and cancers of breast, kidney, colon, stomach, testes, ovary

Lymphoma

• Uncommon

Granulomatous Infection

• Hematogenous dissemination of MTB, coccidioidomycosis, histoplasmosis

1

Multiple Chondrohamartomas

· Rare

Trauma

· With multiple pulmonary hematomas

Nodular Form of *P. Carinii* Pneumonia

· In AIDS patients
· Granulomatous response that sometimes cavitates

MILIARY NODULES (DIAMETER 2 TO 3 TO 10 MM)

FIGURES   F.P.: 4–43, 8–64; A.W.: 6–66, 6–121

Mycobacterium tuberculosis
Fungal infections
    Histoplasmosis
    Coccidioidomycosis
    Blastomycosis
    South American paracocci
Hematogenous metastases
Inhalational lung disease
Viral pneumonias
Multifocal alveolar cell carcinoma
Sarcoidosis
Langerhans' giant cell disease
(histiocytosis X, eosinophilic granuloma of the lung)
Rare causes
    Microlithiasis
    Hemosiderosis
    Amyloidosis

Mycobacterium Tuberculosis

· Hematogenous dissemination
· May or may not have adenopathy

Hematogenous from Metastases

· Thyroid, melanoma, osteogenic sarcoma, choriocarcinoma

Inhalational Lung Disease

· Silicosis
· Pneumoconiosis of coal workers
· Beryllium stannosis

CAVITIES

List five causes of a thick-walled solitary lung cavity.

Thick walled
    Bronchogenic carcinoma
    Primary lymphoma
    Metastasis
    Lung abscess
    Amebic abscess
    Hydatid cyst

Paragonimiasis
Cavitating progressive massive fibrosis
Wegener's granulomatosis
Cavitating rheumatoid nodules

Name five causes of a thin-walled cystic space within the lung.

FIGURES F.P.: 4–49/51; A.W.: 6–32

Thin-walled
Blebs
Bullae
Traumatic lung cyst
Pneumatocele
Excavating bronchogenic cyst
"Congenital" lung cyst
Cavitating metastases
Parenchymal spread of laryngopapillomatosis
Cystic bronchiectasis

FIGURES F.P.: 4–81/82; A.W.: 4–84

General

• Usually multiple, occasionally solitary

Bronchogenic Carcinoma

• Squamous cell common
• Adenocarcinoma rare
• Alveolar cell carcinoma, virtually never
• Small cell carcinoma, virtually never

Primary Lymphoma

• Rare

Metastases

• Squamous cell carcinoma, especially head and neck, cervix, and esophagus
• Choriocarcinoma
• Adenocarcinoma

Lung Abscess

• Causative organisms: anaerobes, staphylococci, *Klebsiella* spp, *Pseudomonas* spp, *E. coli, Legionella* spp
• Tuberculosis: advanced primary or re-infection tuberculosis
• Semi-invasive aspergillosis
• Clinical presentation: hemoptysis, fever, malaise, and brain abscess

Hydatid Cyst

• Usually smoothly marginated with moderately thick wall
• Separation between exocyst and reaction in adjacent lung

Paragonimiasis

• Clusters of moderately thick-walled cysts

Cavitating Progressive Massive Fibrosis

• Incidence of tuberculosis increased with silicosis
• Consider bronchogenic carcinoma, unless stable over years

Cavitating Rheumatoid Nodules

• Smooth inner wall
• Can become thin walled

Cavitating Metastases

• Rarely thin-walled

Parenchymal Spread of Laryngopapillomatosis

• Usually mixed thin walled and thick walled

CAVITY WITH AIR-FLUID LEVEL

Cavitating bronchogenic carcinoma
Tuberculosis
Specific fungal infection, e.g., mycetoma
Pulmonary bulla, infected or noninfected
Infected lung cyst
Lung laceration with liquefied hematoma
Infected sequestration
Necrobiotic nodule in rheumatoid lung disease
Cavitating pulmonary infarct
Infection of preexisting cavity (thin walled cyst)
Wegener's granulomatosis

CONSOLIDATION (LOBAR AND SUBLOBAR)

List five causes of lobar or sublobar consolidation not caused by infection.

Pneumonia
Infarction
Lung contusion
Focal edema
Radiation
Alveolar cell carcinoma
Lymphoma

Pneumonia

• Obscured vessels, air bronchograms, ill-defined margins, pleural margination

Infarction

• Pleural based, hump-shaped, often does not contain air bronchograms
• Composed of edema fluid, hemorrhage, and necrosis

Lung Contusion

• Bleeding into lung without major disruption of tissues

Focal Edema

• Right upper lobe with rupture of anterior leaflet of mitral valve
• Abnormal lung tissue
• Hyperperfusion edema with multiple pulmonary emboli
• Positional edema

Radiation

- Edema phase at 3 to 6 weeks
- Pneumonic phase at 6 weeks to 6 months

Alveolar Cell Carcinoma

- Focal form limited to one lobe

Lymphoma

- Usually multifocal

TUBULAR DENSITIES

Mucoid impaction
AVM
Pulmonary vein varix
Bronchiectasis

Mucoid Impaction

- Especially with allergic bronchopulmonary aspergillosis

FLEETING (RAPIDLY CLEARING) INFILTRATES

List five causes of fleeting infiltrates (multifocal or diffuse).

Allergic reactions
Drugs
Parasites
Inhaled antigens
Löffler's syndrome
Allergic aspergillosis
Recurrent edema
Chronic eosinophilic pneumonia with treatment
Pneumocystis pneumonia bleeding into the lung

DIFFUSE/MULTIFOCAL LUNG DISEASE

DIFFUSE AIR SPACE CONSOLIDATION

Edema ("water")
Pneumonia ("pus")
Hemorrhage ("blood")
Proteinaceous materials
Adult respiratory distress syndrome (ARDS, DAD)

Edema ("water")

What are the two main mechanisms of pulmonary edema production?

What features of the fluid distinguish cardiogenic from noncardiogenic edema?

- "Hemodynamic" or "cardiogenic" ("low protein") type: shows indistinct vessels, hilar haze, vascular enlargement, interstitial lines, pleural effusion, usually cardiomegaly
- "Noncardiogenic" ("high protein") type: caused by capillary leak; indistinguishable from cardiogenic type, although alveolar edema fluid tends to be more peripheral and nondependent

FIGURES   F.P.: 4–6

Pneumonia ("Pus")

· Causes: *Pneumocystis*, fungus, bacteria, or aspiration pneumonia with or without infection

Hemorrhage ("Blood")

· Dissociation between poor radiographic appearance and good oxygenation
· Causes: idiopathic pulmonary hemosiderosis/Goodpasture's syndrome, bleeding diathesis, anticoagulant therapy, renal failure, collagen vascular disease, and trauma

FIGURES F.P.: 4–7

Proteinaceous Materials

· Alveolar proteinosis (phospholipid)

Adult Respiratory Distress Syndrome (ARDS)

· High-protein fluid with membranes

CHRONIC AIR SPACE CONSOLIDATION

List four causes of chronic air space consolidation.

Alveolar proteinosis
Lymphoma
Pseudolymphoma
Bronchoalveolar cell carcinoma
Sarcoidosis
Desquamative interstitial pneumonitis
Chronic specific inflammation
    TB
    Fungus (rare)
Lipoid pneumonia (rare)

FIGURES F.P.: 4–3, 8–21, 17–12; A.W.: 13–54/55

MULTIFOCAL OR DIFFUSE AIR SPACE CONSOLIDATION THAT COMES AND GOES

List five causes of recurrent infiltrates.

Recurrent edema
Recurrent inhalation of toxins
Recurrent exposure to extrinsic allergens ("hypersensitivity pneumonitis")
Recurrent hemorrhage
Intermittent treatment of chronic diffuse consolidation, e.g., sarcoidosis

INTERSTITIAL LUNG DISEASE

CHRONIC SEPTAL THICKENING

· Kerley B lines on chest radiographs
· Interlobular septal lines on HRCT, without architectural distortion
· Causes: chronic pulmonary edema, lymphangitic carcinomatosis, veno-occlusive disease (rare), congenital lymphangiectasia (rare)

FIGURES A.W: 4–92/101

NONCARDIOGENIC PULMONARY EDEMA

List six causes of noncardiogenic pulmonary edema.

- Causes
  - ¶ Aspiration
  - ¶ Raised intracranial pressure
  - ¶ Rapid reexpansion of lung collapsed for more than 72 hours
  - ¶ Drug and blood product reactions
  - ¶ Inhalation of noxious agents
  - ¶ Heroin
  - ¶ Early ARDS with activation of vasoactive pathways, especially as a result of septicemia, shock, or trauma

HONEYCOMB LUNG

Which are five common causes of honeycomb lung? Which collagen vascular diseases can show a honeycomb lung?

- Moderately thick-walled air spaces sharing walls
- Basal peripheral predominance common
- Idiopathic pulmonary fibrosis (fibrosing alveolitis)
  - ¶ 70% of all cases
  - ¶ Striking peripheral distribution
  - ¶ Honeycombing may coexist with features of active inflammation, i.e., ground-glass opacities
- Pneumoconiosis
  - ¶ Asbestosis: 7% of patients with asbestosis have honeycombing with a basal and peripheral predominance
  - ¶ Diatomaceous earth inhalation (acute silicosis)
  - ¶ Alveolar proteinosis initially then can rapidly develop honeycombing
- Langerhans' giant cell granulomatosis (histiocytosis X); honeycombing usually diffuse, may form larger cystic spaces
- Sarcoidosis may have upper and middle lung predominance
- Rheumatoid lung disease
- Other collagen vascular diseases, especially scleroderma, Sjögren's disease, lupus, and mixed connective tissue disease
- Rare causes include amyloid, Gaucher's disease, radiation, gold therapy

FIGURES A.W.: 13–37; F.P.: 17–23/22/25

PREDOMINANTLY UPPER LUNG FIBROSIS AND HILAR ELEVATION

Name three causes of right-sided upper lobe fibrosis.

- Chronic re-infection/reactivation tuberculosis
- Radiation, especially for supraclavicular nodes from breast or head and neck tumors
- Sarcoidosis in chronic destructive phase
- Progressive massive fibrosis (PMF)
  - ¶ Surrounded by peripheral emphysema
  - ¶ Egg-shell calcification
  - ¶ Silicotic nodules in rest of lung
- Histoplasmosis
- Langerhans' giant cell granulomatosis (uncommon)
- Ankylosing spondylitis (rare)

MULTIPLE, ILL-DEFINED NODULES 5 TO 20 MM IN DIAMETER

Name five causes of ill-defined pulmonary nodules.

90% granulomatous disease or metastases
Granulomatous disease can be infectious or noninfectious

1

Noninfectious granulomatous disease: Langerhans' giant cell disease, sarcoidosis; rheumatoid and Wegener's disease usually have fewer nodules

Infectious granulomatous disease: tuberculosis, histoplasmosis, coccidioidomycosis, others; viral pneumonias; metastases; extrinsic allergic alveolitis; pneumoconiosis; drug reaction

INTERSTITIAL LUNG DISEASE WITH PNEUMOTHORAX

- Langerhans' giant cell granulomatosis
- Sarcoidosis
- Any interstitial lung disease
- Cystic fibrosis (pseudointerstitial lung disease)
- Lymphangiomyomatosis

UNILATERAL HYPERLUCENT LUNG

Name five causes of a unilateral hyperlucent lung.

- Technique: patient rotation; decentered tube with focused grid
- Chest wall defects/deformity:
    ¶ Mastectomy
    ¶ Congenital absence of pectoral muscle
- Pulmonary vascular obstruction
    ¶ Proximal interruption/hypoplasia of pulmonary artery
    ¶ Massive emboli
- Airways disease
    ¶ Central airway obstructing lesion with air trapping
    ¶ Bronchiolitis obliterans (Swyer-James/Macleod syndrome)
    ¶ Bullous emphysema
    ¶ Congenital lobar emphysema
    ¶ Atelectasis with compensatory hyperinflation

Which one would be easily diagnosed with a decubitus radiograph?

- Pleural disease
    ¶ Pneumothorax (especially in supine patient)

FIGURES   F.P.: 4–79

COMMON PNEUMOCONIOSES

- With fibrosis
    ¶ Silicosis, caused by silicates
    ¶ Pneumoconiosis of coal workers, caused by coal dust
    ¶ Asbestosis silicate-fibers with length:diameter ratio of more than 3
- Without fibrosis
    ¶ Stannosis, tin
    ¶ Siderosis, iron
    ¶ Barytosis, barium
- Allergenic
    ¶ Berylliosis, beryllium
    ¶ Cadminosis, cadmium
- Organic dusts
    ¶ Farmer's lung, fungi
    ¶ Bagassosis, sugar cane
    ¶ Byssinosis, cotton
    ¶ Bird fancier's lung, proteins from birds
    ¶ Sequoiosis, sequoia tree proteins
    ¶ Many others

PLEURA

PNEUMOTHORAX WITH OTHERWISE NORMAL CHEST RADIOGRAPH

Blebs/bullae
MTB
Trauma
Metastasis (especially osteogenic sarcoma in children)
Asthma
Decompression (diving)
Langerhans' giant cell granulomatosis

SPONTANEOUS PNEUMOTHORAX

What are five causes of a spontaneous pneumothorax?

Blebs
MTB
Metastasis
Asthma
Langerhans' giant cell granulomatosis
Sarcoid
Any interstitial lung disease
Cystic fibrosis

FIGURES F.B.: 18–2/3

UNILATERAL PLEURAL EFFUSION WITH OTHERWISE NORMAL CHEST RADIOGRAPH

List five causes of a unilateral pleural effusion with an otherwise normal chest radiograph. Which of these can relate to infection?

Pleural metastases
Tuberculosis
Collagen vascular disease
Pulmonary embolism
Trauma
Chylothorax
Pancreatitis
Meigs' syndrome
Postpericardiotomy syndromes
Subphrenic abscess
Asbestos-related pleuritis
Peritoneal dialysis
Viral pleuritis
Mesothelioma

FIGURES F.P.: 18–14; A.W.: 15–49 to 60

Pleural Metastases

• Multiple potential sites of origin (most common: breast and lung)

Tuberculosis

• Can be tuberculosis empyema or immunologic response
• Low glucose level, high protein level

Collagen Vascular Disease

· Rheumatoid
· SLE, subdiaphragmatic infection or trauma

Pancreatitis

· High amylase level
· Left side

Meigs' Syndrome

· Most commonly on right side, sometimes left, occasionally bilateral
· Originally described with ovarian fibroma and ascites; now more commonly seen with malignant ovarian tumors

Asbestos-Related Pleuritis

· Seen 7 to 20 years after exposure
· Often bloody
· Can persist
· Many go on to be pleural fibrosis (diffuse pleural thickening)

PREDOMINANTLY LEFT-SIDED PLEURAL EFFUSION

Pulmonary embolism
Constrictive pericarditis
Aortic dissection with rupture
Trauma
Vomiting with esophageal rupture (Boerhaave's syndrome)
Pancreatitis
Traumatic tear of upper thoracic duct
Atypical left heart failure

PREDOMINANTLY RIGHT-SIDED PLEURAL EFFUSION

Which causes of predominantly right-sided effusion are related to infection?

Left heart failure
Liver cirrhosis
After liver transplantation
Subphrenic abscess
Ascites

PLEURAL EFFUSION ASSOCIATED WITH LUNG CONSOLIDATION OR MASS

Bronchogenic carcinoma
Lymphoma
Metastases
Empyema
Pancreatitis
Pneumonia
Pulmonary embolism with infarction
Trauma with hemothorax

Bronchogenic Carcinoma

· 10 to 15% have pleural effusions

Lymphoma

· Especially non-Hodgkin's

Metastases

· Extending across diaphragm or from lung to pleural surface

Empyema/Parapneumonic

· With lung consolidation (pneumonia or abscess)

Pneumonia

· With parapneumonic effusion
· Especially when pneumonia caused by anaerobes, staphylococci, *Klebsiella* spp, fungi, mycoplasma, virus, or amebic abscess

PLEURAL MASS

Name six causes of focal pleural mass.

Mesothelioma
Metastases from extrathoracic neoplasm
Metastatic lung adenocarcinoma
Resolving empyema
Rib lesion
Loculated effusion
Pleural fibroma
Extrapleural lipoma
Postinflammatory fibrin ball
Transpleural extension of invasive thymoma

General

· Can be solitary or multiple
· Must be distinguished from extrapleural masses (may be difficult unless rib involved)
· May be in fissure and away from costal or mediastinal pleura

FIGURES   F.P.: 18–13/14/15; A.W.: 15–67

Pleural Fibroma

· May be mobile and on a stalk

Postinflammatory Fibrin Ball

· May move around chest cavity
· Is the end result of previous exudative effusion

Transpleural Extension of Invasive Thymoma

· Droplet transpleural spread most common to posterior costophrenic angles
· Occurs in 15% of invasive thymomas

1

What are the three most common causes of pleural calcification?

PLEURAL CALCIFICATION

Unilateral
    Asbestos pleural plaques
    Healed bacterial empyema
    Healed tuberculous empyema
    Organized hemothorax
Bilateral
    Asbestosis

Asbestos Pleural Plaques

- Involves parietal pleura predominantly
- Most common over diaphragm or along lateral costal margins between fourth and eighth ribs

Healed Tuberculous Empyema

- May be associated with extensive lung disease, or lungs may appear normal

Organized Hemothorax

FIGURES   A.W.: 15–72/73

Asbestosis

- Only usual cause of bilateral pleural calcification
- Most commonly seen laterally over costal margins, over hemidiaphragms, or paraspinously

PLEURAL THICKENING

Healed empyema
Resolved hemothorax
Resolved asbestos pleuritis
Confluent pleural plaques
Extrapleural fat
Systemic lupus erythematosus
After thoracic surgery

CHEST WALL

UNILATERAL ELEVATED HEMIDIAPHRAGM

Name five causes of an elevated hemidiaphragm.

Subpulmonic effusion (pseudoelevation)
Lobar atelectasis
Postresection
Congenital small lung
Phrenic nerve paralysis
Hypoplastic lung
Subdiaphragmatic abscess, mass
Traumatic rupture of diaphragm
Diaphragmatic tumor
Diaphragmatic hernia
Diaphragmatic eventration

Subpulmonic Effusion

- Lateral diaphragmatic apex
- Obliteration of medial costophrenic angle
- Separation of lung and gastric air bubble on left side (in two projections)

Phrenic Nerve Paralysis

- Idiopathic
- Bronchogenic carcinoma
- Surgery
- Trauma
- Diagnosis by paradoxical motion on fluoroscopy (fluoroscopy in steep oblique position)

Hypoplastic Lung

- Can be from reduced segmentation or reduced vascular supply (e.g., proximal interruption of pulmonary artery)
- Usually on right side

Subdiaphragmatic Disease

- Subphrenic abscess
- Distended stomach or colon on left side
- Tumor mass between liver and diaphragm

Traumatic Rupture of Diaphragm

- Usually at junction of muscular portion of diaphragm and central tendon
- More commonly diagnosed on left side than right side
- Supradiaphragmatic extension of nasogastric tube
- Gastric constriction at site of herniation

Diaphragmatic Tumor

- Lipoma, lymphoma, mesothelioma

Diaphragmatic Hernia

- Bochdalek: posterior (kidney)
- Morgagni: anterior (omentum, colon)
- Medial defect: left side (stomach/kidney)

BILATERAL ELEVATED HEMIDIAPHRAGM

Shallow inspiration
Restrictive lung disease
Obesity/pregnancy/ascites/abdominal mass
Muscle weakness
       Lupus erythematosus
       Myasthenia gravis
       Amyotrophic lateral sclerosis

1

General

- Diaphragm is bilaterally innervated in almost all individuals

CHEST WALL MASS

What are the most common causes of a chest wall mass in children or adults?

Mesodermal tumor
Neurogenic tumor
Bone tumor
Vascular tumor
Hematoma
Infection

General

- Peripheral lung mass with rib lesion much more likely to arise from rib than lung
- No plain radiographic findings reliably distinguish between peripheral lung, pleural mass, and chest wall mass (using GI criteria for chest wall does not work—the lung is too compliant and the chest wall too rigid)

Mesodermal Tumor

- Includes lipoma (most common), desmoid tumor, fibroma, and muscle tumors
- Lipomas are never malignant; should not be resected unless symptomatic

Neurogenic Tumor

- Includes schwannoma, neurofibroma, and neuroblastoma

Vascular Tumor

- Hemangioma/hemangiopericytoma, malignant bone tumor
- In children: Ewing's sarcoma, chondrosarcoma, osteosarcoma, fibrosarcoma,
- In adults: metastases, chondrosarcoma, multiple myeloma

Infection

- Actinomycosis, nocardiasis, blastomycosis, tuberculosis

RIB LESION WITH SURROUNDING SOFT TISSUE MASS

Metastases
Multiple myeloma
Lymphoma
Fibrosarcoma
Neurofibroma
Osteitis
Fracture with hematoma callus
Renal osteodystrophy/Cushing's syndrome
Radiation

Multiple Myeloma

- Expansion of bone
- Older patient
- Usually multiple and bilateral

Osteitis

- Infectious: MTB, mycosis, nocardiosis, blastomycosis

Renal Osteodystrophy/Cushing's Syndrome

- With fractures
- Exuberant callus

MALIGNANT CHEST WALL TUMORS IN CHILDREN

Ewing's sarcoma
Neuroblastoma
Askin's tumor
Rhabdomyosarcoma

Ewing's Sarcoma

- Ribs affected in 10 to 30% (the younger the patient, the more likely to involve ribs)

Askin's Tumor

- Neuroectodermal small cell tumor
- Rib destruction
- Pleural effusion
- May metastasize

Figure References

F.P.: Fraser RG, Paré JAP, Fraser RS, Genereux GP. Diagnosis of the Diseases of the Chest, 3rd edition, vols. 1–4. Philadelphia, WB Saunders, 1988–1991.
A.W.: Armstrong P, Wilson AG, Dee P, Hamsell DM. Imaging of Diseases of the Chest, 2nd edition, St. Louis, CV Mosby, 1995.

THORACIC IMAGING DISEASE ENTITIES

ABSCESS, LUNG

Clinical

- Pus in cavity within lung parenchyma
- Usually caused by pyogenic bacteria
- Organisms: anaerobes (streptococci, fusiform bacteria, and *Bacteriodes* spp), enteric organisms, staphylococci, *Klebsiella* spp
- Predisposing factors: aspiration, decreased level of consciousness, swallowing disorders
- Presentation: fever, cough, foul sputum
- Antecedent pneumonia

Imaging

- Radiographs:
    Air-fluid level in thick-walled cavity, solid mass, usually round

1

- CT:

    Shows mass is within lung and thick walled; useful to distinguish abscess from empyema; good for diagnosing abscess that has not communicated with airway (necrotic, low density center)

- Cavity with a wall:

    Wall less than 1 cm: abscess likely

    Wall more than 1.5 cm: cancer likely

AIDS

Clinical

- Organism: human immunodeficiency virus (HIV) and closely related viruses
- HIV infection is not synonymous with AIDS; infection can be present for 6 to 12 years before AIDS occurs
- AIDS defined by antibodies to HIV, plus certain opportunistic infections and/or specific neoplasms

    Opportunistic Infections
- *Pneumocystis carinii* pneumonia (PCP): by far the most common in North America.

    Presents with cough, fever, and especially hypoxemia; prophylactic antibiotics have changed its frequency and presentation; *See also* **Pneumocystis carinii Pneumonia**

    Cysts: thin-walled cystic spaces common sequelae of PCP; may rupture, causing unilateral or bilateral pneumothoraces, but cysts or pneumothoraces not indicative of active PCP; cysts do not resolve like pneumatoceles

- Cytomegalovirus (CMV) infections can cause symptomatic pneumonia in HIV-positive patients; more frequently found with other infections than alone
- Pyogenic bacteria, especially *Streptococcus pneumoniae*
- Mycobacterial infections

    Incidence: 10 to 15% in North America, but more than 80% in Africa

    Both mycobacterium tuberculosis (MTB) and atypical mycobacterial (MAC) infections common

    Major distinction between HIV-related tuberculosis and non–HIV-related tuberculosis: former frequently disseminated (transbronchial, hematogenous) and can show extensive adenopathy

    High versus low CD4 count probably has little influence on presentation (controversial)

- Fungal pneumonia (including cryptococcus, histoplasmosis and nocardiosis) less common (less than 10% of AIDS-related pneumonias)
- Tumors

    Lymphoma: B-cell lymphomas most common; intrathoracic involvement in less than 15%

    Kaposi's sarcoma (KS): probably requires a concomitant viral infection; common in homosexuals with AIDS, much less common in IV drug abusers with AIDS

- Rare entities

    Lymphocytic interstitial pneumonia (LIP): diagnostic of AIDS in children; uncommon in adults; monoclonal lymphomas in most instances

    Bacillary angiomatosis: presents with skin lesions and visceral involvement; similar in appearance to KS, but is an infection

    Lung cancer: increased incidence not definitely established; aggressive when present

    Bronchiectasis: HIV-related bronchitis and bronchiectasis now most common pulmonary entities; no longer "rare"; presents with chronic productive cough

    Prognosis
- 2 to 12 years from HIV infection to AIDS
- 1 to 5 years from AIDS to death

Imaging

PCP Pneumonia. *See* **Pneumocystis carinii Pneumonia**

CVM *Infection*
- Radiographs:

    Nodular opacities

Pyogenic Bacteria
- Radiographs:
    Usual appearance of bacterial pneumonia with lobar/sublobar consolidation, diffuse consolidation

Mycobacterial Infection
- Radiographs:
    Presentation most frequently similar to that of primary tuberculosis in nonimmunocompromised host

Lymphoma
- Radiographs/CT:
    Frequently atypical with pleural effusions, masses, and adenopathy
    Thoracic adenopathy with marked axillary adenopathy highly suggestive of lymphoma

Kaposi's Sarcoma
- Radiographs:
    Typically show perihilar, interstitial, ill-defined linear opacities (early stage)
    Progress to nodular opacities and disseminated masses with pleural effusions (late stage)
    Adenopathy moderately common

LIP
- Radiographs:
    Nodular/linear opacities

Bronchiectasis
- Radiographs/CT:
    Predominately lower lobe bronchial dilatation and thickening (best seen on CT scans)

ALPHA-1-ANTITRYPSIN DEFICIENCY (A1-AD)

Clinical

- Autosomal recessive disorder of a serum glycoprotein
- Incidence: aproximately 1 in 100,000
- Emphysema (panlobular)
- Ratio of males to females affected is 2:1
- Progressive disease with early death
- Absence of alpha-1-antitrypsin allows proteolytic enzymes to digest lung tissues
- Almost always found with smoking as a cofactor for producing emphysema
- Classic example of panlobular basal emphysema
- Usually emphysema-type symptoms with shortness of breath
- Develops between 35 and 50 years of age
- Symptoms appear 10 years earlier in smokers
- Treatable form of emphysema

Imaging

- Radiographs:
    Striking lower lobe predominance of disease with hyperinflation, vascular attenuation; 5 to 10% do not show lower lobe predominance
- CT:
    More widespread distribution of emphysema, especially in advanced cases
- ? 10 to 20% incidence of bronchiectasis in addition to emphysema
- Diagnosis should be considered in middle-aged smokers with lower lobe emphysema

ALVEOLAR PROTEINOSIS (PULMONARY ALVEOLAR PROTEINOSIS) (PAP)

Clinical

- Accumulation of phospholipid (surfactant) in the air spaces and interstitium of lung
- ? Overproduction of surfactant by type II alveolar cells
- ? Defect in macrophage ingestion of surfactant
- Age 25 to 50 years (rare in childhood and old age)
- Ratio of females to males affected = 3:1

1

- Cough, hemoptysis, dyspnea
- Pulmonary function tests (PFTs) show restriction with decreased diffusing capacity
- Prognosis
     Slow progression 25%
     Stable 50%
     Spontaneous regression 25%
- Predisposition to infections, especially nocardiosis
- Long-term prognosis
     Recovery/improvement 50%
     Death from respiratory failure 33%
     Lingering 17%
- Treatment: bronchopulmonary lavage with large volumes of fluid

Imaging

- Radiographs:
     Usually diffuse, fine, ground-glass to slightly granular opacities more marked at bases than apices
     Spares costophrenic angles
     Unusual presentations: bat-wing; unilateral; dominant interstitial lines, peripheral ground-glass/consolidation
- HRCT:
     Characteristic with ground-glass opacities and undistorted interstitial thickening, often asymmetric
- Differential diagnosis:
     Chronic diffuse lung consolidation (sarcoid, lymphoma group, alveolar cell carcinoma, desquamative interstitial pneumonitis, UIP, hypersensitivity pneumonitis)

AMNIOTIC FLUID EMBOLISM

Clinical

- Common cause of peripartum death
- Woman in prolonged labor
- Labor usually severe
- Shock usually follows delivery
- Amniotic fluid enters circulation through small venous tears or disruption of placental site associated with uterine rupture, placenta previa, or cesarean section
- Presents with dyspnea, hypotension, cyanosis, vomiting, agitation, disseminated intravascular coagulation (DIC), sudden death

Imaging

- Radiographs/CT:
     Noncardiogenic pulmonary edema

AMYLOIDOSIS

Clinical

- Abnormal extracellular deposition of the protein amyloid
- Amyloid divided into systemic or localized
     Systemic is divided into:
          Amyloidosis (AL: light chain amyloid)
          Reactive systemic amyloidosis (AA: amyloid)
          Other forms
- Systemic
     Thoracic involvement limited
     Uncommonly interstitial parenchymal disease and/or lymphadenopathy
- Localized
     Involves lung parenchyma or airways
     Thoracic involvement about 50%
- When limited, may be resected
- Diffuse amyloid can result in respiratory failure

1

Imaging

- Radiographs:
    Trachea or large airways: diffuse or focal narrowing
    Parenchymal nodules: sharp, round, lobulated, irregular, or ill defined; can calcify
    Mediastinal nodal enlargement uncommon

ANKYLOSING SPONDYLITIS

Clinical

- Chronic inflammatory disorder of axial skeleton
- Lung involvement 1 to 2%
- Nonpulmonary features predominate
- Cricoarytenoid joint immobility can produce hoarseness, stridor, or dyspnea

Imaging

- Radiographs/CT:
    Upper lobe fibrosis, retraction, bullae (rare)

ASBESTOS-RELATED DISEASES

- Asbestos is a group of fibrous, naturally-occurring silicates
- Widely used for the first 75 years of this century because of its insulating, fire-resistant, tensile properties
- Fibers longer than 5 microns
- Occupational exposure among workers in mines, mills, construction, insulation, and maintenance
- Types of asbestos: chrysolite, anthophyllite, tremolite, crocidolite, amosite

Asbestosis
- Diffuse or multifocal interstitial fibrosis of the lungs caused by inhalation of asbestos fibers
- Fibers initiate inflammatory response (alveolitis)
- Chronic damage results in scarring and fibrosis (crocidolite and amosite probably more potent than chrysotile in causing asbestosis)
- Diagnosis requires consideration of exposure; latency, i.e., period between exposure and evaluation (asbestosis usually takes more than 15 to 20 years); abnormal imaging study (chest radiographs/CT); restrictive lung disease on pulmonary function tests (PFTs) (small volumes and reduced diffusing capacity); clinical abnormalities (rare)
- Shortness of breath and cough
- Clubbing
- Restriction on PFTs
- Asbestois is present histologically in almost all patients with asbestos exposure and lung cancer

Pleural Disease
- Fibrotic pleural plaques
    Focal areas of hyaline thickening of parietal pleura (uncommonly involves visceral pleura)
    All types of asbestos cause pleural plaques
    Latency usually more than 15 years (prevalence of plaques increases with latency and dose)
    Pleural plaques associated with higher likelihood of functional lung impairment and lung fibrosis
    Plaques may calcify (only a minority do)
    Plaques do not have malignant potential
    Plaques themselves do not cause symptoms (unless massive), but statistically associated with impairment
- Asbestos-related pleuritis (effusion)
    Subacute exudative pleuritis, frequently symptomatic

About 7% of occupationally exposed workers

Latency 5 to 35 years

Usually resolves, causing adhesive fibrothorax

- Diffuse pleural thickening (diffuse fibrosis of the pleura, i.e., fibrothorax)

This appearance can be caused by: confluent pleural plaques, extension of lung fibrosis (asbestosis) to the pleural surface, adhesive fibrothorax after asbestos-related pleuritis, or pseudo-pleural thickening from extrapleural fat

Diffuse pleural thickening usually refers to fibrothorax

Asbestos-related Neoplasms

- Carcinoma of lung

Increased incidence of several neoplasms in occupationally exposed individuals

Most common: bronchogenic carcinoma (histologically indistinguishable from other lung cancers)

More than additive risk from exposure to asbestos (x 6) plus cigarette smoking (x 50 to 90)

Presentation similar to that of other bronchogenic carcinomas

- Mesothelioma

Rare cancer (1500 to 2500 new cases per year in United States)

66% associated with asbestos exposure

All types of fibers causative, especially crocidolite

Unusually long latency (20 to 40 years)

Other cancers: larynx, pharynx, and upper and lower digestive tract; risk of lymphoma statistically significant but small

Benign Lung Masses

- Affect 10% of exposed workers
- Most common: rounded atelectasis, focal mass (more than 5 cm in diameter) of inflammation and enfolding of the lung
- Smaller benign fibrotic masses also common
- Diagnosis of rounded atelectasis:

Fibrothorax (pleural thickening)

Reduced volume of containing lobe

Lentiform mass in continuity with pleural surface

Stability over many years

Biopsy sample should be taken from mass if benignity uncertain

Imaging

Asbestosis

- Radiographs:

Irregular linear opacities in lower lobes (s, t, u, in ILO classification)

Pleural thickening or pleural plaques frequently coexist

CT: 15% of patients with asbestosis do not show plaques on chest radiographs, but almost all patients with asbestosis show plaques on CT

- HRCT:

Interlobular septal thickening, parenchymal bands, centrilobular thickening, subpleural lines, honeycombing, architectural distortion

Strong basal predominance

Asbestos-related Pleuritis/Diffuse Pleural Thickening

- Defined as obliteration of CP angle on chest radiographs or pleural thickening more than 5 x 8 cm on CT

Benign Lung Masses

- CT:

Mass ovoid, not round

Contact between mass and thickened pleura must be unequivocal

Lobe containing mass must be reduced in volume

Calcification uncommon but occurs

Cavitation uncommon but occurs

Mass often enhances with IV contrast

ASPERGILLOSIS

- *Aspergillus fumigatus* is a ubiquitous fungus
- Pulmonary involvement depends on patient's underlying pulmonary and immune status
- Four presentations most common:
      Mycetoma
      Allergic bronchopulmonary aspergillosis (ABPA)
      Invasive aspergillosis
      Semi-invasive aspergillosis
- Rare forms include:
      Acute allergic alveolitis
      Can exist colonizing airways without causing disease, especially in asthmatics
      Tracheobronchial in AIDS

Mycetoma
- Saprophytic growth colonizing preexisting pulmonary cavities, cysts, and other air-containing spaces
- Chronic cough and hemoptysis

ABPA
- Type 1 (Ig-E) plus type 3 (immune-complex) reactions
- Wheezing, eosinophilia, pulmonary opacities, mucus plugs in large airways, elevated IGE, immediate and delayed skin reactions to *Aspergillus,* underlying asthma

Invasive Aspergillosis
- In immunocompromised neutropenic patients (most commonly hematologic malignancies, organ transplantation, or diabetes mellitus)
- The organism is angioinvasive by definition
- High mortality rate

Semi-invasive Aspergillosis
- Indolent focal inflammation, caused by invasion of lung parenchyma
- In mildly immunocompromised middle-aged individuals (e.g., alcoholics) with underlying lung disease
- Chronic fever, malaise, weight loss, cough
- Indolent mass or focal consolidation with or without adjacent pleural thickening
- Predilection for upper lobes
- Can invade chest wall

Imaging

Mycetoma
- Radiographs/CT:
      Fungus ball within cavity
      Typical pleural thickening adjacent to a cavity; air-fluid level within cavity; calcified mass, fixed mass; frond-like appearance on CT
      Superinfection can cause surrounding consolidation

APBA
- Radiographs/CT:
      Central airway dilatation (bronchiectasis) with or without mucus plugs ("finger-in-glove")
      Diffuse bronchiectasis
      Hyperinflation
      Cysts/cavities
      Recurrent or transient parenchymal opacities from allergic pneumonia or recurrent airway obstruction

Invasive Aspergillosis
- Radiographs/CT:
      Rapidly progressive necrotizing pneumonia ("lung balls")
      Peripheral infarcts
      Consolidation

1

CT "halo sign" suggestive of invasive aspergillosis (represents bleeding around infarct)

"Lung ball" represents necrotic lung tissue surrounded by crescent of air (usually seen as white cells return)

ASPIRATION PNEUMONIA

Clinical

- Inhalation of material from the nose, pharynx, or stomach
- Predisposing conditions: impaired consciousness, impaired swallowing, presence of nasogastric or endotracheal tubes, tracheotomy
- Predominates in dependent portions of lungs
- Often considered under headings *acid* or *nonacid* and *infected* or *noninfected*
- Presentation: dyspnea, wheezing, cyanosis, hypotension, hypoxemia
- Can be bland or infected
- Should also be considered among causes of cryptogenic organizing pneumonia/bronchiolitis obliterans organizing pneumonia (BOOP)
- Most common organisms (when infected): staphylococci and *Pseudomonas* spp
- Noninfected aspiration should clear in 96 hours unless ARDS has occurred
- Treatment: antibiotics and support

ASTHMA

Clinical

- Reversible air-flow obstruction caused by bronchoconstriction from airway antigen: antibody reaction
- Has major inflammatory component
- Clinical complex covering numerous diseases with airway hyperirritability
- Dyspnea (reversible, periodic, exercise-induced, cold-induced)
- Cough and sputum
- Function: normal diffusing capacity, variable airflow obstruction

Imaging

Asthma
- Radiographs:
   Normal (most common); hyperinflation
- HRCT:
   Diffuse bronchial wall thickening
   Focal hyperlucency with airtrapping on expiration
   Older asthmatics can have bronchiectasis, emphysema, bronchitis

Complicated Asthma
- Radiographs/CT:
   Allergic bronchopulmonary aspergillosis with mucus plugs
   Pneumonia (consolidation)
   Atelectasis
   Pneumothorax
   Bronchiectasis
   Pneumomediastinum
   Regional hyperlucency/airtrapping

ATELECTASIS (LUNG COLLAPSE)

Clinical

- Congenital or acquired reduction in lung volume
- Most conveniently considered as obstructive or nonobstructive
- Should also be considered on anatomic lines: nonsegmental, subsegmental, segmental, multisegmental, lobar, or whole lung
- Nonobstructive atelectasis: air-bronchograms and volume loss. Increased parenchymal opacity matches the reduced lung volume

- Obstructive atelectasis: absence of air-bronchograms and often retention of fluid and mucus within obstructed, volume-reduced lung
- Lobe can be completely obstructed, airless, and not reduced in volume; similarly, lobe or segment can be completely obstructed and remain aerated (via collateral ventilation)
- Most common causes of obstructive atelectasis: intrinsic neoplasm (malignant and benign), lymphoma, foreign body, inflammatory bronchostenosis (TB, sarcoid, histoplasmosis), aortic or pulmonary artery aneurysm, large nodes
- Varies from asymptomatic to dyspnea, hypoxemia, and hemoptysis (depends on acuteness of atelectasis, extent of continued perfusion of the nonventilated lung, and volume of involvement)

Imaging

- Radiographs:
    Lobar or multilobar collapse
        Primary signs: increased opacity, displaced fissures, crowded vessels and bronchi
        Compensatory signs: hilar movement, hyperinflation, elevated diaphragm, mediastinal shift, shifting granuloma, rib crowding
        Most useful signs: hilar and bronchial elevation/depression, displaced fissures, crowded bronchi/vessels, shifting granuloma or clips
- CT:
    All signs as seen on radiographs
    Can delineate a central mass, especially with IV contrast
    Cannot distinguish between mucosal mass invading outward and mass around bronchus without mucosal tumor (unless distinct cut-off sign)
- Segmental and lobar atelectasis have classic appearances (understand them)
- In most circumstances, collapsed lobes maintain contact with mediastinum and diaphragm, losing contact with chest wall

BEHÇET'S DISEASE

Clinical

- Rare, multisystem chronic vasculitis
- Secondary to immune complex deposition
- Ulcers of mouth and genitalia
- Skin infections and erythema nodosum
- Uveitis
- Arthropathy
- Thrombophlebitis
- Ratio of males to females affected is 2:1
- Thoracic involvement in 5 to 10%
- Hemoptysis, fever, pleuritic chest pain, cough, dyspnea
- Improves with steroids

Imaging

- Radiographs:
    Diffuse pulmonary hemorrhage
    Focal consolidation from hemorrhage
    Pulmonary artery aneurysms and stenoses
    Infarction
    Pleural effusions

BERYLLIOSIS

Clinical

- Caused by inhalation of beryllium powder
- May be acute or chronic

- An allergic reaction causing extrinsic allergic alveolitis/hypersensitivity pneumonitis
- Granulomatous lesions involving skin, kidney, liver, spleen, and lung parenchyma
- Slowly progressive disease with eventual death from respiratory failure

Imaging

- Radiographs:
    - Indistinguishable from sarcoidosis with nodules, reticulonodular opacities, coarse fibrosis and honeycombing, hilar and mediastinal adenopathy
- CT:
    - Very early may show centrilobular opacities

BLASTOMYCOSIS

Clinical

- Fungal infection most common in central and southeastern United States
- Source is soil
- Occurs sporadically or as outbreaks
- Organism: *Blastomyces dermatitidis*
- Middle-aged farmers, lumberjacks
- Fever, cough, myalgia, subcutaneous abscesses that ulcerate
- Asymptomatic pneumonia
- Indolent lung abscess

Imaging

- Radiographs/CT:
    - Ill-defined consolidation, unifocal or multifocal
    - Upper lobes predominate
    - Features similar to fibrocavitatory MTB
    - Multiple nodules
    - Features similar to mass-like bronchogenic carcinoma
    - Pleural effusion/thickening
    - Lytic bone lesions
    - Adenopathy uncommon; not prominent when present

BOERHAAVE'S SYNDROME

Clinical

- Esophageal perforation from vomiting
- Forceful vomiting often in alcoholics
- Tear immediately above diaphragm, usually on left side
- Mucosal to transmural tears
- Hematemesis
- Shock
- Fever, chest pain, subcutaneous emphysema

Imaging

- Radiographs/CT:
    - Pneumomediastinum, subcutaneous emphysema
    - Left pleural effusion/pneumothorax
    - Left lower lobe consolidation
    - Mediastinal mass/abscess
    - Mediastinal widening/obliteration of fat planes
- Esophagogram:
    - Use non-ionic contrast
    - Demonstrates presence of tear
    - Size of tear not accurate from esophagogram

BONE MARROW TRANSPLANTATION

Clinical

- Increasingly used for treatment of hematologic and solid neoplasms as well as myeloma and other conditions
- Complications more frequent than in other transplant recipients
- Pulmonary complications common

Acute Graft-Versus-Host Disease
- Develops in 20 to 100 days
- GI tract, liver, skin most commonly involved

Chronic Graft-Versus-Host Disease
- Develops in more than 100 days to many months
- Lymphocytic infiltration of interstitium
- Bronchiolitis obliterans with larger airway dilatation
- Hyperinflation

Other Entities
- Drug reactions: acute or chronic; ARDS-like appearance
- Diffuse pulmonary hemorrhage: occurs in first days after transplant; high mortality; diffuse lung consolidation with or without hemoptysis
- Infections: viral, especially CMV; PCP; bacterial; fungal, especially aspergillosis and candidiasis; antimicrobial prophylaxis has decreased incidence
- Nonspecific interstitial pneumonitis: obscure cause; diagnosis of exclusion; basal interstitial and patchy air space disease

BRONCHIAL ADENOMA

Clinical

- Group of malignant neoplasms arising in trachea or bronchi from mucosal or submucosal elements
- Two big groups: carcinoid tumors and mixed salivary gland tumors

Carcinoid Tumors
- Group of amine precursor uptake and decarboxylation (APUD) tumors arising from Kulchitsky (neuroendocrine) cells with variable aggressiveness
- Affects young adults to elderly
- Variable growth rate
- More benign variant of small cell carcinoma
- Arises centrally in main, lobar, or segmental bronchi
- Recurrent infection/hemoptysis
- 15% of "typical" carcinoid tumors (Kulchitsky cell carcinoma-I) metastasize
- High percentage of atypical tumors (Kulchitsky cell carcinoma-II) metastasize
- Can secrete adrenocorticotropic hormone (ACTH)

Mixed Salivary Gland Tumors (Cylindromas)
- 90% arise in trachea; 10% in bronchi
- Two most common are adenoid cystic carcinoma and mucoepidermoid carcinoma
- Adenoid cystic carcinoma most malignant and metastasizes most frequently; mucoepidermoid less aggressive
- Presents at ages 30 to 50 years
- Dyspnea, hemoptysis, wheezing

Imaging

Carcinoid Tumors
- Radiographs:
  Bronchial obstruction with atelectasis/airtrapping
  Endobronchial mass

Solitary pulmonary nodule, 1 to 4 cm
Bronchiectasis
Mucoid impaction
- CT:
    Endobronchial mass
    Calcification in 30%, usually when over 2 cm
    Hilar mass
    Contrast enhancing

Mixed Salivary Gland Tumors

- Radiographs/CT:
    Polypoid tracheal mass
    Thickening of tracheal wall
    Can have large extratracheal component
- CT:
    Determine resectability (length of trachea involved: up to 4 to 6 cm can be resected; size of extratracheal component; organ encasement)

BRONCHIAL ATRESIA

Clinical

- Focal interruption of central bronchus in fetal life
- Hypoplastic, hyperinflated distal lung
- Left upper lobe with classic radiographic findings
- Left upper lobe affected more often than right upper lobe, which is affected more often than right middle lobe; lower lobes least often affected
- Often asymptomatic with abnormal chest radiograph
- Usually presents in childhood or young adult life

Imaging

- Radiographs/CT (classic triad):
    Round or ovoid (sometimes branching) central mass formed from dilated mucus-filled bronchi distal to atretic segment
    Hyperinflated distal lung with decreased alveoli (big and black)
    Vessels to region attenuated

BRONCHIECTASIS

Clinical

- Irreversible dilatation of bronchi with inflammation and cartilage destruction
- Most commonly caused by breakdown in defense mechanism of lung
    Congenital: immobile cilia syndrome, cartilage deficiency, mucoviscidosis
    Immune deficiency status: congenital, acquired, AIDS, ABPA
    Postinfection: after childhood infections, including adenoviral infections, MTB, MAC
    Bronchial obstruction: foreign body, tumor
    Immune reactions: bronchiolitis with transplantation
- In many areas, HIV an important cause
- Inflammation in bronchiectasis often extends to involve small airways
- Reid's morphologic classification commonly used but has little clinical significance:
    Cylindrical/fusiform
    Varicose
    Cystic/saccular
- Easier to describe bronchiectasis as either cylindrical or cystic (CT description)
- Cough with sputum, often of years' duration
- Recurrent infections
- Noninfected/"dry" bronchiectasis can be asymptomatic
- Shortness-of-breath/"asthma"

Imaging

- Radiographs:
    "Tram-tracks:" visible bronchial walls
    "Rings:" face-on dilated bronchi
    Tubes: mucus-filled bronchi, may branch
    Variable lung volumes: small, normal, large
    Hyperlucency: usually indicates small airway disease
    Ill-defined or crowded vessels
    Late scarrings, cysts, air-fluid levels
    Segmental/lobar atelectasis
    Normal
    Variation with time
- CT:
    All the positive finding on radiographs
    Invariably asymmetric
    Dilated bronchi readily visible
    CT better than bronchography and has replaced latter for diagnosis
    "Signet-ring" sign: dilated bronchus with adjacent pulmonary artery

BRONCHIOLITIS

Clinical

- Inflammation in small airways (less than 2 mm ID)
- Many different types; important ones:
    Constrictive (bronchiolitis obliterans)
    BOOP (see cryptogenic organizing pneumonia)
    Proliferative (infective, obstructive)
    Smoker's bronchiolitis
    Diffuse panbronchiolitis (Asian panbronchiolitis)
- Clinical presentation: cough, dyspnea
- Many causes:
    Constrictive: after viral infection, certain transplants (lung, heart, bone marrow), certain connective tissue diseases, drugs, idiopathic, noxious gas inhalation, gastric acid aspiration
    Proliferative: infection, especially aspergillosis, AIDS, certain bacterial infections
- Swyer-James syndrome a form of bronchiolitis obliterans

Imaging

- Depends on type

Constrictive
- Radiographs:
    Hyperinflation
    Region of hyperlucency
    Reticulonodular opacities (probably small airway bronchiectasia with panbronchial inflammation)
    Often concomitant bronchiectasis
- HRCT:
    Regional hyperlucency and hypovascularity
    Airtrapping on expiration
    Bronchiectasis

Proliferative
- HRCT:
    Dilated small airways with branching "tree-in-bud" appearance if mucus filled

Smoker's
- HRCT:
  Diffuse ground-glass; interstitial thickening

BRONCHITIS, CHRONIC
Clinical

- Defined clinically as cough and sputum for most days for at least 3 months of at least 2 years' duration
- Relationship to smoking very strong
- Relationship to airflow obstruction weak
- Increased incidence with age
- Pathologic appearance: increases in all mucous layers in large airways
- Some patients have severe airflow obstruction
- Cough and sputum
- Hemoptysis
- Shortness of breath

Imaging

- Radiographs:
  Normal; "dirty" chest; increased bronchial wall visibility
- HRCT:
  Bronchial wall thickening, mild bronchial dilatation, increased visibility of small bronchi

BRONCHOALVEOLAR (BRONCHIOLOALVEOLAR) CELL CARCINOMA
Clinical

- Variant form of adenocarcinoma of lung
- 3% of primary lung cancers and increasing
- Arises from type I pneumocyte
- Two distinct biologic types (forms):
  Focal: slow growing SPN, limited to one lobe, good prognosis
  Diffuse: more than one lobe, rapidly growing, poor prognosis
- Asymptomatic, especially focal form
- Bronchorrhea
- Cough, weight loss

Imaging

- Radiographs:
  SPN
  Multiple ill-defined nodular opacities
  Patchy consolidation
  Lobar/multilobar consolidation
- CT:
  SPN with spiculation, air bronchograms, convergent vessels, pleural tag
  Lobar, sublobar, or multilobar chronic consolidation
  Pleural effusion
  Acinar nodules
  Metastases
  Rarely, if ever, cavitates

BRONCHOGENIC CARCINOMA
Clinical

- Most common fatal malignancy in men and women
- Histologic classification:

Epidermoid	30 to 50%
Adenocarcinoma	30%
Small cell	20 to 30%
Large cell (including giant cell)	10 to 15%

- Staging uses TNM system (*See* Overview, Table 1–6)
- Asymptomatic
- Cough
- Hemoptysis
- Paraneoplastic syndromes
- Metastases
- Weight loss
- Dyspnea/dysphagia
- SVC syndrome

Imaging

- Radiographs:
  - SPN: doubling time (volume) 30 to 450 days (be careful of exceptions)
  - Lobar/segmental bronchial obstruction
  - Cavitation: the thicker the wall the more likely cavity is neoplastic; any cavity wall more than 15 mm highly likely to be malignant
  - Unilateral hilar enlargement
  - Mediastinal mass/widening
  - Pleural effusion
  - Chest wall invasion
  - Mediastinal invasion
- CT/HRCT:
  - All radiographic findings
  - SPN:
    - Absence of benign calcifications
    - Spiculation
    - Air bronchograms
    - Converging vessels
    - Cavity
  - Obstructed bronchus
  - Metastatic hilar/mediastinal nodes (incidence 20 to 25%); more than 10 mm considered abnormal; 10 to 15% of nodal metastases in normal-sized nodes; approximately 5% of nodes more than 10 mm are benign
  - Mediastinal invasion: into mediastinal fat, operable; organ invasion, inoperable
  - Pericardial effusion
  - Pleural effusion
  - Calcification 10%: eccentric, stippled
  - Size of mediastinal nodes on CT not sufficiently accurate to obviate confirmation by biopsy
- Extrathoracic metastases (20 to 30%):
  - Adrenal 5 to 12% (⅔ detectable)
  - Liver   6 to 12% (⅔ detectable)
  - Brain   5 to 10% (½ detectable)
  - Bone   5 to 10% (½ detectable)
- Any suggestion of extrathoracic metastases: look everywhere
- Adenocarcinoma with enlarged mediastinal nodes: metastases should be sought, especially in CNS (incidence more than 40%)

BRONCHOGENIC (BRONCHIAL, FOREGUT) CYST

Clinical

- Should be included with esophageal cysts and called *foregut cyst*
- Mediastinal 70 to 85%; lung 15 to 30%
- 80% within 5 cm of tracheal carina
- Never malignant but can become infected
- May uncommonly communicate with the airway (air-fluid level)
- Asymptomatic
- Dyspnea/dysphagia
- Hemoptysis
- Infection (obstruction)

Imaging

- Radiographs:
    Soft mediastinal/hilar mass
    Lung nodule/mass
    10% lobulated
    Stable, unless infected
- CT:
    Variable density 0 to 100 H
    Thin, smooth inner and outer walls
    Cavitation with air-fluid level
    Curvilinear wall calcification

BRONCHOLITHIASIS

Clinical

- Calcified granular material in airways (sputum) from erosion of inflammatory peribronchial calcified nodes
- Histoplasmosis; tuberculosis; coccidioidomycosis
- Can cause sinus tract, airway obstruction, or bronchoesophageal fistula
- Coughing up granules ("sand")
- Recurrent infection
- Hemoptysis

Imaging

- Radiographs:
    Disappearing calcified lymph nodes, segmental/lobar atelectasis, mucus impaction
- CT:
    Calcified nodes in close proximity to airway lumen; abnormalities distal to airway obstruction (atelectasis, mucus bronchograms, increased density)

BRONCHOPLEURAL FISTULA

Clinical

- Persistent (at least for weeks) communication between bronchus and pleural space
- Usually some reason the communication does not seal
- Causes: barotrauma, abscess, MTB, fungus, bacteria, tumor, AIDS (post PCP), penetrating chest injury, after lung resection, postinfarction (rare), cavitating rheumatoid nodule (rare)
- Cough, fever, chest pain, shortness of breath
- Respiratory impairment
- Persistent air leak from thoracostomy tube
- Treatment options: surgery, cyanoacrylate injection (glue), fibrin sealant, balloon occlusion of airway, pleurodesis

Imaging

- Radiographs and CT:
    Persistent pneumothorax
    Increasing pneumothorax
    Lung cavity/mass
    Pleural fluid with or without infection
    CT enhancement of parietal pleura may or may not be present

BULLOUS LUNG DISEASE

Clinical

- Bullae only or predominant finding (i.e., without generalized emphysema)
- Seen in middle-aged, smoking males; most commonly affected group, African-Americans

1

- May benefit from bullectomy
- If emphysema present, should not be called bullous lung disease
- Severe respiratory impairment
- Bullae function as a mass or pneumothorax, reducing lung volume and causing airways to collapse
- Markedly reduced air flow with preserved diffusing capacity

Imaging

- Radiographs:
    Upper lobe lucent, thin-walled bullae; hyperinflation; no emphysema
- CT:
    Bullae without emphysema

CAPLAN'S SYNDROME

Clinical

- Original description: rheumatoid-like nodules in coal miners
- Now includes coal, silica, asbestos, and aluminum exposure
- Serologic rheumatoid disease; other manifestations of rheumatoid lung disease also included in syndrome
- Asymptomatic
- Symptoms related to the underlying pneumoconiosis

Imaging

- Radiographs/CT:
    Multiple but not innumerable pulmonary nodules 1 to 5 cm
    Stellate scars
    Nodule may calcify, cavitate
    Background of simple/complicated pneumoconiosis

CASTLEMAN'S DISEASE

Clinical

- Also called *giant lymph node hyperplasia; angiofollicular lymph node hyperplasia*
- Two varieties: vascular and plasma cell
- Idiopathic
- ? Some relationship to Kaposi's sarcoma/AIDS
- ? Premalignant
- Cough, dyspnea, hemoptysis, fever
- Anemia, hypergammaglobulinemia
- Lymphadenopathy
- Mistaken for lymphoma

Imaging

- Radiographs:
    Mediastinal mass, usually in middle, less often in posterior, least often in anterior; extrathoracic lymphadenopathy; hilar mass; lung mass
- CT:
    Mass up to 10 to 15 cm in diameter; unusual calcifications; marked contrast enhancement (vascular type)
- Angiography:
    Multiple feeding vessels; marked enhancement (blush) with capillary phase

CHLAMYDIAL PNEUMONIA

Clinical

- Organism: *Chlamydia pneumoniae*
- Responsible for up to 25% of community-acquired pneumonia
- Chlamydial tracheitis/pneumonia in neonates caused by different organism
- Psittacosis from birds caused by different organism

- Fever, cough, headache, chest pain
- Occasionally asymptomatic
- Diagnosis by culture of organism, immunofluorescence, serologic studies

Imaging

- Radiographs:
    Patchy consolidation, lower lobe interstitial opacities

CHRONIC EOSINOPHILIC PNEUMONIA

Clinical

- Idiopathic
- One of the "pulmonary infiltration with eosinophilia" (PIE) syndromes
- Characteristic clinical/radiologic picture
- 50% atopic, 40% asthmatic
- Ratio of females to males affected is 2:1
- Occurs in middle age and later
- Dyspnea, cough, malaise, weight loss
- Hemoptysis (rare)
- 90% have blood eosinophilia, 50% have sputum eosinophilia

Imaging

- Radiographs:
    Chronic, peripheral, nonsegmental, dense consolidation: classic
    Asymmetric and incomplete
    Rapid response to steroids
    Tends to recur at same sites

CHRONIC OBSTRUCTIVE PULMONARY DISEASE

Clinical

- Group of lung diseases that have in common chronic airflow obstruction
- Neoplasms not part of COPD even if they narrow airways and obstruct airflow
- Includes chronic bronchitis, emphysema, bronchiolitis, bronchiectasis, and some types of asthma
- These conditions often overlap, especially in older individuals
- Asthma *See* **Asthma**
- Bronchiolitis *See* **Bronchiolitis**
- Chronic bronchitis *See* **Bronchitis, chronic**

  Emphysema
- Defined pathologically as abnormal permanent enlargement of distal air spaces (increased interalveolar wall distance) without significant fibrosis and with destruction of alveolar walls
- Ratio of males to females affected is 3:1
- Causes include smoking, alpha-1-antitrypsin deficiency, Marfan's syndrome, familial, phosgene inhalation, opium smoking, ? nitrous oxide inhalation
- Pathologic types: panlobular (panacinar), centrilobular, paraseptal (periacinar), and cicatricial (scar)
- Distribution: upper lobes/diffuse in smokers (centrilobular); lower lobes (on radiographs but more diffuse on CT) with alpha-1-antitrypsin deficiency
- Airflow obstruction result of loss of elastic recoil causing narrowing of airways and inflammation in small airways
- Decreased diffusing capacity from loss of alveolar walls
- Dyspnea: with effort or resting
- Hypoxemia without hypercapnia
- Enlarged thorax
- PFTs: decreased FEV_1 and decreased DLCO

Imaging

- Radiographs:
  Hyperinflation: flat diaphragms, increased retrosternal space, "big lungs," splayed ribs, low diaphragms, small heart
  Vascular attenuation: decreased number and size of arteries and veins
  Bullae
  Dirty chest, "increased markings emphysema" occurs with emphysema plus pulmonary hypertension; heart failure; chronic bronchitis; small airways disease; or respiratory bronchiolitis
- CT/HRCT:
  0.5 to 1 cm holes with density equal to air and no walls except interlobular septae
  Diffuse hyperlucency with vascular attenuation
  Bullae: pencil-line walls and air spaces larger than 1 cm
  Vascular distortion around emphysematous spaces

CHYLOTHORAX

Clinical

- Milky pleural fluid containing chylomicrons (from lymph of intestinal origin)
- Must be distinguished from pseudochylothorax, in which fat is cholesterol or lecithin, not triglycerides
- 50% also bloody
- Mechanisms: disruption of thoracic duct, oozing of mediastinal pleural lymphatics, from chylous ascites
- Causes: neoplasm (lymphoma, carcinoma), trauma (penetrating), idiopathy, postoperative, LAM/tuberous sclerosis, inflammation (sclerosing mediastinitis, radiation, pancreatitis)
- Similar to other effusions

Imaging

- Radiographs:
  Effusion, right affected slightly more often than left; bilateral
- CT:
  May show cause; density may be low to high
- Lymphangiogram:
  Documents site of leak in 50% of cases

COAL WORKER'S PNEUMOCONIOSIS

Clinical

- Coal dust can cause lung fibrosis
- Most common lesion: coal macule
- Progressive massive fibrosis (PMF) is rare without silica inhalation
- May lead to a form of centrilobular emphysema
- Most patients asymptomatic and have normal PFTs
- Patients with PMF can have dyspnea

Imaging

- Radiographs:
  Small (1 to 5 mm) dense nodules with an upper lobe predominance
  Indistinguishable from simple silicosis
  PMF shows migrating upper lobe masses
- CT:
  Better defines nodules
  Can detect nodules when radiograph normal
  Centrilobular micronodules, subpleural nodules, masses of PMF, diffuse fibrosis (rare), lymphadenopathy, and calcification of nodes

1

COCAINE ABUSE

Clinical

- Crack lung
- Smoking of cocaine/crack an increasing problem

Imaging

- Radiographs:
    Pneumomediastinum, pneumothorax
    Pulmonary edema
    Pulmonary hemorrhage
    Focal consolidation, subsegmental atelectasis
    Eosinophilic lung disease

COCCIDIOIDOMYCOSIS

Clinical

- Caused by fungus *Coccidioides immitis*
- Found in soil of arid regions
- Inhalation of disturbed soil
- Dissemination in immunocompromised subjects, diabetics
- Usually mild respiratory symptoms
- Hemoptysis
- Skin lesions

Imaging

- Radiographs/CT:
    Limited form
        Progression from focal consolidation to mass to cavity to cyst to clearing
        Ipsilateral adenopathy
        Pleural effusion
    Persistent form
        Chronic pneumonia
        Nodules
        Thick-wall cavity
    Disseminated form
        Miliary nodules
        Contralateral adenopathy
        Upper lobe abnormalities similar to those of MTB with volume loss, cavities, fibronodular opacities

CYSTIC ADENOMATOID MALFORMATION

Clinical

- Rare condition, usually found in neonatal period
- Hamartomatous mass of tissue derived from terminal respiratory elements and containing cystic spaces
- Most commonly one lobe
- Respiratory impairment
- Can rarely present after first year of life as a lung mass

Imaging

- Radiographs:
    Expanded lobe that is opaque mixed with cystic spaces; compressed normal or hypoplastic lung; single cyst
- Appearance can mimic that of bowel protruding through congenital diaphragmatic hernia

CYSTIC FIBROSIS (MUCOVISCIDOSIS)

Clinical

- 1 in 1600 live births; recessive; 1 in 20 carriers
- Upper respiratory tract: sinusitis, polyps
- Lower respiratory tract: bronchiectasis, mucus plugs, abscesses, bronchitis, recurrent pneumonia, atelectasis, pneumothorax, hilar adenopathy, pulmonary hypertension and cor pulmonale, hemoptysis, respiratory failure
- Dyspnea
- Lung infections
- Sinusitis
- Hemoptysis
- Pneumothorax

Imaging

- Radiographs/CT:
    - Upper lobe predominance in adults
    - Hyperinflation, mucus plugs, nodules/masses (abscesses), bronchiectasis, cysts, airtrapping, small airway opacification
- Angiography:
    - For hemoptysis systemic collaterals or hypertrophied bronchial arteries
- Important to recognize and know about this entity

DRESSLER'S SYNDROME

Clinical

- Strictly defined is "post-cardiac injury syndrome" (PCIS) caused by myocardial infarction
- Other causes of PCIS are cardiac surgery, penetrating pericardial injury, closed chest trauma
- Thought to be immunologic
- Fever, pleuritis, pericarditis, 2 to 80 days after event
- High erythrocyte sedimentation rate, with or without leukocytosis
- Largely preventable by nonsteroidal anti-inflammatory agents (e.g., indomethacin)

Imaging

- Radiographs/CT:

Pleural effusion: left, right, bilateral	80%
Enlarged cardiac silhouette (rapid)	50%
Basal consolidation	75%
Normal chest radiograph	10%

DRUG-INDUCED LUNG DISEASE

Clinical

- More than 40 drugs can affect the lungs
- General groups:
    - Toxic reactions, e.g., cytotoxic drugs
    - Hypersensitivity reactions
    - Autoimmune reactions (SLE-like)
    - Vasculitis
    - Phospholipidoses (e.g., amiodarone)
- Reactions vary from acute edema or hemorrhage to chronic infiltrative and fibrotic response
- Variable dyspnea, etc.

1

Imaging

- Radiographs/CT:
    Acute reactions
        Noncardiogenic edema-like, pulmonary hemorrhage, lupus-like
    Chronic reactions
        Fibrosis, infiltration, masses (talc, cytotoxics, amiodarone)
        Adenopathy (phenytoin, methotrexate)
        Nodules (inhalation of oil, gold salts)
        Mediastinal lipomatosis (steroids)

EDEMA, PULMONARY

Clinical

- Increased extravascular, extracellular fluid in the lung
- Quantified experimentally by increase in wet weight:dry weight ratio of lung
- Two mechanisms: increased permeability ("noncardiogenic") (high protein) or hydrostatic ("cardiogenic") (low protein); also may be mixed
- Main causes of increased permeability edema:
    Septicemia, toxins
    Shock, cardiac bypass
    Trauma, radiation, near drowning
    Aspiration
    Inhaled noxious gases, oxygen, metal fumes
    Pancreatitis, uremia
    Drugs (heroin, cocaine, methadone)
    Pneumonia
    Neurogenic, high altitude
    Reexpansion
    Amniotic fluid embolism
- Main causes of hydrostatic edema
    Ischemic left ventricular failure
    Cardiomyopathy
    Valvular disease
    Hypervolemia (overhydration, renal failure)
- Dyspnea, tachypnea, wheezing
- Hypoxemia
- Foamy expectorant
- Differential is ARDS, acid aspiration, hemorrhage, infected aspiration, pneumonia
- Most edema reverses within 24 hours

Imaging

- Radiographs/CT:
    Progression of
        Increase in upper lobe venous caliber (not enough for diagnosis)
        Lower lobe vascular obscuration
        Interstitial lines and cuffs
        Alveolar flooding (fuzzy nodules, consolidation, butterfly pattern, basal predominance, ill-defined hila)
        Pleural effusion
        Distinction between cardiogenic and noncardiogenic edema usually not possible from radiographs

EMBOLISM, PULMONARY

Clinical

- Most common acute catastrophe in hospitalized patient (more than 500,000 per year in United States)
- Causes 10 to 15% of hospital deaths
- Diagnosis missed 30 to 40% of the time
- Predisposing conditions: COPD, cardiac disease, surgery, immobilization, cancer

- Pulmonary infarction ("area packed with RBCs") mass is pleural based, hump-shaped, can cavitate, usually has associated pleural effusion. Infarction occurs in less than 10% of cases of pulmonary embolism
- Dyspnea (80%), tachypnea (70%), pleuritic chest pain (60%), hemoptysis (5%), asymptomatic death (all of these are nonspecific because they are common in hospitalized patients); triad of deep venous thrombosis (DVT), chest pain, hemoptysis uncommon
- Laboratory tests: unreliable or nonspecific; hypoxemia commonly present
- D-Dimer measurements: high negative predictive value; is or may become important screening method

Imaging

- Radiographs:
    Atelectasis (70%)
    Region of increased opacity (30%): focal edema, infarct without necrosis, infarct with necrosis
    Pleural effusion (45%)
    Elevated diaphragm (30%)
    Normal (5%)
    Regional hyperlucency and vascular attenuation (Westermark I less than 5%)
    Large central pulmonary artery (Westermark II less than 5%)
- Radionuclides:
    Normal perfusion scan "precludes" pulmonary embolism
    High probability V:Q scan: about 90% predictive (two or more mismatched segments)
    Low probability V:Q scan: 10 to 15% have emboli; clinical judgment on what to do
    Intermediate probability: should have additional studies but often do not
- Ultrasound of legs:
    Positive compression Doppler plus positive history with or without intermediate V:Q scan = diagnostic enough to treat
    Think "thromboembolic disease" (legs and lungs same diagnosis)
- Transesophageal ultrasound:
    If rapidly available can diagnose large central emboli in patient in shock
- Spiral CT:
    90% accurate
    Can replace V:Q scans and pulmonary angiography in many situations in which clinical suspicion high
    Important unanswered question is predictive value of negative spiral CT scan
    Spiral CT good to the fifth or sixth generation; must be intraluminal filling defects
    Bites out of vessel wall indicate chronic emboli
- Angiography:
    Highest accuracy but less available, uncommonly performed
    Being replaced by spiral CT
    Must see intraluminal defects or vessel cut-off
    Bites out of vessel wall, wall thickening, webs indicate chronic incorporated emboli
- Diagnosis of pulmonary embolism in a state of flux, so have a reasoned position

EMPYEMA

Clinical

- Pus in pleural space
- Most common causes: anaerobic bacteria, MTB, staphylococci, streptococci
- Usually spreads to pleura from pneumonia
- Spiking fever
- Fever of unknown origin
- Pleural mass with fever
- Differentiation of empyema from parapneumonic pleural effusion:
    Fluid shows positive culture or Gram stain

Fluid white blood count more than 20,000 per mL
Fluid glucose level less than 20 mg/dL
pH less than 7.0
- Treatment: thoracentesis, chest tube thoracostomy, or decortication and empyectomy

Imaging

- Radiographs:
  Any pleural fluid collection in patient with pneumonia
  Expanding pleural mass
  Opacity (or fluid level) twice as long in one dimension as in the other suggests that it is within pleural space, not lung
- CT:
  Pleural thickening more than 3 mm
  Pleural effusion with contrast enhancing pleural surface is exudate (seen on parietal side of fluid)

ENDOMETRIOSIS, THORACIC

Clinical

- Rare; two types: pleurodiaphragmatic and bronchopulmonary
- Pleurodiaphragmatic causes catamenial pneumothorax or hemothorax
- Bronchopulmonary: one or more foci of tissue in lung causing hemoptysis, consolidation, mass
- Menses-related pneumothorax or hemothorax
- Menses-related consolidation or hemoptysis

Imaging

- Radiograph:
  Pneumothorax, pleural effusion, lung nodule/mass, consolidation
- CT:
  Hemothorax with varied density from altered blood and soft tissue

EOSINOPHILIC GRANULOMA

Clinical

- Also called *Langerhans' giant cell granulomatosis, histiocytosis X*
- Idiopathic granulomatous disease containing Langerhans' cells
- Spectrum of disease ranges from multisystem to one or two organs
- Lung usually found without bone involvement
- Granulomas 1 to 15 mm in diameter in interstitium or airways
- Fibrosis can lead to end stage lung, especially with honeycombing and large cystic spaces
- 33% asymptomatic
- 33% systemic symptoms
- 66% respiratory symptoms
- 95% (at least) of those with lung disease smoke
- 1 of 7 have pneumothorax at some time

Imaging

- Radiographs:
  Early
    Diffuse fuzzy nodules (1 to 15 mm) and fine lines with somewhat of a middle and upper lobe predominance
    Large nodules/masses
  Late
    Honeycombing
    Large air spaces with upper lobe dominance
    Big lungs (1/3)
    End-stage fibrobullous lung disease

- HRCT:
    Nodules
    Cysts more evident: "geographic," i.e., bizarre shapes characteristic; differential
        lymphangiomyomatosis (DDLAM)
    Other features of interstitial lung disease (ILD) (septal lines, irregular vascular
        margins, architectural distortion)
    Ground-glass opacities
    5 to 10% bone involvement
    Effusions, mediastinal adenopathy, enlarged thymus: all rare

End Note

- Know this disease; it gets shown in conferences a lot

EOSINOPHILIC LUNG DISEASE (ELD)

Clinical

- All disorders of airways or lung parenchyma in which blood or lung eosinophilia,
  or both, present
- Not quite the same as pulmonary infiltrate with eosinophilia (PIE) because
  "infiltrates" may not be present
- Two groups:

Eosinophils important	Eosinophils incidental
Asthma	Some infections, e.g., chlamydial
Idiopathic	Neoplasms
Acute (Loeffler's syndrome)	Irradiation
Chronic eosinophilic pneumonia	Collagen vascular disease
(Carrington's disease)	Sarcoid
Allergic: drugs, parasites, aspergillosis	Hemodialysis
Vasculitis and granulomatosis	
Churg-Strauss	
Bronchocentric granulomatosis	
Wegener's granulomatosis	
Hypereosinophilia syndrome	
Lymphoma	

- Symptoms tend to come and go
- Wheezing
- Steroid responsive
- Systemic symptoms may or may not be present

Imaging

- Radiographs/CT:
    "Flame" or wedge-shaped infiltrates that come and go
    Peripheral homogeneous consolidation especially in upper lungs (chronic eo-
        sinophilic pneumonia)
    Normal chest
    Proximal and distal bronchiectasis, plugs, atelectasis, mycetoma, cysts (allergic
        bronchopulmonary aspergillosis [ABPA])
    Nodules (bronchocentric granulomatosis)
    Diffuse ground-glass opacities
    Cardiomegaly, effusions, pulmonary edema (hypereosinophilia syndrome)

FAT EMBOLISM

Clinical

- Pulmonary and systemic embolization of fat droplets
- Fat usually from bone marrow released by trauma
- Other causes include pancreatitis, decompression (diving), burns
- Diagnosis from fat droplets in blood, urine, retina

1

- Damage is from fat converting to reactive fatty acids
- Delay of 12 to 72 hours
- Dyspnea, fever, hypoxia, petechia, altered mental status (AMS), headache, coma, seizures, stupor, cyanosis, death
- Rash in 2 to 3 days

Imaging

- Radiographs/CT:
  Early: normal
  Late: pulmonary edema, ARDS
  Distribution of edema tends to be peripheral and may be predominantly interstitial or alveolar

FOREIGN MATERIAL EMBOLISM

Clinical

- Many substances can embolize to lungs, including fat droplets, bone marrow particles, amniotic fluid, parasites and ova, tumor, trophoblastic cells, air, talc, mercury, cotton fibers, and iodinated oil (contrast material)
- Response of lung depends on amount of vascular bed obstructed and reactivity of embolized material
- Several small, nonreactive emboli can result in pulmonary arterial hypertension
- Reactive materials can produce pulmonary edema, ARDS, or lung inflammation and fibrosis
- Most common cause of pulmonary arterial hypertension worldwide: embolized ova from schistosomiasis
- Clinical circumstances usually indicate diagnosis; can be anything from sudden death to slow right heart failure

Imaging

- Radiographs/CT:
  Extremely varied; nodules; pulmonary arterial hypertension; talc can cause nodules and upper lobe fibrosis with calcification

FRACTURED BRONCHUS OR TRACHEA

Clinical

- Severe blunt trauma
- Injury to chest wall, lungs, mediastinal vessels, diaphragm may be present as well
- Diagnosis often missed
- Usual site is hilum
- Bronchial wall tear and/or hematoma are the two causes of the abnormal findings
- Pneumothorax with lung not collapsing or not reexpanding after chest tube insertion
- Hypoxia, difficult to correct with ventilation

Imaging

- Radiographs/CT:
  Pneumomediastinum: must always be explained after trauma
  Pneumothorax with possible tension
  Consolidated, non-reexpanding lung after chest tube insertion
  Look for (often missed) diaphragmatic rupture
  "Fallen lung:" rare with total disruption of hilum
  Later, lung becomes airless and consolidated

1

GERM CELL TUMORS

Clinical

- Derived from embryonic germ cells
- Include teratoma (more than one germ layer), dermoid, seminoma, teratocarcinoma, embryonal cell carcinoma, endodermal sinus tumor, choriocarcinoma, mixed
- Most arise in or around thymus
- Benign teratomas constitute 50% of germ cell tumors
- Findings suggesting malignancy: large; infiltration of mediastinum; invasion of lung; symptoms; elevated level of human chorionic gonadotropin (HCG) or alpha fetoprotein (AFP) or both
- 50% asymptomatic
- Airway/vascular compression, e.g., SVC syndrome
- Chest pain, cough, fever
- Trichoptysis (sounds acute but is rare): expectorating hair

Imaging

- Radiographs:
    Anterior mediastinal mass (rarely middle or posterior mediastinum)
    Lobulated, well defined
    Sudden increase in size from hemorrhage
    Invades mediastinum/lung
- CT:
    Mass containing fat, soft tissue, calcium, bone (fat-fluid level)
    Calcification does not indicate benignity
    Cystic degeneration common (large cystic anterior mediastinal mass almost always cystic teratoma)

End Notes

- Main differential is thymoma, occasionally lymphoma
- Almost all intrathoracic goiters are retro-aortic
- Radiologist should ask for HCG and AFP levels when confronted with an anterior mediastinal mass

GOITER (INTRATHORACIC)

Clinical

- Intrathoracic (mediastinal) goiter an extension from benign multinodular goiter in neck
- Defined by extension below top of manubrium
- 95% between trachea and great vessels/ascending aorta
- Most do not compress trachea
- Neck mass
- Positional shortness of breath
- Asymptomatic

Imaging

- Radiographs:
    Well-defined mediastinal mass, most commonly on the right
    Displaces trachea posteriorly and/or to one side
    May compress trachea from both sides
    Sometimes mass between trachea and esophagus
- CT characteristic features:
    Position in mediastinum and well-defined
    Connection with neck goiter
    Inhomogeneous, with high CT density regions, cysts and calcifications (most)
    Delayed enhancement with IV contrast
- CT better for diagnosis than radionuclide studies or MRI

1

GOODPASTURE'S SYNDROME

Clinical

- Diffuse pulmonary hemorrhage with glomerulonephritis from antibasement membrane antibody (occasionally only lung or kidney involved)
- Smooth immune protein deposition, natural killer (NK) cells
- Hemoptysis, dyspnea, anemia, cough
- Young white males most commonly affected

Imaging

- Radiographs/CT:
    Diffuse lung consolidation/ground-glass opacities; blood often has fine granular texture on radiographs; comes and goes with a periodicity of days or weeks
- Minor symptoms and marked diffuse consolidation: think of blood
- Can clear in 1 or 2 days, especially if patient taking steroids
- Severe diffuse pulmonary hemorrhage can occur without hemoptysis

HAMARTOMA (PULMONARY)

Clinical

- Correct term is *chondrohamartoma*
- Benign tumor-like mass consisting of abnormal mix of normal lung elements
- Contains soft tissue, calcification, and often fat
- Asymptomatic
- Unusual to be large enough to compromise structures
- Occasionally endobronchial

Imaging

- Radiographs:
    Solitary (rarely multiple) nodules or masses 1 to 12 cm in diameter; 15% calcify, usually larger ones
- CT:
    Most over 2 cm show calcifications ("popcorn" is classic); 50% contain fat
- Be careful in interpreting fat in hamartoma: hamartomas lobulate, and low CT density can result from partial volume effect from air within surface indentations
- 60% can be diagnosed by HRCT

HEMORRHAGE, DIFFUSE PULMONARY

Clinical

- Diffuse or multifocal hemorrhage (does not include focal bleeding or aspirated blood)
- Can occur without hemoptysis
- Causes:
    Immunologic (antibasement membrane antibody disease; most have kidney involvement)
    Connective tissue diseases (systemic lupus erythematosus [SLE], rheumatoid arthritis, Wegener's granulomatosis, mixed connective tissue disease)
    Idiopathic pulmonary hemosiderosis
    Renal failure
    Anticoagulants
    Drugs, chemicals, inhaled toxins
    Acute bone marrow transplant rejection
    Acute infections (hemorrhagic pneumonia)
    Mechanical (venoocclusive disease, mitral stenosis)
- Anemia, hemoptysis, infiltrates

Imaging

- Radiographs/CT:
    Diffuse increase in lung opacity; tends to be granular, especially when clearing

1

• When opacities out of proportion to respiratory impairment: think of blood
• Granular appearance: think of blood or alveolar proteinosis

HISTOPLASMOSIS

Clinical

• Fungus: *Histoplasma capsulatum*; found in middle North America, in birds and bats
• Classification
    Limited form
        Pneumonia: asymptomatic (80%) or symptomatic
        Histoplasmoma: single or multiple nodules
        Chronic focal cavitary form
        Scattered granulomas in liver and spleen
        Single site end-organ disease, e.g., bone, CNS
        Fibrosing mediastinitis
    Disseminated form (immunocompromised host)
        Miliary pneumonia
        Systematic dissemination
        Widespread adenopathy
• Presentation ranges from asymptomatic (more than 95%) to disseminated infection and death

Imaging

• Radiographs/CT:
    Patchy consolidation ("bronchopneumonia pattern")
    Ipsilateral nodal enlargement
    Multiple nodules with or without calcification (bulls-eye or diffuse)
    Large stable nodules or masses ("giant histoplasmomas")
    Miliary nodules
    Cavitary form with or without fibrosis and retraction (uncommon)

HYDATID DISEASE

Clinical

• Tapeworm *Echinococcus granulosus*
• Humans accidental intermediate hosts instead of cow, sheep, or moose; primary host: wolf or dog
• Ova are ingested, larvae go to liver/lungs where they develop into cysts
• Three layers: endocyst, ectocyst, and host reaction (pericyst)
• Asymptomatic with abnormal radiograph
• Cyst ruptures and becomes infected
• Anaphylaxis
• Eosinophilia

Imaging

• Radiographs/CT:
    Masses: smooth, soft, well-defined, lower lobes, right side
    Lung hydatids rarely calcify
    "Floating lily" sign: cyst ruptures
    "Air crescent" sign: separation between ectocyst and pericyst
    Direct invasion through right hemidiaphragm into pleural space can also occur
• CT:
    Thin-walled, water content, daughter cysts shown as septations; mediastinal cysts rare

End Note

• Many cases are the sylvanic form in and from Alaska

HYPERSENSITIVITY PNEUMONITIS (EXTRINSIC ALLERGIC ALVEOLITIS)

Clinical

• Immune lung reaction to inhaled antigenic material, usually proteins
• Origin of proteins varies from microorganisms to animal and plant proteins; can also be single chemicals or minerals; most common: bird proteins and thermophylic *Actinomyces* spp proteins
• Acute, subacute, and chronic forms
• Symptoms may be respiratory alone or with systemic components

Imaging

• Radiographs/CT:
　　Acute/subacute
　　　　Small nodules, (bronchocentric on HRCT), 1 to 5 mm
　　　　Ground-glass opacities
　　　　Focal, patchy consolidation
　　　　Linear "interstitial" pattern
　　Chronic
　　　　Scarring, honeycombing, architectural distortion
　　　　Bronchiectasis
　　　　Thin-walled cystic spaces
　　　　Small nodules
　　　　Ground-glass opacities of lung fibrosis (HRCT)

End Note

• Exposure history is key; clinician often has not asked correct questions (especially pets and occupation)

HYPOGENETIC LUNG SYNDROME

Clinical

• Also called *venolobar syndrome, scimitar syndrome*
• Congenital maldevelopment of right lung bud
• Involves airways, pulmonary vessels, systemic vessels
• Basic components: small lung from a dropout of segments (often difficult to define remaining segments or lobes)
• Anomalous pulmonary venous return from right upper lobe or whole right lung to inferior vena cava (IVC) hepatic veins
• Can have variable systemic blood supply to lung
• Can have proximal interruption of right pulmonary artery
• Can have cardiac defects, especially ventricular septal defect (VSD), atrial septal defect (ASD)
• Can have diaphragmatic anomalies, especially eventration/hernias
• Most asymptomatic
• Hemoptysis

Imaging

• Radiographs/CT:
　　Small lung that does not trap gas
　　Serpiginous scimitar vein behind heart on lateral view
　　Anomalous systemic artery on CT
　　Proximal interruption of right pulmonary artery on CT
　　CT should be diagnostic

End Note

- Any condition with systemic blood supply to lung is at risk for hemoptysis

IMMOTILE CILIA SYNDROMES

Clinical

- Genetic defect in ciliary function and structure (dynein arms)
- Exactly 50% of patients have dextrocardia; then disease called *Kartagener's syndrome*
- Men infertile; fertility reduced in women
- Increasingly important cause of bronchiectasis
- Sinusitis, bronchitis, recurrent infections, bronchiectasis
- Respiratory failure
- Course more benign than that of cystic fibrosis

Imaging

- Radiographs/CT:
    Bronchiectasis, especially lower and middle lobes; situs inversus; sinusitis

IMMUNE COMPLEX DISEASES (COLLAGEN VASCULAR DISEASES)

- Type III immune complex deposition
- Share clinical features
- Can overlap
- Can share some findings with the granulomatous diseases and have elements of vasculitis
- *See* **Ankylosing Spondylitis**
- *See* **Behçet's Disease**
- *See* **Systemic Lupus Erythematosus**
- *See* **Rheumatoid Lung Disease**
- *See* **Progressive Systemic Sclerosis (PSS)**
- *See* **Sjögren's Syndrome**
- *See* **Relapsing Polychondritis (RP)**

INTERSTITIAL PNEUMONITIDES

Clinical

- Group of idiopathic diseases characterized by interstitial inflammation and fibrosis
- Most require biopsy for diagnosis
- Sometimes overlap with immune-complex diseases

Idiopathic Pulmonary Fibrosis (IPF)
- Also called *usual interstitial pneumonia, fibrosing alveolitis, Hamman-Rich syndrome*
- Idiopathic lung disease characterized by its clinicopathologic features
- Patchy lung inflammation at different stages of maturity with normal lung intervening
- 33% of cases show some features of lung immune-complex diseases, cirrhosis, thyroid disease, ulcerative colitis, etc.
- Incidence 4 to 15 per 100,000 population; wide age range, but especially in older patients of either gender
- Dyspnea, cough, restrictive lung function, clubbing
- Activated lymphocytes on lavage

Desquamative Interstitial Pneumonitis
- Probably a more active variant of IPF
- Alveoli full of macrophages
- Prognosis better than that of IPF
- Presentation same as IPF (more acute course)

Lymphocytic Interstitial Pneumonitis (LIP)
- Confusing entity because diagnosis is histologic
- In some cases, LIP monoclonal and prelymphoma
- Some cases reactive and polyclonal
- Some cases AIDS related
- Lymphocytes in interstitium, not around airways and no granulomas
- Cough, chest pain, fever, weight loss
- Wide age range
- More common in females than in males

Imaging

Idiopathic Pulmonary Fibrosis (IPF)
- Radiographs/CT:
    Interstitial fibrosis pattern with small lungs, linear and reticular opacities; later may show honeycombing
    HRCT:
        Septal lines, thickened core structures, parenchymal bands, subpleural lines, honeycombing, architectural distortion, subpleural nodules
    When advanced, peripheral honeycombing can be striking
    Ground-glass opacities from alveolitis or fibrosis
    Pulmonary arterial hypertension
    Increased incidence of lung cancer
    May show large, thin-walled cystic spaces
    Lymphadenopathy on CT (minor feature)

Desquamative Interstitial Pneumonitis
- Radiographs/CT:
    Can show all features of IPF; may be only interstitial lines and ground-glass opacities; ground-glass with basal or peripheral predominance on HRCT
- Requires biopsy for diagnosis
- If interstitial fibrosis (honeycombing, architectural distortion) seen on HRCT, disease is IPF, not desquamative interstitial pneumonitis
- Is steroid responsive

Lymphocytic Interstitial Pneumonitis (LIP)
- Radiographs/CT:
    Many nodules, small and fuzzy, miliary, acinar
    Patchy consolidation
    Interstitial thickening, ground-glass opacities, patchy consolidation on HRCT
    Can progress to appearance of end-stage lung

LEUKEMIA

Clinical

- Six causes of thoracic abnormalities: infiltration with leukemic cells, lymphadenopathy, infection, treatment (drug reactions), leukostasis (sludging), and hemorrhage
- Varied
- Imaging must be interpreted in clinical context (drugs, bleeding tendency, white cell count must be known)

Imaging

- Radiographs:
    Masses, adenopathy, ground-glass/consolidation, ARDS-like
- Most common causes of lung abnormality: infection and hemorrhage
- Sludging occurs only when white blood cell count more than 250,000/mL
- Radiographs with sludging usually normal or show "edema pattern"

1

LIPOID PNEUMONIA ("PARAFFINOMAS")
Clinical

- Chronic aspiration of oil, usually mineral or vegetable, mainly in women self-treating for constipation
- With or without esophageal reflux
- Asymptomatic
- Fever, dyspnea

Imaging

- Radiographs:
    Bilateral basal linear opacities; basal mass-like opacities
- CT:
    Masses may show striking low density or soft tissue density; chronic consolidation (air bronchograms)
- Triad of appropriate clinical history; slow progression; and basal, mass-like opacities or consolidation
- Other considerations: alveolar cell carcinoma, sarcoid, lymphoma/pseudolymphoma, rounded atelectasis (must have associated fibrothorax), alveolar proteinosis

LIPOMATOSIS, MEDIASTINAL
Clinical

- Can be normal variant
- Found in patients on steroid therapy or with Cushing's syndrome
- Asymptomatic

Imaging

- Radiographs:
    Wide mediastinum; smooth, regular, and low density
- CT:
    Fat density mediastinal widening
- Usually other fat deposits, extrapleural or epicardial
- CT usually not needed for diagnosis

LOBAR EMPHYSEMA (CONGENITAL)
Clinical

- Probably caused by congenital defect in wall of lobar bronchus
- Found in neonatal period to first months of life
- Middle lobe or upper lobes affected
- Respiratory distress
- Can be fatal
- Occasionally patients reach childhood and remain asymptomatic

Imaging

- Radiographs:
    Hyperexpansion of one lobe with a ball-valve effect
    Can completely compress other lobe or lobes on same side and fill hemithorax
    Contralateral displacement of heart/mediastinum
- CT:
    Vessels in hyperexpanded lobe can be identified, eliminating possibility of a pneumothorax
    Compressed lobes can be identified
    CT may be able to exclude mass in or around offending bronchus
- Scintigrams:
    Do not add to CT
- Most patients undergo resection based on diagnosis provided by imaging features
- Some cases in older infants can be followed (carefully)
- Similar appearance found with the rare "polyalveolar lobe"

1

LÖFFLER'S SYNDROME

• *See* **Eosinophilic Lung Disease**

LYMPHANGIOMA (CYSTIC HYGROMA)

Clinical

• Mass-like congenital malformation of lymph channels
• Variable in size, often cystic
• Variable vascular components
• Most common sites: neck, mediastinum, or both
• Asymptomatic and incidental
• Compression of mediastinal structures
• Neck mass

Imaging

• Radiographs:
    Mass or masses in anterior or superior mediastinum; pleural effusion with or without chylous fluid
• CT:
    Water density, fluid-filled cysts; septations frequent; SVC dilation
• Looks like atypical bronchogenic cyst but more anterior and superior, septated, and often extends into neck

LYMPHANGIOMYOMATOSIS (LYMPHANGIOLEIOMYOMATOSIS) (LAM)

Clinical

• Shares many features with pulmonary tuberous sclerosis
• Perilymphatic smooth muscle proliferation with involvement of airways and vessels
• Distinguishing features: females of reproductive age, chylous effusions, pneumothorax, large cystic lungs; renal angiomyolipomas rare, mediastinal nodal enlargement common
• Dyspnea, hemoptysis
• Chylous pleural effusions/ascites
• Airflow obstruction
• Reduced diffusing capacity

Imaging

• Radiographs:
    Large lungs, cysts: geographic, irregular; reticulonodular opacities; pneumothorax (60 to 80%)
• HRCT:
    Multiple, thin-walled cysts, 2 to 50 mm in diameter; rarely nodules; pleural effusion (75%)

LYMPHANGITIC CARCINOMATOSIS

Clinical

• Lymphatic and interstitial permeation of lung by neoplastic cells with interstitial edema from lymphatic obstruction
• 50% back flow from hilar nodes
• 50% break out from small tumor emboli to pulmonary capillaries
• Sites of origin: lung, breast, stomach, pancreas, colon, prostate (common histologically but not clinically)
• Dyspnea, cough

Imaging

• Radiographs:
    Plain films often confusing because of nonuniformity of appearances and nodular air space opacities

Reticulonodular, linear opacities
Unilateral septal lines
Fissural/pleural thickening
Pleural effusion
Blotchy nodular, air space opacities
- HRCT:
Diagnostic in correct clinical setting
Undistorted interstitial thickening ("polygons")
Nodular ("beaded") interstitial thickening (not always)
Patchy air space opacities
Peribronchial thickening
With or without hilar adenopathy

LYMPHOMA

Clinical

- Malignancy from lymphocytes and histiocytes and associated inflammation
- Two groups: Hodgkin's and non-Hodgkin's

Hodgkin's Lymphoma
- Four types: nodular sclerosing, lymphocyte predominance, mixed cellularity, lymphocyte depleted
- Four stages:
  I Single nodal group or extralymphatic site
  II Two nodal groups or one site plus one nodal group, all on same side of diaphragm
  III Nodal regions both sides of diaphragm with or without focal extralymphatic site
  IV Diffuse extralymphatic
- Occurs in second to fourth decades
- Neck swelling
- Systemic symptoms
- Anemia

Non-Hodgkin's Lymphoma
- From specific cell lines: B lymphocytes, T lymphocytes, or histiocytes
- Three grades: low, intermediate, high
- Usually not staged anatomically
- Usually widespread disease at initial presentation
- Presentation similar to that of Hodgkin's disease

Imaging

Hodgkin's Lymphoma
- Radiographs:
  Bulky anterior mediastinal nodal mass
  Mediastinal and hilar nodal enlargement
  Can involve lung (linear, nodular, with or without cavities, peribronchial thickening)
  Can involve pleura (effusion, masses, diffuse thickening)
  Can involve chest wall (mass, rib destruction)
  Can involve vertebra (mass, white vertebrae)
  Can cause endobronchial obstruction
  Nodal calcification: usually after treatment
  Paracardiac nodes: usually a site for recurrence
  Consolidation with appearance of pneumonia
  SVC obstruction
- CT:
  More sensitive for findings
  Nodes can be discrete or matted
  Nodes may show edge enhancement with contrast
  Calcified nodes: diffuse, stippled, eggshell

1

Involvement contiguous; i.e., no "skip" areas
Pericardial effusion

Non-Hodgkin's Lymphoma

- Radiographs/CT:
  Less than half have abnormal chest radiographs at presentation
  May show all the features of Hodgkin's disease
  Adenopathy less characteristically anterior mediastinal
  Skip areas seen
  Parenchymal disease without adenopathy
  Rare primary pulmonary lymphoma
  Endobronchial masses from mucosal lymphoma
  Rare intravascular form with pulmonary hypertension

End Note

- Lymphoma is protean in its presentation; should always be kept in mind

MARFAN'S SYNDROME

Clinical

- One of the four most common congenital disorders of fibrous connective tissue
- Involves eyes, heart, aorta, musculoskeletal system, joints, spine
- Thoracic involvement: pneumothorax (10%), bullae/cysts, emphysema, pectus, kyphoscoliosis, bronchiectasis, upper lobe fibrosis (rare)
- Aortic aneurysm, aortic regurgitation, mitral valve disease
- Dyspnea, chest pain
- Span greater than height

Imaging

- CT/radiographs:
  Aortic root dilatation; enlarged left ventricle; emphysema, pneumothorax, hyperinflation; kyphoscoliosis/pectus

MEDIASTINITIS (FIBROSING)

Clinical

- Most cases result of histoplasmosis, radiation, other fungi, MTB, drugs, or idiopathic
- Progressive fibrosis of mediastinum with increasing obstruction of aerodigestive or vascular systems
- Facial swelling (SVC syndrome), dyspnea, cough, respiratory tract infections, hemoptysis, chest pain

Imaging

- Radiographs:
  Two types
    Focal: lobulated mass
    Diffuse: mediastinal widening
  Mediastinal calcification
  Normal radiograph
  Adenopathy with or without calcifications
- CT:
  SVC obstruction
  Airway or pulmonary artery obstruction
  Esophageal obstruction

Dense calcified mediastinal masses or matted nodes
Diffuse mediastinal increased density and obliteration of fat planes
Collateral venous channels
- MRI:
Low signal intensity masses; vascular abnormalities

MESOTHELIOMA

Clinical

- Two entirely different pleural tumors are often both called *mesotheliomas*; they should be considered separately

Fibrous Tumor of Pleura ("Pleural Fibroma")
- Arises from mesenchymal cells
- 70% benign and slow growing
- Can be very large ("giant pleural fibrosis tumor")
- Pain, fever, osteoarthropathy, hypoglycemia

Mesothelioma
- Always malignant and invariably diffuse
- Rare tumor arising from pleural epithelial cells (50%) or mesenchymal cells (25%); may be mixed (25%)
- 60% of patients have asbestos exposure (occupational or home contact with a worker)
- Risk is exposure to the first power, but latency (time from exposure) to the fourth power (i.e., low dose, lung latency)
- Invariably fatal and untreatable
- Spread by extension, hematogenous, lymphatic
- Chest pain, weight loss, heaviness in thorax

Imaging

Fibrous Tumor of Pleura
- Radiographs:
Pleural mass taking the line of least resistance, i.e., invaginating the lung; noncalcified; rib erosions
- CT:
Well marginated, pleural-based, homogeneous mass; large lesions may show low-density centers; may enhance with contrast

Mesothelioma
- Radiographs/CT:
Diffuse lobular pleural thickening extending into fissures ("encasement" of lung)
Hemithorax reduced in size
Pleural effusion without visible masses
Metastases to chest wall, lung, nodes, pericardium
Pleural plaques may be visible (on contralateral or ipsilateral sides)
- Metastases of other tumors to pleura can produce similar findings but are infrequently as extensive
- Other causes of fibrothorax should be considered in differential diagnosis (infection or blood)

METASTASES, INTRATHORACIC

Clinical

- Most common site for many tumors: lung, breast, colon, kidney, head and neck, uterus, prostate (these sites account for 70% of lung metastases)
- Highest frequency: melanoma, choriocarcinoma, Ewing's sarcoma, osteosarcoma, thyroid, testes, kidney (these all have an incidence of lung metastases of 65 to 75%)
- Asymptomatic
- Dyspnea, effusion, pneumothorax

Imaging

- Radiographic/CT patterns of metastases:
    Nodules
        Multiple, discrete, tend to basal and peripheral
        Multiple, fuzzy
        Multiple with or without cavitating
        Snowstorm: miliary (thyroid, renal, osteosarcoma, melanoma)
        Solitary nodule: 4 to 6% of SPNs are metastases; colon responsible for 60%
            of metastases that present as SPN
        Calcified (rare): osteosarcoma, breast, thyroid, ovarian
    Interstitial
        Lines and dots, blotchy consolidation, pleural effusion (*See* **Lymphangitic Carcinomatosis**)
    Hilar/mediastinal adenopathy (midline tumors)
        Thyroid, renal, head and neck, breast, testes, melanoma
    Tumor emboli
        Present as infarcts (large) or pulmonary hypertension (small)
    Pleural effusion
        Lung, breast, pancreas, ovary, stomach, lymphoma
        Variable size
        50% bloody
        50% positive cytologic studies
    Chest wall/ribs
        Mass
        Destruction
    Endobronchial
        Mass/obstruction (breast, melanoma, kidney, colon)

MIDDLE LOBE SYNDROME

Clinical

- Chronic nonobstructive middle lobe collapse
- Probably postinfectious with scarring
- Formerly thought to be postobstructive resulting from TB adenopathy that had resolved
- Cough, recurrent infection
- Can occur at any age

Imaging

- Radiographs/CT:
    Persistent middle lobe collapse without endobronchial component
- MRI:
    Higher intensity on T2-weighted images with obstructive atelectasis

MUCOID IMPACTION (BRONCHOCELE)

Clinical

- Chronic mucus pooling in dilated bronchi
- With or without proximal obstructing lesion
- Result of asthma, allergic aspergillosis, bronchial atresia, cystic fibrosis, obstruction from tumor or foreign body, benign stenosis, idiopathic
- Asymptomatic
- Cough, fever, wheezing, hemoptysis

Imaging

- Radiographs:
    "Finger-in-glove," drumstick, segmental atelectasis; other findings of underlying disease

- CT:
    If lung airless: mucus bronchograms; if lung air filled: finger-in-glove appearance
- Frequently not considered from radiographs; anticipate atypical findings or ill-defined masslike lesions

MUCORMYCOSIS

Clinical

- One of the *Phycomycetes* fungi
- Pneumonia in immunocompromised patients (usually those with hematologic malignancies) with high mortality
- Angioinvasive organism
- Fever, cough, chest pain, hemoptysis

Imaging

- Radiographs/CT:
    Nodule or mass
    Consolidation
    Paranasal sinus infection
    Infarcts, cavitation
    "Lung balls" from infarcted infected lung
    Pleural effusion

MYCETOMA (FUNGUS BALL)

Clinical

- Coalescent hyphae forming a ball within preexisting air-containing space in lung (cavity, bulla, cyst) or, rarely, in pleura
- Usual organism *Aspergillus fumigatus*
- Diagnosis usually radiologic
- Incidental finding
- Hemoptysis
- Treatment: resection/intracavitary antifungal agents

Imaging

- Radiographs:
    Mobile, soft tissue mass within cavity; air meniscus or air crescent sign; cyst wall can be irregularly thickened; air-fluid level
- CT:
    Visible air spaces in most fungus balls; attachments to cavity wall; early can be incomplete spongy, mass-like ball

MYCOPLASMA PNEUMONIA (PRIMARY ATYPICAL PNEUMONIA)

Clinical

- Eton agent
- Most common nonbacterial cause of community acquired pneumonia
- Occurs in young individuals
- Discrepancy between limited symptoms and marked radiographic findings
- Viral-like syndrome that persists for weeks
- Otitis media with pneumonia; patient should be asked about earache
- Rapid clinical response to erythromycin, rare progressive fatal cases

Imaging

- Radiographs:
    Variable: unilateral, bilateral, patchy, dense consolidation

1

Most common: lobar consolidation
Patchy, multifocal, subsegmental consolidation also common
Small pleural effusion common
Adenopathy uncommon
Clears slowly

NOCARDIAL PNEUMONIA

Clinical

- *Nocardia asteroides*: fungus-like bacillus
- Pneumonia in immunocompromised; debilitated patients; or patients with alveolar proteinosis
- Progression variable
- Patients infected and often very sick

Imaging

- Radiographs/CT:
    Variable
    Lobar/sublobar consolidation
    Multiple nodules, millimeters to 5.0 cm with or without rapid cavitation
    Thick-walled cavity mistaken for bronchogenic carcinoma
    Pleural effusion (50%)
    Hilar adenopathy (30%)

End Notes

- In an immunocompromised patient who has multiple nodules with some cavities when first seen, consider nocardial infection, septic emboli, cryptococcus
- Multiple areas of patchy consolidation ("bronchopneumonia pattern")

PANCOAST'S (SUPERIOR SULCUS) TUMOR

Clinical

- Originally triad of shoulder and arm pain (brachial plexopathy), Horner's syndrome, bone destruction
- Tumor arises at cupula of lung
- Any of the bronchogenic carcinoma cell types
- Key is invasion in any or all directions
- Shoulder/arm pain, muscle wasting

Imaging

- Radiographs:
    Apical mass; any convex, downward, asymmetrical, apical, pleural thickening; bone destruction; regional adenopathy, hilar and mediastinal; vertebral destruction; change in apical cap
- CT/MR:
    Provides useful information on extent, brachial plexus involvement, intraspinal extension, fat plane violation

PLEURAL EFFUSION

Clinical

- Accumulation of fluid in pleural space beyond normal 7 to 15 mL
- Mechanisms of fluid accumulation: hydrostatic, oncotic, permeability, lymph drainage, pleural pressure, transdiaphragmatic passage
- Abnormal fluid enters mainly from visceral but also from parietal pleura
- Fluid content varies: two main groups, transudates and exudates

Transudate
- Specific gravity less than 1.016, protein less than 3 g/dL, lactate dehydrogenase (LDH) ratio less than 0.6, protein less than 0.5 of serum protein
- Causes: hemodynamics (heart failure, pericardial constriction), neoplasm (renal, liver disease, hypoalbuminemia), or local pressure (atelectasis, pulmonary infarction, trauma)

Exudate
- Specific gravity, protein, and LDH ratio all higher than those in transudate
- Causes: neoplasm (metastases, primary lung, primary pleural), almost any infection, irritation (Dressler's syndrome, subphrenic abscess, trauma, pancreatitis, dialysis), or inflammation (collagen vascular disease, drug reactions, asbestos, sarcoid)
- Incidental
- Cause of effusion causes symptoms
- Dyspnea, heaviness

Imaging

- Ultrasound generally suggested for initial evaluation, then CT
- Radiographs:
    Erect
        Meniscus posteriorly
        Meniscus laterally
        General haziness more medially over the lungs
        Fluid in fissures
        Middle lobe step
        Effusion around a lobe
        Azygoesophageal recess displacement to left
        Encapsulated fluid in a fissure
        Encapsulated fluid against mediastinum
        Unilateral opacified hemithorax
        Apical cap
        Arcuate opacity of fluid in major fissure
    Subpulmonic
        High false hemidiaphragm
        Lateral apex of false hemidiaphragm
        Separation of gastric bubble and lung (must be in two projections)
        Absent medial mediastinal-phrenic angle
        Blunted lateral costophrenic angle
    Decubitus
        Lateral position of fluid
        Down lung always at lower volume and pleural thickening without fluid appears thicker (beware!)
        250 to 300 mL per cm depth in this position (adult)
        Apical cap
    Supine
        Hemithorax shows diffuse hazy opacity (less evident towards apex, no air bronchograms, preserved vessels)
        Obscured hemidiaphragm
        Blunted costophrenic angle
        Fluid in minor fissure (right side)
        Widened paraspinous line
        Apical cap
        Elevated false hemidiaphragm
    Tension
        Opaque hemithorax
        Inverted hemidiaphragm
        Contralateral mediastinal shift
- CT:
    All features as on supine radiographs
    Tells more about cause, distribution, underlying lung, etc.

Ascites versus effusion: with effusion, crus displaced anteriorly and laterally, liver/spleen interphase hazy, fluid outside diaphragm

Collapsed lower lobe versus diaphragm: continuity with lung superiorly, air bronchograms, lung thicker superiorly

Contrast-enhancing pleura with fluid: 75% exudates so thoracentesis/biopsy usually necessary, if cause not known

- Ultrasound:
    Sensitive for localization and detection of effusion
    Best method to show septations
    Commonly anechoic and delineated by echogenic line at lung interface
    Echogenic effusion often exudative
    Can separate solid from fluid-containing pleural masses
    Show subpulmonic effusion
    Localizes fluid for aspiration

PNEUMOCYSTIS CARINII PNEUMONIA (PCP)

- *See also under* **AIDS**

Clinical

- Organism a protozoan or primitive fungus
- Asymptomatic infection common; symptomatic disease mostly in T-cell deficiency states
- Atypical presentation now more common than typical
- In those with AIDS, prophylaxis given when CD4 count falls below 200
- Dyspnea, acute or subacute
- Hypoxia, reduced diffusing capacity for carbon monoxide
- Immunodeficient background

Imaging

- Radiographs:
    Typical
        Diffuse ground-glass opacities (often slightly granular appearance), progressing to air-space consolidation
        Perihilar accentuation
        Upper lobes: similar to findings in TB, i.e., with nodular patchy consolidation
        Thin-walled cysts 1 to 10 cm, indicative of prior PCP infection
    Atypical
        One or more nodules with or without cavitation
        Solid mass
        Pneumothorax
        Effusion: rare
        Nodal calcification: rare
        Normal radiograph (15 to 20%)
- CT/HRCT:
    Air-space consolidation/ground-glass opacities more evident
    All other radiographic findings also seen

End Notes

- Low CD4 count, diffuse consolidation: probably PCP; if no hypoxia with this presentation, unlikely to be PCP
- If ground-glass opacities not seen on HRCT, likelihood of active PCP is less than 5%

PNEUMOMEDIASTINUM

Clinical

- Gas in mediastinum from lung, air-containing mediastinal organ, neck, retroperitoneum

- Causes: barotrauma, asthma, esophageal rupture, bronchial injury, thoracic/retroperitoneal surgery, tracheostomy, or instrumentation
- Chest pain: retrosternal or pleuritic
- Crunching sensation, subcutaneous emphysema

Imaging

- Radiographs/CT:
    Air outlining mediastinal structures: thymus, trachea, great vessels, pericardium. Pneumomediastinum is obvious with CT
- Distinguishing between pneumomediastinum and pneumopericardium can be difficult; former is more common; thus, unless air evident around proximal great vessels, it is probably pneumomediastinum
- 15% of patients with pneumomediastinum develop pneumothorax; reverse does not happen
- Distinguishing between pneumomediastinum and medial pneumothorax can be difficult; air should be sought around great vessels

PNEUMOTHORAX, SPONTANEOUS

Clinical

- Gas (rapidly nitrogen) in pleural space
- Causes: blebs (in smokers mainly); asthma; infection (TB formerly); infarction; neoplasm; COPD; all causes of interstitial fibrosis, especially sarcoid and Langerhans' giant cell granulomatosis (eosinophilic granuloma); trauma (many mechanisms); catamenial
- Pleuritic chest pain, dyspnea, asymptomatic, strange sensation in that hemithorax

Imaging

- Radiographs:
    Erect
        Visible lung edge: increase in lung density is less than expected because blood flow decreases
        Distinguish from bullae, blebs, cysts
        Small effusion occurs in 50%; not clinically significant
        Lung collapses downward and medially
        Subpulmonic pneumothorax: rare
        Contralateral shift of mediastinum can be normal on deep inspiration (should return to midline on expiration)
    Supine
        Hyperlucent hemithorax
        Deep sulcus sign
        Medial air mimicking pneumomediastinum
        Sharp hemidiaphragm, cardiac border, mediastinum
        Medial retraction of middle lobe
        Depressed diaphragm, expanded hemithorax
    Tension
        A clinical diagnosis
        Inverted hemidiaphragm
        Contralateral mediastinal shift that increases on expiration
- Diagnosis of loculated pneumothorax and fissural pneumothorax can be difficult
- Air in inferior pulmonary ligament a variant of pneumomediastinum, not pneumothorax
- Increasing sensitivity: erect frontal (inspiratory), erect frontal (expiratory), decubitus (expiratory), CT
- Bilateral pneumothorax from unilateral cause: incomplete anterior junction line (seen in less than 1% of humans, all buffalo), after heart transplantation or other mediastinal surgery

1

PROGRESSIVE MASSIVE FIBROSIS (PMF)

Clinical

- Fibrotic mass 1 to 10 cm in diameter found in silicosis and possibly coal worker's pneumoconiosis
- Result of coalescence of silicotic nodules, usually in upper lobes
- Associated with severe paraseptal scar emphysema around masses and compensating hyperinflation of lower lobes
- Migrate medially and grow in size over years
- Asymptomatic
- Dyspnea
- Mistaken for cancer

Imaging

- Radiographs:
    Sharply marginated masses often without other silicotic nodules
    Unilateral or bilateral
    Can cavitate, then bronchogenic carcinoma or MTB must be excluded
- CT:
    More easily demonstrates PMF; usual but not inevitable paraseptal emphysema around PMF; can show calcification, cavitation
- Appearance different from that of nodules in Caplan's syndrome

PROGRESSIVE SYSTEMIC SCLEROSIS (PSS)

Clinical

- Skin and musculoskeletal disease; Raynaud's phenomenon common
- Deep visceral involvement in approximately 50% of cases
- Lung involvement in approximately 70% of those
- Females affected more often than males; ages range from teens to old age
- Skin thickening, tightening, arthralgia
- Dyspnea, dysphagia
- Restrictive lung disease

Imaging

- Radiographs/CT:
    Lower lobe fibrosis (reticular, linear, honeycombing); pulmonary vasculitis; aspiration pneumonia, esophageal dilatation; bony abnormalities; increased incidence of adeno/alveolar cell carcinoma of lung
- Esophageal air-fluid levels do not occur

PSEUDOLYMPHOMA

Clinical

- Confusing tumorlike lung mass containing lymphocytes
- Most polyclonal and do not develop into malignant lesions
- Minority (15%) prelymphomas or localized lymphoma from the start
- Benign course, often asymptomatic
- Dyspnea

Imaging

- Radiographs/CT:
    Focal, multifocal regions of chronic lung consolidation; round, lobar, sublobar, segmental mass

End Note

- Rare cause of chronic consolidation; more common causes: alveolar proteinosis, alveolar cell carcinoma, lymphoma, sarcoid, lipoid pneumonia, UIP, and DIP

PULMONARY ARTERIAL HYPERTENSION

Clinical

- Persistent raised pulmonary artery pressure above normal upper limit of 30 torr systolic or 18 torr mean
- Many causes, including:
    In lumen: clot, ova, injected material
    In wall: essential, vasculitis, drugs, congenital
    In lung: emphysema, chronic bronchitis, interstitial fibrosis
    In chest wall: scoliosis, obesity, chest wall deformity
    In air: sleep apnea, high altitude
    Chronic increased blood flow (left-to-right shunts)
    Pulmonary venous hypertension
- Poor prognostic sign with restrictive lung disease
- Response of pulmonary arteries to hypertension is dilation of central elastic arteries and constriction of more peripheral muscular arteries
- With severe hypertension, flow becomes slow and in situ thrombosis occurs
- Dyspnea, syncope, asymptomatic, weakness, chest pain
- Hemoptysis
- Cyanosis in late stage
- *Primary pulmonary hypertension* refers to patients with hypertension of unknown cause; many show features suggesting an immune disease (Raynaud's phenomenon, abnormal complement)
- Plexogenic pulmonary arteriopathy is the histologic lesion

Imaging

- Radiographs:
    Dilated central arteries (distal interlobar artery more than 1.6 cm)
    Constricted peripheral arteries (pruned)
    Asymmetric peripheral pruning with thromboembolic disease
    Dilated peripheral vessels when cause of pulmonary hypertension is increased flow
- CT:
    Main pulmonary artery more than 28 mm defines pulmonary hypertension, if shunt not present
    Enlarged intraparenchymal vessels with increased flow
    Regional inhomogeneity with thromboembolic disease (hypovascular and hypervascular regions)

PULMONARY VENOUS HYPERTENSION (SEE ALSO EDEMA, PULMONARY)

Clinical

- Acute: left ventricular failure, atrial myxoma
- Chronic: left ventricular failure, mitral valve disease, atrial myxoma, veno-occlusive disease (involves small veins and presents as pulmonary arterial hypertension with chronic interstitial edema)
- Sequence: increased caliber of upper lobe veins; perivenous edema in lower lobes; interstitial fluid accumulation more widespread; alveolar flooding
- "Redistribution" of flow with inversion of normal ratio of 4 to 5:1 lower:upper lobe flow found only with chronic raised venous pressure
- Upper lobe venous distention by itself too nonspecific (fluid overload, renal failure, high output states) for diagnosis of pulmonary venous hypertension or left heart failure
- Dyspnea, orthopnea

Imaging

- Radiographs/CT:
    Upper lobe venous distention, lower lobe obscuration, interstitial lines and peribronchial cuffs, hilar haze, alveolar flooding, pleural effusions

RADIATION PNEUMONITIS (PNEUMONOPATHY)

Clinical

- Usually found only with doses over 6000 rads
- Time course:

3 to 6 weeks	Edema phase
6 weeks to 6 months	Pneumonic phase
More than 6 months up to 2 years	Fibrotic phase

- Effects limited to radiation field
- Deep pain; cough if trachea included in field
- Dyspnea, depending on volume of lung irradiated
- Hemoptysis

Imaging

- Sequential radiographs:
    Ground-glass/consolidation (6 to 8 weeks)
    Consolidation and volume loss
    Increasing opacity with straight/spiculated borders
    Air bronchograms prominent in fibrotic phase
    Most commonly paramediastinal/parahilar or apical from supraclavicular irradiations
    Marked volume loss a late finding
- CT:
    Same findings as radiographs
    More sensitive in detecting early edema phase
    Vascular pruning (attenuation) in distal subtended lung
    Pericardial fluid
    Increased density of mediastinal fat
    Crowded air bronchograms obvious at late stage
    Pleural thickening

End Notes

- Any increase in size or change in irradiated field after 9 to 12 months is suggestive of tumor recurrence
- In-field recurrence of lymphoma is uncommon; especially rare after 10 to 12 weeks

RELAPSING POLYCHONDRITIS (RP)

Clinical

- Uncommon disease of cartilage
- 50% of patients have upper airway involvement
- Deafness, saddle-back nose, polyarthritis
- Dyspnea, hoarseness
- Occurs in middle age, in both sexes

Imaging

- Radiographs/CT:
    Diffuse, smooth narrowing of trachea and larger bronchi; CT shows dense cartilages; laryngeal narrowing and scarring

1

RHEUMATOID LUNG DISEASE

Clinical

- Lung involvement in 10 to 50% of patients
- Males affected more often than females
- Arthritis almost always present (exception in Caplan's syndrome)
- Arthritis, subcutaneous nodules, dyspnea
- Antinuclear antibodies (ANA), positive Rh factor

Imaging

- Radiographs/CT:
    Pleural effusion: unilateral (90%) or bilateral; waxes and wanes over months, low glucose level that does not increase on glucose loading; exudative; may lead to fibrothorax or pleural thickening
    Interstitial fibrosis: progressive, lower lobes, linear-nodular, obscured vessels, honeycombing, progressive lung shrinkage, older smoking men, poor prognosis
    HRCT findings indistinguishable from those of idiopathic pulmonary fibrosis (IPF); early in disease may have ground-glass opacities of alveolitis
    Nodules of two types:
        Necrobiotic: well defined, in 50% of cases cavitate, 1 to 20 in number ("countable"), 1 to 10 cm in diameter
        Caplan's syndrome: nodules few in number, develop very slowly, can cavitate, can occur before arthritis (with coal or silica) or other minerals
    Infections
    Pulmonary hypertension from vasculitis independent of interstitial drug disease (ILD)
    Bronchiolitis with abnormal airways on HRCT
    Pericardial effusion: usually small and found on echocardiograms
    Rare: bronchocentric granulomatosis, gold toxicity, drug reactions

SARCOIDOSIS

Clinical

- Systemic, idiopathic, noncaseating granulomatous disease
- Classic type IV immune reaction (cellular immunity)
- Sequence: mononuclear alveolitis, granulomas, fibrosis
- Stages:
    I   Mediastinal/hilar adenopathy
    II Adenopathy plus lung nodules (consolidation, masses)
    III Lung nodules (or other features)
    IV End-stage fibrotic lung
- Progression from presentation (over 3 years): one third get better; one third stable; one third get worse
- Often asymptomatic or less symptomatic than expected from severity of radiographs
- Malaise, weight loss, night sweats
- Arthralgia
- Involved organ symptoms
- Erythema nodosa
- Fever
- Laboratory findings: elevated erythrocyte sedimentation rate (ESR), hypercalcemia, elevated angiotensin-converting enzyme, cutaneous anergy, eosinophilia; bronchoalveolar lavage shows activated T-cells
- Young to middle-aged women, African-Americans most commonly affected

Imaging

- Radiographs:
    Adenopathy (80%); "potato nodes"; distribution:
        Bilateral hilar and right paratracheal

Bilateral hilar and mediastinal
Different distributions
Anterior or posterior mediastinum uncommon
Isolated peripheral hilar: good prognosis
Nodes may calcify and have solid, stippled, or eggshell pattern
Lung disease (60%)
Nodules: 2 mm to 2 cm; fuzzy or well defined
Linear opacities
Scarring with volume loss, especially upper lobes
Bullae
Consolidation (10%)
Large masses (2%)
Acinar nodules 1 cm and around consolidation
Pleural effusion rare
Cavitation of nodules rare
Bronchostenosis from fibrosis rare: segmental/lobar atelectasis
Pulmonary arterial hypertension
Pneumothorax
- CT/HRCT:
Same finding as radiographs
Subpleural nodules and septal nodules common
Architectural distortion
Irregular vascular margins
Bronchocentric nodules
Traction bronchiectasis
Polygons: uncommon
Ground-glass opacities: uncommon

End Notes

- Adenopathy will not develop after lung disease becomes evident in untreated patients
- Consolidated lung ("alveolar sarcoid") a good prognostic sign
- Other organs that can be involved: bone, eye, heart, CNS, liver, muscle
- Diagnosis made most commonly by transbronchial biopsy
- Look for superimposed mycetoma in upper lobe cysts

SEPTIC EMBOLI

Clinical

- Cause can be any of several organisms, similar to those causing endocarditis, especially staphylococci and streptococci
- Sources are catheters, clots, prosthetic valves, and dirty needles
- Diagnosis by imaging and blood cultures
- Systemic infection, chest pain, hemoptysis: rare

Imaging

- Radiographs/CT:
Nodules: 1 to 4 cm in diameter, 1 to 10 in number; well-defined to ill-defined
Cavitation (50% on CT)
Ill-defined regions of patchy consolidation with air bronchograms on CT (looks like bronchopneumonia)
Uncommon—larger, peripheral wedge-shaped opacity
- Index of suspicion high in IV drug abusers, immunocompromised patients
- Clot too small to be seen on CT or angiography
- Nodules/cavities multiple but can be counted

SEQUESTRATION, PULMONARY

Clinical

- Intralobar or extralobar (the latter is rare and not included in this discussion)
- Defined by absence of bronchial connection to rest of lung

1

- Ventilated by collateral ventilation and incomplete fissures
- Prone to infection
- Systemic blood supply is persistent fetal lung blood supply: anomalous vessel from thoracic aorta or below diaphragm
- Symptomatic when infected
- Diagnosis usually suggested from radiographs
- Left side and lower thorax most common site

Imaging

- Radiographs:
    Basal opacity: solid mass, ill-defined opacity; abscess/chronic pneumonia/air-fluid levels; hyperlucent region around infected opacity; cysts
- CT:
    Same finding as on radiographs
    Hyperlucency more readily appreciated
    Contrast-enhanced spiral CT may demonstrate abnormal arterial supply
    Ultrasound can sometimes show aberrant artery
    Calcification within sequestered mass is uncommon

End Notes

- Arterial supply is systemic
- Venous return is to pulmonary veins (85%) or systemic veins (15%)
- Differential diagnosis: infected foregut cyst

SILICOSIS (SEE ALSO CAPLAN'S SYNDROME)

Clinical

- Pneumoconiosis caused by inhalation of silica (not silicone)
- Known occupational exposure over many years
- Latency 10 to 30 years
- Basic lesion: silicotic nodule of hyaline fibrous tissue containing silica particles
- Cough, dyspnea, clubbing
- Progressive respiratory impairment
- Increased incidence of MTB, lung cancer

Imaging

- Radiographs:
    Simple silicosis (nodular disease)
        Nodules 1 to 5 mm in diameter (p, q, r by ILO classification)
        Upper lobes predominate, exquisitely well defined
        Minor/no pleural disease (thickening)
        Profusion on a 12-point scale (ILO)
        Calcification of nodules and nodes (eggshell)
    Complicated silicosis (mass disease)
        Conglomeration ("coalescence") of nodules into masses more than 1 cm in diameter, 1 to 15 cm (See also **Progressive Massive Fibrosis**)
        Can cavitate
        Adenopathy not uncommon on CT
    Acute silicosis (silico-proteinosis)
        All of the features of pulmonary alveolar proteinosis
        Can be fatal
- CT/HRCT:
    Increased detection of nodules and calcification in nodules
    Easier detection of conglomerate masses
    Easier detection of cavitation
    Better demonstration of nodes
- Caution should be exercised with the following findings: masses not surrounded

by nodules, any rapid change in size of a mass, and any cavity; TB or lung cancer must be considered in differential diagnosis

SJÖGREN'S SYNDROME

Clinical

- Characteristic findings: dry eyes, mouth, and airways
- Histologic study shows lymphocyte and plasma cell infiltration
- Often has features of other immune-complex diseases, especially rheumatoid arthritis, SLE, PSS
- Affects middle-aged women
- Recurrent infection, ILD, chest pain
- Dysgammaglobulinemia, lymphoma

Imaging

- Radiographs/CT:
    Pleural effusions/thickening: chronic; interstitial fibrosis: reticular nodular opacities; atelectasis and pneumonia; pulmonary artery enlargement from pulmonary hypertension

SOLITARY PULMONARY NODULE (SEE SECTION I, PULMONARY NEOPLASMS)

SWYER-JAMES (MACLEOD) SYNDROME

Clinical

- Also called *unilateral emphysema* and *unilateral hyperlucent lung*
- Hyperinflation of lung parenchyma distal to bronchiolitis obliterans
- Unilateral
- Usually from an adenovirus (others are measles, mycoplasma, pertussis) pneumonia in childhood
- CT scans often show bilateral disease
- Large airways often show bronchiectasis
- "Emphysema" is of type found with obliterative bronchiolitis
- Asymptomatic and incidental
- Symptoms of bronchiectasis (cough and sputum)
- Recurrent infection
- Dyspnea on effort

Imaging

- Radiographs:
    Unilateral hyperlucency and pruned vessels (reduced number and size)
    Ipsilateral small hilum
    Airtrapping on expiratory radiographs with contralateral mediastinal shift
    Ipsilateral lung volume normal or slightly reduced at total lung capacity
- V:Q scan:
    Decreased perfusion and ventilation
- Angiography:
    Small vessels
- CT:
    Hyperlucency, airtrapping: unilateral or bilateral, lobar or patchy
    Pruned vessels
    Bronchial dilatation (as seen with bronchiolitis obliterans) or bronchiectasis
    Regions of scarring
- For cost-effective diagnosis, inspiration:expiration PA radiographs should be used

End Note

- Differential diagnosis includes hypogenetic lung, proximal interruption of PA, absence of chest wall, grid cut-off, patient obliquity

SYSTEMIC LUPUS ERYTHEMATOSUS (SLE)

Clinical

- Most common systemic collagen vascular disease
- Widespread inflammation of vessels, serosal surfaces, connective tissue
- Thoracic involvement in 50% of patients, usually in association with other deep viscera
- Most common skin, muscle, and joint disease
- Affects mostly women
- Skin, joint, muscle findings
- Chest pain, dyspnea
- Positive lupus erythematosus preparation, ANA, rheumatoid arthritis factor, anemia, dysgammaglobulinemia

Imaging

- Radiographs/CT:
    Pleural effusion/residual pleural thickening
    Lupus pneumonitis: focal/diffuse
    Diffuse hemorrhage
    Diffuse parenchymal fibrosis with or without honeycombing
    High diaphragm from muscle dysfunction
    Complications of immunosuppression (e.g., infection)
    Increased incidence of pulmonary embolism (PE)
    Pericardial effusion/cardiomyopathy
    Big pulmonary arteries from pulmonary hypertension (pulmonary vasculitis)

TALCOSIS

Clinical

- Pneumoconiosis caused by inhalation of talc (a magnesium silicate)
- Often contaminated with asbestos or silica, or both
- Pure talc causes a reticulonodular (lines and nodules) pattern in the middle and lower lungs
- Mild symptoms
- Dyspnea on effort

Imaging

- Radiographs:
    Basal and lung reticulonodular opacities; other findings can be ascribed to asbestos or silica contamination in talc

THYMOMA (SEE GERM CELL TUMORS)

THYMOLIPOMA

Clinical

- Unusual benign thymic tumor in which thymic elements not evident on imaging
- Composed predominantly of encapsulated adipose tissue but contains fibrous bands, blood vessels, and involuted thymus
- Soft and large; molds to anterior mediastinum
- Incidental
- Heavy sensation in chest

Imaging

- Radiographs, CT, MRI:
    Large anterior mediastinal mass composed of fat with vessels and fibrous bands; can extend down over diaphragm
- Suspected from chest radiograph and confirmed by CT
- Should not be mistaken for epicardial fat pad

TRACHEOBRONCHOMEGALY (MOUNIER-KUHN SYNDROME)

Clinical

- Rare primary lesion of trachea with marked increase in size and excess collapsibility of trachea
- Invariably associated with bronchiectasis
- Lesion is atrophy of cartilage and muscular elements of entire tracheal wall
- Presentation similar to that of long-standing bronchitis or bronchiectasis (cough and sputum)
- Ineffective cough

Imaging

- Radiographs/CT:
    Trachea more than 26 to 30 mm in diameter
    Main bronchi more than 20 mm in diameter
    Central bronchiectasis with more normal peripheral airways
    Corrugated tracheal appearance
    May show tracheal or bronchial diverticula
- Proximal bronchiectasis should not be mistaken for ABPA
- Saber sheath trachea is large only in AP dimension

TRAUMA (BLUNT)

Clinical

Bony Thorax
- Rib fractures most common
- Fracture of ribs 1 to 3 indicates severe trauma and increased likelihood of great vessel or airway damage
- Fracture of ribs 10 to 12 indicates possible upper abdominal visceral injury
- Absence of rib fractures does not preclude severe internal injury
- Sternal fractures indicate severe trauma
- Spinal fractures can produce large paraspinal hematomas

Pleura
- Pneumothorax most commonly associated with rib fractures, although they may not be evident
- 50% of pneumothoraces have small effusion of no significance
- Large effusion indicates hemothorax that in most circumstances should be drained

Lung Parenchyma
- Three levels of injury can occur:
    Contusion
        Blood in lung without major disruption of lung tissue
        Focal/multifocal, patchy/dense consolidation
        Distribution along lines of shock wave
        Relatively rapid resolution
    Hematoma
        Region of disrupted lung tissue containing blood
        Whenever lung is torn, it tends to form spherical air-spaces ("cyst," "pneumatocele") that may contain blood and are 1 to 15 or more cm in diameter
        Slow resolution
        Can develop air-fluid levels
    Laceration
        Disruption of lung tissue that has not formed cystlike sphere
        Most commonly found paraspinally with crush injuries
        Irregular jagged lesion surrounded by blood
        Slow resolution

- Presentation variable, hemoptysis
- Other injuries usually dominate clinical picture

Trachea/Bronchi See Fractured Bronchus

Mediastinum
- Most common life-threatening injury is to aorta
- Deceleration with avulsion or pinching around insertion of ligamentum arteriosus or aortic root
- Most with such injuries dead on arrival; mortality increases with each passing hour for the first 24 hours, then decreases over weeks
- Contained aortic tear
- Venous bleeding with mediastinal blood more common than aortic tear
- Associated fractures of ribs 1 to 3 in 10 to 20% of patients
- Should always be repaired

Esophagus (See also Boerhaave's Syndrome)
- Blunt trauma rarely causes esophageal rupture
- Penetrating injury/instrumentation more common causes of injury
- Concern is mediastinitis, empyema
- Dysphagia, pain, infection

Thoracic Duct
- Almost always injured during surgery or by penetrating injury
- Presents as chylothorax
- Diagnosis is easy from fluid
- Effusion that can be large

Diaphragm
- Injury is rupture at junction of central tendon and muscle bundles
- Left and right sides affected equally, but left more easily diagnosed, so 70% of diagnosed cases on left
- Only 50% diagnosed or considered
- Diagnosed by herniation of abdominal contents into chest
- Other injuries dominate
- Respiratory compromise
- Abnormal radiograph with delayed diagnosis

Imaging

Bony Thorax
- Radiographs:
    Most self-evident; detailed rib views rarely beneficial or cost effective
- Shoulder girdle should also be considered
- Bony thoracic injury should be used as an indication of possible organ injury

Lung Parenchyma
- Radiographs/CT:
    Patchy/dense consolidation, fluid or air- and fluid-filled cysts; jagged lucencies in consolidated lung; concomitant chest wall, pleural, or mediastinal injury

Mediastinum
- Radiographs:
    Obscured aortic knob
    Separation of trachea and aortic arch
    Left apical cap
    Right displacement of esophageal tube
    Widened left on right paraspinous line
    Left pleural effusion
    Left lower lobe consolidation and atelectasis
- Angiography:
    Obtained when spiral CT shows hematoma and has not diagnosed aortic tear
    Tear; pseudoaneurysm; dissection; mediastinal hematoma

- CT:
  - Obtain spiral CT in most cases if patient is stable
  - If "widened mediastinum" is fat and not hematoma diagnosis is excluded
  - Blood with increased CT density indicates hematoma not site of bleeding
  - Many of same features as radiographs
  - New studies with spiral CT showing flap and pseudoaneurysm can be diagnostic in over 50% of cases
- Transesophageal echocardiography:
  - Should be used if patient is unstable and if readily available; accuracy not established

Esophagus
- Radiographs:
  - Air in mediastinum
  - Mass
  - Widened mediastinum
  - Left or right pleural effusion
  - Pneumothorax
  - Gastrografin swallow can show tear but not its size
  - CT with oral contrast (use non-ionic, sterile contrast) can also show tear and mass

Thoracic Duct
- Radiographs/CT:
  Pleural effusion more common on right side than left; CT density usually not low; can present as apical extrapleural mass (injury during first rib resection for thoracic outlet syndrome)

Diaphragm
- Radiographs:
  - Bowel in left hemithorax
  - Herniated liver in right hemithorax
  - Constriction at level of diaphragm
  - Passage of air from peritoneum into pleural space
- Barium:
  - Constriction of bowel as it enters thorax through tear
  - Gastroesophageal junction in normal position
  - Nasogastric tube extending into thorax
  - Fractured lower ribs
- Spiral CT with reformatted images/MRI:
  Can show abnormalities in sagittal coronal planes

End Note

- Know trauma; it is important and often confusing

WEGENER'S GRANULOMATOSIS

Clinical

- Immune complex disease with both necrotizing granulomas and vasculitis involving arteries and veins
- Bronchi can also be involved
- Difficult to diagnose unless high index of suspicion
- Subacute to chronic course
- Upper airway inflammation
- Renal impairment
- Cough, hemoptysis
- Positive antineutrophil cytoplasmic antibodies (ANCA) (90%)
- Relapsing course

Imaging

- Radiographs/CT:
    Extremely varied
    Discrete or ill-defined nodules (1 to 5 cm)
    Cavitation (2/3) with thick walls
    Focal consolidation
    Recurrence in same site as previously affected (eosinophilic pneumonia similar)
    Air-fluid levels in cavity
    Peripheral infarct-like, wedge-shaped opacities
    Diffuse consolidation from hemorrhage
    Tracheal/bronchial narrowing
    Sinus destruction

End Note

- Diagnosis usually by ANCA and upper airway (nasal or sinus) biopsy

2

Neuroimaging

■ Calvin J. Cruz, M.D., Ph.D.

OVERVIEW

BRAIN IMAGING

Magnetic resonance imaging (MRI) and computed tomography (CT) are the mainstays of modern brain imaging. Because of its multiplanar capabilities, high anatomic resolution, and high sensitivity for the detection of parenchymal pathology, MRI is equivalent or superior to CT for the evaluation of most intracranial pathology. CT is still the examination of choice for evaluation of acute head injury, acute subarachnoid hemorrhage, and suspected bone disease. CT is also helpful in characterizing intracranial calcifications or calcified masses.

Angiography has been performed less frequently since the advent of MRI and magnetic resonance angiography (MRA), but it remains the examination of choice for preoperative evaluation of aneurysms, arteriovenous malformations, and dural arteriovenous fistulas. In certain instances, angiography may be used to evaluate the arterial supply of vascular tumors when preoperative embolization is being considered.

A standard screening brain MRI protocol might consist of T1 sagittal, T2 axial, and T1 axial sequences. The T1 sagittal sequence allows optimal visualization of midline structures, including the sella, pineal region, and foramen magnum. T2 sequences are exquisitely sensitive to parenchymal pathology; in fact, if T2 images are normal in a routine screening examination, it is reasonable to proceed no further. If the screening examination shows abnormalities or if there is a specific clinical question, other sequences are added to the three previously mentioned. For further characterization of signal abnormalities or mass lesions, for example, gadolinium-enhanced T1 images can be obtained, usually in two planes. Other sequences that are helpful in specific situations include the following:

Sagittal T2: This sequence permits optimal evaluation of white matter in the corpus callosum in multiple sclerosis.
Coronal T2: This sequence permits optimal evaluation of the hippocampi and temporal lobes in patients with seizure disorders.

111

Gradient echo: Because of the susceptibility of gradient echo images to local field inhomogeneities, this sequence is more sensitive than spin echo sequences for the detection of calcification and hemosiderin. Gradient echo images are thus useful in evaluation of blood products, calcification, and cryptic vascular malformations.

T1 post-gadolinium with fat saturation: Fat is normally bright on T1 images. When a pulse that "saturates" fat is used, this sequence yields images in which fat is dark rather than bright. Thus, the conspicuousness of gadolinium-enhancing lesions (i.e., lesions bright on T1 post-gadolinium images) that are in or near fat is dramatically increased. This sequence is particularly useful in identifying the exact extent of enhancing tumors that involve the skull base, where the distinction between fatty marrow and enhancing tumor is often unclear. Usually, enhancing tumors or inflammatory diseases that involve the orbit also are visualized better when fat saturation is used to suppress signal from the abundant orbital fat.

Time-of-flight MRA: This is the workhorse MRA technique in the neck and brain; it can provide useful information if clinical history or other imaging evaluation suggests atherosclerotic carotid disease, aneurysm, arteriovenous malformation, dural venous sinus thrombosis, or dural arteriovenous fistula. The other MRA technique currently in use, *phase-contrast MRA,* is more sensitive than time-of-flight MRA for detecting very slow flow. Thus, phase-contrast is occasionally helpful in differentiating very slow flow from thrombosis (for example, in a dural venous sinus).

Approach. There are many ways to approach interpretation of cross-sectional neuroimaging studies; however, almost all share the following four important principles.

1. *Every study must be systematically reviewed, and every image in the study must be examined.* Although this sounds self-evident, failure to carefully scrutinize all images in a study, particularly in an MRI examination that may contain 50 images (and sometimes many more!), is a prescription for disaster. Clearly, the "gestalt" approach is inadequate and inappropriate for neuroradiology.

In every cross-sectional study of the brain, the following structures should be evaluated:

Ventricles, sulci, and cisterns
Cortex and subcortical white matter
Basal ganglia (caudate, putamen, globus pallidus) and thalami
Brain stem (midbrain, pons, medulla)
Cerebellum
Sella and cavernous sinuses
Vascular structures (major intracranial arteries and dural venous sinuses)
Orbits
Paranasal sinuses, mastoid air cells, and nasopharynx

2. *The mass effect associated with an abnormality must be assessed.* The following questions must be answered: Is there no mass effect or only local mass effect (e.g., sulcal effacement without brain herniation)? Is actual brain herniation (subfalcine, uncal, downward, or upward) present? Is there associated hemorrhage that could lead to the rapid development of significant mass effect even if none is present on the initial imaging study?

3. *The location of an intracranial abnormality must be characterized.* This helps limit the differential diagnosis. The two most important questions to be addressed are: Is the abnormality intraaxial (arising from the brain parenchyma) or extraaxial (arising outside the brain parenchyma)? Can the list of diagnostic possibilities be further reduced by placing the abnormality in a compartment for which a limited differential diagnosis exists? Examples of such compartments (which are discussed in detail in the differential diagnosis section of this chapter) include the cerebellopontine angle, sella and suprasellar region, and intraventricular spaces. These compartments have their own limited differential diagnoses, consisting in some instances of both intraaxial *and* extraaxial lesions.

4. The attenuation (CT), signal characteristics (MRI), and enhancement properties of an abnormality must be characterized. These features can, in many instances, help further narrow the differential diagnosis.

SPINE IMAGING

MRI is the study of choice for evaluating pathology of the spinal canal and vertebral column. CT is still important for evaluation of fractures and other bone pathology, but otherwise plays a limited role in spine imaging. In the evaluation of canal stenosis or radiculopathy caused by degenerative disc disease (the most common conditions leading to a request for spine imaging), CT myelography occasionally is used as the primary study when MRI cannot be performed. Likewise, in a patient with suspected canal compromise and cord compression caused by neoplastic disease, CT myelography is an acceptable second-choice imaging study. CT myelography may also be a helpful ancillary examination in confusing cases, particularly in patients whose MRI study is not optimal.

Plain film myelography is reserved for the evaluation of a suspected dural arteriovenous fistula and for patients with instrumentation hardware that produces CT and MRI artifacts. Spinal angiography is necessary for characterization of a dural arteriovenous fistula prior to neurosurgical or neurointerventional therapy.

MRI protocols for screening studies of the spine vary slightly for the cervical, thoracic, and lumbar regions. Although sagittal T1 and T2 sequences are performed for all spine studies, the type of axial sequence depends on the level being examined.

In the cervical spine, where the neural foramina are relatively small, a three-dimensional ("volume") gradient echo (GE) study is usually performed (on GE magnets, the sequence most commonly used is known as 3D-GRASS) in patients with degenerative disc disease. The 3D-GRASS sequence allows the cervical spine to be partitioned into very thin (1 to 2 mm) axial slices, making it less likely that foraminal pathology or a small disc protrusion will be missed as a result of volume averaging.

In the thoracic spine, axial images rarely are performed routinely but instead are used to evaluate specific pathology identified on the screening sagittal sequences.

In the lumbar spine, a T2 axial sequence, which allows optimal evaluation of disc protrusions, is usually performed in patients with degenerative disc disease. A post-gadolinium T1 axial sequence is usually added to the protocol in patients who have undergone back surgery; this sequence helps distinguish recurrent disc protrusion (which should not enhance) from scar (which enhances).

T1 axial sequences, with and without gadolinium, also are used to evaluate inflammatory and neoplastic conditions involving either the bony vertebral column or contents of the spinal canal. Bony metastatic disease, which is typically low in signal on T1 images, often enhances after gadolinium and thus can be indistinguishable from normal fatty marrow on post-gadolinium images. T1 images *without* gadolinium should always be included in the MRI protocol so that metastatic disease is not missed. T1 images post-gadolinium with fat saturation also may be helpful not only in the evaluation of bone pathology, but also in the characterization of lumbar epidural disease (epidural fat is most abundant in the lumbar region).

Approach. In every cross-sectional study of the spine, the following features should be evaluated:

> Vertebral body alignment
> Vertebral body and disc space height
> Bone marrow and disc space signal
> Cord morphology and signal
> Neural foramina
> Epidural space
> Paraspinous soft tissues (esophagus, airway, thyroid gland, cervical and retro-
> peritoneal nodes, posteromedial lungs, kidneys, aorta, and inferior vena
> cava)

In cervical spine studies, the posterior fossa structures and region of the foramen magnum should also be inspected; it is embarrassing to render an impression of

2

"normal C-spine" in a patient who turns out to have a Chiari I malformation or, worse yet, a posterior fossa neoplasm clearly visible on the cervical spine MRI study.

An abnormality involving the spinal column should be placed into the *intramedullary* (i.e., within the substance of the cord), *intradural extramedullary*, or *extradural* compartment. Determining the compartment in which a lesion arises can be difficult, and multiplanar MRI usually is required. However, because each of the three compartments has its own differential diagnosis, this determination is critical.

As is the case with MRI of the brain, the mass effect, signal characteristics, and contrast enhancement of an abnormality should be characterized. In addition, the levels of the spinal cord affected should be described, both to correlate the imaging findings with the presenting neurologic deficits and to let the clinicians know which cord or root levels should receive particular attention on physical examination.

HEAD AND NECK IMAGING

CT and MRI are both used in head and neck imaging; the choice of imaging modality depends on the region of interest and the specific clinical question. Because of the anatomic complexity of this area, multiplanar imaging (usually axial and coronal) almost always is warranted and, in many cases, mandatory.

Approach. Because the head and neck is an anatomically complex region, it intimidates many general radiologists (and more than a few neuroradiologists!). The key to developing competence in head and neck radiology is to become intimately familiar with normal anatomy, the compartmental approach championed by Harnsberger, the differential diagnoses for disease processes affecting each of those compartments, and the imaging features of these disease processes.

Harnsberger divides the head and neck (from a cranial to caudal direction) into the following three regions: (1) skull base to hard palate, (2) hard palate to hyoid bone (suprahyoid neck), and (3) hyoid bone to clavicles (infrahyoid neck).

The head and neck from *skull base to hard palate* comprises the temporal bone, paranasal sinuses and mastoid air cells, orbits, and soft tissues of the face. The *suprahyoid neck* (hard palate to hyoid bone) is subdivided into nine spaces: parapharyngeal, mucosal, retropharyngeal, prevertebral, carotid, parotid, masticator, submandibular, and sublingual. The *infrahyoid neck* (hyoid bone to clavicles) is divided into five spaces, four of which are continuations of spaces in the suprahyoid neck (retropharyngeal, prevertebral, carotid, and posterior cervical) and one of which (the visceral space) is unique to the infrahyoid neck.

Once a clinically detected mass is confirmed by imaging, the radiologist must attempt to determine the space of origin, and then, based on imaging characteristics, give a reasonable differential diagnosis. This approach is discussed in detail by Harnsberger in his excellent *Handbook of Head and Neck Imaging*.

Expertise in head and neck radiology is neither expected on the American Board of Radiology (ABR) board examination nor encountered frequently in clinical practice. Ability to recognize pathologic findings (and to give a short differential diagnosis) and to identify pseudotumors that mimic real pathology are the most important skills to retain, for both the boards and real life. In that spirit, only the most common entities encountered in the various spaces of the head and neck are mentioned in the differential diagnoses listed in the following section.

NEUROIMAGING DIFFERENTIAL DIAGNOSES

Differential diagnoses
Brain
    Mass lesions
    White matter disease
    Stroke, hemorrhage, and vascular disease
    Meningeal disease
    Hydrocephalus
    Miscellaneous conditions

Spine
    Intramedullary lesions
    Intradural, extramedullary masses
    Extradural masses
Head and neck
    Skull base
    Orbits, temporal bones, and paranasal sinuses
    Suprahyoid neck
    Infrahyoid neck

BRAIN

MASS LESIONS

RING-ENHANCING, INTRAAXIAL LESION(S)

What are the most common causes of multiple intraaxial ring-enhancing lesions?

Metastasis
Abscess
Glioma

FIGURES   Osborn: 534, 537, 542

Infarct
Contusion or hematoma
Demyelinating disease
Radiation necrosis

FIGURE   Osborn: 767

Metastasis

- Multiple
- Gray-white junction
- Surrounding vasogenic edema
- Seen in older patients
- History of primary neoplasm
- Metastatic disease, abscess, and glioma the most common causes of multiple intraaxial ring-enhancing lesions

FIGURES   Osborn: 421, 662

Abscess

- Multiple if hematogenously spread; single if direct extension of infection from paranasal sinuses or mastoids
- Smooth ring enhancement that is thicker on the cortical side of the abscess
- Surrounding vasogenic edema
- Ill patient or patient at risk for infection (acquired immune deficiency syndrome [AIDS], immunocompromised, intravenous [IV] drug user)
- Elevated white blood cell count, fever

FIGURES   Osborn: 690–693

Infarct

- Acute onset of neurological deficit ("stroke-like presentation")
- Confined to a vascular territory
- Characteristic evolution of enhancement pattern, signal characteristics, and mass effect on follow-up studies

Contusion/Hematoma

- Characteristic location of posttraumatic hematoma (e.g., frontal lobes, anterior temporal lobes)

FIGURES   Osborn: 162, 195

Demyelinating Disease (Multiple Sclerosis)

- Little or no surrounding vasogenic edema
- Incomplete ring enhancement (i.e., enhancement along one side of lesion)
- Other lesions on T2 images that are characteristic for demyelinating disease (e.g., corpus callosum, periatrial white matter, middle cerebellar peduncle)
- Young or middle-aged patient with history of illness marked by exacerbations and remissions
- Demyelinative cerebrospinal fluid (CSF) profile (myelin basic protein, oligoclonal bands, IgG)

FIGURE   Osborn: 760

LESIONS CROSSING THE CORPUS CALLOSUM

Which common extraaxial lesion can mimic an intraaxial callosal lesion?

Glioblastoma multiforme
Lymphoma
Progressive multifocal leukoencephalopathy
Multiple sclerosis
Parafalcine meningioma

Glioblastoma Multiforme

- Nodular, irregular, heterogeneous enhancement

FIGURES   Osborn: 543, 545

Lymphoma

- Enhancement in nonimmunocompromised patient characteristically homogeneous, an appearance that strongly favors lymphoma over glioblastoma
- Enhancement in immunocompromised patient usually irregular and heterogeneous because of necrosis, an appearance that is indistinguishable from that of glioblastoma
- Most common lesion that crosses the corpus callosum in AIDS patients

FIGURE   Osborn: 622

Progressive Multifocal Leukoencephalopathy

- No mass effect
- No enhancement, except occasionally at leading margin

Multiple Sclerosis

- Characteristic appearance of callosal plaques: multiple ovoid or linear foci of T2 prolongation, oriented orthogonal to the lateral ventricles
- Other characteristic findings of multiple sclerosis (*see Demyelinating disease*)

FIGURES   Osborn: 757–760

Parafalcine Meningiomas

- Can cross the midline and thereby mimic an intraaxial lesion involving the corpus callosum, particularly when viewed in the axial plane
- Meningioma distinguished from true callosal lesions by intense, homogeneous enhancement typical of meningioma and extraaxial location above the corpus callosum (usually seen best in coronal plane)

POSTERIOR FOSSA MASS, IN CHILD

Medulloblastoma
Cerebellar astrocytoma
Ependymoma
Pontine glioma

FIGURES   Osborn: 557; Barkovich: 342–344

Medulloblastoma

What imaging features favor a diagnosis of medulloblastoma in a child with a posterior fossa mass?

- Most common posterior fossa neoplasm in children
- Midline tumor, filling fourth ventricle and producing obstructive hydrocephalus
- Homogeneity of the tumor, intermediate or high attenuation on noncontrast CT, and low to intermediate T2 signal favor medulloblastoma over ependymoma

FIGURES   Osborn: 436, 616, 617; Barkovich: 325–329

Cerebellar Astrocytoma

What is the classic imaging appearance of a juvenile pilocytic astrocytoma?

- Second most common posterior fossa neoplasm in children
- Classic appearance: enhancing nodule or mass associated with a cyst; cyst walls may or may not enhance
- Cerebellar pilocytic astrocytoma associated with cyst having no mural enhancement could closely resemble hemangioblastoma; however, these lesions are rarely confused: childhood pilocytic astrocytomas peak in the first decade, hemangioblastomas usually present in the third or fourth decade

FIGURES   Osborn: 554–557; Barkovich: 334–337

Ependymoma

What imaging feature strongly favors a diagnosis of ependymoma in a child with a posterior fossa mass?

- Caudal tongue-like extension of tumor through fourth ventricular outlet foramina of Luschka and Magendie

FIGURES   Osborn: 457, 570; Barkovich: 339–341

POSTERIOR FOSSA MASS, IN ADULT

Metastasis
Cerebellar astrocytoma
Hemangioblastoma
Medulloblastoma
Hemorrhage

2

What is the most common posterior fossa mass lesion in an adult?

Metastasis

- Most common posterior fossa neoplasm in adults

FIGURE   Osborn: 445

Cerebellar Astrocytoma

- Cystic and solid components
- Wall of cystic portion may or may not enhance

Hemangioblastoma

With which phakomatosis are multiple hemangioblastomas usually associated?

- Associated with von Hippel-Lindau syndrome, in which multiple hemangioblastomas often occur
- Classic appearance: cystic mass with intensely enhancing mural nodule and surrounding flow voids
- Can appear similar to cystic astrocytoma
- Cyst wall does not enhance with hemangioblastoma; enhancement of cyst wall strongly favors astrocytoma

FIGURES   Osborn: 607–609; Barkovich: 311, 313, 314

Medulloblastoma

How does the typical location of cerebellar medulloblastoma differ between adult and pediatric patients?

- In adults usually occurs in *cerebellar hemisphere* rather than in the midline, as is most commonly seen in pediatric medulloblastomas

FIGURE   Osborn: 617

Hemorrhage

- Characteristic imaging features of acute hematoma
- History of hypertension

EXTRAAXIAL MASS

Meningioma
Arachnoid cyst
Epidermoid cyst
Dural metastasis

FIGURES   Osborn: 658, 659

Bone lesion with intracranial extension

FIGURES   Osborn: 657, 658

Empyema, subdural or epidural

FIGURES   Osborn: 684, 685; Barkovich: 609–611

Sarcoidosis

FIGURE   Osborn: 522

Identification of Extraaxial Mass

- Arises outside the brain parenchyma, from the meninges or calvarium; thus brain parenchyma displaced away from rather than expanded by the lesion
- Other clues to extraaxial origin of a mass: broad contact with bone or a meningeal surface, CSF cleft between mass and brain,

and reactive changes in adjacent calvarium (e.g., bony hyperostosis adjacent to a meningioma)
- Multiplanar MRI often necessary to confirm extraaxial origin in difficult cases
- Clinical history, imaging appearance, and location of extraaxial mass often serve to sharply narrow the differential diagnosis
- Certain extraaxial locations (e.g., cerebellopontine angle, suprasellar region, and intraventricular spaces) have their own limited differential diagnosis; recognizing that a lesion is in one of these compartments is therefore helpful

Meningioma

- Most common extraaxial neoplasm
- Intense, homogeneous enhancement
- Variable calcification
- Variable reactive hyperostosis or blistering of adjacent bony surfaces

FIGURES   Osborn: 591–604

Arachnoid Cyst

- Similar to CSF in CT attenuation and MR signal characteristics
- No enhancement
- Displacement of vessels and nerves

FIGURES   Osborn: 64, 456, 641, 642; Barkovich: 450, 452, 453

Epidermoid Cyst

- Similar to CSF in CT attenuation and MR signal characteristics
- No enhancement
- Encasement of vessels and nerves

FIGURES   Osborn: 634; Barkovich: 349–351

CEREBELLOPONTINE ANGLE MASS

Which cerebellopontine angle lesions present as a mass that is similar to CSF in attenuation and signal characteristics?

Acoustic schwannoma
Meningioma
Arachnoid cyst
Epidermoid cyst
Other neoplasm

Acoustic schwannoma

What are the most common lesions to present as a mass in the cerebellopontine angle?
Which imaging features favor a diagnosis of acoustic schwannoma?

- Acoustic schwannoma and meningioma are the most common masses that occur in this location
- Can appear identical to meningioma; however, following findings favor acoustic schwannoma:
    ¶ Heterogeneity with cyst formation or hemorrhage (or both)
    ¶ Extension into the internal auditory canal
    ¶ Widening of the internal auditory canal and erosion of the posterior lip of the acoustic meatus on thin-section axial CT images

FIGURES   Osborn: 441, 629

Meningioma

- Findings that favor meningioma over acoustic schwannoma:
    - ¶ Broad base against the petrous bone
    - ¶ High attenuation on noncontrast CT
    - ¶ Low to intermediate signal on T2

FIGURES   Osborn: 442

Arachnoid cyst

- Similar to CSF in CT attenuation and MR signal characteristics

FIGURES   Osborn: 456, 642

Epidermoid cyst

- Similar to CSF in MR signal characteristics
- Lobular margins and slight hyperintensity to CSF on proton-density images favor epidermoid over arachnoid cyst
- Diffusion-weighted imaging is new MRI technique; may help differentiate epidermoid from arachnoid cyst, by virtue of the lower diffusion coefficient of free water in epidermoid cyst

FIGURES   Osborn: 442, 634, 636

Other neoplasms

- Extension of a fourth ventricular neoplasm (e.g., ependymoma)
- Exophytic growth of an intraaxial neoplasm of the cerebellar hemisphere
- Schwannoma of cranial nerve V
- Glomus jugulare

SELLAR OR SUPRASELLAR MASS

Mnemonic "GATCHMOD"
Germ cell tumor

FIGURES   Osborn: 476, 477, 483; Barkovich: 398, 400, 402

Granuloma (e.g., sarcoid, eosinophilic granuloma)

FIGURES   Osborn: 483; Barkovich: 394

Adenoma

FIGURES   Osborn: 466, 472, 473, 652, 653

Aneurysm

FIGURES   Osborn: 479

Arachnoid cyst

FIGURES   Osborn: 480; Barkovich: 450

Tuber cinereum hamartoma

FIGURES   Osborn: 480; Barkovich: 393, 394

Craniopharyngioma
Cyst of Rathke's cleft

FIGURES   Osborn: 468, 480; Barkovich: 396

Hypothalamic glioma
Meningioma

2

Metastasis

FIGURES   Osborn: 469, 479

Optic (chiasmatic) glioma

FIGURES   Osborn: 559; Barkovich: 384, 385

Dermoid

FIGURES   Osborn: 636, 637

Epidermoid

FIGURES   Osborn: 477, 634, 636

General

- This laundry list of suprasellar pathology is a helpful aid to remembering the entities that can occur in this region; however, almost never will it be appropriate to mention all or even most of them in a given case
- Usually, imaging features or clinical information limits the differential diagnosis
- Five entities account for more than 90% of all sellar and suprasellar pathology: pituitary adenoma, craniopharyngioma, meningioma, glioma (chiasmatic/hypothalamic), and aneurysm
- In children, only three entities account for more than 95% of all suprasellar pathology: craniopharyngioma, chiasmatic/hypothalamic glioma, and germinoma

SUPRASELLAR MASS, IN CHILD

What are the three most common suprasellar masses in the pediatric population?

Craniopharyngioma
Chiasmatic/hypothalamic glioma
Germinoma

Craniopharyngioma

- Most common childhood suprasellar mass
- Cystic or mixed cystic and solid
- Calcifications common

FIGURES   Osborn: 475, 655, 656; Barkovich: 387–393

Chiasmatic/hypothalamic glioma

- Heterogeneous, infiltrative mass
- Homogeneous enlargement of the chiasm more typical of low grade astrocytomas seen in patients with neurofibromatosis (NF) type I

FIGURES   Osborn: 80, 476, 559; Barkovich: 384, 385

Germinoma

Why is MRI screening of the entire neural axis important in patients with germinoma?

- Most common germ cell tumor of the suprasellar region
- Homogeneous enhancement
- No cystic components
- No calcification
- Commonly spreads through the CSF; evidence of leptomeningeal enhancement should be sought in the brain and spine

FIGURES   Osborn: 476, 477, 483; Barkovich: 398, 400

2

SUPRASELLAR MASS, HOMOGENEOUSLY ENHANCING

Homogeneous enhancement of a suprasellar mass usually limits the differential diagnosis to which entities?

Macroadenoma
Meningioma
Aneurysm
Germinoma

Macroadenoma

How does the size of the sella help differentiate pituitary macroadenoma from suprasellar meningioma?

- Sella expanded (because tumor originates there)
- "Hourglass" shape in coronal plane as result of narrowing of the tumor waist at the diaphragma sellae

FIGURES   Osborn: 466, 472, 473; 653

Meningioma

- Sella usually normal (intrasellar meningioma rare)
- Enhancing dural tail extending along the planum sphenoidale or clivus
- Narrowing or occlusion of vessels (e.g., cavernous internal carotid artery)

FIGURES   Osborn: 469, 597

Aneurysm

How can an MRI artifact help establish the diagnosis of aneurysm?

- Flow void on spin-echo MRI
- Pulsation artifact transmitted along the phase-encoding axis
- Confirmation by MRA and catheter angiography

FIGURES   Osborn: 263, 264, 267, 470, 479

SUPRASELLAR MASS, PARTIALLY CALCIFIED

CT evidence of calcification in a suprasellar mass usually limits the differential diagnosis to which entities?

Meningioma
Craniopharyngioma
Aneurysm
Granuloma
Dermoid

SUPRASELLAR MASS, INTRINSIC HIGH ATTENUATION ON CT

High attenuation of a suprasellar mass on noncontrast CT usually limits the differential diagnosis to which entities?

Meningioma
Craniopharyngioma
Adenoma, hemorrhagic
Aneurysm
Glioma

SUPRASELLAR MASS, HYPERINTENSE ON T1 AND T2

Blood products and proteinaceous fluid are the most common causes of high signal on both T1- and T2-weighted images. Therefore, the finding of high signal in a suprasellar mass on both T1 and T2 usually limits the differential diagnosis to which entities?

Adenoma, hemorrhagic
Craniopharyngioma

FIGURES Osborn: 475, 655–656; Barkovich: 387–392

Rathke cleft cyst

FIGURES Osborn: 468, 480; Barkovich: 396

INFUNDIBULAR MASS, IN CHILD

What are the most common causes of an infundibular mass in a child? In an adult?

Common causes
    Germinoma
    Eosinophilic granuloma
    Meningitis
Uncommon causes
    Lymphoma
    Glioma

INFUNDIBULAR MASS, IN ADULT

Common causes
    Metastasis
    Sarcoidosis
    Germinoma
Uncommon causes
    Lymphoma
    Glioma
    Choristoma (granular cell tumor)

CAVERNOUS SINUS MASS

Meningioma

FIGURE Osborn: 499

Schwannoma

FIGURES Osborn: 500–501, 629

Neurofibroma

FIGURES Osborn: 499–500

Aneurysm of the cavernous internal carotid artery
Cavernous sinus thrombosis
Carotid-cavernous fistula

FIGURE Osborn: 239

Metastasis

FIGURE Osborn: 504

Lymphoma

FIGURES Osborn: 505, 506

Macroadenoma
Extension from bone tumors (metastasis, chordoma, chondrosarcoma)

Diagnosis

- Because cranial nerves III, IV, V^1, V^2, and VI traverse the cavernous sinus, unilateral cranial neuropathy involving one or more of these nerves may be the clue to the presence of cavernous sinus mass

CAVERNOUS SINUS MASS, BILATERAL

Macroadenoma
Meningioma
Lymphoma
Metastases

PINEAL REGION MASS

Pineal cyst
Germ cell tumor
  Germinoma
Pineal cell tumor
Metastasis
Glioma
  Tectal glioma
Meningioma
Vein of Galen malformation

Pineal Cyst

- No enhancement or thin rim of mural enhancement
- No obstructive hydrocephalus

FIGURES   Osborn: 413; Barkovich: 406

Germinoma

- Most common germ cell tumor of the pineal region
- Most common pineal region tumor
- Homogeneous enhancement
- Calcification variable
- Commonly spreads through the CSF; evidence of leptomeningeal enhancement should be sought in brain and spine, especially in recesses of the third ventricle

FIGURES   Osborn: 411, 412, 610, 611; Barkovich: 398–401

Pineal Cell Tumor

- Pineocytoma (benign tumor of young adults) or pineoblastoma (malignant tumor of children)
- Commonly spreads through CSF

FIGURES   Osborn: 612, 613; Barkovich: 404

Tectal Glioma

- Usually slow-growing, low-grade tumor
- Bulbous morphology of the tectum
- Effacement of the cerebral aqueduct
- T2 hyperintense
- May show no enhancement

FIGURES   Osborn: 415; Barkovich: 405

Meningioma

- Extraaxial mass arising from the tentorium
- Homogeneous enhancement

FIGURE Osborn: 420

Vein of Galen Malformation

A bruit heard over the head in an infant with congestive heart failure suggests which diagnosis?

- Presentation in infancy with congestive heart failure, macrocephaly, obstructive hydrocephalus, and bruit
- Homogeneous enhancement
- Enlarged feeding arteries or draining veins
- Confirmation by ultrasound, MRA, and catheter angiography

FIGURES Osborn: 321–324

INTRAVENTRICULAR MASS

Meningioma
Metastasis

FIGURE Osborn: 429

Ependymoma
Subependymoma
Choroid plexus papilloma
Colloid cyst
Astrocytoma
Neurocytoma
Medulloblastoma

Meningioma

What is the most common intraventricular mass lesion?

- Most common intraventricular mass
- Tumor of adulthood
- Smooth margins
- Intense, homogeneous enhancement
- Located in atrium of lateral ventricle

Where are intraventricular meningiomas typically located?

FIGURES Osborn: 588; Barkovich: 410

Ependymoma

- Heterogeneous mass
- Most commonly presents as fourth ventricle tumor with variable extension through fourth ventricular outlet foramina

FIGURES Osborn: 429; Barkovich: 338–341

Subependymoma

- Rare, nonenhancing or minimally enhancing tumor of adulthood
- Occurs in either fourth ventricle or frontal horn of lateral ventricle

FIGURE Osborn: 571

Choroid Plexus Papilloma

In what age group does choroid plexus papilloma usually occur?

- Tumor of infancy or early childhood
- Lobulated, frond-like margins

2

- Intense but heterogeneous enhancement
- Located in atrium or body of lateral ventricle; rare adult tumor occurs in fourth ventricle
- Communicating hydrocephalus (caused by overproduction of CSF or arachnoiditis resulting from previous hemorrhages)

FIGURES Osborn: 429, 573–576; Barkovich: 408

Colloid Cyst

Colloid cysts are found in what specific location?

- Located in anterosuperior third ventricle, at foramina of Monro
- No enhancement
- Obstructive hydrocephalus

FIGURES Osborn: 432, 643–645

Astrocytoma

- Can either originate within the ventricular system or invade the ventricles
- *Giant cell astrocytoma* seen in patients with tuberous sclerosis; typically produces obstructive hydrocephalus because of its characteristic location near the foramen of Monro

FIGURES Osborn: 434, 435

Neurocytoma

- Rare, benign tumor of adulthood
- Located in body of lateral ventricle

FIGURE Osborn: 428

Medulloblastoma

- Located in fourth ventricle of children (*See Posterior fossa mass, child*) or cerebellar hemisphere in adults

FIGURES Osborn: 436, 616, 617; Barkovich: 325–329

WHITE MATTER DISEASE
MULTIPLE WHITE MATTER LESIONS

Ischemia
Multiple sclerosis
Acute disseminated encephalomyelitis
Central pontine myelinolysis
Systemic lupus and other collagen vascular diseases
Sarcoid
Lyme disease
Vitamin B_{12} deficiency
Radiation injury

Differential Diagnosis

- Scattered foci of T2 signal hyperintensity in subcortical white matter without associated mass effect or enhancement can result from any one of several causes; narrowing the differential diagnosis can be perplexing
- Certain imaging patterns helpful, but clinical information most useful in development of differential diagnosis

Unilateral or asymmetrical white matter disease involving the centrum semiovale in an elderly patient should suggest what underlying cause?

Ischemia

· In the elderly, most common cause of multiple periventricular white matter signal hyperintensities presumed to be chronic ischemia; this pattern often described as "chronic small vessel ischemic change"
· Work-up not pursued unless clinical suspicion of demyelinating or other inflammatory disease or patient has asymmetrical watershed white matter disease (e.g., unilateral parasagittal white matter disease in the centrum semiovale); the latter suggests possibility of flow-limiting disease in the ipsilateral carotid, requiring appropriate work-up (i.e., carotid ultrasound, MRA, angiography)

Multiple Sclerosis

What are Dawson's fingers?

· Young to middle-aged adults with history of illness marked by exacerbations and remissions
· Characteristic location and appearance of lesions:
  ¶ Multiple linear or ovoid T2 hyperintensities in corpus callosum, oriented orthogonal to the bodies of the lateral ventricles ("Dawson's fingers")
  ¶ Periatrial and other *periventricular* white matter
  ¶ Middle cerebellar peduncle
· Demyelinative CSF profile (myelin basic protein, oligoclonal bands, IgG)

FIGURES   Osborn: 757–760; Barkovich: 79, 80

Acute Disseminated Encephalomyelitis

· History of recent viral illness (e.g., measles, varicella, mononucleosis, mumps)
· *Peripheral,* subcortical white matter
· CSF showing lymphocytic pleocytosis

FIGURES   Barkovich: 81, 82; Osborn: 704, 705

Central Pontine Myelinolysis

· History of rapid correction of a severe electrolyte imbalance
· Characteristic demyelination of the central pons (periphery of pons spared)

FIGURE   Osborn: 763

Radiation Injury

· Lesions confined to radiation ports

STROKE, HEMORRHAGE, AND VASCULAR DISEASE

INFARCT, YOUNG ADULT

Dissection
Drug abuse (e.g., cocaine, amphetamine)
Vasculitis
Basilar meningitis
Fibromuscular dysplasia
Migraine

2

What MRI sequence best shows the subintimal hematoma associated with arterial dissection?

What are the angiographic findings of arterial dissection?

Dissection

- Posttraumatic
- Presentation may be delayed (hours to weeks after trauma)
- Neck pain, cranial neuropathy (IX–XII), and Horner's syndrome may precede or accompany symptoms of stroke
- Evaluation for possible dissection: T1 axial images with fat saturation obtained from the carotid bifurcation through the skull base
    ¶ Crescentic high signal around the vessel lumen (subintimal hematoma) confirms the diagnosis
- Angiography shows eccentric tapering of the contrast column and possibly an intimal flap

FIGURES Osborn: 235–237

Basilar Meningitis

- Infarction occurs because of perivascular inflammation and vasospasm
- Ancillary clinical (e.g., lumbar puncture) or imaging (e.g., leptomeningeal enhancement, communicating hydrocephalus) findings

FIGURE Osborn: 685

What are the angiographic findings in fibromuscular dysplasia?

Fibromuscular Dysplasia

- More common in females
- Usually involves distal internal carotid artery
- Multiple vessel involvement common
- Risk of spontaneous dissection
- Angiogram shows saccular dilated segments alternating with focally narrowed segments ("string of beads")

FIGURE Osborn: 380

GYRIFORM CORTICAL ENHANCEMENT

Stroke
Cerebritis
Postictal state
Hypertensive encephalopathy
Drug effect (e.g., cyclosporin, methotrexate)

Stroke

- Acute onset of neurological deficit
- Enhancement confined to a vascular territory

Cerebritis

- More gradual onset of deficits
- Ancillary clinical and imaging findings of meningitis or local source of infection (e.g., otomastoiditis, sinusitis)

Postictal State

- Patchy occipital or parietooccipital enhancement after seizure, presumably result of transient injury to blood-brain barrier
- Resolution of enhancement in days to weeks

- Similar findings can be seen in hypertensive encephalopathy or cyclosporin toxicity

DURAL VENOUS SINUS THROMBOSIS

Infection (e.g., adjacent otomastoiditis)
Pregnancy

FIGURE   Osborn: 389

Dehydration

FIGURES   Osborn: 393, 394

Sepsis
Neoplasm (e.g., falx meningioma)
Other hypercoagulable states

CONDITIONS ASSOCIATED WITH CEREBRAL ANEURYSMS

Arteriovenous malformation

FIGURE   Osborn: 276

Adult polycystic kidney disease
Fibromuscular dysplasia
Neurofibromatosis
Collagen vascular disease

FIGURE   Osborn: 277

Marfan syndrome
Coarctation of the aorta

ANEURYSM IN UNUSUAL LOCATION

Mycotic
Vasculitis

FIGURE   Osborn: 278

Arteriovenous malformation
Posttraumatic

HEMORRHAGE(S), INTRAAXIAL

Trauma
Hypertension
Aneurysm
Vascular malformation
  Arteriovenous malformation
  Cryptic vascular malformation
Infarct
  Thromboembolic
  Venous
Neoplasm
  Metastasis
  Glioma
Amyloid angiopathy
Cocaine or amphetamine abuse

2

FIGURE   Osborn: 196

Vasculitis

FIGURE   Osborn: 376

Coagulopathy
Encephalitis

Trauma

- Characteristic locations: frontal lobes, temporal lobes above the petrous ridges, anterior temporal lobes
- Other evidence of trauma: scalp soft tissue swelling, skull fracture, extraaxial hematoma

FIGURES   Osborn: 215–221

Hypertension

What are the common locations of hypertensive hemorrhage?

- Characteristic locations: putamen, thalamus, pons, cerebellar hemisphere

FIGURE   Osborn: 176

Aneurysm

- History of sudden onset; "worst headache of life"
- Accompanying subarachnoid blood
- Confirmation by catheter angiogram

FIGURE   Osborn: 261

Arteriovenous Malformation

- Large flow voids in or near the hematoma
- Follow-up imaging or early catheter angiography may be necessary because acute hematoma could obscure a small vascular malformation
- Confirmation by catheter angiography

FIGURES   Osborn: 186–187

Cryptic Vascular Malformation

- Evidence of other cryptic vascular malformations by MRI

FIGURES   Osborn: 187, 313

Infarct, Thromboembolic

- Acute onset of neurological deficit ("stroke-like presentation")
- Confined to a vascular territory
- Characteristic evolution of enhancement pattern, signal characteristics, and mass effect on follow-up studies

FIGURE   Osborn: 180

Infarct, Venous

What are the characteristic locations of parenchymal hematomas caused by dural sinus thrombosis?

- Subcortical hematoma in characteristic location:
    ¶ Temporal lobe (transverse sinus or vein of Labbé thrombosis)
    ¶ Parasagittal subcortical white matter (superior sagittal sinus thrombosis)
    ¶ Bilateral thalami (straight sinus or vein of Galen)

2

• Evidence of venous sinus thrombosis by MRI and MR venography

FIGURES Osborn: 181; Barkovich: 579, 580

Neoplasm

What are the implications of a fluid-fluid level within an intraaxial hematoma?

• Fluid-fluid level in a hematoma (in a patient without coagulopathy) raises the possibility of an underlying mass lesion
• Follow-up imaging after partial resolution of hematoma (about 6 weeks after presentation) helpful to rule out mass lesion

Hemorrhage associated with metastases suggests which primary neoplasms?

• Most common hemorrhagic metastases: melanoma, adenocarcinoma (breast, lung, renal, colon), thyroid carcinoma, choriocarcinoma

Which primary CNS tumors are most commonly associated with hemorrhage?

• Most common hemorrhagic primary neoplasms: glioblastoma, oligodendroglioma

FIGURES Osborn: 171, 189, 191, 192, 663

Amyloid Angiopathy

• Elderly patient
• Lobar hematoma
• Multiple tiny foci of hemosiderin deposition on gradient-recalled echo (GRE) images

HEMORRHAGE, SPONTANEOUS INTRAAXIAL; ELDERLY PATIENT

Hypertension
Amyloid angiopathy
Metastasis

HEMORRHAGE, SPONTANEOUS INTRAAXIAL; YOUNG PATIENT

What are the most common causes of a spontaneous intraaxial hemorrhage in an elderly patient? In a young patient?

Vascular malformation
Aneurysm
Drug abuse
Neoplasm

Vascular Malformation

• Unexplained hemorrhage in a young patient mandates cerebral angiography to rule out an underlying arteriovenous malformation or aneurysm

Drug Abuse

• Street drugs such as cocaine and amphetamine can produce "spontaneous" intracranial hemorrhage in young patients, presumably by inducing transient hypertension
• These drugs able to induce bleeding from preexisting vascular or neoplastic lesions (e.g., arteriovenous malformation, aneurysm); thus, MRI/MRA and cerebral angiography are still mandatory

HEMORRHAGE, MULTIFOCAL INTRAAXIAL

Trauma
Metastases
Amyloid angiopathy
Vasculitis
Venous infarction
Coagulopathy

HEMORRHAGE, SUBARACHNOID

Aneurysm
Trauma
Arteriovenous malformation

Aneurysm

- Unexplained subarachnoid hemorrhage requires further evaluation by conventional "four-vessel" (both vertebral arteries and both internal carotid arteries) cerebral angiography; if both posterior inferior cerebellar artery (PICA) origins can be clearly shown after injection of dominant vertebral artery, the other vertebral artery does not have to be injected

FIGURES   Osborn: 167, 182, 183, 254

Trauma

- Posttraumatic subarachnoid hemorrhage common, both over the hemispheric convexities and in the basilar cisterns
- History of closed head injury and other imaging findings consistent with trauma (e.g., subdural hematoma, contusion)
- If there is any possibility that trauma may have resulted from a ruptured aneurysm, angiography is indicated; occasional patients in this category have a history of "found down" or "fell and hit head"

FIGURE   Osborn: 213

HEMORRHAGE, SUBDURAL OR EPIDURAL

Trauma

FIGURES   Osborn: 159–162, 204, 206–211

Coagulopathy

MENINGEAL AND EPENDYMAL DISEASE

LEPTOMENINGEAL ENHANCEMENT

Metastases
Meningitis
Postsurgical
Subarachnoid hemorrhage
Meningeal angiomatosis in Sturge-Weber syndrome

FIGURES   Barkovich: 306, 308

2

Metastases

Which primary CNS neoplasms most frequently spread via CSF?

- Extracranial primary (e.g., lung, breast, melanoma, lymphoma, leukemia)
- Intracranial primary; certain primary central nervous system (CNS) neoplasms have a propensity for spread via CSF:
  - ¶ Germ cell tumor
  - ¶ Ependymoma
  - ¶ Primitive neuroectodermal tumors (PNET): medulloblastoma, pineoblastoma, retinoblastoma
  - ¶ Glioblastoma
  - ¶ Choroid plexus carcinoma

FIGURES   Osborn: 548, 660, 661; Barkovich: 333

Meningitis

- Leptomeningeal enhancement uncommon in pyogenic or viral meningitis; more common in fungal or mycobacterial meningitis
- Basilar meningeal enhancement suggests tuberculous or fungal meningitis

What are the possible complications of meningitis?

- Always look for a local source of infection (e.g., otomastoiditis, sinusitis) and complications (hydrocephalus, infarction, abscess, extraaxial empyema)

DURAL ENHANCEMENT OR MASS

Iatrogenic
  Postcraniotomy
  Post-lumbar puncture or CSF diversion
Neoplasm
  Meningioma
  Metastases
  Direct spread of primary intracranial tumor
Meningitis
Posthemorrhagic
Spontaneous intracranial hypotension
Sarcoidosis

Iatrogenic

- Postcraniotomy: most common cause of dural enhancement; smooth; focal or diffuse
- Post-lumbar puncture or CSF diversion

Meningioma

- Most common noniatrogenic cause of dural enhancement
- Meningioma with *lobular* morphology rarely mistaken for other entities that produce dural enhancement; meningioma with *en plaque* morphology occasionally leads to confusion
- Characteristic location, calcification, reactive bony changes, or associated vasogenic edema, if present, may support the diagnosis

FIGURES   Osborn: 594–600

2

Metastases

- Breast, prostate, lymphoma
- No calcification
- Solitary dural metastasis could mimic meningioma, but is sufficiently rare that it should not be mentioned unless patient has a known primary or lesion has atypical features (e.g., inhomogeneous enhancement, adjacent calvarial destruction

FIGURES   Osborn: 601, 622, 658, 659

Posthemorrhagic

- History of subdural or epidural hematoma
- Ancillary findings of remote trauma (e.g., frontal encephalomalacia)

Spontaneous Intracranial Hypotension

- Caused by spontaneous CSF leak from lumbosacral root sleeve cyst
- History of severe postural headache
- Diffuse dural enhancement with ancillary MRI findings of:
    ¶ Brain "sagging" with crowding of the posterior fossa and foramen magnum
    ¶ Pituitary enlargement
    ¶ Variable bilateral subdural hematomas
    ¶ Lumbosacral root sleeve cysts
    ¶ CSF leak from root sleeve demonstrated by careful myelography or radionuclide study

EPENDYMAL ENHANCEMENT

Neoplasm
Ventriculitis

Neoplasm

- Direct extension from glioma or lymphoma that abuts a ventricular surface
- CSF spread of intracranial or extracranial primary (*See Leptomeningeal enhancement*)

FIGURE   Osborn: 539

Ventriculitis

- Usually a complication of meningitis or surgery (e.g., post-shunting)
- Cytomegalovirus (CMV) ventriculitis is fairly common in the AIDS population

HYDROCEPHALUS

General

- Hydrocephalus in the neonate has separate differential diagnosis; beyond neonatal period, hydrocephalus first should be characterized as communicating or obstructive

- *Communicating* hydrocephalus implies that ventricles "communicate" freely; i.e., no obstruction to CSF flow exists within ventricles, and ventricles are diffusely and proportionately enlarged
  - ¶ Obstruction in most cases of communicating hydrocephalus presumed to be at level of arachnoid granulations over the cerebral convexities, where CSF is normally resorbed
- *Obstructive* hydrocephalus implies that there is an obstruction to CSF flow within ventricular system, usually from an intraventricular or intraaxial mass lesion, resulting in enlargement of one or more (but not all) ventricles

CONGENITAL HYDROCEPHALUS

What are the most common causes of congenital hydrocephalus?

Idiopathic
Chiari II malformation
Dandy-Walker malformation
Congenital aqueductal stenosis
Perinatal hemorrhage
Perinatal meningitis

Idiopathic

- Diagnosis of exclusion

Chiari II Malformation

- Myelomeningocele at birth
- Imaging manifestations of Chiari II

FIGURES   Osborn: 22, 23, 457; Barkovich: 240

Dandy-Walker Malformation

- If not diagnosed by prenatal ultrasound, presents at 1 to 3 months of life with enlarging head caused by hydrocephalus
- Imaging manifestations of Dandy-Walker malformation

FIGURES   Osborn: 62, 63; Barkovich: 248, 249

Congenital Aqueductal Stenosis

- Diagnosis of exclusion that should be made only after careful MRI evaluation has ruled out an obstructive mass lesion originating in the tectum, suprasellar region, or anterior third ventricle
- Absence of normal CSF-filled aqueduct on sagittal and axial T1 images

COMMUNICATING HYDROCEPHALUS

Meningitis
Subarachnoid hemorrhage
Meningeal carcinomatosis

General

- Because CSF normally resorbed via arachnoid granulations over cerebral hemispheres, any condition that inflames the leptomenin-

2

ges can interfere with CSF resorption and lead to communicating hydrocephalus

MISCELLANEOUS CONDITIONS

PARENCHYMAL CALCIFICATIONS, NEONATE

CMV infection
Toxoplasmosis

FIGURES Osborn: 676; Barkovich: 575

Rubella infection

FIGURE Osborn: 677

Herpes simplex infection
HIV infection

CMV Infection

- TORCH (toxoplasmosis, rubella, cytomegalovirus, herpes simplex) group of infectious agents all can cause congenital meningo-encephalitis and parenchymal calcifications
- CMV infection is the most common congenital meningoencephalitis
- Calcifications predominantly periventricular
- Classic clinical triad: periventricular calcification, hydrocephalus, and chorioretinitis
- Imaging findings (and clinical presentation) of CMV infection, toxoplasmosis, and rubella overlap
- Subependymal tubers of tuberous sclerosis usually do not calcify before the age of 2 years and are associated with other imaging abnormalities on MRI; thus, rarely confused with periventricular calcifications of CMV or other congenital infections

FIGURES Osborn: 675; Barkovich: 570–574

Herpes Simplex Infection

- History of vaginal delivery from a mother infected with herpes simplex virus (HSV)-2
- Severe liquefaction necrosis of widespread areas of brain parenchyma

FIGURES Osborn: 678, 679; Barkovich: 576

HIV Infection

- Calcifications associated with congenital HIV infection occur beyond the newborn period; typically affect the basal ganglia symmetrically

FIGURES Osborn: 679; Barkovich: 596

T1 HYPERINTENSITY; T2 HYPOINTENSITY

General

- Most acute or subacute pathology in the brain appears on non-contrast MRI as lesions that are hypointense on T1 and hyperintense on T2; because relatively few substances can cause T1 hyperintensity or T2 hypointensity, knowledge of these differentials can be helpful

T1 HYPERINTENSITY

Which substances may be responsible for the shortening of the T1 relaxation time (i.e., hyperintensity on a T1-weighted image)?

Blood breakdown products
   Intracellular methemoglobin
   Extracellular methemoglobin
Fat
Proteinaceous fluid
Melanin
Slow blood flow on certain sequences
Calcification (rarely)

T2 HYPOINTENSITY

Which substances may be responsible for shortening of the T2 relaxation time (i.e., hypointensity on a T2-weighted image)?

Vascular flow voids
Blood breakdown products
   Deoxyhemoglobin
   Intracellular methemoglobin
   Ferritin
   Hemosiderin
Calcification or ossification
Proteinaceous fluid
Densely cellular masses
   Meningioma
   Lymphoma
   PNET (medulloblastoma, pinealoblastoma, neuroblastoma)
Metals
   Iron deposition, physiologic (basal ganglia, substantia nigra, red nucleus, dentate nucleus)
   Iron deposition, pathologic

SPINE

INTRAMEDULLARY LESION

What are the most common intramedullary spinal neoplasms?

Neoplasm
   Ependymoma
   Astrocytoma

FIGURES   Osborn: 912, 913; Barkovich: 542, 543

   Hemangioblastoma

FIGURES   Osborn: 915, 916; Barkovich: 313, 314

   Metastasis (rare)
Infarct or ischemia
Hematoma
Demyelinating disease
Myelitis
Cryptic vascular malformation
Syrinx
Contusion
Abscess

Ependymoma

- Most common intramedullary tumor in adults; second most common in children
- Most common primary tumor of the conus medullaris and filum
- Imaging appearance overlaps with astrocytoma; well-demarcated superior or inferior border of the enhancing portion of tumor favors ependymoma

FIGURES   Osborn: 908–911; Barkovich: 542, 543

Metastasis

- Rare
- Very unlikely to be initial presentation of metastatic disease; should be mentioned in differential diagnosis only if patient has known primary neoplasm

Infarct or Ischemia

- Nonspecific imaging features (T1 hypointense, T2 hyperintense, variable enhancement and mass effect)
- In patient with unexplained progressive myelopathy, thecal sac should be carefully inspected for abnormal flow voids that might be a clue to the presence of a *dural arteriovenous fistula* (absence of flow voids does not rule out fistula; ultimately, spinal angiography may be necessary in this setting)

FIGURES   Osborn: 833, 835

Hematoma

- MRI signal compatible with blood
- Other evidence of trauma (epidural hematoma, fractures, subluxation, traumatic disc herniation)

Demyelinating Disease

- Most commonly caused by multiple sclerosis (MS) in young or middle-aged patient
- Clinical history and intracranial MR findings suggestive of MS

FIGURES   Osborn: 827, 829

Myelitis

- Diagnosis of exclusion
- Nonspecific term that comprises postviral and other inflammatory processes

FIGURE   Osborn: 829

Cryptic Vascular Malformation

- Identical appearance to intracranial cryptic vascular malformation

Syrinx

Why is it important to obtain gadolinium-enhanced images in the evaluation of a syrinx?

- Follows CSF in signal
- Gadolinium-enhanced images should always be obtained in imaging work-up of unexplained syrinx to rule out an associated cord neoplasm

Contusion

- Nonspecific imaging features (T1 hypointense, T2 hyperintense, variable enhancement and mass effect)
- Other evidence of trauma (epidural hematoma, fractures, subluxation, traumatic disc herniation)

FIGURE   Osborn: 871

Abscess

- *Intramedullary* abscess is rare
- Usually seen in immunocompromised patients
- Can mimic neoplasm or other enhancing intramedullary lesions

SYRINGOMYELIA

Trauma
Neoplasm
Chiari malformation
Infarct
Arachnoiditis

Trauma

- Focal myelomalacia (thinning of the cord)
- No enhancement

FIGURE   Osborn: 872

Neoplasm

- Expansion of cord
- Virtually always shows some enhancement; for this reason, gadolinium-enhanced images should always be obtained as part of imaging work-up of unexplained syrinx

Chiari Malformation

- Associated imaging findings of Chiari I or Chiari II malformation

FIGURE   Osborn: 815

Infarct

- Focal myelomalacia

Arachnoiditis

- History of meningitis, back surgery, or other potential predisposing condition
- Associated imaging findings of arachnoiditis in the lumbosacral spine: nerve root thickening, clumping, and adherence to sac wall; CSF loculations

FIGURES   Osborn: 860, 861

2

INTRADURAL, EXTRAMEDULLARY LESION

Meningioma
Schwannoma
Neurofibroma
Metastases
Dermoid
Epidermoid

FIGURE   Osborn: 902

Ependymoma
Lipoma

Differential Diagnosis

What are the two most common causes of an intradural extramedullary mass?

How can these two entities be distinguished from each other?

- Most common differential diagnosis in the extramedullary intradural compartment is *meningioma* versus *nerve sheath tumor* (neurofibroma or schwannoma)
- Both of these entities may cause cord or nerve root compression; both may have similar signal characteristics on MRI, including uniform contrast enhancement
- Posterolateral location within the canal favors meningioma over nerve sheath tumors, which tend to be located anterolaterally and often grow into the neural foramen, leading to "dumbbell" morphology
- Most isolated nerve sheath tumors are schwannomas, although an occasional isolated nerve sheath tumor turns out to be a neurofibroma
- Neurofibromas are commonly multiple tumors seen in patients with NF type 1

Meningioma

Multiple meningiomas suggest what underlying condition?

- Solitary, except in NF type 2
- Posterolateral location favors meningioma over schwannoma

FIGURES   Osborn: 900–901

Schwannoma

Multiple schwannomas suggest what underlying condition?

- Solitary, except in NF type 2
- Foraminal location and dumbbell morphology favor schwannoma over meningioma

FIGURES   Osborn: 897–899; Barkovich: 293–294

Neurofibroma

- Multiple tumors in NF type 1
- Associated imaging findings of NF type 1

FIGURES   Osborn: 897–899

Metastases

Which primary CNS tumors are most commonly associated with seeding of the CNS?

- Many tumors may seed the CSF and result in intradural, extramedullary metastatic deposits
- Primary tumors of the neural axis
    - ¶ Germ cell tumors
    - ¶ Ependymoma

¶ Primitive neuroectodermal tumors (medulloblastoma, pineoblastoma, retinoblastoma)
- Extraneural primary tumors
    ¶ Adenocarcinoma
    ¶ Melanoma
    ¶ Lymphoma
    ¶ Leukemia
- Appearance varies, ranging from "frosting" of cord surface and nerve roots with a thin layer of enhancement to nodular, enhancing foci in thecal sac and within the roots of the cauda equina

FIGURES   Osborn: 904–906; Barkovich: 547–550

EXTRADURAL LESION

Degenerative disease
  Disc protrusion
  Osteophyte
  Synovial cyst
Neoplasm
  Metastases to vertebrae
  Other vertebral tumors
    Myeloma

FIGURE   Osborn: 893

    Chordoma

FIGURES   Osborn: 889–891

    Aneurysmal bone cyst

FIGURES   Osborn: 884, 885; Barkovich: 551

    Giant cell tumor

FIGURES   Osborn: 883; Barkovich: 554

    Lymphoma

FIGURES   Osborn: 892; Barkovich: 556

    Leukemia

FIGURES   Barkovich: 564, 565

    Osteoblastoma

FIGURE   Barkovich: 556

    Eosinophilic granuloma

FIGURES   Barkovich: 552, 553

Nerve sheath tumors
  Schwannoma
  Neurofibroma

FIGURES   Barkovich: 559, 560

Ganglion cell tumors
  Ganglioneuroma

FIGURE   Barkovich: 563

    Ganglioneuroblastoma
    Neuroblastoma

FIGURES   Barkovich: 561, 562

Epidural abscess
  Discitis or osteomyelitis

Figures Barkovich: 613–614

Hematoma

Figure Osborn: 870

Disc Protrusion

- Epidural soft tissue contiguous with and isointense to disc
- No enhancement
- Commonly associated with disc space narrowing, desiccation of the parent disc, and signal changes in vertebral end plates adjacent to the parent disc
- Most common in lower cervical or lower lumbar spine

Figures Osborn: 841, 842

Osteophyte

- Most easily distinguished from disc on sagittal images
- Low signal on T2 and GRE images
- No enhancement

Figures Osborn: 844–846

Synovial Cyst

- Round, cystic lesion contiguous with the medial aspect of a diseased (hypertrophic) facet joint
- Occasionally large enough to impinge on lateral thecal sac and exiting nerve roots

Figures Osborn: 852–855

Metastases to Vertebrae

- Epidural tumor most commonly represents extension from bony vertebral metastases (i.e., involvement of epidural space without antecedent bony metastatic disease is rare)
- Several vertebrae involved
- Discs spared
- Extension into vertebral pedicles, epidural tissues, and paraspinous tissues
- Most common primaries: lung, breast, or prostate carcinomas or lymphoma

Figure Osborn: 878

Nerve Sheath Tumors

- Most commonly intradural, extramedullary
- Can occasionally have an extradural component or be exclusively extradural
- Homogeneous enhancement of foraminal nerve sheath tumor distinguishes schwannoma or neurofibroma from foraminal disc protrusion, which does not enhance

Figures Osborn: 897–899

What are the imaging findings of discitis and epidural abscess?

Epidural Abscess

- Epidural abscess or phlegmon is almost always result of spread of infection from a contiguous focus of discitis or osteomyelitis
- Key imaging findings:
    - ¶ Involved disc narrowed, enhanced on T1 post-gadolinium, and hyperintense on T2
    - ¶ Adjacent end plates edematous (T1 hypointense, T2 hyperintense) and enhanced on T1 post-gadolinium
    - ¶ Fluid collections and/or enhancing phlegmonous tissue in epidural, paraspinous, and prevertebral spaces

EPIDURAL LESION, CHILD

Extension of paraspinal or vertebral tumor
Abscess

FIGURES Barkovich: 612–614

Extension of Paraspinal or Vertebral Tumor

- Ganglion cell (neuroblastoma, ganglioneuroblastoma, ganglioneuroma) and nerve sheath (neurofibroma, schwannoma) tumors
- Ewing's sarcoma
- Lymphoma
- Leukemia
- Eosinophilic granuloma
- Other vertebral body tumors (*See Extradural Lesion, Neoplasm*)

FIGURES Osborn: 892; Barkovich: 551–555, 560–565

EPIDURAL LESION EXTENDING OVER MANY LEVELS

Abscess
Hematoma
Metastases
Lymphoma

HEAD AND NECK

SKULL BASE

DESTRUCTIVE MIDLINE, SKULL-BASE LESION

Metastasis
Myeloma
Nasopharyngeal carcinoma

FIGURE Osborn: 504

Chordoma
Chondrosarcoma
Meningioma

FIGURES Osborn: 494, 498

Macroadenoma
Lymphoma
Esthesioneuroblastoma

Aggressive sinusitis
Benign paranasal sinus condition
  Mucocele
  Polyposis

FIGURES   Osborn: 489, 490

Imaging Modality

- For lesions of skull base, CT allows optimal evaluation of the extent of bone and foraminal destruction
- MRI allows optimal evaluation of the extent of disease, including intracranial extension and perineural spread of tumor along cranial nerves

Metastasis

- Most common destructive skull base lesion
- Multiple lesions

FIGURES   Osborn: 460, 504

Myeloma

- Multiple lesions

FIGURE   Osborn: 504

Chordoma

- Midline tumor, centered in region of clivus

FIGURE   Osborn: 502

Chondrosarcoma

- Centered slightly off midline, in the region of the petrooccipital suture
- Chondroid matrix on CT

FIGURE   Osborn: 504

Macroadenoma

- Occasionally grows through the sellar floor into sphenoid sinus
- Centered in and expands sella
- Lobular suprasellar component usually present

FIGURES   Osborn: 497, 498

Esthesioneuroblastoma

- Centered in the anterior midline near the cribriform plate
- Bulk of tumor may be:
  - ¶ Predominantly within the nasal cavity
  - ¶ Predominantly intracranial, in the inferior frontal region
  - ¶ In both the nasal cavity and inferior frontal region, traversing the skull base at the cribriform plate

Aggressive Sinusitis

- Skull base destruction and mass-like intracranial extension with aspergillus infection or mucormycosis

¶ *Aspergillus* sinus infection may be seen in immunocompetent patients
¶ Mucormycosis most common in diabetics and immunocompromised patients
- Fungal sinusitis is characteristically high attenuation on CT and often hypointense on T2 images

FIGURES Osborn: 495, 496

DESTRUCTIVE SKULL-BASE LESION OF ANTERIOR (FRONTAL) MIDLINE

Esthesioneuroblastoma
Metastasis
Meningioma
Sinonasal carcinoma
Lymphoma
Rhabdomyosarcoma
Aggressive sinusitis
Benign paranasal sinus condition
   Mucocele
   Polyposis

DESTRUCTIVE SKULL-BASE LESION OF CENTRAL (BASISPHENOID) MIDLINE

Nasopharyngeal carcinoma
Chordoma
Chondrosarcoma
Metastasis or myeloma
Macroadenoma
Meningioma
Aggressive sinusitis

Nasopharyngeal Carcinoma

- Originates from mucosa in or near the fossa of Rosenmüller
- Commonly produces early eustachian tube obstruction and mastoiditis
- One of the skull base tumors most likely to have associated perineural (usually along the fifth cranial nerve) and perivascular spread

Unilateral mastoiditis in an adult should alert one to the possibility of which diagnosis?

Meningioma

- Also occurs commonly along the sphenoid bone

Aggressive Sinusitis

- Infection from aggressive sinusitis (e.g., aspergillosis or mucormycosis) can involve skull base and spread intracranially
- If patient is known to have diabetes, AIDS, organ transplant, or any immunocompromising condition, it is appropriate to keep infection in the differential diagnosis

JUGULAR FORAMEN MASS

Glomus jugulare
Schwannoma

FIGURES Osborn: 455, 509, 510

Metastasis

FIGURE Osborn: 456

Give some examples of pseudotumors that may occur near the jugular foramen.

Meningioma
Vascular pseudotumor
   Asymmetrical or thrombosed jugular vein
   Ectatic carotid artery
   Carotid pseudoaneurysm

General

How might a patient with a jugular foramen mass lesion present clinically?

- Jugular foramen mass lesions present with lower cranial neuropathies (cranial nerves IX, X, and XI), pulsatile tinnitus, and variable conductive hearing loss

Glomus Jugulare

"Salt-and-pepper" appearance describes which jugular foramen lesion?

What causes the salt-and-pepper appearance on T1 images?

- Most common jugular foramen tumor
- "Salt-and-pepper" appearance on T1 (small foci of hyperintense signal, presumably hemorrhage, and small flow voids)
- Prominent flow voids favor glomus tumor over meningioma or schwannoma

FIGURES Osborn: 455, 507

Vascular Pseudotumor

- Occasionally symptomatic (e.g., carotid pseudoaneurysm) but may be incidental finding that leads to work-up for a jugular foramen tumor
- Heterogeneous, concentric dark and bright signal on spin-echo images should suggest flow-related signal in a vascular pseudotumor
- Consider further evaluation by MRA or catheter angiography

ORBITS, TEMPORAL BONES, AND PARANASAL SINUSES

ORBITAL LESIONS

For the purpose of describing imaging findings and arriving at a differential diagnosis, the orbit can be divided into six compartments: globe, optic nerve sheath, rectus muscles, lacrimal fossa, intraconal compartment, and extraconal compartment (*cone* refers to the extraocular muscle cone). As is the case in the brain, if pathology can be isolated to certain specific locations (e.g., lacrimal fossa, extraocular muscles), the differential diagnosis can be significantly narrowed.

GLOBE LESIONS

Adult
   Uveal melanoma
   Uveal metastasis

2

Choroidal or retinal detachment
Vitreous hemorrhage
Pseudotumor
Pediatric
Retinoblastoma

Uveal Melanoma

- Hyperintense on T1
- Lobular morphology more common
- Unilateral

Uveal Metastasis

- Isointense on T1
- Plaque-like morphology more common

Retinoblastoma

A unilateral or bilateral calcified retinal mass in an infant is pathognomonic of what condition?

- Unilateral or bilateral retinal calcifications on CT
- Presents in infants with leukokoria

FIGURE   Barkovich: 414

OPTIC NERVE OR NERVE SHEATH ENLARGEMENT

Neoplasm
    Optic glioma
    Optic nerve sheath meningioma
    Lymphoma
    Leukemia
    Metastasis
Pseudotumor
Optic neuritis
Sarcoidosis

Optic Glioma

- Presents in childhood
- Imaging findings of NF type 1 may be seen (30% of children with optic glioma have NF 1)
- Fusiform enlargement and kinking of the optic nerve
- Moderate enhancement
- Variable posterior extension into the chiasm, optic tracts, and optic radiations

FIGURES   Barkovich: 382, 383; Osborn: 74, 75

Optic Nerve Sheath Meningioma

- Presents in middle-aged adults
- Linear or globular calcification
- Intense homogeneous enhancement
- Tumors with tubular morphology (growing around and along the optic nerve) show linear "tram track" enhancement in the axial plane; this pattern refers to enhanced tubular tumor surrounding nonenhanced optic nerve

2

Optic Neuritis

- Inflammation of the optic nerve that may be nonspecific or related to demyelinating or inflammatory disease
- Enlarged, enhancing optic nerve
- MRI of the brain should be obtained so that evidence of MS can be sought

RECTUS MUSCLE ENLARGEMENT

Thyroid ophthalmopathy
Pseudotumor
Myositis
Neoplasm
   Metastasis
   Lymphoma
   Others
Vascular congestion
   Mass at orbital apex
   Carotid-cavernous fistula
   Cavernous sinus thrombosis
   Dural arteriovenous malformation

Thyroid Ophthalmopathy

What imaging features help distinguish thyroid ophthalmopathy from orbital pseudotumor?

- Most common cause of rectus muscle enlargement
- Painless, gradual onset
- Imaging features that favor thyroid ophthalmopathy over pseudotumor as cause of rectus muscle enlargement:
    - ¶ Bilaterality
    - ¶ Symmetry
    - ¶ Sparing of tendinous insertions
    - ¶ Characteristic clinical progression, with involvement of inferior rectus early followed by medial rectus, superior rectus, and lateral rectus

Pseudotumor

What clinical features suggest a diagnosis of orbital pseudotumor in a patient with rectus muscle enlargement?

- Painful, rapid onset
- Dramatic improvement with steroids

Myositis

- Usually secondary to extension of infection from paranasal sinuses or pseudotumor
    - ¶ Mucosal thickening or fluid in the ethmoid air cells and thickening of ipsilateral medial rectus muscle suggest spread of sinus infection
    - ¶ Acute, painful onset suggests pseudotumor

Carotid-cavernous Fistula

- Enlargement of rectus muscles caused by venous congestion
- Enlargement of superior ophthalmic vein

FIGURE   Osborn: 239

LACRIMAL FOSSA MASS

Viral infection
Neoplasm

2

Adenoma
Carcinoma
Lymphoma
Metastasis
Dermoid
Pseudotumor
Sarcoidosis
Sjögren's syndrome
Wegener's granulomatosis

Viral Infection

• Self-limited lacrimal gland enlargement
• Occurs in child or young adult

Neoplasm

• Epithelial tumors account for half of all lacrimal fossa masses:
  ¶ Half are pleomorphic adenomas (benign mixed tumor)
  ¶ Half are carcinomas (usually adenoid cystic carcinoma)
• Benign tumors: well circumscribed, erosion of bone is smooth
• Carcinoma infiltrating, bone destroyed
• Dermoid tumor is well demarcated, extraconal mass that contains fat and often calcification; most commonly arises in the lacrimal fossa

LACRIMAL FOSSA MASS, BILATERAL

Lymphoma
Sarcoidosis

INTRACONAL MASS

Congenital
  Cavernous hemangioma (adult)
  Capillary hemangioma (infant)
  Lymphangioma (child)
Inflammatory
  Orbital cellulitis
  Pseudotumor
Vascular
  Varix
  Carotid-cavernous fistula
Neoplasm
  Lymphoma
  Rhabdomyosarcoma
  Metastasis

Cavernous Hemangioma

• Occurs in adults
• Well-demarcated, intensely enhancing mass
• Progressive, painless proptosis

FIGURE   Barkovich: 420

Capillary Hemangioma

• Occurs in infants
• Well-demarcated, intensely enhancing mass

Fluid-fluid levels in a lobular retrobulbar mass in a child suggest what diagnosis?

- Proptosis or periorbital skin discoloration (or both) in the first weeks of life

FIGURE Barkovich: 418

Lymphangioma

- Occurs in children
- Multilocular, moderately enhancing, infiltrative cystic mass with fluid-fluid levels and variable hemorrhage
- Progressive proptosis

FIGURES Barkovich: 418, 419

Orbital Cellulitis

- Evidence of source of infection (ethmoid sinusitis, preseptal cellulitis)
- Infiltration of the orbital fat
- Associated subperiosteal abscess along the medial wall of the orbit

FIGURE Barkovich: 611

Pseudotumor

- Sudden, painful onset
- Dramatic improvement with steroids

Varix

What maneuvers help confirm that a homogeneously enhancing orbital mass is a varix?

- Tubular, well-demarcated, enhancing structure
- Proptosis and increase in size of varix elicited by Valsalva maneuver or prone position

Carotid-cavernous Fistula

Enlargement of the superior ophthalmic vein in a patient with chemosis and proptosis suggests what diagnosis?

- Enlargement of extraocular muscles and superior ophthalmic vein
- Pulsatile exophthalmos

Metastasis

- Most metastases involving the pediatric orbit (e.g., neuroblastoma) are to bone
- Metastases in adult orbit (e.g., breast, lung, prostate, melanoma) can occur to the uvea, rectus muscles, or bone

FIGURE Barkovich: 423

EXTRACONAL MASS

Metastasis to bony orbit
Invasion of adjacent primary neoplasm involving:
    Paranasal sinuses (e.g., squamous cell carcinoma)
    Nasal cavity
    Intracranial meninges (e.g., sphenoid wing meningioma)
Lacrimal fossa mass (*See Lacrimal fossa mass*)
Subperiosteal hematoma or abscess

2

MIDDLE EAR MASS

Inflammatory
    Cholesteatoma
    Inflammatory debris/granulation tissue
    Cholesterol granuloma
Vascular
    Ectopic carotid artery
    Dehiscent jugular bulb
Neoplasm
    Glomus tympanicum
    Glomus jugulare invading middle ear
    ("glomus jugulotympanicum")
    Hemangioma
    Others

Cholesteatoma

- Nonenhancing soft tissue in the epitympanum
- Displacement or erosion of ossicles
- Erosion of scutum
- Features favoring cholesteatoma over granulation tissue: lack of enhancement; mass effect; bone erosion

Cholesterol Granuloma

- Hyperintense on T1 and T2
- No bone erosion

Ectopic Carotid Artery

- Best evaluated by high-resolution, thin-section temporal bone CT
- Carotid artery takes an abnormal course through middle ear

Dehiscent Jugular Bulb

- Best evaluated by high-resolution, thin-section temporal bone CT
- Bony plate that normally separates jugular bulb from middle ear is absent

Glomus Tympanicum

- Intensely enhancing soft tissue mass abutting cochlear promontory

Glomus Jugulotympanicum

- Intensely enhancing mass arising in jugular foramen
- Bone destroyed and middle ear invaded
- "Salt-and-pepper" appearance on T1
- Cranial neuropathies (IX, X, XI)

LESION CAUSING PULSATILE TINNITUS

Congenital vascular lesion
    Ectopic carotid artery
    High jugular bulb or dehiscent jugular bulb
Acquired vascular lesion

Transverse sinus/jugular vein thrombosis
High-grade carotid stenosis
Dural arteriovenous fistula
Neoplasm
Glomus tympanicum
Glomus jugular invading middle ear
("glomus jugulotympanicum")

Dural Arteriovenous Fistula

- CT and MRI findings usually normal
- Catheter angiography required for evaluation

"VASCULAR" RETROTYMPANIC MASS

Congenital vascular
Ectopic carotid artery
High jugular bulb or dehiscent jugular bulb
Neoplasm
Glomus tympanicum
Glomus jugulare invading middle ear
("glomus jugulotympanicum")
Inflammatory
Cholesterol granuloma
Inflammatory/granulation tissue

PARANASAL SINUS MASS

Mucocele
Neoplasm
Squamous cell carcinoma
Adenocarcinoma
Lymphoma

FIGURE   Osborn: 492

Inverted papilloma
Esthesioneuroblastoma

FIGURE   Osborn: 492

Ameloblastoma
Rhabdomyosarcoma
Juvenile angiofibroma

FIGURE   Osborn: 501

Infectious sinusitis

FIGURE   Osborn: 496

Granulomatous sinusitis

FIGURE   Osborn: 492

Osteoma

FIGURE   Osborn: 490

Odontogenic cyst

SUPRAHYOID NECK

PARAPHARYNGEAL SPACE

Contents
  Fat
  Branches of cranial nerve V3
  Salivary gland rests

Infiltrative neoplasm (e.g., squamous cell carcinoma) invading
  from:
  Adjacent pharyngeal mucosal space
  Parotid space
  Masticator space
Abscess extension from:
  Pharyngeal mucosal space (tonsillar abscess)
  Masticator space (odontogenic abscess)

PHARYNGEAL MUCOSAL SPACE

Contents
  Mucosa
  Waldeyer's ring (lymphoid tissue)
  Eustachian tube opening
  Minor salivary glands, muscles

Squamous cell carcinoma
Non-Hodgkin's lymphoma
Abscess (tonsillar)

MASTICATOR SPACE

Contents
  Muscles of mastication (medial and lateral pterygoid muscles,
    masseter muscle, temporalis muscle)
  Mandibular ramus
  Branches of cranial nerve V3

Abscess (odontogenic)
Neoplasm arising from mandible (e.g., osteogenic sarcoma)
Neoplasm arising from muscle (e.g., rhabdomyosarcoma)
Invasion from squamous cell carcinoma or other infiltrative
  neoplasm arising in adjacent pharyngeal mucosal or parotid
  space
Non-Hodgkin's lymphoma

RETROPHARYNGEAL SPACE

Contents
  Fat, nodes

Abscess
Reactive adenopathy
  Often normal finding in children
  Upper respiratory infection
  Tonsillitis
Invasion from squamous cell carcinoma arising in pharyngeal
  mucosal space
Nodal metastases
  Pharyngeal squamous cell carcinoma
  Non-Hodgkin's lymphoma

2

PREVERTEBRAL SPACE

Contents
    Muscles (prevertebral, paraspinal, and scalene)
    Brachial plexus roots
    Phrenic nerve
    Vertebrae
    Vertebral arteries

Discitis/osteomyelitis
Metastases
Primary vertebral body tumor

CAROTID SPACE

Contents
    Internal carotid artery
    Internal jugular vein
    Cranial nerves IX, X, XI, XII
    Nodes

Nerve sheath tumor
    Schwannoma
    Neurofibroma
Glomus tumor
    Glomus jugulare
    Carotid body tumor
Meningioma of jugular foramen
Nodal metastases
Vascular pseudotumor
    Asymmetrical or thrombosed jugular vein
    Ectatic carotid artery
    Carotid pseudoaneurysm

PAROTID SPACE

Contents
    Parotid glands
    Intraparotid lymph nodes
    Branches of cranial nerve VII
    External carotid artery

Benign neoplasm
    Pleomorphic adenoma (benign mixed tumor)
    Warthin's tumor
Malignant primary neoplasm
    Mucoepidermoid carcinoma
    Adenoid cystic carcinoma
    Non-Hodgkin's lymphoma
Nodal metastases
    Squamous cell carcinoma
    Non-Hodgkin's lymphoma
    Melanoma
Abscess
Lymphoepithelial cysts (AIDS)
Hemangioma or lymphangioma (children)

General

- Most parotid space lesions present as a lump in the cheek detected by patient
- Mass that is hard on palpation or associated with injury to cranial

2

nerve V or VII likely to be malignant, but absence of these features does not imply benignity

Pleomorphic Adenoma

- Benign epithelial tumor of middle or old age
- Most common parotid neoplasm
- Well demarcated, variably enhancing intraparotid mass
- Hyperintense on T2

Warthin's Tumor

- Benign tumor of middle or old age
- Derived from heterotopic salivary gland tissue within parotid lymph nodes
- Well-demarcated, enhancing, frequently heterogeneous (cystic areas and foci of hemorrhage) intraparotid mass
- 10% bilateral

Malignant Primary Neoplasm

- Infiltrative, enhancing parotid mass
- Small mucoepidermoid carcinomas can be well demarcated, mimicking pleomorphic adenoma

PAROTID LESIONS, MULTIPLE OR BILATERAL

Warthin's tumors
Nodal metastases
   Squamous cell carcinoma
   Non-Hodgkin's lymphoma
   Melanoma
Lymphoepithelial cysts (AIDS)

SUBMANDIBULAR AND SUBLINGUAL SPACE

Contents
   Salivary glands (submandibular and sublingual)
   Mylohyoid muscle
   Anterior tongue
   Nodes
   Branches of cranial nerves V_3, VII, IX, XII

General

What structure separates the submandibular and sublingual spaces?

- Mylohyoid muscle separates submandibular space (inferolateral) from sublingual space (superomedial)

SUBMANDIBULAR SPACE

Malignant neoplasm
   Nodal metastases
Direct invasion from squamous cell carcinoma
   Non-Hodgkin's lymphoma
   Salivary gland neoplasm
Benign neoplasm
   Dermoid or epidermoid
   Cystic hygroma
   Hemangioma

2

Salivary gland neoplasm
Inflammatory
  Abscess
  Lymphadenitis
Second branchial cleft cyst
Thyroglossal duct cyst
Diving ranula

Dermoid or Epidermoid

· Well-demarcated, unilocular, fat- (dermoid) or fluid- (epidermoid) density mass

Cystic Hygroma

· Multilocular cystic mass; can occur in the posterior triangle of the neck, submandibular/sublingual space, or mediastinum
· Presents usually in infancy or early childhood, occasionally in young adults

Second Branchial Cleft Cyst

· Unilocular, congenital cyst anteromedial to sternocleidomastoid muscle at angle of jaw
· May be associated with sinus or fistula tract

Thyroglossal Duct Cyst

· Unilocular, congenital midline cyst near the hyoid bone
· More commonly infrahyoid than suprahyoid

Ranula

What is the difference between a simple ranula and a diving ranula?

· Fluid-density retention cyst of sublingual gland
· Simple ranula is cyst confined to sublingual space
· Diving ranula is cyst that extends posteroinferiorly into the submandibular space

SUBMANDIBULAR SPACE, CYSTIC MASS

Second branchial cleft cyst
Cystic hygroma
Epidermoid or dermoid
Thyroglossal duct cyst
Diving ranula
Abscess or necrotic neoplasm

SUBLINGUAL SPACE

Neoplasm
  Invasive squamous cell carcinoma arising in tongue
  Salivary gland neoplasm
  Dermoid or epidermoid
Inflammatory
  Dilated Wharton's (submandibular gland) duct
  Abscess
    Odontogenic
    Complication of sialadenitis
Dermoid or epidermoid
Ranula
Cystic hygroma

SUBLINGUAL SPACE, CYSTIC MASS

Epidermoid or dermoid
Ranula
Cystic hygroma
Abscess or necrotic neoplasm

INFRAHYOID NECK

The infrahyoid neck is mentioned here for the sake of
    completeness, but many, if not most, of the fine points of
    infrahyoid imaging are beyond the scope of this review. As
    already mentioned, the visceral space is the only space unique
    to the infrahyoid neck; the others (retropharyngeal,
    prevertebral, carotid, posterior cervical) are continuations of
    spaces in the suprahyoid neck.
Pathology that is common in the suprahyoid neck (lymphoma,
    squamous cell carcinoma, neoplastic or inflammatory nodal
    disease, and abscess) is also common in the infrahyoid neck,
    and the imaging appearance is similar in both regions.

VISCERAL SPACE LESION

Contents
    Thyroid and parathyroid glands
    Esophagus
    Larynx and trachea
    Recurrent laryngeal nerve
    Nodes

Neoplasm
    Squamous cell carcinoma of larynx
    Thyroid neoplasm
    Esophageal carcinoma
    Nodal metastases or lymphoma
    Salivary gland neoplasm
    Dermoid or epidermoid
Inflammatory
    Reactive adenopathy
    Abscess
Laryngocele

Figure References

Barkovich AJ. Pediatric Neuroimaging, 2nd ed. New York: Raven Press, 1995.
Osborn AG. Diagnostic Neuroradiology. St. Louis: Mosby–Year Book, 1994.
*The following texts are well illustrated and provide many examples of cases frequently given on the
    ABR oral board examination:*
Castillo M. Neuroradiology Companion: Methods, Guidelines, and Imaging Fundamentals.
    Philadelphia: J.B. Lippincott, 1995.
Grossman RI, Yousem DM. Neuroradiology: The Requisites. St. Louis: Mosby–Year Book,
    1994.
Runge VM. Magnetic Resonance Imaging of the Brain. Philadelphia: J.B. Lippincott, 1994.
Runge VM, Awh MH, et al. Magnetic Resonance Imaging of the Spine. Philadelphia: J.B.
    Lippincott, 1995.
Yock DH. Imaging of CNS Disease: A CT and MR Teaching File, 2nd ed. St. Louis: Mosby,
    1991.
Yock DH. Magnetic Resonance Imaging of CNS Disease: A Teaching File. St. Louis:
    Mosby–Year Book, 1995.

2

NEUROIMAGING DISEASE ENTITIES

TUMORS AND TUMOR-LIKE CONDITIONS

Intraaxial Brain
Extraaxial Brain
     Sellar/suprasellar region
     Pineal region
     Intraventricular
     Miscellaneous
Intramedullary Spine
Extramedullary Intradural Spine
Epidural Spine
Head and Neck
     Paranasal sinuses
     Orbit
     Temporal bone and skull base
     Pharynx

Intraaxial Brain

Astrocytoma

Clinical
- Most common glioma, accounting for about 70% of gliomas (oligodendrogliomas and ependymomas make up most of the rest)
- Can be classified, based on pathological features, as low-grade (most "benign"), anaplastic, or glioblastoma multiforme (most malignant)
- Higher grade astrocytomas tend to occur in older patients

Imaging
- CT and MRI: variable; although high-grade tumors tend to have more heterogeneity, enhancement, mass effect, and vasogenic edema, none of these features necessarily predicts tumor grade

Astrocytoma, Juvenile Pilocytic (JPA)

Clinical
- Subtype of astrocytoma that is a benign, slow-growing, noninvasive tumor that accounts for majority of pediatric astrocytomas
- May be associated with neurofibromatosis type 1
- Common locations: optic chiasm/hypothalamus, cerebellum, brain stem
- Presents in first decade with cerebellar symptoms or with obstructive hydrocephalus resulting from mass effect on fourth ventricle
- Does not undergo transformation to more aggressive astrocytomas

Imaging
- CT and MR: *Posterior fossa JPA* is predominantly cystic, well-demarcated posterior fossa mass, often arising near the midline, with enhancing mural nodule and/or other solid components
- Cyst wall of posterior fossa JPA may or may not enhance; nonenhancement of cyst wall suggests that the cyst is nonneoplastic (in this instance, only solid components need to be resected)
- T2 hyperintensity of a solid infratentorial tumor favors JPA over medulloblastoma (solid JPAs are uncommon, however)

Ependymoma

Clinical
- Second most common glioma
- Most commonly occurs in posterior fossa in children, where it typically grows within fourth ventricle, often extending inferiorly and inferolaterally through the fourth ventricular outlet foramina of Magendie and Luschka
- Posterior fossa tumor presents in early childhood with cerebellar symptoms and obstructive hydrocephalus

- Other locations include supratentorial ventricles and brain parenchyma; ependymomas are also common intramedullary spinal neoplasms

Imaging
- CT: heterogeneous, lobulated posterior fossa mass; moderate, heterogeneous enhancement; cyst formation, calcification, and hemorrhage; obstructive hydrocephalus
- MRI:
  - T1: heterogeneous mass with isointense solid portions; centered in fourth ventricle, often extending into the foramen magnum through fourth ventricular outlet foramina; foci of low signal as result of necrosis or calcification
  - T2: hyperintense solid portions; foci of bright signal result of cyst formation, necrosis, or hemorrhage; foci of low signal result of calcification or hemosiderin
- Tends to spread via CSF; therefore, all newly diagnosed patients should have screening MR of the spine before surgery, because postoperative blood in the CSF can be confused with leptomeningeal spread of tumor
- Supratentorial ependymoma cannot be differentiated from astrocytoma by imaging

Ganglioglioma

Clinical
- Slow growing, usually supratentorial, most common in temporal lobe; associated with good prognosis
- Composed of neuronal and glial elements
- Tumors of this histological type include *ganglioglioma* (glial elements predominate) and *ganglioneuroma* (neuronal elements predominate)
- Presents in childhood or young adulthood with seizures

Imaging
- CT and MR: well-circumscribed, solid or partially cystic mass; focal calcification common; enhancement variable
- Nonenhancing tumor can be confused with neuronal heterotopia; unlike heterotopia, ganglioglioma should not be exactly isointense to gray matter on all three spin-echo sequences

Glioblastoma Multiforme

Clinical
- Most malignant grade of astrocytoma; most common primary brain neoplasm
- Accounts for about half of all intracranial gliomas
- Presents in middle-aged to elderly adults
- Supratentorial
- Frequently enters the contralateral hemisphere via white matter pathways (corpus callosum, anterior commissure, posterior commissure) and spreads via CSF and direct extension to leptomeninges and ependyma
- Aggressive tumor with a very poor prognosis

Imaging
- MRI:
  - T1: isointense, heterogeneous mass showing irregular, heterogeneous enhancement; thickening and enhancement of meninges or ependyma; areas of hypo- and hyperintensity may be present, corresponding to necrosis and hemorrhage, respectively
  - T2: hyperintense mass with extensive surrounding vasogenic edema
- Neither T2 signal abnormality nor contrast enhancement accurately predicts extent of tumor infiltration
- Glioblastoma occasionally presents as "butterfly glioma," a midline mass involving the corpus callosum and medial cerebral hemispheres; primary differential diagnosis is lymphoma

Hemangioblastoma

Clinical
- Most common primary posterior fossa tumor in adults
- Presents in young adulthood or middle age

2

- Symptoms related to posterior fossa mass effect (progressive ataxia and obstructive hydrocephalus at the level of the fourth ventricle)
- Vision disturbance related to associated retinal angiomas (von Hippel-Lindau syndrome)
- Acute presentation can result from obstructive hydrocephalus or hemorrhage
- Majority sporadic, but 15% associated with von Hippel-Lindau syndrome
- Solitary, except in patients with von Hippel-Lindau syndrome
- About half of patients with von Hippel-Lindau syndrome have posterior fossa hemangioblastoma; about half of von Hippel-Lindau patients with hemangioblastoma have multiple tumors
- Although usually occurs in cerebellum, hemangioblastoma also can occur in brain stem and spinal cord

Imaging
- CT and MRI: cystic, well-demarcated posterior fossa mass with enhancing mural nodule that abuts a pial surface; adjacent large vessels; 10% of hemangioblastomas consist of an enhancing pial nodule only (i.e., no associated cystic component)
- Angiography: intense staining of mural nodule; occasional arteriovenous shunting
- Enhancement of cyst wall is not a feature of hemangioblastoma; instead, should suggest astrocytoma, medulloblastoma, or cystic metastasis

Lymphoma

Clinical
- CNS lymphoma may be either primary or metastatic
- Most common histology is B-cell, non-Hodgkin's lymphoma
- Primary CNS lymphoma most common in immunocompromised patients, including AIDS patients and transplant recipients; also occurs in immunocompetent elderly adults
- Presents with neurological deficits resulting from mass effect or leptomeningeal disease
- Very poor prognosis

Imaging
- CT: hyperdense (result of dense cellularity); areas of low-attenuation necrosis common in immunocompromised patients
- MRI:
  - T1: masses abutting ependymal surfaces, often involving periventricular white matter, deep gray nuclei, and corpus callosum; hypointense to isointense; homogeneous enhancement (nonimmunocompromised patients); ring or heterogeneous enhancement (immunocompromised patients); enhancement along ventricular lining represents subependymal spread of tumor
  - T2: isointense to hyperintense
- Primary CNS lymphoma and toxoplasmosis both commonly present in end-stage AIDS patients as multiple ring-enhancing, intraaxial mass lesions; usually cannot be differentiated by imaging, but hemorrhage favors toxoplasmosis, ependymal enhancement favors lymphoma
- Secondary lymphoma may present as either leptomeningeal and ependymal disease (with or without parenchymal metastases) or dural disease

Medulloblastoma

Clinical
- Most common posterior fossa tumor of childhood
- Highly malignant tumor composed of poorly differentiated small, round cells
- Grouped by many pathologists with other primitive neuroectodermal (PNET) tumor
- Peaks at age 4 to 8 years and again in young adulthood
- Presents with nausea, vomiting, headaches, vision disturbance, or gait abnormality
- Childhood tumor is midline lesion that fills part or all of the fourth ventricle and commonly produces obstructive hydrocephalus; adult tumor is more commonly lateral (i.e., in the cerebellar hemisphere)

- Tends to spread via CSF; therefore, all newly diagnosed patients should have a screening MRI of the spine before surgery, because postoperative blood in CSF can be confused with leptomeningeal spread of tumor
- Rare skeletal metastases

Imaging
- CT: Hyperdense, well-demarcated, homogeneously enhancing vermian mass; diffuse enhancement; obstructive hydrocephalus; variable cystic change or partial calcification
- MRI:
  - T1: hypointense; homogeneous enhancement; leptomeningeal and ependymal enhancement may be present as a result of CSF spread
  - T2: isointense to mildly hyperintense

Oligodendroglioma

Clinical
- Well demarcated, supratentorial, hemispheric glial neoplasm
- Accounts for 5 to 10% of intracranial gliomas
- Presents in young to middle-aged adults, often with seizure

Imaging
- CT and MRI: heterogeneous, well-demarcated mass; *calcification* common; variable enhancement

Extraaxial Brain

Sellar/suprasellar region
Pineal region
Intraventricular
Miscellaneous

Sellar/Suprasellar Region

Adenoma, Pituitary

Clinical
- Most common sellar lesion
- Benign neoplasm derived from the anterior pituitary

Imaging
- Optimal evaluation of the pituitary requires four MRI sequences:
  - Sagittal T1
  - Coronal T1
  - Sagittal T1 post-gadolinium
  - Coronal T1 post-gadolinium

Macroadenoma

Clinical
- Mass lesion of more than 10 mm; centered in and expands the sella; extends into suprasellar cistern
- Presents as result of mass effect (usually not hormonally active) on the optic chiasm: bitemporal hemianopsia; diplopia; other visual complaints

Imaging
- MRI modality of choice
- Homogeneous, isointense, or slightly hyperintense mass expanding the sella and extending into the suprasellar cistern
- Homogeneous enhancement
- Can extend laterally into the cavernous sinuses or inferiorly through the bony floor of the sella into the sphenoid sinus
- "Hourglass" shape in the coronal plane caused by narrowing of the tumor waist at the diaphragma sellae
- Cavernous internal carotid artery may be encased, but narrowing or occlusion is rare (this complication is seen more frequently in parasellar meningioma)
- Heterogeneous signal with areas of intrinsic T1 hyperintensity suggests hemorrhage or cyst formation

- *Pituitary apoplexy* is not synonymous with pituitary hemorrhage; it is a clinical syndrome of acute visual disturbance caused by hemorrhage into a macroadenoma and compression of the optic chiasm; this condition is a neurosurgical emergency

Microadenoma

Imaging
- Measures less than 10 mm and typically does not distort sella
- Prolactinoma accounts for the majority; growth hormone- and ACTH-secreting tumors make up most of the rest
- Presents at a relatively small size because of hormonal activity
- Prolactinoma: amenorrhea, galactorrhea, impotence, serum prolactin more than 150 ng/mL
- Growth hormone microadenoma: acromegaly
- ACTH microadenoma: Cushing's syndrome

Imaging
- MRI modality of choice
- Focal, well circumscribed lesion within the pituitary gland
- *Decreased enhancement relative to normal pituitary* immediately after gadolinium administration
- Secondary signs: deviation of the infundibulum away from the lesion; focal convexity of the dorsal surface of the pituitary

Craniopharyngioma

Clinical
- Benign neoplasm derived from epithelial rests along Rathke's cleft; usually centered in the suprasellar region
- Most common childhood suprasellar mass; peak incidence at 5 to 10 years
- Second, late peak occurs at 50 to 60 years
- Presents as result of mass effect (increased intracranial pressure, visual disturbance, diabetes insipidus, pituitary insufficiency)

Imaging
- CT: heterogeneous cystic or cystic and solid suprasellar mass; *cystic components* and *calcifications,* either globular or curvilinear, in 90%
- MRI:

  T1: heterogeneous cystic or cystic and solid mass; solid portions and margins enhance; cystic portion usually hyperintense or isointense; foci of low signal because of calcification

  T2: cystic portion usually hyperintense

Dermoid

Clinical
- Congenital, usually midline tumor that results from inclusion of cutaneous ectodermal elements with neuroectoderm during neural tube closure
- Both dermoid and epidermoid are derived from cutaneous ectoderm; pathological distinction is made by the presence of *dermal appendages* (e.g., hair follicles, sebaceous glands, sweat glands) found in dermoid but not in epidermoid
- Cyst is lined by squamous epithelium and filled with fat and dermal appendages
- Common locations:

  Posterior fossa (fourth ventricle or vermis)

  Suprasellar region

  Lumbosacral spine
- Presents in third decade with symptoms as result of mass effect (e.g., visual disturbances or hydrocephalus in the case of suprasellar tumors)
- Rupture leads to subarachnoid fat (best seen on CT as low attenuation in the subarachnoid spaces) and can present as severe chemical meningitis
- Presence of a nasoethmoidal or occipital dermal sinus tract should be suspected in the setting of midline intracranial dermoid, particularly if evidence of superimposed infection exists

Imaging
- CT: lobulated, heterogeneous midline mass; predominantly fat-attenuation, but can have soft-tissue attenuation components; no enhancement; variable calcification

- MRI: signal characteristics similar to fat (T1 hyperintense, T2 hypointense)

Germinoma (see also Pineal Region)
- Suprasellar region is second most common location of intracranial germinoma (majority occur in pineal region)
- Males and females equally affected (i.e., the marked male predominance seen with pineal germinomas is not seen with suprasellar germinomas)
- Presents commonly with diabetes insipidus
- Other presenting symptoms may be result of pituitary dysfunction (e.g., precocious puberty) or mass effect (visual changes, hydrocephalus)

Imaging
- CT: isodense to hyperdense, well-circumscribed, homogeneously enhancing midline mass centered in the suprasellar/flood of third ventricle region
- MRI:
  - T1: hypointense to isointense, lobulated, homogeneously enhancing, predominantly or entirely solid mass
  - T2: usually hyperintense; T2 hypointensity is unusual in other tumors and should suggest the diagnosis
- Absence of cystic and calcific components helps distinguish germinoma from craniopharyngioma
- Tends to spread via CSF; all newly diagnosed patients should have screening MRI of the spine before surgery, because postoperative blood in the CSF can be confused with leptomeningeal spread of tumor

Glioma, Chiasmatic/Hypothalamic

Clinical
- Site of origin (optic chiasm versus hypothalamus) often impossible to determine, either by imaging or pathology
- Presents with decreased vision or increased intracranial pressure (or both) in young children or, uncommonly, in adults
- Typically aggressive tumor that infiltrates surrounding structures; however, gliomas originating in the optic nerve and involving the chiasm and optic tracts by posterior extension typically are low-grade tumors (often juvenile pilocytic astrocytomas) seen in patients with neurofibromatosis type 1; these are more indolent tumors with a better prognosis
- Increased incidence in *neurofibromatosis type 1* (about 30% of patients have neurofibromatosis type 1)

Imaging
- MRI:
  - T1: hypointense or isointense, lobulated mass centered in the region of the optic chiasm/hypothalamus; heterogeneous enhancement; cystic regions common in large tumors
  - T2: hyperintense

Hamartoma, Tuber Cinereum

Clinical
- Rare, congenital malformation of neural tissue, typically a few millimeters to 2 cm in size, projecting from the tuber cinereum of the hypothalamus into the posterior suprasellar or interpeduncular cistern
- Presents in infancy or early childhood with *precocious puberty,* seizures, or both
- Does not enlarge or invade adjacent structures

Imaging
- MRI:
  - T1: isointense, well-demarcated mass between the infundibulum and mamillary bodies; no enhancement
  - T2: isointense

Rathke's Cleft Cyst

Clinical
- Congenital cyst derived from epithelial remnants of Rathke's cleft, the embryologic precursor of pars intermedia of anterior pituitary
- Usually an incidental finding and asymptomatic

• Majority centrally located within the sella or suprasellar region

Imaging
• MRI:
> T1: smooth-margined intrasellar or intrasellar/suprasellar cyst; isointense to hyperintense, depending on cyst contents; no enhancement
> T2: hypointense to isointense, depending on cyst contents
• Intrasellar location and absence of enhancement help in differentiation from craniopharyngioma

Pineal Region

Germinoma (see also Sellar/Suprasellar Region)

Clinical
• Most common pineal region mass, accounting for about half of all pineal region masses
• Most common of a number of germ cell tumors (including teratoma, choriocarcinoma, endodermal sinus tumor, embryonal carcinoma) that occur in the pineal and suprasellar regions
• Pineal region is the most common location of intracranial germinoma
• Marked male predominance (90%) with *pineal* region germinomas is not seen with germinomas in other locations (e.g., suprasellar germinoma)
• Presents in older children or young adults with endocrine abnormalities (precocious puberty, diabetes insipidus), hydrocephalus caused by aqueductal compression, and/or Parinaud's syndrome (upward gaze palsy, failure of convergence, and dissociation of light and accommodation responses)

Imaging
• CT: hyperdense, well-demarcated mass; marked homogeneous enhancement
• MRI:
> T1: hypointense; leptomeningeal and ependymal enhancement caused by CSF spread of tumor can occur anywhere, but particularly common in the recesses of the third ventricle; local parenchymal invasion may occur
> T2: isointense to hyperintense
• Spread via CSF is common; all newly diagnosed patients should have screening MRI of the spine before surgery, because postoperative blood in the CSF can be confused with leptomeningeal spread of tumor
• Calcified pineal mass in a male is most likely germinoma; in a female, pineocytoma

Pineal Cyst

Clinical
• Common pineal region lesion ranging in size from a few millimeters to several centimeters
• Usually asymptomatic, even when large enough to exert mass effect on the dorsal midbrain
• Asymptomatic lesion with the characteristic imaging features of pineal cyst can be followed or dismissed as an incidental finding

Imaging
• MRI:
> T1: round, smoothly marginated, homogeneous hypointense pineal mass; cyst wall may show thin rim of enhancement
> T2: hyperintense

Pineoblastoma

Clinical
• Together with pineocytoma, accounts for about 15% of pineal region masses
• Malignant tumor of young children, made up of poorly differentiated pineal gland cells
• Similar histologically to primitive neuroectodermal tumors (e.g., medulloblastoma)
• Rare, inherited variant associated with unilateral or bilateral retinoblastoma(s) sometimes referred to as *trilateral retinoblastoma*

Imaging
- CT and MRI: large, lobulated mass, often with parenchymal invasion; heterogeneous enhancement; leptomeningeal and ependymal enhancement result of CSF spread of tumor
- As with germinomas, spread via CSF is common; all newly diagnosed patients should have screening MRI of the spine before surgery, because postoperative blood in CSF can be confused with leptomeningeal spread of tumor

Pineocytoma

Clinical
- Together with pineoblastoma, accounts for about 15% of pineal region masses
- Benign, slow-growing tumor of young adults, derived from pineal gland cells

Imaging
- CT and MRI: imaging features nonspecific; when small, can resemble pineal cyst; when large, can resemble germinoma or pineoblastoma

Intraventricular
Choroid Plexus Papilloma

Clinical
- Rare, benign intraventricular neoplasm derived from choroid plexus epithelium
- Majority are tumors of early childhood or infancy, occurring in the atrium or body of the lateral ventricle
- Rare, adult tumor occurs more commonly in the fourth ventricle
- Presents with communicating *hydrocephalus*, thought to be caused by CSF overproduction, arachnoiditis (as result of repeated low-level hemorrhage into the ventricles), or both

Imaging
- CT: predominantly isodense intraventricular mass; intense, homogeneous enhancement; calcification occasionally present; hydrocephalus
- MRI:
    - T1: well-demarcated, isointense, intraventricular mass; irregular, frond-like margins; asymmetrical, communicating hydrocephalus; blood products and vascular flow voids occasionally present
    - T2: isointense
- Imaging features that intuitively might be associated with malignancy (e.g., local parenchymal invasion or metastases via CSF pathways) cannot reliably differentiate choroid plexus papilloma from the much rarer choroid plexus carcinoma

Colloid Cyst

Clinical
- Rare, benign congenital cyst that arises from primitive epithelium
- Located in the anterosuperior third ventricle at the foramina of Monro
- Ranges in size from a few mm to several cm
- Enlarges slowly, usually presenting in adulthood with postural headaches caused by intermittent obstructive hydrocephalus

Imaging
- CT: round, smoothly marginated mass in anterosuperior third ventricle; isodense to hyperdense; rim may be enhanced
- MRI: Two signal patterns have been described:
    - *T1 hyperintense, T2 hypointense*: may be result of cholesterol or metal ions within the cyst; cysts with these MRI characteristics often have high attenuation on CT
    - *T1 isointense, T2 hyperintense* (similar to CSF): cysts with these MRI characteristics often have low attenuation on CT

Neurocytoma

Clinical
- Benign, slow-growing tumor of adulthood
- Located in the body of the lateral ventricle

Imaging
- CT: well-demarcated, isodense, mildly heterogeneous mass; variable mild, heterogeneous enhancement; low attenuation foci representing cystic components
- MRI:
    T1: isointense; variable mild enhancement
    T2: isointense to mildly hyperintense

Miscellaneous

Arachnoid Cyst

Clinical
- Congenital, thin-walled, extraaxial cyst containing CSF
- Common locations: middle cranial fossa, sylvian fissure, suprasellar cistern, quadrigeminal plate cistern, cerebellopontine angle, superior cerebellar cistern
- Presents with symptoms related to local mass effect

Imaging
- CT: smooth-bordered, extraaxial mass; homogeneous and isodense to CSF; no enhancement; variable smooth erosion of adjacent calvarium
- MRI:
    T1: isointense to CSF; displacement of vessels and nerves
    T2: isointense to CSF; proton density isointense or hyperintense to CSF
- Diffusion-weighted MRI may help differentiate arachnoid cyst from epidermoid (which may appear identical to arachnoid cyst on routine spin-echo sequences)

Dermoid

Clinical
- Congenital, benign, cystic tumor that results from inclusion of ectodermal elements and dermal appendages during neural tube closure
- Intracranial dermoids are much less common than epidermoids
- Cyst is lined by squamous epithelium and contains liquid fatty material
- Presents in early to middle adulthood
- May rupture into subarachnoid space or ventricles, causing chemical meningitis
- Most common location is the lumbosacral spine, where the cyst is often associated with a dermal sinus tract
- Common intracranial locations include the suprasellar/parasellar region, posterior fossa midline (fourth ventricle, cisterna magna), lateral and third ventricles

Imaging
- CT: extraaxial, heterogeneous, lobulated midline mass; focal areas of fat, calcification, or bone; no enhancement; very low (fat) attenuation in the subarachnoid spaces and/or fat/fluid levels in the ventricles if rupture has occurred
- MRI: imaging features reflect fat content
    T1: hyperintense; foci of low signal on T1 and T2 images result of calcification
    T2: hypointense

Epidermoid

Clinical
- Congenital tumor that results from inclusion of cutaneous ectodermal elements (but not dermal appendages) with neuroectoderm during neural tube closure
- Both dermoid and epidermoid are derived from cutaneous ectoderm; pathologic distinction is made by the presence of *dermal appendages* (e.g., hair follicles, sebaceous glands, sweat glands) found in dermoid but not in epidermoid
- Cyst is lined by squamous epithelium and filled with keratin and cholesterol
- Presents in early adulthood with symptoms caused by mass effect (e.g., hydrocephalus, cranial neuropathies)
- Common locations: cerebellopontine angle; suprasellar region; pineal region; middle cranial fossa; calvarium

Imaging
- Imaging usually cannot differentiate epidermoid from arachnoid cyst; diffusion-weighted MRI may be helpful in distinguishing between them

- CT and MRI: attenuation and signal characteristics similar to those of arachnoid cyst; encasement of vessels and nerves

Meningioma

Clinical
- Most common extraaxial mass lesion and most common nonglial primary brain tumor
- Majority are benign
- Derived in most cases from arachnoid meningothelial cells
- More common in women than in men (2:1)
- Multiple meningiomas and childhood meningiomas are seen in patients with neurofibromatosis type 2
- Symptomatic tumors present in middle-aged and elderly patients (except in patients with neurofibromatosis type 2) as result of mass effect and occasionally because of vascular encasement and narrowing
- Common locations: parasagittal (falcine); hemispheric convexities; sphenoid wing; olfactory groove; suprasellar/parasellar region; cerebellopontine angle; tentorium; atrium of lateral ventricle

Imaging
- CT: homogeneous, hyperdense, well-demarcated extraaxial mass lesion; intense, homogeneous enhancement; occasional thin layer of dural enhancement ("dural tail") extending away from the tumor; variable surrounding low attenuation caused by vasogenic edema (50%); hyperostosis or "blistering" of adjacent bone (5%); calcifications (20%) and small cysts (20%)
- MRI:
  - T1: isointense, homogeneous, extraaxial mass; lobular or flat ("en plaque") morphology; CSF cleft demarcating tumor from underlying brain; foci of very low signal on T1 and T2 images may represent calcifications or flow voids due to tumor vascularity
  - T2: isointense to mildly hyperintense; variable surrounding hyperintense signal as a result of vasogenic edema
- Angiography: supply from meningeal branches of the external carotid artery with variable pial supply from the internal carotid artery circulation; early, prolonged vascular blush ("mother-in-law" sign)
- Nonspecific features suggestive of the diagnosis include enhancing, thickened dura at the margins of a lesion ("dural tail"); hyperostosis of adjacent bone; encasement and narrowing of vessels (rather than displacement)
- Imaging cannot distinguish benign from malignant meningiomas

Schwannoma

Clinical
- Benign, encapsulated, slow-growing nerve sheath tumor derived from Schwann cells
- Solitary lesion of older adults except in patients with neurofibromatosis type 2, who may have multiple schwannomas in young adulthood
- Presents with cranial neuropathies (e.g., sensorineural hearing loss associated with a vestibular schwannoma, facial pain and numbness associated with a trigeminal schwannoma) early; and symptoms resulting from mass effect (obstructive hydrocephalus, brain stem compression) later
- Common intracranial locations: cerebellopontine angle and/or internal auditory canal (IAC) (90%) (vestibular division of vestibulocochlear nerve, cranial nerve VIII); prepontine cistern/cavernous sinus (5%) (trigeminal nerve, cranial nerve V)
- Most common cerebellopontine angle mass, accounting for 80% of the masses in this region
- Malignant transformation rare

Imaging
- CT: isodense, homogeneous or heterogeneous, well-demarcated extraaxial mass; intense enhancement of solid portions; foci of low attenuation, representing cystic change within the tumor or loculated CSF collections; widening of the internal auditory canal on bone windows (vestibular schwannoma); atrophy of muscles of mastication (trigeminal schwannoma)

- MRI:
    T1: isointense; homogeneous, intense enhancement
    T2: hyperintense; foci of bright signal representing cysts
- Bilateral vestibular schwannomas pathognomonic of neurofibromatosis type 2
- *Cerebellopontine angle tumor:* tumor heterogeneity, extension of tumor into internal auditory canal, acute angles with petrous bone, and clinical history of progressive sensorineural hearing loss favor vestibular schwannoma over meningioma

Intramedullary Spine

Astrocytoma

Clinical
- Most common intramedullary tumor in children; second most common in adults

Imaging
- MRI:
    T1: localized fusiform expansion of cord, possibly with associated cysts; hypo-intense or isointense; enhancement often more irregular than that seen with ependymoma
    T2: hyperintense tumor with surrounding hyperintense vasogenic edema

Ependymoma

Clinical
- Most common intramedullary tumor in adults; second most common in children
- Most common primary tumor of the conus medullaris and filum
- Presents in middle age (i.e., later than intracranial ependymoma) with back and leg pain and mild neurological deficits

Imaging
- MRI:
    T1: localized fusiform expansion of cord, possibly with associated cysts; hypo-intense or isointense; heterogeneous or homogeneous enhancement, often with well-demarcated superior or inferior border
    T2: hyperintense tumor with surrounding hyperintense vasogenic edema
- Ependymomas, especially the myxopapillary subtype, have a propensity to bleed and can occasionally present as an unexplained communicating hydrocephalus

Hemangioblastoma (see also Intraaxial Brain Neoplasms)

Clinical
- Uncommon spinal cord tumor
- Majority are solitary; multiple tumors occur in association with cerebellar hemangi-oblastomas in von Hippel-Lindau syndrome
- Presents in young adulthood
- Usually intramedullary (60%), but can be extramedullary, intradural or, very rarely, extradural

Imaging
- MRI: intramedullary mass, often cystic; densely enhancing tumor nodule; extensive surrounding vasogenic edema; variable flow voids caused by enlarged feeding arteries or draining veins
- Angiography: dense tumor blush; enlarged draining veins

Metastases, Spinal Cord

Clinical
- Intramedullary metastatic lesions are rare; much less common than either epidural or leptomeningeal metastatic disease
- Primaries include lung, breast, melanoma, lymphoma, and leukemia

Imaging
- MRI:
    T1: hypointense lesion(s); focal cord expansion; ring enhancement
    T2: hyperintense lesion; surrounding hyperintense vasogenic edema

Syringohydromyelia

Clinical
- Fusiform cavitation of the spinal cord
- Differentiation between syringomyelia (eccentric, fusiform cavitation of the cord) and hydromyelia (dilatation of the central canal) difficult and not clinically important
- Multiple possible causes: intramedullary neoplasm; Chiari I or II malformation; trauma; arachnoiditis
- Presents with pain, dissociated sensory deficit (preserved touch; loss of pain and temperature sensation), weakness, and limb atrophy
- Posttraumatic syrinx often presents years after spinal trauma

Imaging
- MRI: fusiform intramedullary lesion on sagittal images; isointense to CSF on both T1 and T2; cord can be expanded, normal in caliber, or atrophic; certain imaging findings can suggest cause of syrinx:
    - Contrast-enhancing lesion suggests neoplasm
    - Cerebellar tonsillar ectopia suggests Chiari I malformation
    - Arachnoid loculations in the thecal sac suggest prior arachnoiditis
- As part of the evaluation of unexplained syrinx:
    - Contrast-enhanced images should always be obtained to rule out intramedullary neoplasm
    - Region of the foramen magnum should be evaluated to rule out Chiari I malformation or mass lesion interfering with CSF flow

Extramedullary Intradural Spine

Dermoid and Epidermoid *(see also Suprasellar)*

Clinical
- Congenital cystic tumors that result from inclusion of cutaneous ectodermal elements with neuroectoderm during neural tube closure
- Presence of dermal appendages (e.g., hair follicles and sweat glands) distinguishes dermoid from epidermoid
- Epidermoid can, rarely, be acquired via implantation of cutaneous ectoderm into thecal sac during lumbar puncture
- Presents in children or young adults with symptoms related to cord tethering (progressive lower extremity weakness/spasticity and bowel and bladder symptoms)
- Most common in lumbosacral region
- Extramedullary intradural (50%) or intramedullary (50%)
- May be associated with spinal dysraphism and dermal sinus tract (20%)

Imaging
- CT and MRI: variable appearance; dermoid often follows fat in attenuation and signal, epidermoid often follows CSF; no enhancement; associated spinal dysraphism and vertebral segmentation anomalies

Meningioma, Spinal Canal

Clinical
- Most common extramedullary intradural mass
- Usually solitary and extramedullary intradural; a small percentage have both intradural and extradural components or are exclusively extradural
- Presents in middle age with pain and radiculopathy
- Female predominance (4:1)
- Most commonly involves thoracic spine (80%)

Imaging
- MRI:
    - T1: isointense; dense, homogeneous enhancement
    - T2: isointense
- The most common differential diagnosis of a homogenously enhancing intradural, extramedullary mass is meningioma versus nerve sheath tumor (schwannoma or neurofibroma)

Metastases, Leptomeningeal

Clinical
- Leptomeningeal enhancement along the cord surface or nodular, enhancing extra-medullary intradural foci (or both)
- Most common in the lumbosacral thecal sac
- Can result from CSF spread of either a primary CNS neoplasm (e.g., glioblastoma, ependymoma, medulloblastoma, germ cell tumor, pineoblastoma) or seeding of the CSF by a primary tumor outside the CNS ("leptomeningeal carcinomatosis") (e.g., lung, breast, melanoma, lymphoma)

Imaging
- MRI:
    - T1: contrast-enhanced T1 images are most sensitive for detection of leptomeningeal metastatic disease; nodular isointense thickening of cauda equina roots; enhancement along the cord surface or within tumor along the cauda equina roots; heterogeneously increased signal within the CSF in advanced disease
    - T2: nodular thickening of cauda equina roots; much less sensitive than contrast-enhanced T1 images
- Normal MRI examination does not exclude CSF spread of tumor; correlation with CSF cytology is important if clinical suspicion of leptomeningeal carcinomatosis exists

Neurofibroma

Clinical
- Benign nerve sheath tumor composed of Schwann cells and fibroblasts that is inseparable from nerve of origin
- Usually multiple and in patients with neurofibromatosis type 1 (solitary, sporadic neurofibromas uncommon)

Imaging
- MRI: imaging characteristics similar to those of schwannoma

Schwannoma

Clinical
- Benign nerve sheath tumor composed of Schwann cells that arises extrinsic to the nerve of origin (i.e., can be dissected away from the nerve)
- Much more common than neurofibroma in the setting of a solitary extramedullary, intradural mass
- Usually solitary and extramedullary intradural; small percentage have both intra-dural and extradural components or are exclusively extradural
- Presents in adulthood with pain and radiculopathy
- Multiple tumors are seen in neurofibromatosis type 2

Imaging
- MRI:
    - T1: isointense, lobulated mass; dense, homogenous enhancement; hemorrhage, cyst formation, and heterogeneous enhancement can occur; "dumbbell" mor-phology, with extension through and widening of the ipsilateral vertebral foramen
    - T2: hyperintense; variable central focus of hypointensity
- Malignant degeneration uncommon

Epidural Spine

Metastases

Clinical
- Epidural compartment is most frequent site of metastatic disease that involves the spine
- Usually represents local extension of bone metastasis that involves vertebral bodies or posterior elements

Imaging
- MRI:
    - T1: foci of low signal in multiple vertebrae; enhancing epidural tissue impress-

ing on the thecal sac; cord compression can occur as result of epidural metastatic disease or pathologic vertebral body collapse with posterior displacement of bone fragments into the spinal canal

T2: effacement of thecal sac; variable hyperintense cord signal at sites of cord compression

Head and Neck

Paranasal sinuses
Orbit
Temporal bone and skull base
Pharynx

Paranasal Sinuses

Screening CT of the sinuses, performed in the coronal plane with 3-mm collimation, is an appropriate first examination in the patient with suspected paranasal sinus pathology. If the patient is unable to maintain the position necessary for direct coronal imaging, axial CT images with 1- or 3-mm collimation should be performed; coronal images can be reconstructed from the axial data set. Contrast is not used routinely for screening examinations but can be helpful if evidence exists of neoplastic disease or complicated inflammatory disease.

MRI is helpful in further characterizing a mass lesion identified on CT. Although the imaging characteristics of most paranasal sinus masses are nonspecific, making it very difficult to distinguish inflammatory from neoplastic disease, the following features, when present, suggest neoplasm: intermediate signal intensity on T2 (inflammatory paranasal sinus disease is usually hyperintense on T2), destruction of bone, intracranial extension, or extension into surrounding soft tissue.

Angiofibroma, Juvenile

Clinical
- Rare, benign, locally aggressive, highly vascular tumor of adolescent males, centered in the posterior nasal cavity, nasopharynx, or pterygopalatine fossa
- Presents with epistaxis or nasal obstruction

Imaging
- CT: homogeneous, densely enhancing mass; expansion of the pterygopalatine fossa; destruction or remodeling of adjacent bone; can extend into the sphenoid sinus, infratemporal fossa (via pterygomaxillary fissure), orbit (via inferior orbital fissure), or middle cranial fossa (via superior orbital fissure)
- MRI:
    T1: isointense; variable rounded foci of low signal corresponding to flow voids; marked, homogeneous enhancement
    T2: hyperintense
- Angiography: enlarged, feeding arteries, usually branches of the internal maxillary artery; embolization may be used as a temporizing measure in patients with severe epistaxis and preoperatively to minimize blood loss at surgery

Inverted Papilloma

Clinical
- Mass abutting superolateral nasal wall and centered at the hiatus semilunaris
- Nasal epithelium inverts and grows into underlying mucosa
- Risk of malignant degeneration to squamous cell carcinoma

Imaging
- MRI:
    T1: unilateral, isointense mass against the superolateral nasal wall; centered near the hiatus semilunaris; moderate enhancement
    T2: intermediate intensity

Mucocele

Clinical
- Expansile paranasal sinus mass occurs as a result of obstruction of sinus drainage and accumulation of mucus

- Presents with headache; displacement of the globe also may be present with frontoethmoidal mucoceles
- Most common in frontal sinuses (frontal sinus affected more often than ethmoid, which is affected more often than maxillary; sphenoid least often affected)

Imaging
- Two common imaging patterns:
    Inspissated mucus
        CT: high attenuation, nonenhancing, expansile paranasal sinus mass
        MRI: T1 hypointense, T2 hypointense
    Hydrated mucus
        CT: low to intermediate attenuation
        MRI: T1 isointense to hyperintense, T2 hyperintense

Polyposis, Sinonasal

Clinical
- Hyperplastic mucosa acquired as result of chronic allergic sinusitis (adults) or cystic fibrosis (children)
- Presents with chronic sinusitis and history of allergies

Imaging
- CT and MRI: multiple round and ovoid soft tissue masses filling the paranasal sinuses; high attenuation on CT; heterogeneous signal on MRI; thinning of sinus walls; occasional erosion of the skull base, mimicking aggressive neoplasm

Orbit
Hemangioma

Cavernous Hemangioma

Clinical
- Benign, encapsulated orbital tumor of adulthood
- Most common vascular orbital mass in adults
- Presents with progressive, painless proptosis

Imaging
- CT: well-demarcated, lobular, intraconal mass; hyperdense; intense, homogeneous enhancement; variable extraconal components; calcified phleboliths
- MRI:
    T1: isointense; blood products
    T2: hyperintense

Capillary Hemangioma

Clinical
- Benign, nonencapsulated orbital/periorbital tumor of infancy
- Most common orbital mass in neonates and infants
- Presents with proptosis or periorbital skin discoloration in the first weeks of life
- Increases in size during the first year, then gradually involutes

Imaging
- CT: isodense; intense enhancement
- MRI:
    T1: fairly well-demarcated isointense mass involving orbital or periorbital tissues
    T2: hyperintense

Lymphangioma

Clinical
- Benign, nonencapsulated, orbital/periorbital tumor of childhood
- Most common orbital mass in children (aged 1 to 15 years)
- Presents with slowly progressive proptosis, possibly exacerbated by hemorrhage

Imaging
- MRI:
    T1: heterogeneous infiltrative mass involving lids, conjunctivae, and/or intraconal tissue; foci of high signal because of methemoglobin; cystic spaces with fluid-fluid levels; moderate enhancement

2

T2: hyperintense

Melanoma, Uveal

Clinical
- Primary, unilateral, malignant neoplasm arising in the uvea (choroid, ciliary body, and iris), the vascular layer between the sclera and retina
- Metastases to brain and viscera

Imaging
- CT: hyperdense, well-demarcated intraocular mass; moderate, homogeneous enhancement
- MRI:
  T1: hyperintense, lobular intraocular mass; variable associated retinal detachment; subretinal fluid demarcated anteriorly by V-shaped sensory layer of retina, with apex of the V at optic disc; invasion of sclera or retrobulbar tissue
  T2: hypointense
- Main differential diagnosis is uveal metastasis or hemangioma; intrinsic T1 hyperintensity of melanoma is most helpful distinguishing feature
- Metastases from mucinous adenocarcinoma may be hyperintense on T1, mimicking typical uveal melanoma
- Amelanotic melanoma may be isointense on T1, mimicking typical metastasis

Neurofibroma, Plexiform

Clinical
- Transspatial, infiltrative mass always associated with neurofibromatosis type 1
- Intracranial extension occurs along the course of cranial nerves
- Malignant transformation in 10%

Imaging
- CT: isodense; erosion of skull base
- MRI:
  T1: isointense; variable enhancement
  T2: hyperintense

Optic Nerve Glioma

Clinical
- Most commonly low-grade, slow-growing astrocytoma (juvenile pilocytic astrocytoma) of early childhood, often in children with neurofibromatosis type 1, that causes diffuse optic nerve enlargement
- Optic gliomas presenting in adulthood rare and more aggressive
- Presents with loss of visual acuity and proptosis
- Tends to spread retrograde to the chiasm, optic tracts, and optic radiations

Imaging
- CT: fusiform or globular optic nerve enlargement; isodense to brain; no calcification
- MRI:
  T1: fusiform, isointense optic nerve enlargement; kinking of the optic nerve (best seen in sagittal or oblique sagittal plane); homogeneous enhancement
  T2: hyperintense; high signal along paths of intracranial spread (chiasm, optic tracts, optic radiations)
- Bilateral optic nerve gliomas pathognomonic of neurofibromatosis type 1

Optic Nerve Sheath Meningioma

Clinical
- Benign neoplasm histologically identical to intracranial meningiomas, arising from arachnoid of optic nerve sheath
- Presents in middle age with progressive vision loss and papilledema

Imaging
- CT: hyperdense mass growing along optic nerve; variable morphology:
  Fusiform enlargement of optic nerve sheath complex, resulting from circumferential growth of tumor
  Lobular mass displacing the optic nerve, resulting from eccentric growth of

tumor; linear or globular calcification; dense, homogeneous enhancement of tumor

"Tram-track" pattern of enhancement refers to enhancing tubular tumor surrounding nonenhancing optic nerve

- MRI: T1 images with fat saturation and gadolinium enhancement best demonstrate intracranial extension through the optic canal

T1: isointense tumor surrounding or abutting optic nerve

T2: isointense

Retinoblastoma

Clinical

- Malignant neoplasm derived from retinal neuroectoderm
- Most common globe lesion of infants; almost always presents before age 3 years
- Bilateral in 30%; small percentage of bilateral tumors associated with pineal region tumor ("trilateral retinoblastoma")
- Presents in infancy with leukokoria (white pupillary reflex), strabismus, vision loss, glaucoma
- Pathways of spread include direct invasion of retrobulbar tissues and leptomeningeal spread by extension to the CSF space in the optic nerve sheath

Imaging

- Performed to confirm diagnosis, evaluate contralateral globe, and determine extent of tumor spread
- CT: initial examination of choice because of its sensitivity for calcification; unilateral or bilateral retinal calcifications (>90%); enhancement; variable morphology:

Lobular mass extending through the retina into the vitreous

Focal thickening of the posterior globe wall with associated progressive retinal detachment

Plaque-like growth along the globe wall

- *Calcified mass in the globe of an infant or young child is a retinoblastoma until proven otherwise*
- Radiation-induced neoplasm, especially sarcoma, a delayed complication that appears years after therapy
- Other lesions that present with leukokoria have clinical and imaging features that usually allow differentiation from retinoblastoma:

Retinopathy of prematurity (retrolental fibroplasia)

Calcification is rare

History of premature birth requiring prolonged ventilator support

Microphthalmia in end stage

Sclerosing endophthalmitis (granulomatous infection with *Toxocara cani*, found in dog excrement)

No calcification

Dense vitreous is most common CT appearance

Focal mass is rare

Coats's disease (retinal telangiectasias)

No calcification

Presents after age 3 years

Persistent hyperplastic primary vitreous (persistence of vascular embryonic tissue in the vitreous)

Calcification is rare

Microphthalmia

Temporal Bone and Skull Base
Cholesteatoma, Acquired

Clinical

- Middle ear soft tissue debris surrounded by stratified squamous epithelium and capable of aggressive bone destruction
- Presents with conductive hearing loss or other complications; history of chronic otitis media is common
- Complications related to aggressive bone erosion: conductive hearing loss; labyrinthine fistula; facial nerve palsy; meningitis, subdural empyema, brain abscess; dural venous sinus thrombosis

2

Imaging
- High-resolution CT of the temporal bone in the coronal and axial planes essential for diagnosis; contrast not necessary
- MRI not necessary routinely in uncomplicated cholesteatoma, but may be helpful in advanced cases with extensive temporal bone destruction and suspected intracranial complications
- CT: homogeneous soft tissue mass arising in Prussak's space (epitympanic recess between the neck of the malleus and the scutum) or the facial nerve recess; either the scutum (superior bony attachment of the tympanic membrane) or the auditory ossicles eroded
- Bone erosion (scutum and auditory ossicles) and absence of contrast enhancement support the diagnosis of cholesteatoma over postinflammatory granulation tissue

Cholesterol Granuloma

Clinical
- Acquired, slowly expansile, cystic lesion of the petrous apex, filled with cellular debris and blood breakdown products from recurrent hemorrhage
- In most cases, probably caused by repeated inflammatory disease (petrous apicitis) and poor drainage of petrous air cells
- Presents with variable cranial neuropathies caused by local mass effect; cranial nerves VI and VII most commonly affected

Imaging
- CT: well-demarcated, expansile lesion of the petrous apex; no enhancement or thin rim of enhancement
- MRI:
  - T1: hyperintense
  - T2: hyperintense; hypointense foci may be seen as result of hemosiderin
- Only lesion of petrous apex that tends to be hyperintense on T1; this feature a helpful differentiating point between cholesterol granuloma and congenital cholesteatoma of the petrous apex

Chondrosarcoma

Clinical
- Slow-growing, malignant tumor that, in the head and neck, often originates at the skull base
- Derived from cartilage or endochondral bone

Imaging
- CT: destructive skull base mass, usually centered off the midline at the petrooccipital suture; chondroid calcifications
- MRI:
  - T1: hypointense; heterogeneity of signal on T1 and T2 is the result of calcifications; heterogeneous enhancement
  - T2: hyperintense

Chordoma

Clinical
- Tumor of notochordal (and therefore midline) tissue, most common in sacrum (50%) and clivus (35%); 15% vertebral (C2–C4 most common)
- Slow-growing but locally aggressive tumor with very high recurrence rate after therapy
- Clivus chordoma peaks at 20 to 40 years of age
- Clivus chordoma usually a bulky mass that can directly invade both anterior nasopharynx and middle and posterior cranial fossas; its appearance may be mimicked by chondrosarcoma and other destructive skull-base lesions
- Chondrosarcoma usually arises laterally in region of petrooccipital fissure, a helpful differentiating feature from chordoma, which usually arises in the midline

Imaging
- CT: destructive midline skull-base lesion; isodense to brain; bone fragments or calcification; moderate, heterogeneous enhancement
- MRI:
  - T1: isointense; foci of low signal on T1 and T2 because of calcification or bone fragments

2

T2: hyperintense

Esthesioneuroblastoma

Clinical
- Malignant tumor that arises in the olfactory mucosa in the upper nasal cavity
- Derived from olfactory sensory cells and also known as *olfactory neuroblastoma*
- Peak incidence in young adults

Imaging
- CT and MRI: expansile, heterogeneously enhancing mass centered near the cribriform plate; may be confined to nasal cavity, involve nasal cavity and paranasal sinuses, or extend intracranially through cribriform plate
- Even if the mass appears confined to the upper nasal cavity, involvement of both sides of cribriform plate must be presumed

Glomus Jugulare Tumor (Paraganglioma, Chemodectoma)

Clinical
- Most common tumor of jugular foramen, accounting for 80% of jugular foramen masses
- One of a group of histologically identical tumors that arise from chemoreceptor cells in the neck and skull base
- Multiple in small percentage of patients
- Glomus tumors named according to location:

Jugular foramen	glomus jugulare
Jugular foramen with extension into middle ear	glomus jugulotympanicum
Middle ear	glomus tympanicum
Carotid bifurcation	carotid body tumor
Vagus nerve	glomus vagale

- Glomus jugulare/jugulotympanicum presents with pulsatile tinnitus, conductive hearing loss, cranial neuropathies (e.g., hoarseness, dysphagia, facial paralysis); cranial nerves IX, X, and XI, which exit skull base through jugular foramen, are most commonly affected; large tumors can also affect cranial nerve VII because of destruction of the mastoid bone and cranial nerve XII as result of extension of mass to hypoglossal canal

Imaging
- CT: mass centered in jugular foramen; erosion of jugular foramen and jugular spine; intense, homogeneous enhancement
- MRI:
    T1: isointense; small flow voids and small foci of hyperintense signal (presumably foci of hemorrhage) account for the classic "salt-and-pepper" appearance on T1 images
    T2: hyperintense
- MR venography: helpful to assess patency of ipsilateral jugular vein
- Angiography: may be performed if preoperative embolization is contemplated; dense tumor blush
- Prominent flow voids favor paraganglioma over meningioma or schwannoma (other common lesions that occur in jugular foramen)

Glomus Tympanicum

Clinical
- Presents with pulsatile tinnitus and a vascular retrotympanic mass at otoscopy

Imaging
- CT: rounded, enhancing soft tissue in the middle ear, arising near the cochlear promontory
- MRI: usually not required if the diagnosis of glomus tympanicum is clear-cut; may be helpful in confusing cases if there is suggestion of tumor extension into the region of the jugular foramen; signal characteristics similar to those of other glomus tumors

Rhabdomyosarcoma

Clinical
- Most common primary pediatric neoplasm to involve central skull base
- Sites of origin in head and neck include orbit, nasopharynx, nasal cavity, and paranasal sinuses

Imaging
- CT: bulky, destructive soft tissue mass
- MRI:
    T1: isointense; enhancement; perineural spread can occur
    T2: hyperintense

Pharynx
Carcinoma, Nasopharyngeal

Clinical
- Most common primary neoplasm to involve the central skull base
- 85% squamous cell, 15% adenocarcinoma
- Higher prevalence in Asian populations
- Originates in mucosa in or near the fossa of Rosenmüller (cartilaginous eustachian tube orifice) and therefore commonly produces early eustachian tube obstruction and mastoiditis (i.e., in the absence of a large mass)
- Clinical presentation varies, depending on tumor size and extent, ranging from mastoiditis in early disease to cranial neuropathy and ischemic brain injury caused by carotid encasement
- Intracranial extension can occur via direct invasion through bone or perineural spread (usually through foramen ovale along branches of trigeminal nerve)

Imaging
- CT: allows optimal characterization of bone destruction
- MRI: allows optimal characterization of the extent of disease, including intracranial extension and perineural spread
    T1: isointense mass centered in nasopharynx and central skull base; homogeneous enhancement; initial lymphatic spread to lateral retropharyngeal node; perineural spread along trigeminal nerve best visualized on coronal T1 and coronal T1 post-gadolinium with fat saturation as nerve thickening and enhancement
    T2: hyperintense; atrophy of the muscles of mastication (decreased size and high T2 signal) a clue to presence of perineural tumor spread along trigeminal nerve
- *Unilateral serous otomastoiditis should always prompt a careful evaluation of the ipsilateral nasopharynx to rule out early nasopharyngeal carcinoma*

INFLAMMATORY DISEASE

Brain
Spine
Head and Neck

Brain

Abscess, Parenchymal

Clinical
- Round or ovoid, encapsulated collection of pus
- Pyogenic abscesses most common, but fungal and mycobacterial abscesses not rare
- Causes:
    Direct spread of infection (via septic thrombophlebitis) from the middle ear, mastoid air cells, or paranasal sinuses
    Hematogenous dissemination of infection originating outside CNS
    Complication of meningitis
    Iatrogenic or posttraumatic
- Presents with altered mental status, fever, and focal neurologic deficits
- Four stages of intracranial abscess development: early cerebritis (days), late cerebritis (weeks), early capsule (more than 2 weeks), late capsule (several weeks to months)

Imaging
- Imaging findings range from subtle lesion without mass effect or enhancement in early cerebritis to ring-enhancing mass lesion with associated vasogenic edema after capsule formation has begun

- CT: focus of low attenuation; smooth ring enhancement once capsule formation has begun; enhancement often thicker on the cortical side of abscess, presumably because of greater vascular supply to the capsule from cortical vessels; surrounding low attenuation caused by vasogenic edema; variable mass effect
- MRI:
  - T1: ill-defined hypointense focus; capsule isointense to hyperintense
  - T2: hyperintense; capsule hypointense; surrounding hyperintense vasogenic edema

Cryptococcus

Clinical

- Common fungal infection that involves CNS by hematogenous spread from lungs
- Occurs in immunocompetent individuals as well as in patients with AIDS, transplant recipients, etc.
- Presents with meningitis
- Cryptococcal antigen in CSF, present in majority of patients, confirms diagnosis
- Imaging features of CNS disease include enhancing leptomeninges, gelatinous pseudocysts (dilated perivascular spaces filled with *Cryptococcus* organisms), and parenchymal cryptococcomas

Imaging

- CT and MRI:
  - Leptomeningeal disease: meningeal enhancement may be seen, particularly in the basilar cisterns, but is unusual; communicating hydrocephalus
  - Gelatinous pseudocysts: low-attenuation, well-demarcated, round cystic (T1 hypointense, T2 hyperintense) lesions in the basal ganglia; no enhancement or mass effect
  - Cryptococcomas: multiple small, homogeneously or ring-enhancing parenchymal nodules

Cysticercosis

Clinical

- Parasite that infects the CNS by hematogenous dissemination of oncospheres (primary larvae of the pork tapeworm, *Taenia solium*) that invade the GI tract
- Presents with seizures (90%) or, uncommonly, obstructive hydrocephalus due to intraventricular disease
- Common in immigrants from Mexico and South America
- Cysticerci (secondary larvae) that develop in the brain can involve parenchyma, leptomeninges, ventricles, and basilar cisterns

Imaging

- CT and MRI:
  - Parenchymal lesions
    - Single or multiple small lesions near the gray/white junction that vary in appearance with the chronicity of the infection:
    - *Acute:* focal edema (inflammatory response elicited by death of the secondary larvae) without enhancement or significant mass effect
    - *Subacute:* focal homogeneous or ring enhancement
    - *Chronic:* focal calcification on CT without edema or enhancement; or normal scan
    - Evolution of imaging changes from acute to chronic spans at least 1 year
  - Leptomeningeal disease
    - Nodular enhancement of basilar meninges
  - Intraventricular cysts
    - Isodense (CT) or isointense (MRI) to CSF; 1 to 2 cm; no enhancement; mural nodule (scolex) may be identified by MRI; most common in fourth ventricle
  - Basilar cistern cysts
    - Multilobular, "racemose" cysts; most common in cerebellopontine angle, suprasellar cistern, and basilar cisterns

Cytomegalovirus

Clinical

- Can produce encephalitis in both neonates and immunocompromised adults
- High rate of subclinical infection in pregnant women and other adults

In Utero Infection
- Most common cause of congenital CNS infection
- Hematogenous (transplacental) infection occurs in utero, resulting in a wide spectrum of insults, depending on the timing of the infection relative to gestational age
- Clinical features include microcephaly, hepatosplenomegaly

Immunocompromised Adults
- Reactivation of latent viral infection, rather than de novo infection
- Common cause of meningoencephalitis and ventriculitis in AIDS patients

Imaging

In Utero Infection
- CT: parenchymal calcifications with periventricular predominance; atrophy
- MRI: atrophy; cortical dysplasia

Immunocompromised Adults
- MRI: T1 often normal; variable enhancement of nerve roots, leptomeninges, or ependyma

Empyema, Subdural or Epidural

Clinical
- Noniatrogenic extraaxial empyemas usually caused by paranasal sinus (frontal or ethmoid) or middle ear infection that directly involves intervening bone or spreads via retrograde septic thrombophlebitis (bridging emissary veins)
- Potentially life-threatening condition that can present with meningismus, seizures, focal deficits, and rapid deterioration

Imaging
- CT and MRI: unilateral, extraaxial collection with enhancing dura; most common over hemispheric convexity or along falx; associated source of infection (e.g., paranasal sinus disease, middle ear infection, or mastoiditis)

Herpes Simplex Encephalitis

Clinical
  Neonates
- Herpes simplex virus (HSV)-2 acquired during vaginal delivery of an infected mother; brain is involved in 30%
- This devastating illness results in severe liquefaction necrosis of widespread areas of brain parenchyma; no temporal lobe predilection

  Children and Adults
- Herpes encephalitis is the result of HSV-1, via either primary infection or reactivation of latent virus in the trigeminal ganglion
- Temporal lobes and inferior frontal lobes preferentially affected; involvement of insular and subinsular white matter with sparing of putamen characteristic
- Unilateral or bilateral

Imaging
  Neonates
- CT: initially patchy low attenuation involving cortex and subcortical white matter; cortex eventually high in attenuation
- MRI:
    T1: hypointense cortex and subcortical white matter as result of edema; cortex eventually hyperintense and may remain so for weeks
    T2: hyperintense cortex and subcortical white matter as result of edema

  Children and Adults
- CT: patchy low attenuation in the temporal and inferior frontal lobe(s)
- MRI:
    T1: subtle hypointensity (edema) and mass effect; foci of bright signal are the result of hemorrhage; patchy gyral enhancement post-gadolinium
    T2: hyperintense cortex and subcortical white matter (edema) in temporal and inferior frontal lobes

2

Human Immunodeficiency Virus Encephalitis

Clinical
- Common subacute encephalitis in AIDS population; occurs as result of brain infection with human immunodeficiency virus (HIV)
- Atrophy, demyelination, and gliosis
- Presents with altered mental status

Imaging
- Relative symmetry and hazy, ill-defined nature of the T2 signal abnormality help differentiate HIV encephalitis from progressive multifocal leukoencephalopathy
- CT: confluent areas of low attenuation in the subcortical white matter
- MRI:
    - T1: atrophy; no enhancement or mass effect
    - T2: relatively symmetrical, confluent, ill-defined hyperintensity in white matter of corona radiata and centrum semiovale

Meningitis

Clinical
- Infection of the leptomeninges, because of either extension from a contiguous infection (e.g., otitis media, frontal sinusitis) or hematogenous spread
- Bacterial meningitis presents as an acute illness with headache and meningismus
- Mycobacterial and fungal meningitides present as a subacute or chronic illness
- Viral meningitis usually self-limited, benign illness, except in immunocompromised patients
- Usually diagnosed clinically

Imaging
- Imaging most helpful in evaluating complications of meningitis:
    - Hydrocephalus, either communicating (resulting from impaired resorption of CSF) or obstructive (resulting from inflammatory changes in lining of cerebral aqueduct)
    - Subdural or epidural effusions or empyema
    - Cerebritis
    - Abscess
    - Infarction caused by perivascular inflammatory changes and subsequent vasospasm
- CT: may be normal; variable sulcal (leptomeningeal) enhancement; complications:

Ventricular enlargement	hydrocephalus
Cortical low attenuation	cerebritis or infarction
Low to intermediate attenuation/extraaxial collection with enhancing margins	subdural effusion or empyema abscess
Ring-enhancing intraaxial mass	

- MRI: more sensitive than CT; variable sulcal (leptomeningeal) enhancement; evidence of complications
- Normal imaging examination does not rule out meningitis
- Frontal sinusitis in patient with altered mental status or suspected meningitis should prompt careful inspection of frontal and interhemispheric extraaxial spaces for possible subdural empyema
- Tuberculous meningitis tends to involve basilar cisterns

Toxoplasmosis

Clinical
- Ubiquitous protozoan *Toxoplasma gondii* can affect developing fetus or immunocompromised adults

In Utero Infection
- Hematogenous (transplacental) infection occurs in utero, resulting in wide spectrum of insults, depending on the timing of infection relative to gestational age
- Infection may result in no symptoms, mild symptoms (e.g., seizures later in childhood, mild developmental delay), or severe brain injury
- Clinical and imaging findings may be similar to those of other congenital infections in the TORCH (toxoplasmosis, rubella, cytomegalovirus, herpes simplex) group

2

Immunocompromised Adults
- Most common cause of ring-enhancing mass lesion(s) in AIDS population; main differential diagnostic consideration in these patients is primary CNS lymphoma
- Presents with symptoms caused by mass effect (e.g., focal deficits, altered mental status, headache)
- Although certain imaging features can favor either toxoplasmosis or lymphoma, most patients are given a trial of antitoxoplasmosis therapy and imaged again in several weeks. Interval improvement leads to a presumptive diagnosis of toxoplasmosis; failure to improve leads to a presumptive diagnosis of lymphoma, which can be confirmed by brain biopsy prior to radiation therapy.

Imaging
In Utero Infection
- CT: intracranial calcifications that may involve periventricular white matter, deep gray nuclei, or cortex; microcephaly, atrophy, and hydrocephalus in severely affected infants

Immunocompromised Adults
- CT: multiple mass lesions with surrounding edema, involving deep gray nuclei and hemispheric gray/white junction; homogeneous or ring enhancement (lesions larger than 1 to 2 cm almost always show ring enhancement); high attenuation may be caused by associated hemorrhage or calcification (common in treated toxoplasmosis)
- Imaging features that favor toxoplasmosis over lymphoma:
  Hemorrhage
  Multiplicity of lesions
  Peripheral location
  Eccentric nodule of enhancement within a ring-enhancing lesion, or "cluster of grapes" ring-enhancing lesions
- Imaging features that favor lymphoma over toxoplasmosis:
  Corpus callosum involvement
  Solitary lesion
  Periventricular location
  Ependymal enhancement
  Homogeneous enhancement in a lesion larger than 2 cm

Ventriculitis

Clinical
- Inflammation of the ependyma, usually iatrogenic (e.g., complication of shunting or ventricular drain placement) or complication of meningitis
- Common complication of CMV meningitis in AIDS patients; differential diagnosis in this population includes opportunistic neoplasm (lymphoma)

Imaging
- CT and MRI: enhancement of ependymal surfaces and possibly periventricular parenchyma; edema in periventricular parenchyma; intraventricular septations/arachnoid loculations; fluid/debris layer within the ventricles; communicating or obstructive hydrocephalus

Spine

Abscess, Epidural

Clinical
- Most often direct extension of infection from adjacent focus of discitis/osteomyelitis
- Populations at increased risk: intravenous drug abusers and elderly patients with occult infection (e.g., low-grade pneumonia) that spreads hematogenously to a disc space
- Medical or neurosurgical emergency: rapid deterioration may occur secondary to cord compression or septic thrombophlebitis

Imaging
- MRI:
  T1: loss of disc space; low signal in adjacent vertebral end plates; partial

collapse of adjacent vertebral bodies; contiguous hypointense epidural fluid collection centered at disc space and impressing thecal sac; enhancement of disc space, adjacent end plates, and margins of epidural collection; epidural collection and enhancing phlegmonous tissue can extend over several vertebral body levels in epidural and anterior subligamentous spaces; infection commonly extends to paraspinous soft tissues

T2: hyperintense disc space; contiguous hyperintense epidural fluid collection centered at the disc space and impressing ventral thecal sac

- Collapsed, degenerated discs desiccated and low in signal on T2 images; *high signal in a collapsed disc on T2 images should always suggest the possibility of disc space infection*

Head and Neck

Orbital Cellulitis

Clinical
- Infection involving postseptal orbital tissues
- Orbital septum a circumferential band of connective tissue extending from bony walls of anterior orbit to tarsal plates of eyelids; septum helps limit spread of superficial periorbital (preseptal) cellulitis into the orbit
- Presents with swelling and erythema of periorbital soft tissues, fever, and pain
- Differentiation from preseptal cellulitis is critical, because preseptal infection is treated medically, whereas orbital (i.e., postseptal) cellulitis is a potential surgical emergency
- Usually caused by spread of infection originating in adjacent paranasal sinuses (especially ethmoid air cells) or skin
- Complications:
    Septic thrombophlebitis with thrombosis of superior ophthalmic vein or cavernous sinus
    Intracranial extension leading to cerebritis, abscess, or epidural empyema

Imaging
- CT: infiltration of postseptal orbital fat; subperiosteal abscess, typically along medial orbital wall adjacent to ipsilateral ethmoid air cell disease

Orbital Pseudotumor

Clinical
- Poorly understood lymphocytic inflammatory condition
- Most common cause of intraorbital mass lesion in adults; second most common cause (after Graves' disease) of unilateral proptosis
- Presents with rapid onset of unilateral pain, limitation of eye movement, and proptosis
- Often a presumptive diagnosis, made after characteristic dramatic improvement with steroids

Imaging
- CT and MRI: extremely variable imaging features, many of which may not be present in an individual patient:
    Infiltration of orbital fat (80%)
    Extraocular muscle enlargement (60%); principal feature of myositic subtype of pseudotumor
    Optic nerve sheath enlargement (40%)
    Uveal/scleral thickening (30%)
    Lacrimal fossa mass (5%); enhancing mass in the lacrimal fossa or elsewhere in the orbit is principal feature of tumefactive subtype of pseudotumor
- Myositic pseudotumor must be distinguished from thyroid ophthalmopathy; tumefactive pseudotumor must be distinguished from true orbital neoplasm

Sinusitis

Clinical
- Acute or chronic inflammatory disease of the paranasal sinuses
- Presents with headache, facial pain, nasal drainage, or fever
- Chronic sinusitis often associated with allergic rhinitis and polyposis

Imaging
- Should be reserved for patients with recurrent, atypical (e.g., sinusitis in an immunocompromised patient), or suspected complicated sinusitis
- Direct coronal CT without contrast is the preferred screening examination of the sinuses; contrast-enhanced CT (axial and coronal) and MRI are the preferred examinations for complicated sinusitis
- Complications of sinusitis: osteomyelitis, intracranial extension (empyema, abscess, or cerebritis; dural venous sinus thrombosis; cavernous sinus thrombosis), intraorbital extension (orbital cellulitis; orbital abscess), mucocele, polyposis
- CT:
  - *Uncomplicated sinusitis:* mucosal thickening; fluid-fluid levels; opacification of one or more sinuses; opacification of the osteomeatal units
  - *Complicated sinusitis:* bone destruction; extraaxial fluid collection or abscess in the frontotemporal region; high attenuation in thrombosed dural venous sinus on noncontrast images; orbital cellulitis or abscess (usually along the medial orbital wall, adjacent to ethmoidal sinus disease); mucocele (*see Mucocele*); polyposis
- MRI:
  - *Complicated sinusitis*
    - See CT findings above
    - Intermediate T2 signal in paranasal sinus mass suggests neoplasm; hyperintense T2 signal suggests inflammatory sinus disease
    - Mass that is intermediate signal on T1, very low signal on T2, and high attenuation on CT raises the possibility of fungal sinusitis
    - MR venography may be helpful to evaluate patency of the dural venous sinuses

Thyroid Ophthalmopathy (Graves' Disease)

Clinical
- Autoimmune disease that affects the thyroid gland and orbital soft tissues
- Presents in middle-aged or elderly adults with slowly progressive, painless proptosis; decreased range of globe motion; and diplopia
- More common in women (4:1)
- Most common cause of unilateral or bilateral proptosis in an adult
- Thyroid ophthalmopathy a clinical diagnosis; imaging used to evaluate extent of extraocular muscle involvement, optic nerve compression near the orbital apex, and response to therapy
- Often bilateral and symmetrical; single or multiple muscles

Imaging
- Extraocular muscle enlargement and proptosis are the main imaging findings
- Extraocular muscle enlargement usually occurs in predictable order: inferior rectus affected earliest and most frequently, followed by medial rectus, superior rectus, lateral rectus, and obliques (mnemonic: I'm slow)
- CT: enlargement of extraocular muscles (best shown by coronal images); sparing of tendinous insertions (best shown by axial images)
- MRI T1: enlarged extraocular muscles (best shown by coronal T1 with fat saturation and gadolinium)

WHITE MATTER DISEASE

MRI is always the imaging modality of choice in evaluating white matter disease, because of the high sensitivity of T2 images for the detection of white matter injury. T2 images show areas of white matter injury as hyperintense foci. T1 images show areas of white matter injury as hypointense foci. T1 images are inferior to T2 images for evaluation of the presence, size, and distribution of lesions, but can be helpful with gadolinium contrast, because enhancement can reflect an active phase of a demyelinating illness.

CT is much less sensitive than MRI for white matter disease and should be reserved for patients who cannot have an MRI examination. CT shows white matter injury as low attenuation foci.

2

Acute Disseminated Encephalomyelitis

Clinical
- Subacute, autoimmune, inflammatory demyelination that follows a viral illness
- Presents with seizures and neurological deficits that appear several weeks after viral illness or vaccination
- Clinical features: history of recent viral illness (e.g., measles, varicella, mononucleosis, mumps); CSF showing lymphocytic pleocytosis; resolution of deficits in weeks to months; complete recovery in majority of patients, but permanent deficits or death can occur
- Common locations: subcortical white matter; deep gray nuclei (basal ganglia and thalamus); brain stem; spinal cord

Imaging
- MRI:
  - T1: variable enhancement
  - T2: multiple, hyperintense foci; bilateral but asymmetrical; well demarcated or poorly defined

Central Pontine Myelinolysis

Clinical
- Acute demyelination affecting white matter of the central pons and, in some cases, other regions also, including the midbrain, thalami, basal ganglia, and subcortical white matter
- Rapid correction of severe electrolyte imbalance (e.g., hyponatremia) often implicated as precipitating event
- Presents with quadriplegia, "locked-in" state, pseudobulbar palsy, or altered mental status
- Most common in alcoholics and children

Imaging
- MRI:
  - T1: hypointense central pons; no enhancement or mass effect
  - T2: hyperintense central pons; area of signal abnormality may have a triangular shape and characteristically spares the periphery of the pons; variable foci of high signal elsewhere, reflecting sites of "extrapontine" demyelination

Multiple Sclerosis (MS)

Clinical
- Idiopathic demyelinating disease that can affect the white matter of both brain and spinal cord
- Presents in young adulthood or middle age with visual complaints, gait disturbance, and motor or sensory deficits
- More common in women
- Clinical diagnosis with specific criteria that must be met:
  - Clinical course marked by remissions and relapses
  - Anatomically separate lesions documented by neurological examination or MRI
  - Demyelinative CSF profile (myelin basic protein, oligoclonal bands, IgG)

Imaging
- MRI:
  - T1: hypointense foci that may be ill defined or well defined, depending on size and age of plaque; enhancement (at margin of plaque only or homogeneous) may reflect active inflammation (i.e., acute or subacute demyelination)
  - T2: multiple round or ovoid foci of well-demarcated T2 hyperintensity, often in characteristic locations:
    - Periventricular and especially periatrial white matter
    - Corpus callosum
    - Middle cerebellar peduncles
    - Periaqueductal midbrain
    - Pons
  - *Sagittal* T2 images should be included in every examination to evaluate the callosal white matter; *Dawson's fingers* refers to the linear bands of T2 hyper-

intensity in the corpus callosum, oriented orthogonal to the axis of the callosum, which are highly characteristic of MS; *spinal cord* plaques usually elongated and tend to involve dorsal columns; their imaging features otherwise similar to those of brain lesions

- Atypical locations of lesions are fairly common
- Tumefactive MS plaque with mass effect and enhancement along a portion of its margin can mimic neoplasm; to avoid an unnecessary biopsy of a tumefactive MS plaque, have a high index of suspicion in young or middle-aged patients, especially if their MRI examination shows multiple white matter lesions

Progressive Multifocal Leukoencephalopathy

Clinical
- Viral demyelinating disease seen in end-stage AIDS and in other diseases that severely compromise the immune system
- Caused by infection with group B papovavirus
- Presents with visual loss, altered mental status, and dementia
- Rapid deterioration to profound deficits; death usually occurs within 6 months of diagnosis
- Common locations: subcortical white matter; corpus callosum; brain stem; deep gray nuclei

Imaging
- MRI:
    T1: occasional enhancement of the leading edge of demyelination; no mass effect
    T2: focal, confluent region of hyperintensity in subcortical white matter, usually sparing cortical ribbon
- Must be distinguished from HIV encephalopathy, which usually affects white matter of centrum semiovale diffusely and symmetrically and has much better prognosis

Radiation Injury

Clinical
- White matter changes result from effects of radiation
- Location corresponds to region of brain that was irradiated
- Divided into acute and delayed (or chronic) injury
    Acute (days to weeks after radiation): transient vasogenic edema resulting from direct toxic effects of radiation on white matter; asymptomatic
    Chronic (more than 6 months after radiation): demyelination and necrosis resulting from radiation vasculopathy; presents with focal neurological deficits, altered mental status, or new lesions on follow-up imaging examinations; confluent or multiple discrete foci of demyelination; variable enhancement
- Chemotherapy (e.g., methotrexate) alone can injure white matter but can also potentiate effects of radiation

Imaging
- MRI:
    Acute
        T1: no enhancement; no mass effect
        T2: hazy, confluent hyperintensity in the white matter
    Chronic
        T1: variable homogeneous or ring enhancement; variable mass effect; atrophy in late stages
        T2: hyperintense regions of white matter (representing demyelination or necrosis); confluent or multiple discrete foci
- Differentiation of radiation necrosis from recurrent tumor in a new enhancing lesion(s) is a frequent problem
    Features that favor radiation necrosis:
        Distribution limited to radiation field
        Hypometabolism on fluorodeoxyglucose PET scan
    Features that favor recurrent tumor:

New enhancement not in keeping with expected time course of radiation necrosis

New enhancement in regions of brain remote from radiation field

Hypermetabolism on fluorodeoxyglucose PET scan

VASCULAR DISEASE

Amyloid Angiopathy

Clinical
- Common cause of spontaneous intraaxial hematoma in elderly patients
- Deposition of amyloid in walls of small and medium-sized cortical and leptomeningeal vessels

Imaging
- MRI: gradient echo sequences, by demonstrating multiple tiny foci of hemosiderin deposition near gray-white junction, can help suggest amyloid angiopathy as cause of spontaneous lobar hematoma in an elderly patient

Aneurysms

Clinical
- Most common sites: anterior communicating artery (30%), posterior communicating artery (30%), middle cerebral artery bifurcation (20%), basilar tip (5%); posterior inferior cerebellar artery, anterior inferior cerebellar artery, or superior cerebellar artery (5%)
- Multiple in 20% of patients
- Increased incidence in polycystic kidney disease, neurofibromatosis, collagen vascular disease, Marfan's syndrome, coarctation of the aorta, fibromuscular dysplasia
- Classic presentation after rupture: sudden onset of "worst headache of life" (attributable to leptomeningeal irritation from acute subarachnoid hemorrhage); hydrocephalus (communicating or obstructive due to intraventricular clot); intraparenchymal hematoma with deficits related to mass effect may also occur; ipsilateral third nerve palsy may occur in posterior communicating artery aneurysm
- If aneurysm has not ruptured, cumulative risk of bleeding is 1 to 2% per year
- If aneurysm has ruptured and bled, risk of bleeding again 20 to 50% in the first 2 weeks; 50% in the first 6 months

Imaging
- CT: noncontrast CT is the examination of choice for evaluation of possible acute subarachnoid hemorrhage; distribution of subarachnoid hemorrhage can be a clue to location of ruptured aneurysm:

    Symmetrical bihemispheric subarachnoid hemorrhage or blood limited to the interpeduncular fossa favors a midline aneurysm (anterior communicating artery or basilar tip)

    Sylvian cistern hemorrhage or inferior frontotemporal hematoma favors an ipsilateral middle cerebral artery bifurcation aneurysm

    Fourth ventricular hemorrhage suggests a posterior inferior cerebellar artery (PICA) aneurysm

    Delayed complications of subarachnoid hemorrhage: infarction secondary to vasospasm; communicating or obstructive hydrocephalus

- MRI: not as sensitive as CT for detection of acute subarachnoid hemorrhage; abnormal contour of intracranial vascular flow void, especially if associated with phase artifact (artifact propagated along the phase axis due to vascular pulsation), should suggest aneurysm
- MRA: capable of detecting most aneurysms more than 3 mm in size; considered by most neurosurgeons to be inadequate alone for preoperative evaluation (i.e., diagnostic MRA study does not obviate cerebral angiogram)
- Angiography: four-vessel cerebral angiogram mandatory for visualization of both vertebrobasilar and internal carotid circulations; vertebrals should be visualized proximal to PICA origins; if multiple aneurysms identified, angiographic findings that favor one aneurysm over another as the source of bleeding include:

    Proximity to intraaxial or extraaxial hemorrhage identified on CT

    Large size

Spasm
Beaking of aneurysm contours
Frank extravasation of dye during the angiogram (rare)
Some angiographers evaluate both external carotid circulations if no aneurysm is found initially; rarely, dural arteriovenous fistula supplied by external carotid branches can be the source of subarachnoid hemorrhage

Aneurysm, Mycotic

Clinical
- Small peripheral aneurysm(s), caused by infection and subsequent mural weakening of peripheral arteries
- Most common in patients with bacterial endocarditis
- Presents with hemorrhage or altered mental status

Imaging
- CT: foci of low attenuation near the gray-white junction that show variable enhancement
- MRI:
    T1: small foci of enhancement near the gray-white junction
    T2: small peripheral hyperintense foci
- Angiography: aneurysm(s) in unusual location, usually in small, peripheral arteries

Angiographic Arterial Anatomy
- External carotid artery branches (proximal to distal)
    Ascending pharyngeal
    Superior thyroidal
    Lingual
    Facial
    Occipital
    Posterior auricular
    Superficial temporal
    Internal maxillary
        Middle meningeal is the largest branch of internal maxillary
- Internal carotid artery segments (proximal to distal):
    Cervical
    Petrous
    Cavernous
    Supraclinoid
- Carotid "siphon" refers to S-shape of cavernous and supraclinoid segments of distal internal carotid seen on lateral view; the siphon has four important branches (mnemonic: MOPA):
    Meningohypophyseal
    Ophthalmic
    Posterior communicating
    Anterior choroidal
- Terminal (supraclinoid) segment of internal carotid artery bifurcates to form A1 segment of anterior cerebral artery and M1 segment of middle cerebral artery
- Middle cerebral artery (MCA) segments
    M1 (MCA origin to the MCA bifurcation)
        Lateral lenticulostriate arteries
    M2 (insular branches)
    M3 (opercular branches)
- Anterior cerebral artery (ACA) segments
    A1 (ACA origin to the anterior communicating artery)
        Medial lenticulostriate arteries
        Recurrent artery of Heubner
    A2 (anterior communicating artery to the pericallosal artery origin)
        Orbitofrontal artery
        Frontopolar artery
        Bifurcates to form pericallosal and callosomarginal arteries
- Vertebral artery branches
    Each vertebral artery takes off from ipsilateral proximal subclavian artery and ascends to run within transverse foramina of cervical vertebrae

Extracranial branches: spinal, muscular, and meningeal arteries
Intracranial branches: PICA, anterior spinal artery
Vertebrals come together anterior to the lower brain stem to form basilar artery
- Basilar artery branches
Basilar artery branches are paired vessels; one emitted from either side of basilar
Anterior inferior cerebellar artery (AICA)
Numerous small pontine perforating arteries
Superior cerebellar artery (SCA)
Posterior cerebral artery (PCA) (basilar bifurcation)
- Posterior cerebral artery segments
P1 (peduncular) (origin to posterior communicating artery)
P2 (ambient) (posterior communicating artery to bifurcation)
Medial posterior choroidal artery
Lateral posterior choroidal artery
P3 (quadrigeminal) segment

Angiographic Technique

- With improvements in equipment, many neuroradiologists rely almost exclusively on digital subtraction angiography for most diagnostic angiograms
- Contrast used at our institution: iohexol (Omnipaque 300), nonionic iodinated dye that contains 300 mg iodine per 100 mL; 50% dilution for digital angiography; full strength for cut film angiography
- Catheters used at our institution for routine diagnostic cerebral angiography include 5 and 7 French Norman, Berenstein, and Simmons; Simmons is particularly useful in studying carotid bifurcation and cervical internal carotid in elderly patients with tortuous vascular anatomy
- Common carotid run: catheter tip positioned in proximal common carotid artery; typical injection, 6 mL/second for a total volume of 6 mL; common carotid, bifurcation, and cervical internal and external carotid vessels filmed in anteroposterior (AP), lateral, and oblique projections as necessary
- Internal carotid run: catheter tip positioned in distal cervical internal carotid approximately at level of C1–C2; typical injection 6 mL/second for a total of 8 mL; intracranial vessels filmed in AP, lateral, and oblique projections as necessary
- Vertebral run: catheter tip positioned in proximal dominant (usually the left) vertebral artery; typical injection 5 mL/second for a total of 7 mL; intracranial posterior circulation filmed in AP (straight AP, Waters, Towne), lateral, and oblique projections as necessary
Waters view allows optimal visualization of basilar tip and basilar artery branches
Towne view allows optimal visualization of posterior cerebral arteries and their branches
- External carotid run: catheter tip positioned in proximal external carotid; typical injection 3 mL/second for a total of 5 mL

Arteriovenous Malformation

Clinical

- Congenital malformation of abnormal, enlarged feeding arteries and draining veins that communicate directly (i.e., no intervening capillary bed)
- Presents with parenchymal hemorrhage, seizure, or focal neurologic deficit
- Risk of hemorrhage 2% per year; risk of hemorrhage increases if angiography shows associated feeding vessel aneurysms, deep venous drainage, or venous restriction (narrowing of draining veins)

Imaging

- CT: contrast-enhanced scan shows tubular areas of enhancement representing enlarged feeding arteries and draining veins; variable calcification; variable encephalomalacia; no mass effect in the absence of hemorrhage
- MRI:
T1: tubular flow voids corresponding to enlarged feeding arteries and draining veins; contrast not usually necessary
T2: tubular flow voids; surrounding hyperintensity caused by gliosis or ischemia

- Angiography: enlarged, feeding arteries; early draining, enlarged veins that may drain to superficial cortical veins or sinuses, deep veins, or both; possible feeding vessel or nidus aneurysms
- Hematoma can obscure an arteriovenous malformation; angiography therefore is necessary for complete evaluation of unexplained hematoma

Carotid-Cavernous Fistula

Clinical
- Abnormal communication between the internal carotid artery and cavernous sinus
- Causes include trauma, atherosclerosis, congenital defect of the media, internal carotid artery (ICA) aneurysm rupture
- Presents with acute pulsating exophthalmos, orbital bruit, and visual loss

Imaging
- CT and MRI: dilation of cavernous sinus and superior ophthalmic vein; enlargement of rectus muscles
- Angiography: internal carotid injection shows premature filling of dilated cavernous sinus, orbital veins, and inferior petrosal sinus
- Interventional neuroradiologists can occlude carotid cavernous fistulas by deploying detachable balloons

Cryptic (Occult) Vascular Malformation

Clinical
- Includes both *cavernous hemangiomas* and *capillary telangiectasias,* malformations usually not detected by angiography and therefore "occult" or "cryptic"
- Cavernous hemangiomas (no intervening normal brain parenchyma) and capillary telangiectasias (intervening normal brain parenchyma) can be distinguished pathologically, but not always by imaging; therefore, they are usually grouped together as cryptic vascular malformations
- Both malformations can occur anywhere in the brain; capillary telangiectasias are most common in the pons
- Cavernous hemangioma presents with hemorrhage, seizure, or focal neurologic deficit; capillary telangiectasia usually an incidental finding

Imaging
- CT: very insensitive compared with MRI; focal calcification

Cavernous Hemangioma
- MRI:
  - T1: ill-defined small focus of heterogeneous signal, usually containing some central hyperintense signal (methemoglobin) and a rim of low signal (hemosiderin); frequently multiple; variable enhancement; occasionally associated with anomalous draining vein (venous angioma); no mass effect in the absence of hemorrhage
  - T2: heterogeneous focus containing areas of lobular hyperintense signal (methemoglobin) against hypointense background (hemosiderin staining); appearance of lobular hyperintense signal often referred to as classic "popcorn" or "mulberry" appearance of cavernous hemangioma
  - Gradient-recalled echol (GRE): most sensitive sequence for the detection of cryptic malformations; increase in hypointense signal compared with T2, referred to as "blooming" (result of increased susceptibility of GRE sequences to local field inhomogeneities created by blood product deposition)

Capillary Telangiectasia
- MRI:
  - T1: noncontrast scan can appear similar to that of cavernous hemangioma but is occasionally normal; faint, well-demarcated homogeneous contrast enhancement; no mass effect
  - T2: normal; faint hyperintense signal; or hypointense signal (hemosiderin staining)
  - GRE: "blooming" of hypointense signal

2

Dural Venous Sinus Thrombosis

Clinical
- Presents with increased intracranial pressure or venous ischemia
- Causes include adjacent infection (e.g., otomastoiditis, meningitis) or neoplasm (e.g., falx meningioma), dehydration, sepsis, or other hypercoagulable state

Imaging
- CT: much less sensitive than MRI; noncontrast examination may, rarely, show hyperdense clot within superior sagittal or transverse sinuses; postcontrast scan may show filling defect in central portion of superior sagittal sinus ("delta sign")
- MRI T1: *sagittal and coronal planes* most helpful for evaluating dural venous sinus patency; hyperintense or isointense signal replacing the normal sinus flow void; contrast-enhanced scan may show enhancement around margins of acute clot, although intrinsic high signal of acute clot can make post-gadolinium images confusing; location of venous infarction (possibly with associated hemorrhage), if present, provides clue to the sinus involved:

Parasagittal frontoparietal lobes	superior sagittal sinus thrombosis
Temporal lobe	transverse sinus
Thalamus	straight sinus (rare)

- MRV: 2D time-of-flight (TOF) MR venography provides a volumetric rendering of venous sinus anatomy and may help confirm suspected thrombosis; phase-contrast MR venography is more sensitive to slow flow and can be used in questionable cases to confirm absence of flow in thrombosed sinus

Hemorrhage, MRI Imaging Features at 1.5 T
- Most intracranial hematomas follow logical evolution from oxyhemoglobin (rarely seen on imaging studies) to deoxyhemoglobin to methemoglobin to hemosiderin
- These blood breakdown products have different magnetic properties and hence different signal intensities on T1 and T2 images
- Signal changes occur first at margins of hematoma and proceed centrally as hematoma evolves
- Hyperacute hemorrhage (minutes to a few hours)
    Oxyhemoglobin: T1 hypointense, T2 hyperintense
- Acute hemorrhage (hours to days)
    Deoxyhemoglobin: T1 isointense, T2 hypointense
    Methemoglobin (intracellular): T1 hyperintense, T2 hypointense
- Subacute hemorrhage (days to weeks)
    Methemoglobin (extracellular): T1 hyperintense, T2 hyperintense
- Chronic hemorrhage (weeks to months)
    Hemosiderin: T1 hypointense, T2 hypointense

Infarction, Arterial

Clinical
- Irreversible injury of brain tissue caused by prolonged ischemia
- Most common cause is atherosclerosis that leads to large vessel occlusion
- Presents with sudden onset of focal neurologic deficit(s)
- May be caused by large vessel occlusion, small vessel occlusion, emboli, vasospasm, or vasculopathy

Large vessel occlusion	atherosclerosis; trauma with dissection
Small vessel occlusion ("lacunae")	hypertensive vasculopathy; diabetes; atherosclerosis
Vasospasm	subarachnoid hemorrhage; drug abuse (amphetamine, cocaine)
Emboli	atrial fibrillation; atherosclerosis
Vasculopathy	vasculitis of any cause

- Major causes of arterial infarction: thromboembolic disease resulting from atherosclerosis; hypoperfusion (e.g., flow-limiting carotid disease); vasculitis; trauma; anoxia
- Hallmark of arterial infarction is involvement of parenchyma within a specific vascular or watershed territory; therefore, familiarity with cerebral vascular and watershed territories is critical

Imaging
- CT: noncontrast CT is the initial examination of choice; most important task of radiologist in evaluation of early infarction is to *rule out hemorrhage or significant mass effect*; particularly important with cerebellar infarcts, because of the possibility of brain stem compression and rapid deterioration of patient
- MRI may be the preferred initial examination in the setting of possible infarction of the brain stem or posterior fossa, because CT of these regions is plagued by beam-hardening artifact

Acute Cortical Infarction
- Loss of gray-white differentiation and effacement of sulci, usually detectable by 12 to 24 hours; stasis of blood flow, seen as asymmetrical enhancement of cortical vessels on contrast-enhanced images; three signs of early middle cerebral artery (MCA) infarction:
  - Insular ribbon sign: loss of gray-white differentiation at the insular cortex (very common)
  - Loss of gray-white differentiation in basal ganglia (in proximal MCA infarction caused by occlusion of thalamostriate vessels)
  - Dense MCA sign: dense clot within proximal MCA (uncommon)

Subacute Cortical Infarction
- "Gyriform enhancement" over the cortical surface
  - Rule of threes: enhancement appears at about 3 days, peaks at about 3 weeks, and resolves by 3 months
- Hyperdense cortex resulting from petechial hemorrhage or laminar necrosis

Chronic Infarction
- Encephalomalacia
- Wallerian degeneration (e.g., decreased size of cerebral peduncle ipsilateral to large MCA territory infarction)

Moyamoya Syndrome

Clinical
- Progressive occlusion of the distal intracranial ICA with formation of multiple collaterals
- May be idiopathic (moyamoya disease) or caused by an underlying vasculopathy (atherosclerosis, sickle cell disease, neurofibromatosis type 1, fibromuscular dysplasia, Marfan or Ehler-Danlos syndrome, radiation injury)
- Idiopathic form most common in Japan
- Presents with ischemia

Imaging
- CT: ischemic injury
- MRI: enlarged flow voids of collateral vessels; ischemic injury
- Angiography: occlusion of the supraclinoid ICA; multiple tiny "puff-of-smoke" collaterals near the distal ICA; multiple other collateral vessels

Venous Angioma

Clinical
- Common venous anomaly that drains normal brain parenchyma, often in cerebellum or frontal lobe
- Collection of radially oriented venous tributaries emptying into a large draining vein
- Drainage may be to cortical or subependymal veins
- No arterial component
- Usually asymptomatic, incidental finding; hemorrhage rare and, when present, may be from associated cavernous hemangioma

Imaging
- CT and MRI: nonenhanced scans usually normal; MRI may show abnormal parenchymal flow void; single, enhancing, enlarged draining vein; small, enhancing, radially oriented tributaries ("Medusa head")
- T2 images: usually show no parenchymal abnormality; occasionally, hyperintense

signal in surrounding parenchyma may be seen, possible reflecting chronic ischemia or gliosis

Vein of Galen Malformation

Clinical
- Group of malformations that have in common arteriovenous shunting between midline arteries and massively enlarged vein of Galen
- Presents usually in neonatal period with congestive heart failure, macrocephaly, obstructive hydrocephalus, and bruit

Imaging
- Ultrasound (US): cystic posterior midline mass, with flow by color Doppler; hydrocephalus
- CT: homogeneous, slightly hyperdense, posterior midline mass; obstructive hydrocephalus; homogeneous enhancement; enlarged, enhancing feeding arteries
- MRI: hypointense to hyperintense on T1 and T2, depending on degree of flow and presence of partial thrombosis
- Angiography: early filling and delayed emptying of enlarged vein of Galen; enlarged feeding anterior and posterior circulation arteries; venous restriction may be present

TRAUMA

CT is the imaging examination of choice for evaluation of acute trauma because it is sensitive for detection of hemorrhage and fractures and can be performed more easily and rapidly than MRI.

Avulsion of Nerve Root

Clinical
- Results from traction injury; brachial plexus injury during vaginal delivery; injury of other nerve roots in high-speed motor vehicle accidents

Imaging
- MRI is the examination of choice and has largely replaced myelography for the evaluation of nerve root avulsion
    T2: pseudomeningocele (round or ovoid CSF collection adjacent to nerve root sleeve); visualized best on coronal and axial T2

Contusion/Hematoma

Clinical
- Focal intraaxial edema or hemorrhage involving cortex and underlying white matter
- Results from inertial impact at site opposite coup injury (contrecoup), movement of the brain over rough portions of the inner table (e.g., petrous ridge) or, less commonly, direct impact (coup injury)
- Common locations: anterior temporal lobes; midtemporal lobes above petrous ridge; frontal poles; gyrus rectus; parasagittal convexity

Imaging
- CT: focus of heterogeneous high attenuation (acute blood) at the coup or contrecoup site; variable surrounding low attenuation (edema)
- Resolving contusions can show ring enhancement days to weeks after injury, thereby mimicking abscess, infarction, or neoplasm

Diffuse Axonal Injury

Clinical
- Multifocal white matter injury caused by axonal fiber stretching or transection produced by shearing forces
- Results from acceleration/deceleration in high-speed motor vehicle accidents
- Common locations: parasagittal white matter near the gray-white junction; corpus callosum (splenium more often affected than body, which is more often affected than genu); dorsolateral pons and midbrain; posterior limb internal capsule

Imaging
- MRI more accurately depicts the severity of diffuse axonal injury
- GRE sequences, because of their sensitivity to blood product–induced local field inhomogeneities, are more helpful than routine spin echo sequences for confirming diffuse axonal injury
- CT: small, round, low-attenuation foci in characteristic locations; high-attenuation foci (hemorrhage) in 30%
- MRI:
  - T1: focal hypointense (edema) or hyperintense (methemoglobin) signal acutely
  - T2: focal hyperintense signal acutely (edema or methemoglobin); focal hypointense signal chronically (hemosiderin)
  - GRE: focal hypointense signal

Hematoma, Epidural (EDH)

Clinical
- Extraaxial blood collection between the inner table of calvarium and outer layer of dura
- Usually results from fracture of temporal squamosa and laceration of middle meningeal artery, but can also result from laceration of dural venous sinus
- Much more common at coup site than at contrecoup site
- Common locations: frontotemporal convexity; posterior fossa; occipital convexity
- Epidural hematomas *do not cross sutures* because the outer dural layer is tightly adherent to sutural margins
- Epidural hematomas resulting from laceration of the superior sagittal sinus commonly *cross the midline*
- Capable of rapid expansion; usually a neurosurgical emergency

Imaging
- CT: *biconvex* extraaxial collection; skull fracture common; brain herniation common

Hematoma, Subdural (SDH)

Clinical
- Extraaxial blood collection between inner layer of dura and arachnoid
- Usually caused by tearing of bridging cortical veins
- More common at contrecoup site than at coup site, but can occur at either
- Common locations: hemispheric convexity; tentorium (usually along the superior margin); interhemispheric fissure
- Subdural hematomas *cross sutures but do not cross the midline*

Imaging
- CT: wide windows are necessary (e.g., level 75, window 150) for evaluation of extraaxial hematomas; subtle SDH can be missed on routine brain windows; evolves from hyperdense in the acute stages (less than 1 week) to isodense (1 to 3 weeks) to hypodense (more than 3 weeks); initially homogeneous, but can be heterogeneous in several settings:
  - Hyperacute SDH containing unclotted blood
  - Evolution of SDH with clot retraction
  - Recurrent bleeding
  - Associated arachnoid tear with CSF leakage into the SDH
  - Morphology varies with location:

Hemispheric convexity	crescentic
Interhemispheric	thickening of falx
Supratentorial	thickening of tentorium; effacement of underlying sulci; associated brain herniation (subfalcine, uncal)

Temporal Bone Fracture

Clinical
- Two types, classified according to the orientation of the fracture line relative to the long axis of petromastoid portion of temporal bone:
  - *Longitudinal*
    - Parallel to the long axis of petromastoid bone
    - More common (75%)
    - Facial paralysis uncommon; often delayed and incomplete

Ossicular dislocation and tympanic membrane rupture common

Conductive or mixed hearing loss

Transverse

Perpendicular to the long axis of the petromastoid bone

Less common

Facial paralysis common; often immediate and permanent (transection of the facial nerve)

Ossicular dislocation and tympanic membrane rupture uncommon

Sensorineural hearing loss

- Presents with hemotympanum, CSF otorrhea or rhinorrhea, injury of cranial nerves VII and VIII
- Complications: hearing loss (tympanic membrane rupture; hemotympanum; ossicular dislocation; transection of cochlear division of cranial nerve VIII or injury to the cochlea; perilymph fistula); facial palsy; vertigo (injury of the labyrinth or vestibular division of cranial nerve VIII); CSF leak; meningitis

Imaging
- CT: High-resolution CT of temporal bones (1 mm collimation, bone algorithm) in axial and direct coronal planes mandatory

Fracture line(s) (relation to IAC, labyrinth, and jugular foramen)

Fluid in mastoid air cells and middle ear

Pneumocephalus

Ossicular chain disruption

Pneumolabyrinth

Air in condylar fossa of temporomandibular joint

CONGENITAL AND DEVELOPMENTAL DISORDERS

Aqueductal Stenosis

Clinical
- May be congenital or acquired (meningitis, subarachnoid hemorrhage, neoplasm)
- One of the three most common causes (Chiari II malformation, Dandy-Walker malformation, congenital aqueductal stenosis) of congenital hydrocephalus
- Endocrine dysfunction in 20%; presumably result of compression of hypothalamic/pituitary axis by enlarged infundibular recess of third ventricle

Imaging
- CT and MRI: dilated lateral and third ventricles with normal-sized fourth ventricle; tectum may be distorted but should not be bulbous or high in signal on T2 images (features that raise the possibility of tectal glioma)
- Aqueductal stenosis a diagnosis of exclusion that should be made only after careful MRI evaluation has ruled out an obstructive mass lesion originating in the tectum, suprasellar region, or anterior third ventricle

Callosal Agenesis

Clinical
- Callosum develops in anterior to posterior fashion (except rostrum, the anteroinferior tip of the callosum, develops last)
- Depending on timing of developmental insult, callosum may be completely (agenesis) or partially (hypogenesis) absent; in callosal hypogenesis, more anterior portions of callosum are usually present (because that part of callosum forms first) and more posterior portions are absent
- Agenesis of corpus callosum may be isolated, but in 80% of patients is associated with other brain anomalies (Chiari II, Dandy-Walker, lipoma, neuronal migration disorders, holoprosencephaly)

Imaging
- CT and MRI: widely separated, parallel lateral ventricles that have a "steer horn" configuration in the coronal plane; continuity of high third ventricle with interhemispheric fissure to form an "interhemispheric cyst"; longitudinal white matter bundles ("bundles of Probst") indenting the medial aspect of the frontal horns; colpocephaly (dilatation of trigones and occipital horns)

2

Chiari I Malformation

Clinical
- Congenital hindbrain dysplasia characterized by pointed or "peg-like" cerebellar tonsils that project more than 5 mm below foramen magnum
- Can be asymptomatic or can present with findings related to brain stem compression (*exertional headache*, neck pain, nystagmus, lower cranial nerve palsies) or an associated *syrinx* (weakness, atrophy, and decreased sensation in arms and hands)
- Associated abnormalities: syrinx (70%); hydrocephalus (20%); basilar invagination (25%); Klippel-Feil anomaly; atlantooccipital fusion

Imaging
- MRI: sagittal T1 and T2 images of brain and cervical spine best demonstrate tonsillar ectopia and any associated syrinx

Chiari II Malformation

Clinical and Imaging
- Congenital brain and spine malformation characterized by:
  Lumbar Spine
  > Myelomeningocele: neural placode and meninges protrude through open (i.e., no skin covering) midline defect in lower back
  Infratentorial brain and cervical spine
  > Small posterior fossa with low insertion of tentorium cerebelli on occipital bone
  > Inferior displacement and compression of cerebellar vermis, fourth ventricle, brain stem, and upper cervical spine with associated *cervicomedullary kinking* and *tectal beaking*
  > Enlarged foramen magnum with scalloped erosion of petrous bones
  > Syrinx (50%)
  Supratentorial brain
  > Hydrocephalus
  > Interdigitation of paramedian cortical sulci through hypoplastic or fenestrated falx
  > Dysgenesis of corpus callosum
- Presents at birth with myelomeningocele
- One of the three most common causes (Chiari II malformation, Dandy-Walker malformation, congenital aqueductal stenosis) of congenital hydrocephalus

Dandy-Walker Malformation

Clinical
- Congenital hindbrain malformation characterized by:
  > Large posterior fossa with high insertion of tentorium cerebelli
  > *Hypoplastic or absent cerebellar vermis*; variable hypoplasia of cerebellar hemispheres
  > Large fourth ventricle that communicates dorsally with *posterior fossa cyst*
  > Hydrocephalus
- Presents at 1 to 3 months of life with enlarging head caused by hydrocephalus
- One of the three most common causes (Chiari II malformation, Dandy-Walker malformation, congenital aqueductal stenosis) of congenital hydrocephalus
- Associated abnormalities: callosal dysgenesis (25%), neuronal migration disorders (10%), occipital encephalocele (5%)
- Prognosis related to presence of other (supratentorial) anomalies and control of hydrocephalus

Imaging
- MRI: lateral splaying of cerebellar hemispheres by the cyst on axial images

Diastematomyelia

Clinical
- Congenital abnormality characterized by sagittal division of portion of spinal cord into two hemicords, most commonly in the lumbar region
- Presents usually in childhood or adolescence as result of worsening cord tethering
- Hemicords may be contained in a single dural sac (50%) or in two separate dural

2

sacs (50%); a cartilaginous or bony septum that can lead to cord tethering is usually present in the latter
- Hemicords typically reunite below the division
- Associated abnormalities: vertebral body anomalies and scoliosis; cord tethering by the septum that divides the hemicords; myelomeningocele; syrinx; bridging neural tissue adhesions between hemicord and surrounding dura

Imaging
- CT: more sensitive than MRI for demonstration of cartilaginous or bony septum
- MRI: coronal and axial T1 and T2 images define extent of cord abnormality and also allow evaluation of conus position; axial GRE images most sensitive for detection of bony septum

Heterotopia

Clinical
- Heterotopic foci of gray matter between the ventricular surface and cortex
- Results from developmental arrest of normal migration of neuronal precursors from germinal matrix lining ventricles to cortex
- Locations: subependymal; subcortical white matter
- Presents with seizures and variable developmental delay

Imaging
- MRI: multiple round subependymal nodules or foci in subcortical white matter that are isointense to gray matter on all sequences; no enhancement, mass effect, or surrounding T2 abnormality
- *Band heterotopia* is a rare condition in which a band of abnormal gray matter, separated by white matter from the overlying cortex, is seen subjacent to the cortex of both hemispheres (hence the name *double cortex*)

Holoprosencephaly

Clinical
- Disorder of absent or incomplete hemispherization
- Clinical features: midline facial abnormalities (e.g., hypotelorism, cleft palate); trisomy 13 (50%); spontaneous abortion in most severe forms; seizures, retardation, or developmental delay in milder forms
- Spectrum of abnormality, from most severe (alobar holoprosencephaly) to least severe (lobar holoprosencephaly):
  Alobar
    Horseshoe-shaped forebrain
    Falx and interhemispheric fissure absent
    Corpus callosum absent
    Thalami and basal ganglia fused; third ventricle absent
    Optic tracts and olfactory bulbs are absent
    Monoventricle (surrounded by the horseshoe-shaped forebrain) continuous with a large dorsal cyst
  Semilobar
    Falx and interhemispheric fissure partially formed posteriorly
    Splenium of corpus callosum formed
    Thalami partially separated; third ventricle small
    Temporal and occipital horns of lateral ventricles partially formed
  Lobar
    Falx and interhemispheric fissure formed, except for the most anterior portions
    Splenium and body of the corpus callosum formed
    Thalami separated; third ventricle normal
    Lateral ventricles more fully formed
- Main differential diagnosis severe hydrocephalus or hydranencephaly, both of which have distinguishing features:
    Hydrocephalus: widely separated thalami as result of enlarged third ventricle; thin, compressed cortical mantle underlying all parts of the calvarium
    Hydranencephaly: cerebral hemispheres absent

Imaging
- Obstetric ultrasound that shows a normal cavum septum pellucidum excludes all forms of holoprosencephaly

Neurofibromatosis Type I (NF-I; von Recklinghausen disease)

Clinical
- Most common phakomatosis (group of congenital malformations with cutaneous, visceral, and central nervous system abnormalities)
- Bilateral optic nerve gliomas, resulting in fusiform enlargement and kinking of the optic nerves, a radiological hallmark of NF-I
- Clinical features: presents in childhood with café au lait spots and axillary freckling; incidence: 1 in 4,000 (ten times more common than neurofibromatosis type II); autosomal dominant inheritance or sporadic (50%); many cutaneous neurofibromas; intracranial and spinal tumors in 15%

Imaging
- MRI:
  Gliomas
  Optic pathway gliomas and other (e.g., brain stem, basal ganglia, chiasm/hypothalamus) intracranial gliomas
  Many of the gliomas in NF-I are juvenile pilocytic astrocytomas or other low-grade astrocytomas
  Hamartomas
  Multiple foci of T2 hyperintensity involving the brain stem, cerebellum, internal capsule, and basal ganglia
  Appear in infancy, increase in size and number in childhood, resolve by early adulthood
  Distinguished from gliomas by absence of mass effect or enhancement
  Plexiform neurofibroma of the face or scalp
  Sphenoid wing dysplasia
  Neurofibromas of spinal and peripheral nerves
  Lateral thoracic meningocele
- Additional imaging features of NF-I include kyphoscoliosis, posterior scalloping of vertebral bodies because of dural ectasia, bony dysplasias involving appendicular skeleton, and vascular dysplasias

Neurofibromatosis Type II (NF-II)

Clinical
- One of the phakomatoses
- *Bilateral acoustic schwannomas* are a radiological hallmark of NF-II
- Clinical features: presents in young adulthood; incidence: 1 in 50,000 (i.e., much less common than neurofibromatosis type I); autosomal dominant inheritance; paucity of cutaneous lesions; intracranial and spinal tumors

Imaging
- MRI: acoustic schwannomas and other cranial or spinal schwannomas; multiple meningiomas, intracranial and spinal; ependymomas of spinal cord

Neuronal Migration Disorders
Imaging
- MRI the study of choice for evaluation of all neuronal migration disorders
- *See specific disorder (Heterotopia, polymicrogyria, schizencephaly)*

Polymicrogyria (Cortical Dysplasia)

Clinical
- Focal cortical disorganization, leading to thickening of cortex and blurring of gray-white junction
- Any region of cortex can be involved, but perisylvian region is most commonly affected
- Associated in some cases with congenital CMV infection
- Presents with seizures

Imaging
- MRI the modality of choice
- Three-dimensional, gradient echo, thin-section T1 images a critical part of imaging examination because of high resolution and multiplanar re-formation capability
- Findings include cortical thickening and blurring of the gray-white junction, abnormal gyral folding, isointensity to gray matter on all sequences; no enhancement or mass effect; occasional linear T2 signal abnormality subjacent to the cortical abnormality, extending toward the ventricle; commonly associated venous angioma

Schizencephaly

Clinical
- Transcerebral cleft extending from cortical surface (often near the central sulcus) to lateral ventricle
- Polymicrogyric gray matter lines the cleft and allows differentiation from encephalomalacia or porencephalic cyst
- *Closed-lip* (walls of cleft closely apposed) and *open-lip* (walls of cleft separated) describe the appearance of the schizencephalic cleft and have some prognostic significance (closed-lip generally carries better prognosis)
- Presents with seizures, developmental delay, and motor deficits
- Associated abnormalities include gray matter heterotopia, contralateral cortical dysplasia, and septooptic dysplasia

Imaging
- CT and MRI: gray matter–lined cleft extending from cortical surface to lateral ventricle; may be bilateral

Sturge-Weber Syndrome
Clinical
- One of the phakomatoses
- Angiomas involving face, pia, choroid plexus, and ocular choroid
- "Tram-track" cortical calcifications on plain film or CT and focal leptomeningeal enhancement, often parietooccipital, with associated cortical atrophy, are radiological hallmarks of Sturge-Weber syndrome
- Presents in early infancy with seizures
- Clinical features: facial hemangioma ("port-wine" stain) in the distribution of one or more divisions of the trigeminal nerve; unilateral or bilateral; seizures; hemiparesis, hemianopsia; buphthalmos (marked globe enlargement resulting from in utero glaucoma); retardation

Imaging
- Skull film: "tram-track" linear cortical calcifications
- CT: "tram-track" linear cortical calcifications subjacent to the pial venous angioma; ipsilateral focal or diffuse atrophy; ipsilateral paranasal sinus enlargement
- MRI:
  - T1: leptomeningeal enhancement resulting from pial venous angioma, ipsilateral to the facial hemangioma; ipsilateral focal or diffuse atrophy as result of chronic ischemia, presumed secondary to a vascular steal phenomenon involving the pial venous angioma; choroid plexus hypertrophy resulting from choroid plexus hyperplasia or angioma, ipsilateral to facial hemangioma; large subependymal flow voids
  - T2: low signal in the subcortical white matter subjacent to the pial angioma, caused by calcification or long-standing ischemia

Tethered Cord Syndrome

Clinical
- Congenital low-lying conus (below L2–L3 disc space) as result of abnormal anchoring of distal cord or filum terminale
- Differential growth of bony spine and spinal cord leads to cord traction and ischemia
- Presents in children or young adults with progressive gait disturbance, lower extremity weakness and sensory deficit, and bowel and bladder dysfunction
- Conditions responsible for cord tethering include:

Fibrolipoma of the filum terminale with thickened (more than 2 mm at L5–S1), fatty filum

Lipomyelomeningocele: neural placode, attached dorsal lipoma, and meninges protrude through closed (i.e., skin-covered) midline bony defect in lumbosacral spine

Lipoma, dermoid, or epidermoid

Diastematomyelia

Scarring after myelomeningocele repair

Imaging
- MRI: T1 axial images are necessary to accurately determine conus position; conus below L2–L3 level; variable mild hydromyelia in the distal cord that frequently resolves after surgical release of tethered cord

Tuberous Sclerosis

Clinical
- One of the phakomatoses
- Hamartomas of brain, retina, kidneys, skin, and heart
- Hamartomas ("tubers") of cortex, subcortical white matter, and subependymal region of lateral ventricles are the radiological hallmark of tuberous sclerosis
- Clinical features: presents in infancy or early childhood with seizures; incidence: 1 in 100,000; triad of seizures, retardation, and adenoma sebaceum (nodular facial angiofibroma); ash leaf spots (depigmented macules); autosomal dominant inheritance or sporadic (50%)

Imaging
- Three types of lesions are identifiable on imaging examinations: *hamartomas (tubers)* located in cortex, subcortical white matter, and subependymal region of lateral ventricles; *linear T2 signal hyperintensities* in the periventricular white matter; *giant cell astrocytomas* (10%) at the foramen of Monro
- CT:

    Bilateral subependymal nodules (tubers) along the margins of the lateral ventricles

    Usually located along bodies of lateral ventricles and near foramen of Monro

    Commonly calcified after age 2 years

    Variable enhancement

    Enlargement and increasing enhancement of a subependymal tuber near foramen of Monro raises the possibility of degeneration into giant cell astrocytoma, a low-grade neoplasm that can cause obstructive hydrocephalus

    Foci of low attenuation in subcortical white matter, most commonly in frontal and parietal regions, corresponding to cortical/subcortical tubers; expansion of gyrus; variable associated calcification

- MRI: signal characteristics of tubers relative to white matter vary depending on degree of myelination and presence of calcification

    T1: subependymal tubers isointense to hyperintense; cortical tubers hypointense to hyperintense

    T2: subependymal tubers isointense or hypointense; cortical tubers hyperintense; linear hyperintensity in periventricular white matter, radiating from ventricles to cortex

- Additional imaging features of tuberous sclerosis can include renal cysts and angiomyolipomas, interstitial lung disease, cardiac rhabdomyoma

von Hippel-Lindau (VHL) Syndrome

Clinical
- One of the phakomatoses
- Multiple cerebellar and spinal cord hemangioblastomas are a radiological hallmark of VHL
- Autosomal dominant inheritance, but often sporadic
- Presents in young adulthood or middle age with visual problems or symptoms related to posterior fossa mass effect (e.g., progressive ataxia and obstructive hydrocephalus at the level of the fourth ventricle)

2

- Additional features variably present in VHL include retinal angiomas, renal cell carcinoma, pheochromocytoma, pancreatic carcinoma, and visceral cysts (most commonly renal or pancreatic)

Imaging
- CT and MRI: *See Hemangioblastoma*

DEGENERATIVE AND MISCELLANEOUS CONDITIONS

Arachnoiditis

Clinical
- Leptomeningeal and nerve root inflammation that is a delayed complication of a number of conditions
- Presents with back pain, asymmetrical radicular symptoms, or both
- Diverse causes: surgery; meningitis; subarachnoid hemorrhage; trauma; intrathecal injections; Pantopaque myelography

Imaging
- MRI and CT myelography:
    Loss of nerve root sleeve filling
    Clumping and thickening of nerve roots
    Adherence of roots to walls of thecal sac ("empty sac sign")
    Variable nerve root enhancement
    Abnormal soft tissue within the thecal sac
    Arachnoid loculations
    Variable syringomyelia

Degenerative Disc Disease
Disc Protrusion
- *Disc protrusion, disc herniation,* and *focal disc bulge* are terms used by different radiologists to describe focal (as opposed to broad-based or circumferential) extension of disc material beyond the normal confines of the annulus fibrosis
- Common in lower cervical and lower lumbar spines; symptomatic disc protrusion is rare in thoracic spine
- Levels most commonly involved: lower cervical spine (C5–C6 and C6–C7) and lower lumbar spine (L4–L5 and L5–S1)
- Correlation with history and examination is essential to establish clinical relevance, because even large protrusions can be asymptomatic
- Paracentral or lateral disc protrusion presents as a unilateral radiculopathy; central disc protrusion presents as myelopathy in cervical spine or radiculopathy in lumbar spine
- Numbered *cervical spine* nerve roots exit *above* the corresponding numbered pedicle (e.g., C5 spinal nerve roots exit above C5 pedicle via C4–C5 foramen; C7 spinal nerve roots exit above C7 pedicle via C6–C7 foramen); *lateral or foraminal* disc protrusion at C4–C5 results in C5 radiculopathy
- Numbered *lumbar spinal* nerve roots exit *below* the corresponding numbered pedicle (e.g., L5 spinal nerve roots exit below the L5 pedicle via the L5–S1 foramen); *lateral or foraminal* disc protrusion at L5–S1 results in L5 radiculopathy; *central* disc protrusion at L5–S1 usually results in S1 radiculopathy
- *Disc extrusion:* more extensive herniation that can migrate several centimeters in epidural space superiorly or inferiorly from parent disc
- *Free disc fragment:* herniated disc material that has separated from the parent disc; both free fragments and disc extrusions are important to recognize, because the presence of either may alter the surgical approach
- After anterior cervical discectomy and fusion, increased stress is placed on disc levels adjacent to fused segments, increasing the likelihood of disc protrusion or other degenerative changes at those levels

Spinal Stenosis
- Acquired narrowing of spinal canal
- *Cervical stenosis* presents with progressive myelopathy; *lumbar stenosis* presents with chronic low back pain and neurogenic claudication (leg and buttock pain and paresthesias that are exacerbated by walking)

- Commonly multifactorial: broad-based disc bulge or central disc protrusion; facet and ligamentum flavum hypertrophy; spondylolisthesis; congenitally short pedicles

Imaging
- MRI the preferred imaging modality for evaluation of degenerative spine disease
- CT myelography is a more invasive alternative that is very close to MRI in terms of sensitivity and specificity; main disadvantage is the inability to evaluate intrinsic cord abnormality
- Plain film myelography reserved for patients with fixation hardware that would cause pronounced artifacts on both CT and MRI
- MRI findings:
  Disc space narrowing
  Disc dehydration (T2 hypointense)
  Signal changes in vertebral end plates adjacent to degenerated disc range from edema (Modic I) to fatty signal (Modic II) to sclerosis (Modic III)
    Modic I: T1 hypointense, T2 hyperintense
    Modic II: T1 hyperintense, T2 isointense
    Modic III: T1 hypointense, T2 hypointense
  Focal disc protrusion on axial images:
    Epidural tissue isointense to and contiguous with disc space
    No enhancement
  Uncovertebral osteophytes (cervical spine) and facet joint hypertrophy (cervical and lumbar spine) contribute to foraminal narrowing and exacerbate effects of small lateral recess or foraminal disc protrusion
- Gadolinium contrast is not routinely necessary but may be helpful in distinguishing nonenhancing recurrent disc protrusion from enhancing scar in postoperative lumbar spine (disc material and scar may have similar signal characteristics on noncontrast images)

Mesial Temporal Sclerosis

Clinical
- Most common cause of intractable complex partial seizures
- Results in neuronal cell loss and gliosis in hippocampal cortex
- May be bilateral but almost always is strikingly asymmetrical, with the most severely affected side typically on the side of the seizure focus

Imaging
- Key imaging correlates are *atrophy* in hippocampus and mesial temporal lobe and *T2 signal hyperintensity*
- Coronal high-resolution T2 images are the most important part of imaging evaluation
- MRI:
  T1: normal signal; volume loss in hippocampus, and possibly temporal lobe, may be apparent
  T2: high signal in hippocampal cortex, often accompanied by volume loss in hippocampus or entire temporal lobe

Musculoskeletal Imaging

■ **Charles G. Peterfy,** M.D., Ph.D.

■ **Alan Laorr,** M.D.

OVERVIEW

Among the myriad imaging modalities available today, radiography remains the mainstay of musculoskeletal imaging. Despite their unsurpassed spatial resolution, low expense, and wide availability, radiographs are limited in a number of ways, and in several situations must be supplemented with other modalities. A detailed discussion of these alternatives is beyond the scope of this chapter, but a few generalizations bear mention.

One major limitation of radiography is its poor depiction of noncalcified tissue. Fat and gas may be detected in soft tissues, and joint effusions and some masses occasionally can be detected by the displacement of local fat planes. Little additional detail is usually available. Even bone injuries are visible only when there is an actual break in the cortex and some degree of displacement. Overlapping osseous structures or immobilizing cast material can further obscure bony detail and conceal fractures and focal lesions. Occult fractures of the scaphoid and hip are particularly problematic, because they carry a significant risk of avascular necrosis if not immobilized. Conventional radiographs are especially insensitive to isolated destruction of cancellous bone, and losses of as much as 30 to 50% of trabecular bone frequently eludes detection. For this reason, osteopenia caused by trabecular bone loss, as in postmenopausal osteoporosis, is evaluated by dual x-ray absorptiometry (DXA) or quantitative computed tomography (QCT).

Conventional CT overcomes the problem of overlapping structures but generally is limited to imaging in the axial plane. Transverse fracture lines through long bones or the odontoid process may be missed. Multiplanar reformatting is possible, but limited resolution in the slice-select direction and spatial misregistration caused by patient movement between acquisitions degrade the images. Spiral CT partially obviates this problem. CT shows a greater dynamic range in terms of soft-tissue contrast but is still an x-ray–based modality and thus has only limited scope for discriminating noncalcified soft tissues other than fat.

Scintigraphy with "bone-seeking" agents such as technetium 99m phosphates provides unique information about bone turnover and repair. It is more sensitive

3

than radiography or CT for detecting obscured or undisplaced fractures, early osteomyelitis, or metastatic disease. It also has, however, a number of limitations. Impaired delivery of the radiotracer to the bone by vascular insufficiency or thrombosis can conceal some abnormalities. Sluggish bone repair in the elderly can delay detection of radiographically occult fractures for up to 48 hours. Increased uptake of radiotracer is itself a relatively nonspecific finding, and the images offer relatively poor spatial resolution.

Magnetic resonance imaging (MRI) has unparalleled and unprecedented capabilities for imaging musculoskeletal disease. It is free of ionizing radiation and capable of direct multiplanar imaging without the need for reformatting. Because of its unique ability to depict soft tissues and fluid collections, MRI offers a noninvasive means of directly examining muscles, tendons, ligaments, nerves, vessels, fascial connective tissue, menisci, articular cartilage, soft-tissue tumors, and hematomas. MRI is also useful for imaging bone. For example, it is highly sensitive for radiographically occult fractures, contusions, or stress reactions, as well as early osteomyelitis, avascular necrosis, and primary and secondary neoplasms. Although the sensitivity of MRI for detecting these bone abnormalities is unsurpassed, appearances often are nonspecific. Metal within the body (e.g., vascular clips or a pacemaker) can result in injury to the patient from an MRI scan, and artifacts from prosthetic and fixation hardware degrade image quality. The high cost of an examination often is raised as a limitation of MRI, but this expense must be viewed in light of the unique information that MRI often provides and balanced against the costs of management without this information. MRI has been shown actually to reduce total patient management costs for a number of specific clinical indications.

As mentioned earlier, MRI is probably the most sensitive modality for detecting bone lesions, but often is nonspecific. Conventional radiographs are more specific but rarely pathognomonic. It is important, therefore, to consider a variety of differential possibilities in each case. Healing stress fractures or osteomyelitis, for example, can mimic malignant neoplasms. A useful way to conceptualize the different radiographic patterns produced by bone lesions is in terms of their apparent aggressiveness at the level of the interface between the lesion and normal cancellous bone, cortex, periosteum, and adjacent soft tissues.

Slow-growing, nonaggressive focal processes tend to show sharp margins with adjacent normal bone and allow sufficient time for the bone to encase the lesion in a well-formed cortex. The cortex remains intact and there is no periosteal reaction. A solitary bone cyst is an example of a lesion with these nonaggressive features. An otherwise nonaggressive lesion that continues to grow may appear to expand the bone locally through endosteal resorption and periosteal apposition (e.g., aneurysmal bone cyst, enchondroma). When aggressiveness is increased and growth is more rapid, cortication of the margins of the lesion can no longer take place, although the interface may still appear sharp (e.g., giant cell tumor). More aggressive features, as seen with malignant neoplasms and acute osteomyelitis, include indistinctness of the lesion's margins, permeation of the cortex, and stimulation of periosteal reaction.

Although numerous patterns of periosteal reaction have been described, the appearances are largely nonspecific. The most aggressive lesions may progress so rapidly that there is no opportunity for a periosteal reaction to develop. However, mechanical stimulation caused by stripping back of periosteum by an aggressive lesion that has broken through the cortex and tented up the periosteum centrally can produce triangular buttresses of periosteal bone at either end of the lesion (Codman's triangles). Pathologic fracture through a benign lesion (e.g., enchondroma or fibrous dysplasia) can have an aggressive appearance as fracture healing promotes callus formation and periosteal reaction. Biopsy specimens from such lesions, including simple stress fractures, can show features of malignancy and confuse the diagnosis, sometimes with tragic consequences. Moreover, some highly aggressive lesions, such as metastases from renal or thyroid carcinoma, can present a nonaggressive pattern on radiographs.

Whenever subarticular abnormalities are observed in a bone, the other side of the joint must be carefully scrutinized in order to exclude the possibility of arthritis. Although radiography has been the principal modality for imaging arthritis, it is actually quite limited in this regard. Radiographs can visualize directly only bone changes in arthritis, and these tend to occur late in the disease course. Joint effusions and synovitis can be seen only indirectly by the displacement of intraarticular fat pads. Cartilage loss, which is fundamental to the loss of joint function, can be inferred only from narrowing of the joint space. MRI is the only noninvasive method capable of directly evaluating all of these articular components, as well as ligamentous and musculotendinous involvement, which is consistent with current views of arthritis as a disease affecting the joint as a whole organ. However, development of this application of MRI is still in its infancy and, at present, radiographs remain the principal imaging method for evaluating patients with arthritis.

Arthritis can be loosely divided into inflammatory, degenerative, and metabolic/tumoral patterns. Although all components of the joint are important to its functional integrity, and disruption of one component necessarily affects all others, the radiographic patterns associated with these various arthritides reflect differences in the way in which these individual components are affected. Inflammatory arthritides tend to be dominated by the effects of erosive synovitis. Rheumatoid arthritis and seronegative arthritides (e.g., psoriasis and Reiter's syndrome) are associated with erosion of cartilage and subarticular bone, varying degrees of subarticular osteopenia, and, in the case of seronegative arthritis, proliferative changes that cause whiskering of bone erosions, periosteal calcification, and articular fusion. These proliferative features are the most reliable radiographic criteria for discriminating rheumatoid arthritis from seronegative arthritis. Most forms of juvenile chronic arthritis show radiographic features that are similar to those of the seronegative arthritides. Superimposed on these are growth disturbances, such as epiphyseal overgrowth, premature physeal fusion, and bone shortening.

Infectious arthritis also exhibits inflammatory features on radiographs. Pyogenic arthritis should be considered in any inflammatory monoarticular arthritis that shows very rapid progression. Tuberculosis also shows an inflammatory pattern, with juxtaarticular lucencies and osteopenia, although joint-space narrowing is usually a late feature.

Gout can have inflammatory features but is dominated by erosions with sclerotic margins and overhanging edges that form around tophaceous deposits in the juxtaarticular soft tissues. Joint-space narrowing is characteristically late. Tumoral joint conditions, such as pigmented villonodular synovitis and synovial osteochondromatosis, are also characterized by preserved joint space and juxtaarticular pressure erosions.

The radiographic appearance of degenerative arthritis is dominated by proliferative changes and bone remodeling in association with cartilage loss (manifested radiographically as joint-space narrowing). These adaptive changes include subchondral sclerosis, expansion of articular surface area by chondro/osteophyte formation, and increased congruency of the articulating surfaces. Additional changes include subarticular cyst (geode) formation and joint malalignment. Osteoarthritic changes seen directly by MRI include cartilage loss, synovial hyperplasia, joint effusion, subarticular bone marrow edema, ligamentous laxity and rupture, and muscle atrophy. Osteoarthritis is the common end point of several etiopathologic pathways. The severity and distribution of changes in each case is governed by the balance between systemic predisposition and local biomechanical factors. Known systemic risk factors include old age, female gender, and obesity. Biomechanical risk factors include local trauma, chronic overuse, neuropathic disease, cartilage deposition disease (e.g., chondrocalcinosis, hemochromatosis, ochronosis, Wilson's disease), cartilage overgrowth (acromegaly), recurrent hemarthrosis (hemophilia), and articular dysplasias (spondyloepiphyseal dysplasia, multiple epiphyseal dysplasia, developmental dysplasia of the hip).

MUSCULOSKELETAL DIFFERENTIAL DIAGNOSES

3

Long bones
Well-defined lytic lesion
Ill-defined lytic lesion
Expansive lytic lesion
Multiple lytic lesions
Epiphyseal lytic lesion
Well-defined sclerotic lesion
Ill-defined sclerotic lesion
Lesion with sequestrum
Focal periostitis/cortical hyperostosis
Diffuse periostitis
Excessive callus formation
Erlenmeyer flask deformity
Enlarged bone
Short metacarpal or metatarsal
Erosion/absence of distal clavicle
Lucent metaphyseal bands
Dense metaphyseal bands
Epiphyseal irregularity
Epiphyseal overgrowth
Acroosteolysis
Acetabular protrusion
Diffuse osteosclerosis
Expansive lytic posterior element lesion
Coarse trabeculation
Regional osteopenia
Cortical striation/tunneling
Premature closure of the physis
Well-formed bone spurs
Poorly defined bone spurs

Joints
Monoarticular arthritis
Purely erosive arthritis
Erosive and proliferative arthritis
Arthritis with preserved joint space
Accelerated osteoarthritis
Destructive arthritis with sclerosis and debris
Calcified intraarticular loose body
Joint fusion
Ulnar deviation of metacarpophalangeal joints
Sacroiliitis
Arthropathy with soft tissue masses
Periarticular soft tissue calcifications
Chondrocalcinosis
Spine spondylolisthesis
Atlantoaxial subluxation
Paravertebral calcification/ossification
Disc calcification
Ivory vertebra
Enlarged vertebra
Posterior scalloping of vertebra
Anterior scalloping of vertebra
Absent pedicle
Dense pedicle
Dense vertebral end plate

Bone scintigraphy
Cold (photopenic) lesions on bone scan
Diffuse increased uptake ("superscan")

LONG BONES

WELL-DEFINED LYTIC LESION

List five well-defined lytic lesions not generally seen in patients older than 30 years of age.

Metastasis
Multiple myeloma
Giant cell tumor
Enchondroma (digits)
Clear cell chondrosarcoma
Desmoplastic fibroma (desmoid)
Fibrous dysplasia
Brown tumor
Hemophiliac pseudotumor
Subacute osteomyelitis (Brodie's abscess)
Osteoblastoma

Only in Patients Under 30 Years of Age

Aneurysmal bone cyst
Solitary bone cyst
Nonossifying fibroma
Chondroblastoma
Chondromyxoid fibroma
Eosinophilic granuloma

Metastasis

Which metastases can have a benign appearance?

- Usually ill defined and aggressive looking but can be remarkably benign in appearance; this is especially true with thyroid and renal carcinoma, which may also be expansive.
- Typically multiple, but 15% are solitary

FIGURES Resnick: 1080, 1083

Multiple Myeloma

- Usually ill defined, but occasionally sharply marginated and "bubbly," especially in the ribs; solitary plasmacytomas often appear well defined.

FIGURES Resnick: 597–600

Giant Cell Tumor

- Typically well defined and purely lytic without sclerotic margins
- Lesions are eccentric and intramedullary and abut the articular cortex of long bones; most commonly around knee and distal radius
- Almost always present after closure of physis

FIGURES Resnick: 1031–1035

Enchondroma

At which site are enchondromas often not calcified?

- Typically well defined with sharply corticated margins
- May be expansive
- Almost always contain typical chondroid-matrix calcifications, but those in the digits are usually not calcified

FIGURES Resnick: 1010, 1011

Clear Cell Chondrosarcoma

- Epiphyseal lesion resembling chondroblastoma, but in an adult patient

FIGURE   Resnick: 1025

Desmoplastic Fibroma (Desmoid)

- Typically bubbly and lytic in appearance
- Benign, but may have areas that appear aggressive

FIGURE   Resnick: 1029

Fibrous Dysplasia

- Often purely lytic, but intralesional calcification may produce "ground-glass" appearance
- May be expansive
- No periosteal reaction unless complicated by pathologic fracture
- Single or multiple lesions

FIGURES   Resnick: 1206–1210

Brown Tumor

- Never calcifies
- Margins usually corticated
- Look for other evidence of hyperparathyroidism

FIGURE   Resnick: 558

Hemophiliac Pseudotumor

- May be purely lytic and relatively well defined
- May be expansive
- May have a large soft tissue component

FIGURE   Resnick: 643

Subacute Osteomyelitis

- Purely lytic with surrounding sclerosis
- May be associated with periosteal reaction
- May have a serpiginous tract extending toward epiphysis
- Exclude associated pyogenic arthritis if near an articular surface

FIGURE   Resnick: 655

Osteoblastoma

- Benign lytic lesion, usually associated with sclerosis of surrounding bone
- Lytic nidus may calcify
- Most common in posterior vertebral elements

FIGURES   Resnick: 999, 1000

Aneurysmal Bone Cyst

- Benign expansive hemorrhagic lesion
- Usually found in children

FIGURES   Resnick: 1052, 1053

Solitary Bone Cyst

- Proximal humerus and proximal femur are most common sites
- Sharply corticated margins
- No periosteal reaction unless complicated by pathologic fracture
- Dependent fragments of cortical bone within a fractured lesion ("fallen fragment" sign) are virtually pathognomonic

FIGURES Resnick: 1048–1050

Nonossifying Fibroma

- Subcortical, metaphyseal lesion with thin, sclerotic, lobulated margins
- Occasionally mildly expansive
- No matrix calcification, but scleroses during involution

FIGURES Resnick: 1028, 1029

Chondroblastoma

- Epiphyseal lesion usually seen in patients under the age of 20 years
- May be purely lytic, but up to 50% contain chondroid matrix calcifications

FIGURES Resnick: 1013, 1014

Chondromyxoid Fibroma

- Lytic lesion usually seen in patients under the age of 20 years
- Not calcified
- Resembles aneurysmal bone cyst

FIGURES Resnick: 1014, 1015

Eosinophilic Granuloma

- Highly variable radiographic appearance, ranging from geographic to permeative
- May contain sequestrum

FIGURES Resnick: 616, 617

ILL-DEFINED LYTIC LESION

Name three poorly defined lytic lesions in a child.

List three benign conditions that can appear to be ill defined.

Metastasis
Multiple myeloma
Ewing's sarcoma
Acute osteomyelitis
Eosinophilic granuloma
Leukemia
Lymphoma
Telangiectatic osteosarcoma
Malignant fibrous histiocytoma
Fibrosarcoma
Hemangioma

Metastasis

- Most skeletal metastases are ill defined, reflecting their aggressive nature
- Typically, periostitis is absent or minimal

3

FIGURES Resnick: 1080–1089

Multiple Myeloma

- Wide spectrum of radiographic appearances, including moth-eaten and permeative; occasionally appears well defined and expansive

FIGURES Resnick: 597–599

Ewing's Sarcoma

- Malignant neoplasm of childhood
- Typically produces a permeative pattern with aggressive periostitis, cortical erosion, and a soft tissue mass

FIGURES Resnick: 1057–1059

Acute Osteomyelitis

- Typically produces aggressive pattern in bone
- Metaphyses most commonly involved
- May have involucrum (young patient) or sequestrum

FIGURES Resnick: 653, 654

Eosinophilic Granuloma

- Highly variable radiographic appearance includes ill-defined focal lesion or permeative pattern

FIGURES Resnick: 616, 617

Leukemia

- Variable radiographic appearance, including permeative pattern, focal ill-defined lesions and, occasionally, more well-defined lesions

FIGURES Resnick: 626–629

Lymphoma

- Typically has an aggressive appearance in bone
- May be lytic or sclerotic (especially Hodgkin's disease)
- May have periostitis

FIGURES Resnick: 630–632

Telangiectatic Osteosarcoma

- Highly aggressive, nonsclerosing form of osteosarcoma
- Usually in metaphyses of children
- Occurs most commonly around the knee

FIGURE Resnick: 1005

Malignant Fibrous Histiocytoma

- Malignant lesion, usually with moth-eaten or permeative pattern in metaphysis of long bone

FIGURE Resnick: 1037

Fibrosarcoma

- Most commonly in metaphysis of long bone
- Variable appearance, but often moth-eaten or permeative
- No matrix calcification but may contain sequestered bone fragments

FIGURE Resnick: 1030

Hemangioma

- Long bone involvement is uncommon
- Lytic lesion with characteristic lattice-like or web-like, coarse trabecular pattern
- The appearance may seem permeative and mimic malignancy or infection

FIGURE Resnick: 1040–1042

EXPANSIVE LYTIC LESION

Name three important differences between giant cell tumor and aneurysmal bone cyst.

Which malignancies can be lytic and expansive?

Metastasis
Multiple myeloma
Aneurysmal bone cyst
Giant cell tumor
Hemophiliac pseudotumor
Brown tumor
Enchondroma
Nonossifying fibroma
Fibrous dysplasia

Metastasis

- Metastases from renal and thyroid carcinoma may be relatively well defined and expansive, thus mimicking benign lesions

FIGURE Resnick: 1080

Multiple Myeloma

- May result in expansive lesion, especially in ribs

FIGURE Resnick: 599

Aneurysmal Bone Cyst

- Benign, expansive lesion with thin, corticated margins
- Usually in patients under the age of 30 years
- Typically shows fluid levels on CT or MRI

FIGURES Resnick: 1052, 1053

Giant Cell Tumor

- Well defined with nonsclerotic margins
- Produces cortical thinning and occasionally some mild expansion
- Extends to subarticular surface
- Usually benign but may be malignant

FIGURES Resnick: 1031–1035

Hemophiliac Pseudotumor

- Well-defined expansive lesion with sclerotic margins caused by intraosseous hemorrhage
- Occurs in less than 2% of hemophiliacs
- May be intraosseous, subperiosteal, or within soft tissues

FIGURES Resnick: 643, 644

Brown Tumor

- Benign reparative lesion seen in hyperparathyroidism
- Usually well defined with sclerotic margins
- May be expansive and trabeculated
- Other features of hyperparathyroidism

FIGURE Resnick: 558

Enchondroma

- Benign chondroid neoplasm with well-defined, sclerotic margins
- May be expansive, especially in enchondromatosis (Ollier's disease)
- Usually contains chondroid-matrix calcifications, except in the digits, where it may be purely lytic

FIGURES Resnick: 1010, 1011

Nonossifying Fibroma

- Benign fibroosseous lesion with lobulated, sclerotic margins
- Typically occurs in metaphysis of long bones, abutting the endosteal surface
- Larger lesions may show cortical thinning and osseous expansion

FIGURES Resnick: 1028, 1029

Fibrous Dysplasia

- Benign fibroosseous lesion
- Larger lesions are typically expansive and prone to pathologic fracture

FIGURES Resnick: 1206–1210

MULTIPLE LYTIC LESIONS

Name four causes of multiple lytic lesions.

Metastases
Multiple myeloma
Osteomyelitis
Fibrous dysplasia
Brown tumors
Eosinophilic granuloma
Leukemia
Lymphoma
Enchondromatosis (Ollier's disease)

Metastases

What are the primary sites of four tumors that produce lytic metastases?

- Multiple lesions in 85% of cases
- Most common sources are breast, prostate, lung, and renal cell carcinomas

• Predominate in the axial skeleton, but any bone may be affected

Figures Resnick: 1080–1089

Multiple Myeloma

• Axial skeleton is the predominant site of involvement, but any bone may be affected
• Classically presents with numerous, well-marginated lytic lesions of similar size, which is unusual in skeletal metastasis

Figures Resnick: 597–599

Osteomyelitis

• Multiple lesions common in hematogenous osteomyelitis

Figures Resnick: 653–656

Fibrous Dysplasia

• May have solitary or multiple lesions in one, few, or many bones
• About 25% of cases are polyostotic
• Polyostotic cases are usually predominantly one sided

Figures Resnick: 1206–1209

Brown Tumors

• May be solitary or multiple

Figure Resnick: 558

Eosinophilic Granuloma

• Multiple lesions are less common than solitary lesions
• Highly variable radiographic appearance

Figures Resnick: 616, 617, 619

Leukemia

• Lytic lesions (multiple or solitary) are seen in approximately 50% of cases

Figures Resnick: 626–628

Lymphoma

• Bone involvement is present in approximately 20% of lymphoma cases (most commonly non-Hodgkin's)
• Multiple lesions are more common than solitary lesions
• May calcify

Figures Resnick: 630–632

Enchondromatosis (Ollier's Disease)

• Multiple enchondromas, many of which may show chondroid-matrix calcifications
• Affected bones are often short and deformed
• Malignant transformation occurs in approximately 20% of cases

Figure Resnick: 1011

What is the most likely cause of multiple lytic bone lesions on only one side of the skeleton?

3

Name the three lytic epiphyseal lesions most common in childhood.

EPIPHYSEAL LYTIC LESION

Geode
   Osteoarthritis
   Calcium pyrophosphate arthropathy
   Rheumatoid arthritis
   Osteonecrosis
Intraosseous ganglion
Giant cell tumor
Chondroblastoma
Clear cell chondrosarcoma
Eosinophilic granuloma
Infection

Geode

- Also termed *subchondral cyst*
- Geographic lytic lesion with sclerotic margins
- Caused by pulsion of synovial fluid through a defect in the subchondral or marginal cortex or possibly by focal subarticular osteonecrosis and cystic resorption
- Seen in association with osteoarthritis, calcium pyrophosphate arthropathy, rheumatoid arthritis, and osteonecrosis

FIGURES Resnick: 847, 849

Intraosseous Ganglion

- Similar to geode but without associated joint abnormality
- Common sites include the medial malleolus, femoral head, carpus, and acetabulum

FIGURE Resnick: 326

Giant Cell Tumor

- Extends from metaphysis to articular surface
- Usually seen in mature skeleton after closure of the physeal plate
- Most common sites are around the knee and in the distal radius
- Margins discrete but nonsclerotic
- No matrix calcification

FIGURES Resnick: 1031–1035

Describe three radiographic differences between chondroblastoma and giant cell tumor.

Chondroblastoma

- Occurs in epiphysis or apophysis
- Usually seen in immature skeleton, before closure of the physeal plate
- Most common sites are femur, humerus, and tibia
- Margins well defined and sclerotic
- Calcified in up to 50% of cases

FIGURES Resnick: 1013, 1014

Clear Cell Chondrosarcoma

- Rare, low-grade malignancy
- Usually occurs in patients between the ages of 20 and 50 years
- Occurs in epiphysis, with a distribution similar to that of chondroblastoma
- Appearance similar to that of chondroblastoma but seen in patients older than 20 years of age

• Pathologic fracture in 25% of cases

FIGURE Resnick: 1025

Eosinophilic Granuloma

• Epiphysis less commonly involved than diaphysis and metaphysis

FIGURES Resnick: 616, 617

Infection

• Hematogenous osteomyelitis may involve the epiphysis in those under 1 year and over 16 years of age
• Look for associated joint effusion/septic arthritis

FIGURES Resnick: 653, 654

WELL-DEFINED SCLEROTIC LESION

What are two common sites of stress fracture?

Where might noncalcified enchondromas be found?

Metastasis
Bone island
Osteoid osteoma
Osteoblastoma
Mature bone infarct
Enchondroma
Low-grade chondrosarcoma
Fibrous dysplasia
Healing stress fracture
Involuting lytic lesion

Metastasis

• Usually ill defined, but may be well defined in some cases
• Sclerotic metastases most commonly from prostate and breast carcinomas

FIGURES Resnick: 1080–1089

Bone Island

• Usually aligned with the long axis of bone
• "Feathery" or "thorny" bone spicules extending from the periphery of the lesion and blending into the surrounding trabeculae are characteristic

FIGURES Resnick: 1211, 1212

Osteoid Osteoma

• Benign osteoid neoplasm, usually in diaphysis of long bones and posterior vertebral elements
• Typically associated with marked sclerosis of surrounding bone
• Occasionally the otherwise lytic nidus calcifies

FIGURES Resnick: 993–998

Osteoblastoma

• Variable radiographic appearance, but may resemble a "giant osteoid osteoma"
• Less sclerosis of surrounding bone than with osteoid osteoma

3

• Otherwise lytic nidus often calcifies

FIGURE   Resnick: 999

Mature Bone Infarct

• Appears as serpiginous sclerotic lesion, typically in metadia-physis of long bones
• Differential diagnosis includes enchondroma and low-grade chondrosarcoma

FIGURE   Greenspan: 18.26

Enchondroma

• Identification of chondroid-matrix calcification or endosteal scal-loping differentiates this lesion from bone infarct
• Most enchondromas calcify, except occasionally those in the digits

FIGURES   Greenspan: 16.14; Resnick: 1010, 1011

Low-grade Chondrosarcoma

• Difficult to differentiate from enchondroma radiographically and histologically
• The presence of pain is a helpful clinical finding

FIGURES   Resnick: 1022, 1023

Fibrous Dysplasia

• May be sclerotic or mixed lytic-sclerotic
• Solitary or multiple lesions
• Polyostotic lesions usually involve only one side of the skeleton

FIGURES   Resnick: 1206–1209

Healing Stress Fracture

• Healing callus may mimic an aggressive osteoblastic process
• Typical sites include metatarsal shafts, calcaneus, tibia, femur, pubis, and sacrum

FIGURE   Resnick: 727

Involuting Lytic Lesion

• Examples include nonossifying fibroma/fibrous cortical defect, aneurysmal bone cyst, solitary bone cyst, and chondroblastoma

FIGURE   Greenspan: 17.2

ILL-DEFINED SCLEROTIC LESION

What are the most common sources of osteoblastic metastases?

What is the prevalence of Paget's disease?

Metastasis
Immature bone infarct/osteonecrosis
Osteosarcoma
Chondrosarcoma
Lymphoma
Chronic osteomyelitis
Stress fracture
Paget's disease

Metastasis

- May be ill defined or well defined
- Sclerotic metastases most commonly from prostate and breast carcinomas

FIGURES Resnick: 1080–1089

Immature Bone Infarct/Osteonecrosis

- Early lesion appears as patchy sclerosis

FIGURE Resnick: 946

Osteosarcoma

- Aggressive appearance; most commonly mixed sclerotic-lytic; less often is purely sclerotic or lytic
- Commonly associated with a soft tissue mass

FIGURES Resnick: 1002–1004

Chondrosarcoma

- High-grade neoplasms typically have an aggressive appearance with less-pronounced matrix calcifications and a prominent lytic component

FIGURE Greenspan: 15.9

Lymphoma

- Variable appearance including sclerotic, lytic, and mixed; Hodgkin's is more commonly sclerotic than is non-Hodgkin's
- Commonly ill defined

Chronic Osteomyelitis

- May show considerable sclerosis

FIGURES Resnick: 656; Greenspan: 19.4

Stress Fracture

- Healing callus may mimic an aggressive osteoblastic process
- Typical sites include calcaneus, metatarsals, tibia, femur, pubis, and sacrum

FIGURES Resnick: 725–727

Paget's Disease

- Chronic disorder characterized by areas of excessive and abnormal bone remodeling
- Seen in 3% of population over the age of 40 years
- Common sites include the pelvis, spine, femur, skull, and tibia
- Always starts at an articular end of long bone (exception tibia) and advances toward the diaphysis

FIGURES Resnick: 527–535

Name three malignant lesions that may be associated with sequestration of bone.

Which of these lesions typically shows beveled edges in the skull?

LESION WITH SEQUESTRUM

Osteomyelitis
Eosinophilic granuloma
Fibrosarcoma
Malignant fibrous histiocytoma
Desmoplastic fibroma
Lymphoma
Metastasis
Osteoid osteoma ("pseudosequestrum")

Osteomyelitis

• Sequestrum common in infantile and childhood osteomyelitis; less common in adulthood

FIGURE   Resnick: 655

Eosinophilic Granuloma

• In skull lesion, "button" sequestrum with beveled edges is classic but not common

FIGURES   Resnick: 616, 617

Fibrosarcoma

• Variable appearance (geographic to permeative)
• No matrix calcification but sequestered fragments common

FIGURE   Resnick: 1030

Malignant Fibrous Histiocytoma

• Malignant lesion arising in bone de novo or in association with other lesions (e.g., Paget's disease, chronic osteomyelitis, osteonecrosis, radiation osteitis)
• Usually moth-eaten or permeative pattern in metaphysis of long bone

FIGURE   Resnick: 1037

Desmoplastic Fibroma

• Benign but locally aggressive lytic lesion found in mandible, pelvis (ilium), and metaphyses of long tubular bones

Lymphoma

• May have sequestrum

Metastasis

• Sequestra are rare

FIGURES   Resnick: 1081, 1082

Osteoid Osteoma ("Pseudosequestrum")

• Calcification of lucent nidus may resemble a sequestrum

FIGURES   Resnick: 993–997

FOCAL PERIOSTITIS/CORTICAL HYPEROSTOSIS

Name three nonneoplastic causes of focal cortical hyperostosis.

How can parosteal osteosarcoma be differentiated from myositis ossificans?

Osteoma
Osteoid osteoma
Osteoblastoma
Brodie's abscess
Stress fracture
Parosteal osteosarcoma
Cortical desmoid
Parosteal lipoma
Melorheostosis

Osteoma

· Benign periosteal nodule of mature bone
· Usually located in the skull and facial bones (especially the frontal sinus), but may occur in tubular bones
· Multiple lesions found in Gardner's syndrome

FIGURE   Resnick: 1213

Osteoid Osteoma

· Diaphyseal lesions in long bones are typically intracortical and appear as a central lucency with surrounding sclerosis and cortical thickening
· Periosteal lesions evoke a particularly exuberant periosteal response; medullary lesions are associated with relatively less sclerosis

FIGURE   Resnick: 993

Osteoblastoma

· May be predominantly lytic but often associated with intracortical sclerosis and focal periostitis, resembling a "giant osteoid osteoma"

FIGURE   Resnick: 999

Brodie's Abscess

· Intracortical lesion, appearing as a central lucency with surrounding sclerosis and occasionally periostitis, may resemble osteoid osteoma or stress fracture

FIGURE   Resnick: 655

Stress Fracture

· Focal periostitis with a central linear (usually transverse) lucency in cortex

FIGURE   Resnick: 727

Parosteal Osteosarcoma

· Malignant neoplasm most commonly arising along the posterior aspect of the distal femoral metaphysis
· Appears as a mass attached to the underlying cortex, with osteoid-matrix calcifications
· Lesion is calcified centrally, in contrast to myositis ossificans, which calcifies peripherally

3

FIGURE   Resnick: 1007

Cortical Desmoid

- Occurs at the posteromedial aspect of the supracondylar linea aspira of the distal femur and represents a stress reaction at the adductor magnus insertion in children and adolescents
- Appears as a small cortical defect with adjacent sclerosis and periostitis
- May be bilateral
- Appearance and location are virtually diagnostic

Parosteal Lipoma

- Soft tissue lipoma adherent to the underlying bone, which may result in focal hyperostosis or periostitis
- Rare lesion typically in the femur and proximal radius
- In contrast to osteochondroma, bony outgrowth does not contain marrow confluent with the normal medullary space

Melorheostosis

- Wavy cortical hyperostosis resembling dripping candle wax is seen on one side of one or more bones
- Findings are characteristic and often limited to one limb; the lower extremity is more frequently affected than the upper

FIGURES   Resnick: 1216, 1217

DIFFUSE PERIOSTITIS

Which findings are most suggestive of child abuse?

What is the most common disorder associated with hypertrophic osteoarthropathy?

Name four causes of diffuse periostitis in a child.

Adult
    Hypertrophic osteoarthropathy
    Pachydermoperiostosis
    Thyroid acropachy
    Venous stasis
    Fluorosis
Child
    Physiologic
    Caffey's disease
    Child abuse
    Malignancy
    Congenital syphilis
    Hypervitaminosis A
    Scurvy

Hypertrophic Osteoarthropathy

- Benign or aggressive periostitis is initially seen in the proximal and distal diaphyses of long and short tubular bones
- Seen in association with a variety of pulmonary, gastrointestinal, and cardiac conditions, most frequently bronchogenic carcinoma
- Periostitis may progress into the metaphyses but typically spares the epiphyses

FIGURE   Resnick: 1222

Pachydermoperiostosis

- Also called *primary hypertrophic osteoarthropathy*
- In contrast to secondary hypertrophic osteoarthropathy, periostitis commonly extends into the epiphyses

• Has ill-defined bone outgrowths, further differentiating it from secondary hypertrophic osteoarthropathy

FIGURE   Resnick: 1219

Thyroid Acropachy

• Occurs in about 1% of hyperthyroid patients
• Typically seen after disease treatment when the patient is euthyroid or hypothyroid
• Feathery periostitis is usually seen in the diaphyses of the metacarpals, metatarsals, and phalanges

FIGURE   Resnick: 548

Venous Stasis

• Appears as benign, undulating periostitis
• Nearly always affects the lower extremities
• Predominantly involves metaphysis and diaphysis

FIGURE   Resnick: 1225

Fluorosis

• May have undulating periostitis affecting various long and short tubular bones
• Also associated with osteosclerosis, vertebral osteophytosis, and ligamentous and tendinous calcification/ossification

Physiologic

• Seen from 1 to 6 months of age
• Incidence reported to be as high as 35%
• Appears as symmetric diaphyseal periostitis

Caffey's Disease

• Also termed *infantile cortical hyperostosis*
• Uncommon, idiopathic disorder beginning in infancy and resolving by 6 months to 1 year
• Appears as periostitis affecting the diaphysis and metaphysis
• One or several bones may be involved, most commonly the mandible, clavicles, and ribs

FIGURE   Resnick: 1226

Child Abuse

• Multiple fractures in various states of healing in otherwise skeletally normal child is highly suspicious
• Periostitis from subperiosteal hemorrhage
• Metaphyseal corner fracture ("bucket-handle" fracture) is relatively specific

FIGURE   Resnick: 755

Malignancy

• Examples include acute childhood leukemia, neuroblastoma metastasis, and multicentric osteosarcoma

FIGURES   Resnick: 574, 626, 627

3

Congenital Syphilis

- Manifestations include osteochondritis, diaphyseal osteomyelitis, and periostitis
- Dense periosteal apposition along anterior tibia produces "saber-shin" appearance

FIGURE   Resnick: 699

Hypervitaminosis A

- Wavy diaphyseal periostitis in the ulna and metatarsals is typical; other tubular bones may be involved
- Radiographic changes usually appear around the age of 1 year
- Metaphyseal and epiphyseal deformities also may be present

FIGURE   Resnick: 908

Scurvy

- Results from chronic dietary vitamin C deficiency
- Subperiosteal hemorrhage results in periostitis
- Other findings include dense metaphyseal band, lucent metaphyseal band ("scurvy" line), metaphyseal beaks, subepiphyseal infractions, dense shell around epiphysis (Wimberger's sign)

FIGURE   Resnick: 910

EXCESSIVE CALLUS FORMATION

What are the most common radiographic features of osteogenesis imperfecta?

What does marginal condensation *refer to?*

Steroids (exogenous or Cushing's disease)
Inadequate fracture immobilization
Paralysis
Osteogenesis imperfecta

Steroids (Exogenous or Cushing's Disease)

- Radiographic manifestations include osteopenia, osteonecrosis, and vertebral compression and rib fractures that may be associated with excessive callus formation
- Exuberant callus along the superior and inferior end plates of collapsed vertebrae, known as *marginal condensation,* is characteristic of steroid toxicity

FIGURE   Resnick: 573

Inadequate Fracture Immobilization

- May result in excessive callus formation or nonunion, which may be hypertrophic

Paralysis

- Heterotopic ossification is most commonly associated with paraplegia secondary to spinal cord injury, although it may be seen with various neuromuscular disorders

FIGURE   Resnick: 917

Osteogenesis Imperfecta

- Inherited disorder of abnormal collagen synthesis
- Radiographic findings most commonly include osteopenia; thin,

gracile bones; bowing of bones; and multiple fractures of different ages
- Fracture healing is usually normal, but excessive callus may form

FIGURE Resnick: 1117

ERLENMEYER FLASK DEFORMITY
(undertubulation of long bones)

Name three causes of Erlenmeyer flask deformity.

Which cause is associated with a "hair-on-end" calvarial pattern?

Gaucher's disease
Thalassemia/other anemias
Niemann-Pick disease
Osteopetrosis
Metaphyseal dysplasia (Pyle's disease)

Gaucher's Disease

- Rare, inherited disorder of lipid metabolism with accumulation of cerebroside in macrophages (Gaucher's cells) in bone marrow and other tissues
- Radiographic features include Erlenmeyer flask deformities, medullary expansion, diffuse osteopenia, focal lytic lesions, and avascular necrosis

FIGURES Resnick: 609, 610

Thalassemia/Other Anemias

- Beta-thalassemia and other severe anemias result in Erlenmeyer flask deformities and medullary expansion from marrow hyperplasia
- Other radiographic features of beta-thalassemia include osteopenia and widening of the diploic space, producing a "hair-on-end" pattern in the skull
- Typical "rodent facies" seen almost exclusively in thalassemia is a sign of severe anemia

FIGURES Resnick: 589–591

Niemann-Pick Disease

- Rare, inherited disorder with lipid accumulation in the bone marrow and other tissues
- Radiographic findings include Erlenmeyer flask deformities, medullary expansion, and diffuse osteopenia

FIGURE Resnick: 612

Osteopetrosis

- Rare, inherited disorder of osteoclast failure
- Metaphyseal expansion is seen in the presence of diffuse osteosclerosis

FIGURE Resnick: 1140

Metaphyseal Dysplasia (Pyle's Disease)

- Rare, inherited disorder characterized by metaphyseal expansion of tubular bones
- Increased bone fragility

FIGURE Resnick: 1145

ENLARGED BONE

Generalized bone enlargement is most suggestive of which disease?

What is the most common cause of bone enlargement in the elderly?

Paget's disease
Neurofibromatosis
Acromegaly
Hemangioma
Macrodystrophia lipomatosa

Paget's Disease

- Chronic disorder of bone remodeling
- Bone becomes widened/enlarged in the inactive (sclerotic) phase
- Bone enlargement differentiates Paget's disease from osteoblastic metastases

FIGURE   Resnick: 530

Neurofibromatosis

- Hemihypertrophy of long bones is common in children with this disorder
- Anterolateral bowing of tibia or pseudarthrosis formation also is seen

FIGURES   Resnick: 1202, 1226, 1227

Acromegaly

- Skeletal manifestations of generalized tissue overgrowth include enlargement of the distal tufts, sesamoids, vertebrae, paranasal sinuses, mastoid air cells, and mandible

FIGURES   Resnick: 539–542

Hemangioma

- Benign vascular neoplasm may arise within soft tissues or bone
- Bone lesions may be expansive with a striated or reticular pattern
- Soft tissue lesions may result in overgrowth of the adjacent bone

FIGURE   Resnick: 1041

Macrodystrophia Lipomatosa

- Rare, congenital form of localized gigantism with increased fibroadipose tissue and progressive overgrowth of a digit

FIGURES   Resnick: 1126, 1127

SHORT METACARPAL OR METATARSAL

What additional radiographic signs would point to juvenile chronic arthritis as a cause?

Which cause is associated with delayed skeletal maturation?

Idiopathic
Juvenile chronic arthritis
Turner's syndrome
Pseudohypoparathyroidism
Trauma
Sickle cell anemia

Juvenile Chronic Arthritis

- Both overgrowth (caused by hyperemia) and undergrowth (caused by premature closure of physis) can occur
- Additional radiographic findings include osteopenia, erosions,

joint space narrowing, ankylosis, periostitis, and growth abnormalities

Turner's Syndrome

- Characterized by XO sex chromosome configuration
- Radiographic findings include short metacarpals (especially the fourth) and metatarsals, osteopenia, proximal tibia deformity, and delayed skeletal maturation

FIGURE   Resnick: 1153

Pseudohypoparathyroidism

- Inherited disorder with end-organ resistance to parathyroid hormone; associated with short metacarpals, metatarsals, and phalanges
- Pseudopseudohypoparathyroidism is a normocalcemic form of the disorder

FIGURE   Resnick: 569

Trauma

- Growth disturbance may result from a fracture involving the physis

Sickle Cell Anemia

- Short metacarpals, metatarsals, or phalanges may result from sickle cell dactylitis (bone infarction), which typically occurs in patients between 6 months and 2 years of age

FIGURES   Resnick: 583, 584

EROSION/ABSENCE OF DISTAL CLAVICLE

Which causes typically affect both sides of the acromioclavicular joint?

What inherited disorder is this a feature of?

Hyperparathyroidism
Rheumatoid arthritis
Posttraumatic osteolysis
Cleidocranial dysplasia
Metastasis/multiple myeloma
Infection

Hyperparathyroidism

- Resorption is typically bilateral and symmetric

Rheumatoid Arthritis

- Distal clavicle may appear "penciled"
- The adjacent acromion is also affected
- Changes may be unilateral or bilateral
- Additional findings in the shoulder girdle include articular changes in the glenohumeral joint and evidence of a torn rotator cuff (high-riding shoulder)

FIGURES   Resnick: 218, 219

3

Posttraumatic Osteolysis

- Occurs after local trauma, including minor repetitive stress such as weightlifting
- Resorption may also involve the acromion to a lesser degree
- May appear 2 weeks to several years after the insult

FIGURES Resnick: 1233, 1234

Cleidocranial Dysplasia

- Autosomal dominant disorder associated with absence of the distal or middle portions of the clavicle
- Additional radiographic findings include poor skull ossification, Wormian bones, wide cranial sutures and fontanelles with delayed closure, and delayed ossification of the pubis producing widening of the symphysis pubis

FIGURE Resnick: 1138

Metastasis/Multiple Myeloma

- Look for additional lesions

Infection

- Acromioclavicular joint is a common site of infection in intravenous (IV) drug abuse
- Both sides of the joint typically are affected (i.e., septic arthritis)

FIGURE Resnick: 686

LUCENT METAPHYSEAL BANDS

Which nutritional deficiencies are associated with lucent metaphyseal bands?

Name two malignancies that can present lucent metaphyseal bands.

Severe illness
Leukemia
Neuroblastoma metastasis
Normal variant
Scurvy
Congenital infection (toxoplasmosis, rubella, cytomegalovirus, herpes simplex [TORCH])
Juvenile chronic arthritis
Rickets

Severe Illness

- Lucent lines secondary to defective osteogenesis

Leukemia

- Lucent lines caused by inhibition of osteogenesis, not by leukemic infiltrates

FIGURE Resnick: 626

Neuroblastoma Metastasis

- Bone metastases are frequent at the time of diagnosis
- Bilateral metaphyseal lesions are typical

FIGURE Resnick: 574

Scurvy

- Vitamin C deficiency leads to cessation of endochondral bone formation because of osteoblast failure
- Metaphyseal lucency (Trümerfeld zone) represents a local decrease in trabeculae
- Loss of epiphyseal trabeculae accentuates the cortex (Wimberger's sign)
- Additional radiographic signs include osteopenia, dense zone of provisional calcification, metaphyseal corner fractures (Pelkan spurs), and painful periosteal reaction
- Osteopenia is usually the only sign in adults

FIGURE Resnick: 910

Congenital Infection (TORCH)

- Lucent band is caused by a disturbance in endochondral ossification

FIGURES Resnick: 698, 699

Juvenile Chronic Arthritis

- Lucent band may be caused by a disturbance in endochondral ossification (because of severe systemic illness), metaphyseal hyperemia, or both

Rickets

- Decreased density at the zone of provisional calcification
- Other radiographic findings include physeal widening and metaphyseal fraying and cupping

FIGURE Resnick: 518

DENSE METAPHYSEAL BANDS

Name two causes that are probably of no clinical concern.

Which malignancy can cause this?

Growth arrest lines/stress lines
Heavy metal poisoning
Osteopetrosis
Cretinism
Hypervitaminosis D
Leukemia
Rickets
Scurvy
Congenital infection (TORCH)
Osteopathia striata
Hypoparathyroidism

Growth Arrest Lines/Stress Lines

- Also known as *Park lines* or *Harris lines*
- Commonly observed in children and adults
- Probably related to a variant of normal growth patterns

FIGURE Resnick: 913

Heavy Metal Poisoning

- May result from lead, arsenic, bismuth, mercury, etc.
- Calcium deposition is responsible for the appearance, although

lead (or other heavy metal) is also deposited in the metaphysis in much smaller amounts

FIGURE Resnick: 914

Osteopetrosis

- Linear striations are part of the bone-within-bone appearance often seen in these patients

Cretinism

- Infantile thyroid deficiency
- Also results in delayed skeletal maturation and irregular epiphyses

FIGURE Resnick: 550

Hypervitaminosis D

- Dense metaphyseal bands (alternating with lucent bands) represent prominence of the provisional zone of calcification
- Also associated with lobulated masses of soft tissue calcification (tumoral calcinosis)

Leukemia

- Dense bands may be seen adjacent to lucent metaphyseal zones, reflecting disrupted bone growth

FIGURE Resnick: 626

Rickets

- Dense bands seen with healed rickets

Scurvy

- Metaphyseal dense line represents prominent zone of provisional calcification (line of Frankel) and is seen adjacent to a lucent metaphyseal line (Trümerfeld zone)

FIGURE Resnick: 909

Congenital Infection (TORCH)

- Dense vertical metaphyseal lines may produce a "celery stalk" appearance in infants with transplacental infections such as toxoplasmosis, syphilis, rubella, cytomegalovirus, and herpes

FIGURE Resnick: 708

Osteopathia Striata

- Voorhoeve's disease
- Rare disorder characterized by asymptomatic longitudinal striations extending from metaphyses to the diaphyses of long bones
- Pelvic striations may have a radial distribution
- Bone scintigraphy negative
- May coexist with osteopoikilosis, melorheostosis, or osteopetrosis

FIGURE Resnick: 1215

Hypoparathyroidism

- Osteosclerosis and calvarial thickening also may be present

EPIPHYSEAL IRREGULARITY

Name an endocrine cause of epiphyseal irregularity.

Avascular necrosis
Congenital infection (TORCH)
Hypothyroidism
Dysplasia epiphysealis multiplex
Spondyloepiphyseal dysplasia
Trisomy 18 and 21
Normal variant

Avascular Necrosis

- MRI is most sensitive for diagnosis of early osteonecrosis
- Patchy sclerosis in an epiphysis usually precedes articular surface collapse
- Bilateral in 50% of cases

FIGURES   Resnick: 943–957

Congenital Infection (TORCH)

- Additional findings may include dense or lucent metaphyseal bands, metaphyseal abnormalities, periostitis, and osteomyelitis

Hypothyroidism

- Radiographic findings include delayed skeletal maturation, Wormian bones, epiphyseal irregularity or deformity (or both), osteopenia, and slipped capital femoral epiphysis

FIGURE   Resnick: 550

Dysplasia Epiphysealis Multiplex

- Includes chondrodysplasia punctata and Meyer's dysplasia

FIGURES   Resnick: 1122–1125

Spondyloepiphyseal Dysplasia

- Radiographic findings include epiphyseal irregularity and platyspondylisis or vertebral beaking

FIGURE   Resnick: 1131

Trisomy 18 and 21

- May have accessory epiphyses

EPIPHYSEAL OVERGROWTH

Name a cause of epiphyseal overgrowth that is restricted to males.

Which two causes can be indistinguishable radiographically?

Hemophilia
Juvenile chronic arthritis
Paralysis

Hemophilia

- The knee is most frequently affected
- Radiographic features include epiphyseal overgrowth, osteopenia, dense effusions, and secondary osteoarthritis with subchondral cysts, pseudotumors, and osteonecrosis

FIGURE   Resnick: 642

Juvenile Chronic Arthritis

- Radiographic findings may be indistinguishable from those of hemophilia (knowing whether the patient is female is therefore helpful)
- Radiographic features include epiphyseal overgrowth, osteopenia, soft tissue swelling, joint space loss, erosions and subchondral cysts, periostitis, ankylosis, and growth disturbances

FIGURE   Resnick: 241

Paralysis

- Radiographic findings include epiphyseal widening, osteopenia, heterotopic ossification, and growth disturbances

FIGURE   Resnick: 917

ACROOSTEOLYSIS

Which arthritides are associated with tuft erosion?

Define Raynaud's phenomenon.

Scleroderma
Injury
Hyperparathyroidism
Psoriasis
Raynaud's phenomenon/disease
Neuropathic arthropathy
Epidermolysis bullosa
Congenital erythropoietic porphyria
Polyvinyl chloride exposure
Pyknodysostosis
Acroosteolysis of Hajdu and Cheney

Scleroderma

- Radiologic findings include acroosteolysis, soft tissue wasting, and subcutaneous calcifications

FIGURE   Resnick: 299

Injury

- Causes include frostbite, burns, and electrical injury
- May be associated with soft tissue loss or contracture, osteopenia, periostitis, joint abnormalities, soft tissue calcification, and bone destruction
- With frostbite, thumb may be spared as a result of protective clenched-fist position

FIGURES   Resnick: 885–887

Hyperparathyroidism

- Associated subperiosteal bone resorption is a characteristic but insensitive finding

FIGURES   Resnick: 554, 555

Psoriasis

- Radiographic diagnosis depends on presence of other manifestations of psoriatic arthritis (e.g., joint-space narrowing, proliferative erosions, periostitis, joint fusion, etc.)

FIGURES   Resnick: 1232, 1233

Raynaud's Phenomenon/Disease

- Painful attacks of pallor followed by cyanosis, then redness of digits caused by arterial vasoocclusion precipitated by cold or stress and relieved by heat
- Condition may be idiopathic (Raynaud's disease) or associated with various diseases (e.g., scleroderma, rheumatoid arthritis, systemic lupus erythematosus, thoracic outlet syndrome, methysergide intoxication, myxedema, trauma, etc.)

Neuropathic Arthropathy

- Underlying conditions include diabetes, syringomyelia, and especially congenital indifference to pain
- Associated joint abnormalities should be sought

FIGURES   Resnick: 936, 937, 939

Epidermolysis Bullosa

- Rare, inherited skin disorder
- Additional radiographic findings include flexion contractures, digital webbing, and osteopenia

FIGURE   Resnick: 1268

Congenital Erythropoietic Porphyria

- In the hand, radiologic findings resemble those of scleroderma and include acroosteolysis, soft tissue wasting, soft tissue calcifications, and osteopenia

Polyvinyl Chloride Exposure

- Characterized by band-like resorption of terminal phalanges
- Involvement of the hand, especially the thumb, predominates

FIGURES   Resnick: 1232, 1233

Pyknodysostosis

- Autosomal recessive disorder associated with short stature
- Radiographic findings include acroosteolysis, osteosclerosis, hypoplastic mandible, and Wormian bones

FIGURE   Resnick: 1142

Acroosteolysis of Hajdu and Cheney

- Disorder with short stature, recessed mandible, joint laxity, and osteoporosis
- Acroosteolysis involves hands and feet

FIGURE   Resnick: 1234

ACETABULAR PROTRUSION

Which finding on a radiograph of the pelvis showing acetabular protrusion would differentiate ankylosing spondylitis from rheumatoid arthritis as a cause?

Name four causes of bilateral protrusion.

3

Osteomalacia
Rheumatoid arthritis
Ankylosing spondylitis
Infection
Osteoarthritis (medial migration pattern)
Paget's disease
Trauma
Radiation
Familial acetabular protrusion (Otto's pelvis)

Osteomalacia

- Additional radiographic features include osteopenia with coarsened trabeculae, Looser's transformation zones, and bowed long bones

Rheumatoid Arthritis

- Acetabular protrusion is common with severe rheumatoid arthritis of the hip

FIGURE Resnick: 228

Ankylosing Spondylitis

- Typically bilateral and symmetric
- The presence of osteophytes is characteristic
- Ankylosed sacroiliac joints are usually evident within the field of view

FIGURES Resnick: 256, 257

Infection

- Chondral destruction results in axial femoral head migration and may eventually lead to protrusion

Osteoarthritis (Medial Migration Pattern)

- Medial migration of the femoral head is atypical in osteoarthritis, occurring about 10% of the time

FIGURE Resnick: 342

Paget's Disease

- Pelvic involvement is commonly asymmetric
- Additional findings include osteosclerosis, bone expansion, thickened trabeculae, cortical thickening

FIGURE Resnick: 528

Trauma

- Protrusion may occur after acetabular fracture

Radiation

- Radiation weakens bone, causing protrusion

FIGURE Resnick: 895

Familial Acetabular Protrusion (Otto's Pelvis)

- Bilateral involvement

DIFFUSE OSTEOSCLEROSIS

Which metastases can cause diffuse osteosclerosis?

Which cause of osteosclerosis is also associated with avascular necrosis?

Metastasis
Renal osteodystrophy
Sickle cell anemia
Osteopetrosis
Pyknodysostosis
Paget's disease
Mastocytosis
Myelofibrosis
Fluorosis

Metastasis

- Severe cases of prostate and breast carcinoma

FIGURES Resnick: 1080–1083

Renal Osteodystrophy

- Associated findings include vascular calcifications, vertebral end plate sclerosis (rugger-jersey spine), and widening of the sacroiliac joints and symphysis pubis

FIGURES Resnick: 560, 561

Sickle Cell Anemia

- Osteosclerosis results from medullary infarction
- Additional radiographic features include H-shaped vertebrae, marrow hyperplasia/expansion, isolated infarcts, osteonecrosis, and dactylitis

FIGURES Resnick: 583, 584

Osteopetrosis

- Rare, inherited disorder of osteoclast failure
- Radiographic features include diffuse osteosclerosis, metaphyseal expansion, multiple fractures of different ages, bone-within-bone appearance, "sandwich" vertebra

FIGURES Resnick: 1140, 1141

Pyknodysostosis

- Additional radiographic findings include acroosteolysis, hypoplastic mandible, and Wormian bones

FIGURE Resnick: 1142

Paget's Disease

- Associated bone expansion, thickened trabeculae, cortical thickening, and bowing deformities

FIGURES Resnick: 527, 528

3

Mastocytosis

- Rare disorder in which mast cells accumulate in several organs
- Skin lesions are known as *urticaria pigmentosa*
- Radiographic features include osteosclerosis or osteopenia (or both), abnormal bowel loops, and hepatosplenomegaly

FIGURE   Resnick: 634

Myelofibrosis

- Uncommon disorder with sclerotic bone marrow and extramedullary hematopoiesis
- Associated hepatosplenomegaly and lobulated paravertebral thoracic masses (representing extramedullary hematopoiesis) should be sought

FIGURE   Resnick: 636

Fluorosis

- Radiographic findings include osteosclerosis, ligamentous and tendinous calcification, vertebral osteophytosis, and periostitis

FIGURE   Resnick: 903

EXPANSIVE, LYTIC POSTERIOR ELEMENT LESION

Name three causes of lytic expansion of the posterior elements of the spine.

Osteoblastoma
Aneurysmal bone cyst
Tuberculosis

What is the most common cause in a child?

Osteoblastoma

- One third of osteoblastomas occur in the spine, usually in the posterior elements, with frequent extension into the vertebral body
- Appears as a "blown-out" lytic lesion in this location

FIGURE   Resnick: 1000

Aneurysmal Bone Cyst

- Spinal lesions tend to arise in the posterior elements and appear expansive
- Fluid levels may be seen on CT and MRI

FIGURE   Resnick: 1053

Tuberculosis

- May appear expansive in the posterior vertebral elements

COARSE TRABECULATION

Name two causes of coarse trabeculae in the elderly.

Paget's disease
Osteopenia
Hemangioma

Which two causes of coarse trabecular pattern are associated with hepatosplenomegaly?

Thalassemia
Gaucher's disease

Paget's Disease

- Trabecular thickening and disorganization is a manifestation of abnormal bone turnover and remodeling
- Changes restricted to involved bones (five sites on average)

FIGURES   Resnick: 529–535

Osteopenia

- Loss of horizontal trabeculae accentuates the appearance of remaining vertical trabeculae
- Vertical striations finer than those seen with hemangioma and more often associated with biconcave deformities resulting from insufficiency fractures
- In osteomalacia, unmineralized osteoid covering on residual trabeculae adds a "smudged" appearance to cancellous bone

FIGURE   Resnick: 500

Hemangioma

- Removal of secondary transverse trabeculae and compensatory hypertrophy of residual primary vertical trabeculae in vertebral body produces characteristic vertical striations ("corduroy vertebra")
- Extraspinal lesions show radial or web-like trabecular pattern

FIGURES   Resnick: 501, 983, 1040

Thalassemia

- Hematopoietic marrow hyperplasia caused by chronic anemia results in osteoporosis and trabecular resorption, which, along with compensatory hypertrophy of residual trabeculae, produces an irregularly coarsened pattern
- Unlike Paget's disease and hemangiomas, changes in thalassemia are diffuse
- Obliteration of paranasal sinuses and dental malocclusion produce "rodent" facies not seen in Paget's disease or other anemias

FIGURES   Resnick: 589–591

Gaucher's Disease

- Rare, inherited lipid storage disease characterized by infiltration of liver, spleen, lymph nodes, bone marrow, and other tissues by lipid-laden macrophages (Gaucher's cells)
- Marrow infiltration results in trabecular and endosteal bone resorption, with coarsening of the residual trabecular pattern
- Additional skeletal findings include Erlenmeyer flask deformities of the femora, multifocal osteonecrosis, and osteolytic lesions

FIGURES   Resnick: 609, 610

REGIONAL OSTEOPENIA

How is disuse osteopenia differentiated from reflex sympathetic dystrophy syndrome?

How is transient osteoporosis of the hip differentiated from avascular necrosis?

Disuse osteoporosis
Reflex sympathetic dystrophy syndrome
Arthritis
Transient regional osteoporosis
  Transient osteoporosis of the hip
  Regional migratory osteoporosis

Acute avascular necrosis
Ill-defined lytic lesion
  Osteomyelitis
  Neoplasm
  Lytic Paget's disease

Disuse Osteoporosis

- Osteopenia due to bone resorption during local remodeling secondary to decreased use
- Linear or speckled rarefaction of the subcortical region of articular bones is characteristic, but changes most commonly involve the bones diffusely
- Cortical striations usually are present
- Radiographic changes develop slowly, usually over 2 to 3 months
- Common causes include immobilization in a cast or splint or paralysis

FIGURE Resnick: 496

Reflex Sympathetic Dystrophy Syndrome

- Also called *Sudeck's atrophy* or *shoulder-hand syndrome*
- Soft tissue swelling, pain, and vasomotor changes associated with a variety of conditions, including trauma, infection, calcific tendinitis, and myocardial infarction
- Most commonly affects entire upper limb, usually bilaterally
- Radiographs show regional osteopenia with cortical tunneling and occasionally subperiosteal resorption
- In contrast to what occurs in disuse osteoporosis, radiographic changes develop rapidly and are accompanied by soft tissue swelling
- Periarticular osteopenia can simulate arthritis but lacks significant bone erosion or joint-space narrowing
- Regional increased uptake on bone scintigraphy may precede clinical and radiographic findings

FIGURES Resnick: 497, 498

Arthritis

- Periarticular osteopenia characteristic in rheumatoid arthritis and septic arthritis, less common in seronegative arthritis or gout, but can be seen in severely inflamed cases
- Unlike other causes of regional osteopenia, inflammatory and septic arthritis are associated with progressive joint-space narrowing and bone erosion

FIGURES Resnick: 199, 664

Transient Regional Osteoporosis

- Rapidly developing, self-limited, reversible periarticular pain and osteoporosis of several months' duration without identifiable cause
- Transient osteoporosis of the hip presents in middle-aged men and pregnant women and may be bilateral
- Regional migratory osteoporosis successively affects joints, usually of the lower extremity, for several months at a time
- Radiography shows rapidly progressive but completely reversible periarticular osteopenia
- Increased uptake on bone scintigraphy and findings of marrow edema on MRI precede radiographic changes

- Imaging findings may be indistinguishable from early avascular necrosis
- In contrast to inflammatory or septic arthritis, no joint-space narrowing or bone erosion occurs

FIGURES Resnick: 498, 499

Acute Avascular Necrosis

- Intense local inflammation associated with acute avascular necrosis can produce local osteopenia on radiographs, increased radiotracer uptake on bone scintigraphy, and marrow edema on MRI
- Changes predominate in one articular component of a joint
- Development of patchy sclerosis and osseous collapse on radiography or emergence of characteristic serpiginous margins around lesion on MRI are distinctive of avascular necrosis

FIGURE Resnick: 499

Ill-defined Lytic Lesion

- Osteomyelitis usually develops in the metaphysis of children but can extend to the articular surface in infants or toddlers after closure of the physis
- Periostitis may be seen and sclerosis usually develops in subacute and chronic osteomyelitis
- Aggressive neoplasms such as telangiectatic osteosarcoma can mimic other causes of regional osteopenia
- Lytic Paget's disease almost always begins in subarticular bone and should be considered in elderly patients

FIGURES Resnick: 527, 655, 1005

CORTICAL STRIATION/TUNNELING (a sign of rapid bone turnover)

What does cortical tunneling signify?

Name two endocrine causes.

Thyrotoxicosis
Reflex sympathetic dystrophy syndrome
Disuse osteoporosis
Hyperparathyroidism
Paget's disease

Thyrotoxicosis

- Generalized increased bone turnover results in diffuse osteopenia with cortical tunneling
- Changes more pronounced in cortical bone than in trabecular bone
- Osteoporosis can result in pronounced biconcavity of vertebrae
- Feathery periostitis along diaphyses of tubular bones of digits occurs rarely (in 1% or less) after therapy (thyroid acropachy)

FIGURES Resnick: 547, 548

Reflex Sympathetic Dystrophy Syndrome

- Associated soft tissue swelling and rapid development of osteopenia and cortical tunneling distinguish this from disuse osteoporosis
- Usually involves both upper extremities, but changes are asymmetric

FIGURE Resnick: 497

3

Disuse Osteoporosis

- Localized bone resorption in immobilized or paralyzed limb
- Cortical tunneling and subarticular trabecular bone resorption are characteristic, but diffuse rarefaction of articular bones is the most common pattern

FIGURE   Resnick: 496

Hyperparathyroidism

- Excess parathyroid hormone directly stimulates osteoclasts in cortical haversian canals to produce intracortical striations
- Radiographic diagnosis relies on additional findings, such as subperiosteal bone resorption, resorption of distal clavicle, or presence of brown tumors

FIGURE   Resnick: 557

Paget's Disease

- Involved bones may contain osteolytic cortical clefts, which can be more pronounced than those from other causes of increased bone turnover
- Cortical clefts fill in with successful bisphosphonate therapy

FIGURE   Resnick: 530

BONE BOWING

How is osteogenesis imperfecta differentiated from rickets?

Name two hereditary conditions associated with bone bowing.

Paget's disease
Osteogenesis imperfecta
Osteomalacia/rickets
Fibrous dysplasia
Growth plate injury
Neurofibromatosis
Physiologic bowing (tibial)

Paget's Disease

- Woven bone produced during abnormal and excessive turnover is softer than normal laminar bone

FIGURE   Resnick: 530

Osteogenesis Imperfecta

- Production of abnormal collagen renders all bones weak and fragile
- Associated with diffuse osteopenia
- In tarda form (90%), appendicular bones are thin and gracile; short, thick bones indicate severe congenital form
- Fractures heal with exuberant callus formation
- In contrast to what occurs in rickets, growth plate is not widened

FIGURES   Resnick: 1115, 1116

Osteomalacia/Rickets

- Bones are soft because osteoid remains unmineralized
- Bowing in rickets is also the result of epiphyseal displacement by asymmetric musculotendinous pull
- Associated with diffuse osteopenia

- Radiographic diagnosis relies on identification of pseudofractures (specific but rare), widened growth plate (rickets), or smudged appearance of trabeculae

FIGURES Resnick: 517, 518

Fibrous Dysplasia

- Fibrodysplastic bone is softer than normal
- Bowing of proximal femur produces characteristic "shepherd's crook" deformity
- Monoostotic or polyostotic

FIGURE Resnick: 1209

Growth Plate Injury

- Injury to the outer portion of the physis disturbs normal growth of bone and produces bowing convex to the opposite side
- Severity of bowing depends on the amount of potential growth remaining at the time of injury
- Causes include trauma (especially Salter-Harris V fractures) and iatrogenic injury (e.g., anterior cruciate ligament repair)

FIGURE Resnick: 746

Neurofibromatosis

- Long bones may show bowing, pathologic fracture, and pseudarthrosis
- Manifestation of the mesodermal dysplasia
- Tibia most commonly affected, with anterolateral bowing evident in early childhood

FIGURES Resnick: 1202–1204

Physiologic Bowing

- Congenital anomaly of tibia
- In contrast to neurofibromatosis, functional bowing of tibia is usually convex posteriorly

PREMATURE CLOSURE OF THE PHYSIS

Name two endocrine causes of premature physeal fusion.

How might the radiographic pattern associated with these endocrine causes differ from those seen with other causes?

Trauma
Juvenile chronic arthritis
Hemophilia
Accelerated skeletal maturation

Trauma

- Fractures involving the growth plate, especially Salter-Harris V fractures, can lead to fibrous or bony bridging across the physis
- Central physeal fusion results in limb-length discrepancy
- Fusion of outer portion of physis results in bowing
- Severity of growth disturbance depends on how much additional growth remains at the time of injury

FIGURE Resnick: 746

Juvenile Chronic Arthritis

- Local inflammation and hyperemia can result in either overgrowth of a bone or premature physeal fusion and stunted growth
- Distribution of this effect is heterogeneous
- Hypoplasia of cervical vertebrae or mandible is characteristic

FIGURES Resnick: 237, 239–244

Hemophilia

- Premature physeal closure is the result of local hyperemia

Accelerated Skeletal Maturation

- Precocious puberty, as in McCune-Albright syndrome (precocious puberty, cafe au lait spots, and polyostotic fibrous dysplasia), can result in premature physeal fusion and bone shortening
- Hyperthyroidism is another endocrine cause of this disorder
- Bone shortening is diffuse

WELL-FORMED BONE SPURS

Name a key radiographic difference between fluorosis and DISH.

What endocrine abnormality is associated with enthesophytes?

Degenerative enthesopathy
Diffuse idiopathic skeletal hyperostosis (DISH)
Fluorosis
Acromegaly
Ankylosing spondylitis

Degenerative Enthesopathy

- Enthesophyte formation is considered by some to be a normal adaptive change of aging
- Common sites include vertebral end plates (vertebral osteophytes), calcaneal insertions of Achilles tendon and plantar aponeurosis, and ischial tuberosities
- May in some cases actually be related to DISH

FIGURE Resnick: 351

Diffuse Idiopathic Skeletal Hyperostosis (DISH)

- Flowing ossification along anterolateral aspect of the spine spanning four or more vertebral bodies is an essential diagnostic criterion
- Usually accompanied by diffuse enthetic ossification
- Seen in elderly patients

FIGURES Resnick: 379–389

Fluorosis

- Most salient feature is diffuse, chalky sclerosis of axial skeleton (not seen in DISH)
- Enthetic ossifications also occur

FIGURE Resnick: 903

Acromegaly

- Diffuse enthetic ossification accompanies generalized bone and soft tissue overgrowth

FIGURES   Resnick: 539–543

Ankylosing Spondylitis

- Enthetic spurring is often subtle
- Early, ill-defined proliferative erosion at entheses, typical of other seronegative spondyloarthropathies, may mature into well-formed bone spurs
- Fine calcification of outer annulus fibrosus of intervertebral disc (syndesmophytes) is most common pattern
- Syndesmophyte formation preceded by proliferative erosion at insertion of Sharpey's fibers of annulus, producing "shiny corners" and "squaring" of vertebral bodies

FIGURE   Resnick: 248

POORLY DEFINED BONE SPURS (mixed proliferative and erosive enthesitis)

Name a group of arthritides associated with "fuzzy" bone spurs.

Which cause is associated with conjunctivitis?

What is a noninflammatory cause of proliferative changes at a tendon insertion?

Psoriatic spondyloarthropathy
Reiter's syndrome
Ankylosing spondylitis
Avulsion injury

Psoriatic Spondyloarthropathy

- "Whiskered" or "fuzzy" spur formation at entheses is an expression of proliferative inflammation at these sites
- Proliferative enthesitis at capsular insertions of interphalangeal joints produces "mouse ears" appearance
- Calcaneal insertion of plantar aponeurosis is a common site of involvement

FIGURES   Resnick: 267–270

Reiter's Syndrome

- Radiographically indistinguishable from psoriatic spondyloarthropathy but shows greater propensity for the lower extremities

FIGURES   Resnick: 275–279

Ankylosing Spondylitis

- Enthesopathy initially ill defined but may eventually heal into well-defined bone spurs

FIGURE   Resnick: 248

Avulsion Injury

- Callus formation during healing can resemble proliferative enthesitis but is more commonly mistaken for neoplasm (e.g., "cortical desmoid" at insertion of adductor magnus, "hurdler's fracture" at insertion of hamstrings)

3

Which cause of monoarticular arthritis is clinically most urgent?

How do pigmented villonodular synovitis and synovial osteochondromatosis differ on radiographs? On MRI?

JOINTS

MONOARTICULAR ARTHRITIS

Trauma
Infection
   Pyogenic arthritis
   Tuberculosis
Neoplasm
   Pigmented villonodular synovitis
   Synovial osteochondromatosis
Inflammatory arthritis
   Rheumatoid arthritis
   Seronegative arthritis
   Juvenile chronic arthritis
Crystal-induced arthritis
   Gout
   Calcium pyrophosphate dihydrate deposition
   Calcium hydroxyapatite deposition

Trauma

- A common cause of synovitis and joint effusion

Pyogenic Arthritis

- *Gonococcus* is the most common cause of monoarthritis in young adults
- Wrist is the most common site, but any joint can be involved
- Staphylococcal infections common in IV substance abusers, often affecting the sternomanubrial, acromioclavicular, and sacroiliac joints
- It is critical to consider pyogenic arthritis before significant radiographic changes become apparent
- Earliest findings are juxtaarticular osteopenia and local soft tissue swelling
- Joint space narrowing denotes cartilage destruction, which progresses more rapidly than that in rheumatoid arthritis
- Late stages marked by severe joint destruction and bony fusion

FIGURES   Resnick: 663–666

Tuberculosis

- Slower progression and less symptomatic than pyogenic arthritis
- Any joint can be affected, but large joints are most commonly involved
- Early disease characterized by juxtaarticular osteopenia and cyst formation with slow progression of joint-space narrowing (Phemister's triad)
- Less bone proliferation or periostitis than with pyogenic arthritis
- Fibrous ankylosis is common, but osseous fusion is less frequent than with pyogenic arthritis
- In renal tuberculosis, joints are usually seeded hematogenously from the chest, but chest radiographs are often negative

FIGURES   Resnick: 694, 695

Pigmented Villonodular Synovitis

- A rare cause of arthritis, but always monoarticular
- Usually affects large joints, most commonly the knee

3

- Recurrent hemarthrosis results in hemosiderin-stained synovial proliferation and juxtaarticular erosions
- MRI is characteristic: hemosiderin-stained synovitis shows low signal intensity on all pulse sequences; indistinguishable from MRI appearance of hemophilia
- Radiographic changes also resemble those of hemophilia
- Similar process affecting synovial lining of tendon sheaths is called *giant cell tumor of the tendon sheath*

FIGURE Resnick: 646

Synovial Osteochondromatosis

- Usually affects large joints (e.g., knee, hip)
- Nodular chondroid metaplasia of synovium produces juxtaarticular erosions and joint-space widening on radiographs
- Calcified or ossified osteochondral bodies are directly visible on radiographs
- Noncalcified components show water signal on MRI
- Osteochondral bodies may contain marrow fat that is visible on MRI

FIGURES Resnick: 1069, 1070, 1253

Inflammatory Arthritis

- Although rheumatoid seronegative and juvenile chronic arthritis are usually polyarticular, both can also be monoarticular

Crystal-induced Arthritis

- Gout and calcium pyrophosphate dihydrate deposition usually are polyarticular but can be monoarticular
- Calcium hydroxyapatite deposition is usually monoarticular

FIGURES Resnick: 397–407, 412–421, 426–435

PURELY EROSIVE ARTHRITIS

What radiographic features differentiate rheumatoid arthritis from pyogenic arthritis?

What features differentiate tuberculous arthritis from pyogenic arthritis?

Rheumatoid arthritis
Pyogenic arthritis
Tuberculosis

Rheumatoid Arthritis

- Proliferative changes such as periostitis are uncommon; however, carpal or tarsal bones occasionally fuse

FIGURES Resnick: 213–220

Pyogenic Arthritis

- Acute changes usually purely erosive
- Proliferative changes, such as local sclerosis, periostitis, and bony fusion, often emerge with time

FIGURES Resnick: 663–666

Tuberculosis

- Proliferative changes uncommon
- More indolent course than pyogenic arthritis

FIGURES Resnick: 694, 695

EROSIVE AND PROLIFERATIVE ARTHRITIS

What are the most common proliferative manifestations in ankylosing spondylitis?

What finding in the cervical spine is characteristic of juvenile chronic arthritis?

Psoriatic spondyloarthropathy
Reiter's syndrome
Ankylosing spondylitis
Juvenile chronic arthritis
Pyogenic arthritis

3

Name four proliferative manifestations of erosive arthritis.

General

• Characterized by proliferative erosions, periostitis joint fusion, and endosteal bone formation

Psoriatic Spondyloarthropathy

• Proliferative erosions typically appear "whiskered" or "fuzzy" on radiographs
• Tenosynovitis may be associated with periostitis along diaphyses of phalangeal bones, and "sausage-finger" soft tissue swelling
• Bony ankylosis of interphalangeal joints
• Distribution usually asymmetric

FIGURES Resnick: 267–270

Reiter's Syndrome

• Can be indistinguishable from psoriatic spondyloarthropathy but shows greater propensity for the lower extremities

FIGURES Resnick: 275–279

Ankylosing Spondylitis

• Proliferative sacroiliitis and sacroiliac fusion are the most common proliferative manifestations
• Proliferative erosion at the enthetic attachments of the annulus fibrosus on the discovertebral margin produces characteristic "shiny corners" and "squaring" of the vertebral bodies
• Bridging syndesmophytes ultimately may fuse the spine
• Changes are highly symmetric

FIGURES Resnick: 248–259

Juvenile Chronic Arthritis

• Most common proliferative manifestations are diaphyseal periostitis and joint fusion
• Fusion of growing cervical spine produces characteristic undergrowth of the vertebral bodies

Pyogenic Arthritis

• Periostitis, endosteal sclerosis, and ultimately joint fusion are seen in subacute and chronic infections
• Usually monoarticular
• Ideally, correct diagnosis and institution of appropriate therapy should begin before the appearance of such changes

FIGURES Resnick: 663–666

ARTHRITIS WITH PRESERVED JOINT SPACE

List three features that distinguish the robust form of rheumatoid arthritis from classic rheumatoid arthritis.

In which inflammatory arthritis is joint space relatively preserved?

Gout
Tuberculosis
Juvenile chronic arthritis
Hemophilia
Amyloidosis
Synovial osteochondromatosis
Robust (cystic) rheumatoid arthritis
Reactive synovitis

Gout

- The joint space is typically preserved until late in the course of the disease, unless there is severe synovial involvement

FIGURES   Resnick: 397–406

Tuberculosis

- Preservation of joint space until late disease is a measure of the indolent nature of this infection

FIGURES   Resnick: 694, 695

Juvenile Chronic Arthritis

- The lack of salient joint-space narrowing distinguishes this disorder from other inflammatory arthritides

Hemophilia

- Recurrent hemarthrosis causes synovitis and joint destruction in load-bearing joints (e.g., ankles, knees, shoulders)
- Radiographs show epiphyseal overgrowth and subchondral cyst formation; joint-space narrowing is a relatively late sign
- Can be radiographically indistinguishable from juvenile chronic arthritis
- On MRI, hemosiderin-laden synovial hyperplasia appears low in signal intensity and may be indistinguishable from pigmented villonodular synovitis

FIGURES   Resnick: 642, 643

Amyloidosis

- Deposition of amyloid in synovium and other articular tissues produces a nodular polyarthropathy with osteopenia and joint-space widening

FIGURES   Resnick: 604, 605

Synovial Osteochondromatosis

- Osteochondral metaplasia or synovium typically widens the joint space on radiographs
- Calcified osteochondral bodies and articular and periarticular erosions usually visible on radiographs
- Noncalcified chondroid bodies directly visualized by MRI

FIGURES   Resnick: 1069, 1070, 1253

Robust (Cystic) Rheumatoid Arthritis

- Characterized by more pronounced subchondral cyst formation (geodes) and milder clinical and radiographic course than in classic rheumatoid arthritis
- Most common among stoic manual laborers who continue to work with their hands despite arthritis

Reactive Synovitis

- Joint swelling and pain associated with synovitis and effusion in patients with certain infections, neoplasms, or inflammatory bowel disease
- Not destructive
- Usually affects large joints of the lower extremities and may migrate from joint to joint
- In Crohn's disease and ulcerative colitis, the activity of the synovitis correlates with the timing and severity of the bowel disease
- May be one pattern of enteropathic arthropathy

ACCELERATED OSTEOARTHRITIS

Which endocrine disorder is associated with premature osteoarthritis?

Articular trauma
Calcium pyrophosphate dihydrate deposition
Ochronosis
Acromegaly
Articular dysplasias
    Spondyloepiphyseal dysplasia
    Multiple epiphyseal dysplasia
    Developmental dysplasia of the hips

Articular Trauma

- Alteration of the congruency of the articular surface of a joint by fracture can lead to rapidly progressive osteoarthritis

Calcium Pyrophosphate Dihydrate Deposition

- Usually associated with chondrocalcinosis
- Unusual distribution of severe osteoarthritis (e.g., shoulder, elbow, metacarpophalangeal, isolated patellofemoral or radiocarpal involvement)

FIGURES Resnick: 414–421

Ochronosis

- Deposition of pigment in articular tissues produces arthropathy by fourth decade
- Radiographic changes are those of osteoarthritis but with more severe sclerosis, collapse, and fragmentation of articular bone
- Presence of multiple intraarticular bodies is characteristic
- Only minor osteophyte formation
- Associated vertebral disc calcification and degeneration

Acromegaly

- Cartilage overgrowth (joint-space widening) eventually outstrips its diffusional nourishment from synovial fluid, resulting in cartilage breakdown and osteoarthritis

FIGURES Resnick: 542–544

Articular Dysplasias

- Incongruency of the articular surfaces causes predisposition to early osteoarthritis

DESTRUCTIVE ARTHRITIS WITH SCLEROSIS AND DEBRIS

Which cause of destructive arthritis is frequently associated with joint fusion?

What radiographic finding in calcium pyrophosphate dihydrate deposition can help distinguish it from other causes of severely destructive osteoarthritis?

Name an endocrine, an infectious, and a primary neurologic cause of neuropathic arthropathy.

Neuropathic arthropathy
Calcium pyrophosphate arthritis
Chronic pyogenic arthritis
Ochronosis

Neuropathic Arthropathy

- "Charcot joint"
- Arthritis is typically severely destructive and accompanied by marked sclerosis of the articular bones, joint distention, and considerable intraarticular debris
- Ankylosis is uncommon
- Causes include diabetes mellitus, syphilis, syringomyelia, and congenital insensitivity to pain

FIGURES   Resnick: 932–937

Calcium Pyrophosphate Arthritis

- More destructive appearance than usually seen with degenerative joint disease
- Chondrocalcinosis and pronounced subcortical cyst formation are characteristic
- Can closely mimic neuropathic arthropathy
- Patients usually elderly

FIGURES   Resnick: 414–421

Chronic Pyogenic Arthritis

- Subcortical cyst formation is less pronounced than with either neuropathic arthropathy or calcium pyrophosphate dihydrate deposition
- Joint fusion is more common than with the other two possibilities
- Usually monoarticular

FIGURES   Resnick: 663–666

Ochronosis

- Appendicular arthropathy usually associated with severe sclerosis and fragmentation of articular bone but only small osteophytes
- Multiple intraarticular bodies
- Associated sacroiliac involvement and severe intervertebral disc calcification and degeneration

3

CALCIFIED INTRAARTICULAR LOOSE BODY

Name a metabolic disorder associated with severe destructive arthropathy and loose intraarticular bodies.

Which neoplasm is associated with loose intraarticular bodies?

Synovial osteochondromatosis
Detached chondroosteophytes
Acute osteochondral fracture
Osteochondritis dissecans
Ochronosis

Synovial Osteochondromatosis

• Multiple loose osteochondral bodies are a result of chondral and osseous metaplasia of the synovium

FIGURES   Resnick: 1069, 1070, 1253

Detached Chondroosteophytes

• A common cause of loose bodies in osteoarthritic joints
• Suggested by the presence of osteophytes and other signs of osteoarthritis
• Loose bodies often collect in popliteal cysts

FIGURE   Resnick: 348

Acute Osteochondral Fracture

• A host site for the osteochondral fragment should be sought

Osteochondritis Dissecans

• Usually caused by chronic repetitive trauma, although acute trauma may be responsible in some cases
• The articular surface of the femur in the knee is the most common site of involvement, followed by the talar dome of the ankle

FIGURE   Resnick: 734

Ochronosis

• Congenital deficiency in homogentisic acid oxidase results in pigment deposition in articular tissues
• Severe, degenerative-like arthropathy with marked sclerosis and fragmentation results in multiple intraarticular loose bodies

JOINT FUSION

Name two radiographic features that distinguish inflammatory osteoarthritis from conventional osteoarthritis.

Name two causes of joint fusion in children.

What are the two most common sites of tarsal coalition?

Which is the most common seronegative arthritis to cause interphalangeal joint fusion?

Surgical arthrodesis
Previous trauma
Pyogenic arthritis
Coalition
Psoriatic spondyloarthropathy
Reiter's syndrome
Ankylosing spondylitis
Inflammatory (erosive) osteoarthritis
Rheumatoid arthritis (carpal or tarsal)

Surgical Arthrodesis

• Performed primarily for pain control
• Often used at sites where arthroplasty is less effective (e.g., the ankle)

Previous Trauma

• Evidence of prior internal fixation (e.g., screw holes) is helpful

FIGURE   Resnick: 1173

Pyogenic Arthritis

• Usually accompanied by deformity and sclerosis as evidence of prior infection

FIGURE   Resnick: 663

Coalition

• Developmental failure of joint formation
• Often bilateral
• Tarsal coalition is most common; talocalcaneal and calcaneonavicular joints involved in 90% of cases
• Osseous coalitions are seen well on radiographs, but nonosseous coalitions (fibroosseous and fibrocartilaginous or those in immature skeleton) may require CT or MRI
• Calcaneonavicular coalition radiographically best seen on oblique anteroposterior (AP) view of foot
• Harris-Beath view displays subtalar joints
• Carpal coalition also common
• Coalition of bones in different carpal rows is usually associated with congenital malformation syndrome, whereas fusion within a carpal row usually is isolated

FIGURE   Resnick: 1174

Psoriatic Spondyloarthropathy

• Osseous ankylosis usually affects interphalangeal or metacarpophalangeal joints of hands

Reiter's Syndrome

• Intraarticular ankylosis may occur but is less common than in psoriatic spondyloarthropathy and ankylosing spondylitis

FIGURES   Resnick: 275–279

Ankylosing Spondylitis

• Ankylosis usually affects the sacroiliac joints
• Changes are highly symmetric

FIGURES   Resnick: 249, 259

Inflammatory (Erosive) Osteoarthritis

• Severe inflammatory form of osteoarthritis of the hands
• Usually seen in women
• Distinguished radiographically by presence of central erosions and interphalangeal fusion

FIGURE   Resnick: 352

Rheumatoid Arthritis

• Osseous fusions occasionally develop but usually are restricted to intercarpal and intertarsal joints

FIGURE   Resnick: 199

3

ULNAR DEVIATION OF METACARPOPHALANGEAL JOINTS

Name the three classic causes of ulnar deviation of the metacarpophalangeal joints.

Which cause is also associated with avascular necrosis?

Which cause may be seen in childhood?

Rheumatoid arthritis
Systemic lupus erythematosus
Jaccoud's arthropathy

Rheumatoid Arthritis

- Seen in 25 to 50% of cases
- Caused by ligamentous disruption and ulnar deviation of extensor tendons
- Usually accompanied by marginal erosions

FIGURE Resnick: 215

Systemic Lupus Erythematosus

- Ligamentous laxity results in Jaccoud-like, reversible, nondisabling deformities of the joints of the hands
- Unlike rheumatoid arthritis, erosions and joint space narrowing usually not present

FIGURE Resnick: 292

Jaccoud's Arthropathy

- Ligamentous laxity resulting from capsular inflammation and fibrosis associated with rheumatic fever results in reversible joint deformities
- As in lupus, bone erosion and joint space narrowing are rare
- Juvenile chronic arthritis is more commonly associated with radial deviation

FIGURES Resnick: 318, 319

SACROILIITIS

Name three causes of sacroiliitis that may be unilateral.

Which cause of sacroiliitis is associated with ulcerative colitis?

Ankylosing spondylitis
Psoriatic spondyloarthropathy
Reiter's syndrome
Enteropathic arthropathy
Infection

Ankylosing Spondylitis

- Sacroiliac involvement always bilateral and symmetric
- Ultimately, sacroiliac joints fuse
- Sacroiliac joints are usually first site of involvement in men, followed by lumbar spine; in women and children, appendicular joints usually affected first

FIGURES Resnick: 249, 259

Psoriatic Spondyloarthropathy

- Classically unilateral but most often bilateral and asymmetric sacroiliitis
- Most common in HLA-B27–positive patients

- Ankylosis less common than with ankylosing spondylitis or enteric spondylitis

FIGURES   Resnick: 269, 270

Reiter's Syndrome

- Sacroiliitis is common and similar to that seen in psoriatic spondyloarthropathy
- Usually bilateral but, in contrast to ankylosing spondylitis, typically asymmetric

FIGURES   Resnick: 278, 279

Enteropathic Arthropathy

- Spondyloarthropathy associated with various gastrointestinal disorders (ulcerative colitis, Crohn's disease, Whipple's disease)
- Swelling and pain migrate among different large joints but are usually monoarticular at any one time
- Clinical severity of appendicular arthritis correlated with severity of gastrointestinal symptoms, but only minimal radiographic changes
- Sacroiliitis and spondylitis, which can be indistinguishable from ankylosing spondylitis, do not correlate with severity or timing of gastrointestinal manifestations
- 90% of patients with sacroiliitis and spondylitis are HLA-B27 positive

FIGURES   Resnick: 282–283, 285–287

Infection

- Usually unilateral
- Pyogenic and fungal infections are seen
- Common among intravenous substance abusers
- Early changes are predominantly lytic and anteroinferior
- Sclerosis and fusion develop later

FIGURES   Resnick: 680–682

ARTHROPATHY WITH SOFT-TISSUE MASSES

Name two features of multicentric reticulohistiocytosis that are not common in rheumatoid arthritis.

Gout
Amyloidosis
Nodular rheumatoid arthritis
Multicentric reticulohistiocytosis

Gout

- Gouty tophi that accumulate in the periarticular soft tissues stimulate local erosion and proliferation of adjacent bones
- Erosions in gout typically show sclerotic margins; the characteristic "overhanging edges" of these erosions buttress the tophi
- Calcification of tophi is uncommon

FIGURES   Resnick: 397–406

Amyloidosis

- Polyarticular joint disease results from amyloid deposition in bone, synovium, and periarticular tissues

3

- Radiographic changes include soft tissue nodules, osteopenia, erosions, and joint-space widening
- Amyloid deposits may show low signal intensity on T2-weighted MRI
- Polyarticular involvement and osteopenia distinguish amyloidosis from pigmented villonodular synovitis

FIGURES   Resnick: 604, 605

Nodular Rheumatoid Arthritis

- Subcutaneous nodules seen in 25% of patients with rheumatoid arthritis
- Most commonly form at pressure points along extensor surfaces (e.g., elbow)

Multicentric Reticulohistiocytosis

- Erosive polyarthritis caused by histiocytic proliferation in synovium is usually earliest manifestation
- Bilateral and symmetric with predilection for joints of hand and wrist
- Erosions are well defined, as in gout
- In contrast to rheumatoid arthritis, no osteopenia is present, and the distal interphalangeal joints frequently are involved
- No periostitis

FIGURE   Resnick: 613

PERIARTICULAR SOFT TISSUE CALCIFICATIONS

Which form of periarticular calcification may be seen in some patients with peptic ulcer disease?

Which cause of periarticular calcifications may also be associated with esophageal dysmotility?

Hydroxyapatite deposition
Gout
Scleroderma
Tumoral calcinosis

Hydroxyapatite Deposition

- Hydroxyapatite crystals tend to accumulate in soft tissues near tendinous insertions (calcific tendinitis)
- Early calcifications may be ill defined, but usually become well-formed, globular collections
- Can mimic ossicles or fracture fragments, but differentiated by lack of cortical and trabecular morphology or disappearance of the lesion after antiinflammatory medication

FIGURES   Resnick: 428–435

Gout

- Gouty tophi occasionally develop cloud-like calcification

FIGURES   Resnick: 398–400

Scleroderma

- Dystrophic subcutaneous calcifications are a feature of certain connective tissue disorders, such as scleroderma, especially CREST syndrome (calcinosis, Raynaud's phenomenon, esophageal dysmotility, sclerodactyly, and telangiectasia)
- Calcifications are usually periarticular and small but can become "tumoral"

- Subcutaneous calcifications also occasionally are seen in systemic lupus erythematosus and overlap syndromes

FIGURES Resnick: 299–302

Tumoral Calcinosis

- Large, flocculant periarticular collections of calcium, usually adjacent to large joints
- Usually associated with hypercalcemic states (e.g., milk-alkali syndrome, hyperparathyroidism, hypervitaminosis D, sarcoidosis, etc.)
- Radiographic appearance is distinctive

FIGURES Resnick: 562, 563

CHONDROCALCINOSIS

Which cause of chondrocalcinosis is associated with skin discoloration?

Name three common sites of chondrocalcinosis in calcium pyrophosphate dihydrate deposition.

Calcium pyrophosphate dihydrate deposition
Hemochromatosis
Hyperparathyroidism
Gout

Calcium Pyrophosphate Dihydrate Deposition

- Calcification usually involves fibrocartilage (coarse or punctate pattern) of meniscus, triangular cartilage of wrist, symphysis pubis, or labrum
- Hyaline articular cartilage calcification is fine, linear, and parallel to articular cortex
- Capsular structures (linear pattern) and synovium (cloud-like pattern) also may calcify

FIGURES Resnick: 414–421

Hemochromatosis

- Chondrocalcinosis occurs in 40% of cases
- Degenerative-like arthritis is indistinguishable from pyrophosphate arthropathy but less rapidly progressive
- May be associated with bronze skin discoloration

FIGURES Resnick: 439–441

Hyperparathyroidism

- Chondrocalcinosis occurs in 20 to 40% of cases
- Most common in primary hyperparathyroidism but occasionally also seen in renal failure
- Associated articular changes include subchondral resorption and collapse, mild periarticular erosion, and subligamentous bone resorption

FIGURE Resnick: 557

Gout

- Seen in less than 30% of cases
- Usually in fibrocartilage: menisci of knee, triangular cartilage of wrist, or symphysis pubis

FIGURES Resnick: 403, 404

SPINE SPONDYLOLISTHESIS

Name two causes of spondylolisthesis other than spondylolysis.

How can spondylolysis be differentiated from other causes of spondylolisthesis with the use of a lateral radiograph?

Spondylolysis
Facet degeneration
Degenerative disc disease
Trauma
Ligamentous laxity
   Marfan's syndrome
   Ehlers-Danlos syndrome

Spondylolysis

- Bilateral pars interarticularis defects usually result in anterior subluxation of the vertebral body with the proximal spinal column and posterior displacement of the spinous process with the distal spinal column
- L5–S1 and L4–L5 are the two most common locations
- Radiographic diagnosis depends on oblique views
- CT and MRI are most sensitive modalities

FIGURE   Resnick: 365

Facet Degeneration

- Facet laxity and remodeling with degenerative disease can result in spondylolisthesis, but in distinction to that associated with spondylolysis, the spinous process moves forward with the subluxing vertebra
- Spinal stenosis more frequently is a problem in facet degeneration than in spondylolysis

FIGURE   Resnick: 366

Degenerative Disc Disease

- Because of the oblique orientation of the facets, loss of intervertebral space because of disc narrowing results in posterior subluxation of the vertebral body (retrolisthesis)
- Retrolisthesis is a cause of spinal stenosis

FIGURES   Resnick: 365, 366

Trauma

- Unstable fractures or ligamentous disruption of the spine can result in spondylolisthesis
- Flexion-extension radiographs may be necessary to demonstrate the instability, particularly in the cervical spine

FIGURES   Resnick: 805, 806

Marfan's Syndrome

- Autosomal dominant connective tissue disorder associated with joint laxity and scoliosis
- Instability associated with ligamentous laxity may require flexion-extension radiographs

FIGURE   Resnick: 1111

Ehlers-Danlos Syndrome

- Group of familial connective tissue disorders associated with hyperelasticity and fragility of skin, joint laxity, and bleeding diathesis

FIGURES   Resnick: 1112–1114

3

ATLANTOAXIAL SUBLUXATION

Name three congenital conditions associated with atlantoaxial subluxation.

Which technique is useful for demonstrating atlantoaxial subluxation in the absence of odontoid fracture?

Trauma
Arthritis
   Rheumatoid arthritis
   Seronegative arthritis
   Multicentric reticulohistiocytosis
Adjacent infection
Congenital
   Down's syndrome
   Morquio's syndrome
   Congenital hypoplasia of dens/os odontoideum
   Occipitalization of C1
Ligamentous laxity
   Marfan's syndrome
   Ehlers-Danlos syndrome

General

- Atlantoaxial interval greater than 3 mm in adults or 5 mm in children; increases with flexion

Trauma

- Usually associated with odontoid fracture
- Isolated widening of the atlantoaxial interval indicates disruption of the transverse ligament
- Demonstration of atlantoaxial subluxation in the absence of odontoid fracture may require radiography in flexion and extension

FIGURES   Resnick: 797–799, 801–803

Rheumatoid Arthritis

- Ligamentous disruption is an occasional complication of rheumatoid or seronegative arthritis; may require flexion-extension radiography to demonstrate
- Synovitis at the atlantoaxial joint can also cause erosion of the dens
- In addition to atlantoaxial widening, the dens can subluxate cephalad into the foramen magnum
- MRI shows the synovitis directly and can evaluate associated cord compression

FIGURES   Resnick: 225–227

Multicentric Reticulohistiocytosis

- Atlantoaxial subluxation may be an early manifestation
- Can be more severe than in rheumatoid arthritis

3

Adjacent Infection

- Pharyngitis or tonsillitis can inflame and rupture the ligaments about the dens
- Associated with marked prevertebral soft tissue swelling

Down's Syndrome

- Odontoid hypoplasia and congenital weakening of the surrounding ligaments

Morquio's Syndrome

- Associated with odontoid hypoplasia

FIGURE   Resnick: 1156

PARAVERTEBRAL CALCIFICATION/OSSIFICATION

How do paravertebral calcifications in ankylosing spondylitis differ from those in psoriatic spondyloarthropathy?

How do they differ from those in enteropathic arthropathy?

Which cause of paravertebral calcification can be associated with intervertebral disc space narrowing and loss of definition of the vertebral end plates?

Asymmetric
   Psoriatic spondyloarthropathy
   Reiter's syndrome
Symmetric
   Ankylosing spondylitis
   Enteropathic arthropathy
Anterior
   Diffuse idiopathic skeletal hyperostosis (DISH)
Focal mass
   Tuberculosis

Psoriatic Spondyloarthropathy

- Coarse, asymmetric paravertebral calcifications and syndesmophytes are common in psoriatic spondyloarthropathy, especially in patients who are HLA-B27 positive
- Symptoms are usually mild unless there is cervical spine involvement

FIGURES   Resnick: 269, 270

Reiter's Syndrome

- Asymmetric paravertebral ossification is similar to that seen in psoriatic spondyloarthropathy but occurs less commonly and is typically less pronounced

FIGURES   Resnick: 274, 275

Ankylosing Spondylitis

- Fine, symmetric syndesmophytes are best seen on AP projection
- Changes almost always preceded by sacroiliitis
- Diffuse ankylosis can produce a "bamboo spine" appearance

FIGURES   Resnick: 250–254

Enteropathic Arthropathy

- Sacroiliitis and spondylitis, which can be indistinguishable from ankylosing spondylitis, do not correlate with severity or timing of gastrointestinal manifestations

· 90% of patients with sacroiliitis and spondylitis are HLA-B27 positive

FIGURES   Resnick: 282, 283, 285–287

Diffuse Idiopathic Skeletal Hyperostosis (DISH)

· Flowing calcification or ossification along anterolateral aspect of the spine spanning four or more vertebral bodies is an essential diagnostic criterion
· Strict diagnostic criteria also exclude any significant disc degeneration
· Paravertebral calcifications more coarse and asymmetric than in ankylosing spondylitis
· Prevertebral ossification in the cervical spine can cause dysphagia
· Usually accompanied by diffuse enthetic ossification
· Seen in elderly patients

FIGURES   Resnick: 379–386

Tuberculosis

· Calcified paravertebral soft tissue mass spanning two or three vertebral levels
· Associated with discitis and vertebral end plate erosion
· Chest radiographs may be clear

FIGURES   Resnick: 690, 691

DISC CALCIFICATION

Name two causes of disc calcification associated with chondrocalcinosis elsewhere.

Which cause of disc calcification is associated with brown discoloration of urine left to oxidize in the open air?

Degenerative disc disease
Ochronosis
Calcium pyrophosphate dihydrate deposition
Surgical fusion
Ankylosing spondylitis
Hemochromatosis

Degenerative Disc Disease

· Disc calcification is often seen in association with intervertebral narrowing and osteophytosis
· Calcification is presumably dystrophic

Ochronosis

· Severe disc calcification and degeneration (especially in the lumbar spine) associated with vertebral body osteopenia in young adults
· Usually only small osteophytes

Calcium Pyrophosphate Dihydrate Deposition

· Severe degenerative disc disease with disc calcifications, marked end plate irregularity, and osteophytosis occasionally is seen
· Calcification initially appears in the outer annular fibers and may resemble syndesmophytes in ankylosing spondylitis
· Associated with chondrocalcinosis elsewhere and pyrophosphate arthropathy, most commonly of the metacarpophalangeal joints, wrist, shoulder, or knee

FIGURE   Resnick: 421

3

Surgical Fusion

- Disc calcification is restricted to the level of the spinal fusion, unless there are additional causes
- The pathogenesis is not known but speculated to be a response to immobility at the disc

Ankylosing Spondylitis

- Central disc calcification is usually restricted to levels that are ankylosed

FIGURES Resnick: 253–255

Hemochromatosis

- Calcification of outer fibers of annulus fibrosus

IVORY VERTEBRA

Name two neoplastic causes of vertebral body sclerosis.

What radiographic feature might differentiate Paget's disease from other possible causes of ivory vertebra?

Metastasis
Paget's disease
Lymphoma
Chronic infection
Discogenic sclerosis

Metastasis

- Blastic metastases are most commonly from either breast or prostate carcinoma
- Usually multiple lesions

FIGURES Resnick: 373, 1082

Paget's Disease

- Bone enlargement is a characteristic feature of Paget's disease and distinguishes it from other causes of focal bone sclerosis, such as blastic metastases
- Elderly patients (i.e., same age group as those with metastases)
- Spine is second most common site; pelvis most common
- Can be solitary (10 to 30%), but usually several skeletal sites are affected
- Cortical thickening produces "picture frame" appearance to vertebral body
- Trabeculae are thickened and coarse

FIGURES Resnick: 527–535

Lymphoma

- Bone lesions can be lytic or sclerotic
- Hodgkin's disease is the most common variety to cause osteosclerosis
- Usually multiple lesions
- Bone involvement usually denotes advanced disease and is accompanied by secondary symptoms (fever, night sweats, etc.)

FIGURES Resnick: 630, 631

Chronic Infection

- As elsewhere in the skeleton, chronic osteomyelitis of the spine produces sclerosis in addition to local destruction
- Usually involves adjacent vertebrae and is accompanied by marked intervertebral narrowing caused by associated discitis

FIGURES   Resnick: 677, 678

Discogenic Sclerosis

- Usually associated with disc-space narrowing, vacuum phenomenon, osteophytosis, and other evidence of degenerative disc disease
- Several vertebrae usually are involved

ENLARGED VERTEBRA

What radiographic feature differentiates Paget's disease from other causes of vertebral enlargement?

What is the most common cause of enlarged vertebra in children?

Name an endocrine cause of generalized vertebral enlargement.

Paget's disease
Aneurysmal bone cyst
Acromegaly

Paget's Disease

- The spine is commonly affected by Paget's disease
- Both the vertebral body and posterior elements can be involved, but the former are most noticeable on radiographs
- Unlike most other causes of vertebral enlargement, Paget's disease also is associated with local sclerosis
- Other radiographic features in the spine include cortical thickening ("picture framing") and trabecular coarsening

FIGURE   Resnick: 529

Aneurysmal Bone Cyst

- Lesions in the spine are usually situated in the posterior elements and have an appearance similar to that of appendicular lesions
- Patients usually are less than 30 years of age

FIGURE   Resnick: 1053

Acromegaly

- Vertebral bodies are enlarged in AP and transverse dimensions and show posterior scalloping

FIGURES   Resnick: 541–543

POSTERIOR SCALLOPING OF VERTEBRA

Which cause is associated with caudal narrowing of interpediculate distance in the lumbar spine?

Which cause is also associated with diabetes mellitus and premature osteoarthritis?

Increased spinal pressure
  Spinal canal neoplasm
  Syringomyelia
  Hydrocephalus
Dural ectasia
  Neurofibromatosis
  Marfan's syndrome
  Ehlers-Danlos syndrome
Achondroplasia
Acromegaly

3

Spinal Canal Neoplasm

- Scalloping may be focal as a result of direct pressure resorption adjacent to a neoplasm or more diffuse as a result of increased spinal pressure
- Most common neoplasms are lipomas, neurofibromas, and ependymomas

Syringomyelia

- Most commonly seen in thoracic vertebrae

Hydrocephalus

- Vertebral scalloping is seen only in severe, long-standing cases

Neurofibromatosis

- Scalloping most commonly caused by dural ectasia, but focal pressure erosions may develop adjacent to neurofibromas
- Associated neural foraminal widening is usually caused by lateral meningoceles

Achondroplasia

- Commonly associated with spinal stenosis
- Other spinal features include caudally narrowing interpedicular distance in the lumbar spine and anterior vertebral beaking at the thoracolumbar junction
- Characteristic pelvic morphology (horizontal sacral orientation, "champagne glass" pelvic cavity, and squared iliac wings) often is visible on lumbar spine radiographs

Acromegaly

- Diffuse posterior scalloping is associated with AP and lateral enlargement of vertebrae

FIGURES   Resnick: 541–543

ANTERIOR SCALLOPING OF VERTEBRA

Name a malignant condition that may be associated with anterior scalloping of vertebrae.

Which cause may be associated with a calcified paravertebral mass?

Aortic aneurysm
Lymphadenopathy
Tuberculosis

Aortic Aneurysm

- Broad scalloping caused by pressure resorption from the adjacent aneurysm
- Vertebral cortex remains well defined
- Mural calcifications often delineate the aneurysmal aorta

Lymphadenopathy

- Vertebral cortex usually remains well defined
- Intervertebral discs not affected

3

Tuberculosis

- Scalloped anterior cortex and vertebral end plates usually are ill defined
- An associated paravertebral mass (occasionally calcified) may be present

FIGURE Resnick: 690

ABSENT PEDICLE

What radiographic feature differentiates congenital absence of a pedicle from metastatic destruction?

Name two causes that may be seen in children.

Metastasis
Aneurysmal bone cyst
Congenital absence

Metastasis

- Most common cause
- Destruction of a pedicle is often the first radiographic evidence of vertebral metastasis
- Characteristically, no compensatory enlargement or sclerosis of the contralateral pedicle occurs

FIGURES Resnick: 1082–1089

Aneurysmal Bone Cyst

- Spinal lesions most commonly involve the posterior elements
- May progress sufficiently slowly to allow some compensatory changes in contralateral pedicle

FIGURE Resnick: 1053

Congenital Absence

- Hypertrophy of the contralateral pedicle is a specific associated radiographic sign

DENSE PEDICLE

Name a nonneoplastic cause of a dense vertebral pedicle.

What radiographic feature differentiates osteoid osteoma from osteoblastic metastasis?

Congenital absence of contralateral pedicle
Osteoblastic metastasis
Osteoid osteoma
Osteoblastoma

Osteoblastic Metastasis

- Usually accompanied by additional skeletal lesions

Osteoid Osteoma

- Rare in the spine, but usually these involve the posterior elements
- Pain may cause a positional scoliosis that is concave ipsilaterally
- A lucent nidus may be difficult to identify on spinal radiographs because of overlapping structures; CT is more useful unless the nidus is fully calcified
- Patients almost always are under the age of 30 years

FIGURE Resnick: 997

3

Osteoblastoma

- Patients usually are under the age of 30 years
- Posterior elements of the spine are a common location for this lesion
- Even though the nidus is often large and lucent, the sclerotic component of the lesion may be the most conspicuous feature on spine radiographs

FIGURES   Resnick: 999, 1000

DENSE VERTEBRAL END PLATE

Which cause is also associated with increased risk of avascular necrosis?

Which cause is associated with vascular calcifications?

Degenerative disc disease
Renal osteodystrophy
Excess steroids

Degenerative Disc Disease

- Adaptive sclerosis in response to altered biomechanics of degenerating disc; process is analogous to subchondral sclerosis in osteoarthritic joints
- Accompanied by other degenerative changes, such as osteophytosis and disc-space narrowing

FIGURES   Resnick: 366, 373

Renal Osteodystrophy

- Radiographic changes are caused by the combination of secondary hyperparathyroidism, vitamin D deficiency, and elevated serum phosphorus and calcium concentrations
- Vertebral end plate sclerosis produces a pattern of alternating dense and lucent horizontal bands called *rugger-jersey spine*
- Associated radiographic findings may include insufficiency fractures, "smudged" trabecular pattern, subperiosteal bone resorption, resorption of the distal clavicles, widening of the sacroiliac joints and the symphysis pubis, brown tumors, and vascular calcifications
- No disc-space narrowing and osteophytosis unless concurrent degenerative disc disease exists

FIGURE   Resnick: 560

Excess Steroids

- Skeletal changes associated with excess steroids include generalized osteopenia, insufficiency fractures, exuberant callus formation, and avascular necrosis
- Even without overt vertebral fracture, stress reaction or microfracture at the vertebral end plates often produces sclerosis called *marginal condensation*
- Disc-space narrowing or osteophytosis is seen only if concurrent degenerative disc disease exists
- Most common causes of excess exogenous steroids are organ transplantation, systemic inflammatory disorders (e.g., rheumatoid arthritis or systemic lupus erythematosus), and asthma
- Excess endogenous steroids are usually the result of Cushing's disease

BONE SCINTIGRAPHY

COLD (PHOTOPENIC) LESIONS ON BONE SCAN

Name three neoplasms that may appear falsely negative on bone scintigraphy.

Infarct/avascular necrosis
Certain metastases
Neoplasms
Osteomyelitis
Radiation
Artifact

Infarct/avascular Necrosis

· Photopenia occurs in early stages
· Later stages usually include patchy sclerosis

Certain Metastasis

· Especially with renal cell carcinoma, thyroid carcinoma, neuroblastoma, and anaplastic neoplasms

FIGURE Mettler: 218

Neoplasms

· Including multiple myeloma, eosinophilic granuloma, lymphoma, and neuroblastoma

Osteomyelitis

· Photopenia occurs in early stages, especially in pediatric patients
· May be related to vascular thrombosis or tamponade

Radiation

· Caused by vascular occlusion

Artifact

· From overlying density such as orthopedic hardware, pacemaker, barium, etc.

DIFFUSE INCREASED UPTAKE ("SUPERSCAN")

What neoplastic condition can cause a generalized increase in radiotracer uptake?

What do brown tumors complicating hyperparathyroidism appear as?

Renal failure
Hyperparathyroidism
Metastasis
Hematologic disorders

Renal Failure

· May be accentuated by effects of secondary hyperparathyroidism

Hyperparathyroidism

· Occurs in primary or secondary forms
· Focal areas of intense uptake may represent brown tumors

Metastasis

- Seen with widespread metastasis most often from prostate, breast, lymphoma, lung, and bladder primary malignancies
- Prostate carcinoma metastasis is the leading cause of a superscan

FIGURE Mettler: 216

Hematologic Disorders

- Conditions include myelofibrosis and mastocytosis

Figure References

Greenspan A: Orthopedic Radiology, 2nd ed. Philadelphia: Lippincott-Raven, 1995.
Mettler F, Guiberteau M: Essentials of Nuclear Medicine, 3rd ed. Philadelphia: W. B. Saunders, 1991.
Resnick D: Bone and Joint Imaging, 2nd ed. Philadelphia: W. B. Saunders, 1996.

MUSCULOSKELETAL IMAGING: DISEASE ENTITIES

ACROMEGALY

Clinical

- Effects of elevated growth hormone after skeletal maturity (hyperpituitary giantism before skeletal maturity)
- Usually caused by pituitary adenoma
- Usually presents in third or fourth decade with deepened voice, characteristic facies, thickened skin, visceromegaly, and generalized tissue overgrowth
- Endocrine abnormalities include diabetes mellitus and adenomas of pancreatic islet cells and parathyroid glands
- Other complaints include fatigue, weakness, headaches, visual disturbance, diminished libido, amenorrhea, backache, compression neuropathy, and joint pain

Imaging

- Associated with enlargement of the distal tufts, sesamoids, vertebra, paranasal sinuses and mastoids, and mandible
- Other radiographic findings include cranial vault thickening, heel pad thickening and soft tissue hypertrophy, posterior vertebral scalloping
- Cartilage overgrowth initially results in joint-space widening, but as the thickened cartilage outstrips its diffusional supply of nutrients from the synovial fluid, cartilage breaks down and osteoarthritis develops

ANEURYSMAL BONE CYST

Clinical

- Vast majority occur in patients under 20 years of age
- May be primary or secondary (most commonly arise from chondroblastoma, giant cell tumor, fibrous dysplasia)
- Presents with pain and swelling

Imaging

- Lytic, expansive ("aneurysmal") lesion with thinly corticated margins
- Usually metaphyseal in long bones
- Fluid levels on CT or MRI are characteristic but nonspecific

ANKYLOSING SPONDYLITIS

Clinical

- Chronic spondyloarthropathy affecting primarily the axial skeleton
- Most commonly affects men between the ages of 15 and 35 years
- Insidious onset of sciatic pain is the most common presentation, occasionally with anorexia and fever
- Proximal appendicular joints may become involved in some patients
- Less than 20% progress to significant disability

Imaging

- Bilaterally symmetric sacroiliitis is the earliest finding; ultimately, the sacroiliac joints show intraarticular ankylosis
- Changes in the spine usually follow those in the sacroiliac joints
- Proliferative erosion at discovertebral junctions results in "shiny corners" and "squaring," most noticeably in the lumbar spine
- Calcification of the annulus fibrosus produces fine, bilaterally symmetric syndes-mophytes, eventually leading to a "bamboo spine" appearance
- Mild synovitis in appendicular joints may resemble rheumatoid arthritis, with mild joint-space narrowing and bone erosion; however, juxtaarticular osteopenia is less common
- In contrast to rheumatoid arthritis, subchondral sclerosis, periostitis, and intraar-ticular osseous ankylosis are common
- As in other seronegative arthritides, ill-defined erosion occurs at entheses; however, the enthesitis may mature into well-defined spurs

AVASCULAR NECROSIS (AVN)

- Causes of AVN (also known as *osteonecrosis, ischemic necrosis, aseptic necrosis*) can be remembered by the mnemonic ASSEPTIC RAG:
  - Alcohol
  - Steroids
  - Sickle cell anemia
  - Embolism (caisson disease, fat)
  - Pancreatitis
  - Trauma
  - Idiopathic (Legg-Calvé-Perthes disease, spontaneous)
  - Collagen vascular disease (lupus, scleroderma, rheumatoid arthritis)
  - Radiation
  - Amyloid
  - Gaucher's disease
- Radiographic stages:
  - I   Normal radiograph, abnormal bone scintigraphy/MRI
  - II Osteopenia, patchy sclerosis
  - III Subchondral crescentic lucency ("crescent" sign)
  - IV Subchondral collapse with flattening
  - V Secondary osteoarthritis
- MRI is most sensitive but can be nonspecific in early osteonecrosis (local marrow edema)
- Mature osteonecrosis shows characteristic serpiginous margin of reparative bone at the interface between devitalized bone and adjacent viable tissue

BONE ISLAND

Clinical

- Also termed *enostosis*
- Benign, asymptomatic lesion composed of normal compact bone

Imaging

- Single or multiple sclerotic lesions with feathery, radiating spicules
- May increase or decrease in size; rarely, lesions disappear
- Bone scan usually normal, but 5% show increased uptake

CALCIUM PYROPHOSPHATE DIHYDRATE DEPOSITION

Clinical

- Affects middle-aged men and women
- Most common clinical pattern is bilateral large joint osteoarthritis with intermittent inflammatory episodes
- Patients in 10 to 20% of cases present with acute, self-limited attacks of pain and swelling mimicking gout (pseudogout); 5% present with continuous inflammation (pseudorheumatoid arthritis)
- May be asymptomatic
- May be hereditary or sporadic

Imaging

- Chondrocalcinosis most commonly involves fibrocartilage (e.g., menisci, triangular cartilage of the wrist, symphysis pubis, annulus fibrosus, glenoid labrum) and appears coarse; hyaline articular cartilage calcification is fine and linear
- Synovial and capsular calcifications are also common
- Pyrophosphate arthropathy may appear without chondrocalcinosis; changes include bilaterally symmetric degenerative-like arthritis, with joint-space narrowing (but relatively uniform), subchondral sclerosis and collapse, prominent subchondral cysts, and variable osteophyte formation
- Distribution of arthritis atypical for degenerative joint disease (e.g., metacarpophalangeal joint, radiocarpal joint, elbow, shoulder)
- Changes often rapidly progressive and destructive
- May mimic neuropathic joint disease

CHONDROBLASTOMA

Clinical

- Benign cartilaginous lesion
- Presents with local pain, swelling, and tenderness
- Vast majority seen in patients younger than 20 years of age

Imaging

- Occurs most commonly in epiphyses of long bones, especially the femur, humerus, and tibia
- 50% contain chondroid-matrix calcifications

CHONDROMYXOID FIBROMA

Clinical

- Very rare benign cartilaginous neoplasm
- Usually seen in patients younger than 20 years of age

Imaging

- Lytic lesion with sharply marginated, sclerotic borders and eccentric expansion
- Most commonly in proximal tibial metaphysis
- May resemble aneurysmal bone cyst
- Calcification uncommon

CHONDROSARCOMA

Clinical

- Malignant chondroid neoplasm may arise de novo or secondarily in preexisting chondroid lesion (e.g., enchondroma, osteochondroma)
- Peak incidence in those aged 30 to 60 years
- Characteristically presents with pain

Imaging

- Aggressive lytic lesion with variable amount of chondroid-matrix calcification
- Secondary lesions may appear as foci of aggressive radiographic appearance in a lesion that otherwise has a benign appearance
- Common sites are pelvis, femur, humerus, and rib
- Most long bone lesions are metaphyseal
- Metastatic lesions often not calcified

CORTICAL DESMOID

Clinical

- Also known as *periosteal* or *juxtacortical desmoid*
- Occurs at the posteromedial aspect of the supracondylar portion of the distal femur and represents a stress reaction to the adductor magnus insertion
- Typically affects those aged 15 to 20 years
- Usually asymptomatic; may be bilateral

Imaging

- Lytic/sclerotic cortical lesion of the distal medial linea aspera femoris
- May simulate malignancy radiographically and histologically and should not be sampled for biopsy

DESMOPLASTIC FIBROMA (DESMOID)

Clinical

- Rare, benign but locally aggressive lesion characterized by abundant collagen content
- Lesions often recur after surgical resection

Imaging

- Typically found in mandible, pelvis (ilium), or long bone metaphyses
- Lesions are lytic with internal trabeculations but no matrix calcifications
- Central localization in bone differentiates desmoplastic fibroma from nonossifying fibroma
- May have aggressive appearance simulating malignancy (e.g., fibrosarcoma, thyroid, or renal metastasis)

DIFFUSE IDIOPATHIC SKELETAL HYPEROSTOSIS (DISH)

Clinical

- Ossifying diathesis at skeletal sites of stress, particularly the entheses and the anterior longitudinal ligament of the spine
- Also shows propensity for heterotopic bone formation after surgery (e.g., hip arthroplasty) and in association with coexisting rheumatic disorders
- Clinical symptoms (e.g., spinal stiffness, cervical dysphagia) are mild or obscured by associated disorders
- Seen in elderly patients

Imaging

- Flowing calcification or ossification of the anterolateral perivertebral tissues of at least four contiguous vertebral bodies is an essential diagnostic criterion
- Absence of significant degenerative disc disease or intraarticular ankylosis of the sacroiliac or apophyseal joints is an additional criterion necessary for specific diagnosis
- Extraspinal manifestations are proliferative changes at entheses, including well-formed bone spurs and periarticular osteophytes

ENCHONDROMA

Clinical

- Benign chondroid neoplasm most often in the diaphyses of tubular bones
- Rarely undergo malignant transformation to chondrosarcoma with pain and local destruction
- Lesions painless unless complicated by pathologic fracture or malignant transformation
- Multiple enchondromas are seen in Ollier's disease and in association with hemangiomas in Maffucci's syndrome

Imaging

- Lytic lesion with thin, tightly lobulated sclerotic margins
- Typically diaphyseal, may be expansive
- Long bone lesions usually contain chondroid-matrix calcifications, but lesions in the short tubular bones may be purely lytic
- CT may be useful in delineating matrix calcifications in lesions that are obscured on radiographs by overlapping structures

EOSINOPHILIC GRANULOMA

Clinical

- Mildest and most common (70%) form of histiocytosis X, a benign proliferation of reticuloendothelial cells (Langerhans cells) seen in white boys usually under 7 years of age
- Eosinophilic granuloma shows primarily bone involvement
- Clinical symptoms include bone pain and local swelling
- Bone lesions may be multifocal, but usually less than four are present
- Can involve any bone
- Other forms of histiocytosis X include Hand-Schüller-Christian disease (in patients 1 to 3 years of age; bone and visceral involvement) and Letterer-Siwe disease (in patients younger than 1 year; most acute form, primarily visceral)
- May resolve spontaneously

Imaging

- Variable radiographic appearance, ranging from well-defined, lucent lesions with sclerotic margins to ill-defined, aggressive-appearing lesions with periostitis and soft tissue mass
- May contain sequestra
- May cause "floating tooth" appearance in mandible
- Skull lesions typically show beveled edges
- Severe vertebral collapse (vertebra plana) can completely reverse with healing
- Bone scintigraphy is less sensitive than radiography

EWING'S SARCOMA

Clinical

- Malignant neoplasm composed of small, round cells, similar histologically to lymphoma and neuroblastoma

- 90% occur in patients between 5 and 30 years of age
- Almost exclusively seen in whites
- Presents with local pain, swelling, and fever
- Usually affects pelvis and lower extremities (femur most common)

Imaging

- Moth-eaten or permeative lucency, typically associated with cortical erosion (intracortical striations, external saucerization) and laminated or "onion-skin" periosteal reaction
- 40% of lesions are diaphyseal
- Commonly associated with a soft tissue mass
- Can be indistinguishable from osteomyelitis or eosinophilic granuloma
- Osteosclerotic lesions (uncommon) may mimic osteosarcoma or lymphoma
- MRI is optimal for evaluating periosseous extension

FIBROSARCOMA

Clinical

- Rare malignant neoplasm occurring most frequently in the third to sixth decades
- May be primary or may develop in preexisting areas of Paget's disease, chronic osteomyelitis, osteonecrosis, or radiation osteitis

Imaging

- Purely lytic lesion with geographic, moth-eaten, or permeative appearance, usually in metaphysis of long bones
- Radiographically similar to malignant fibrous histiocytoma
- May have sequestra

FIBROUS DYSPLASIA

Clinical

- Painless, benign fibroosseous lesion
- Usually incidental and monostotic
- Very rare malignant transformation, particularly after irradiation
- McCune-Albright syndrome typically affects females and consists of polyostotic fibrous dysplasia, endocrine dysfunction (precocious puberty), and café au lait spots (with irregular, ragged "coast of Maine" borders)

Imaging

- Can be purely lytic, sclerotic, or mixed, depending on the proportions of fibrous and osseous matrices
- Polyostotic form usually unilateral
- Polyostotic fibrous dysplasia has a predilection for the skull, facial bones, pelvis, spine, and shoulder, although any bone may be affected

FLUOROSIS

Clinical

- Acute fluoride intoxication is associated with severe gastrointestinal symptoms and toxic nephritis
- Chronic exposure leads to joint pain and stiffness

Imaging

- Diffuse chalky osteosclerosis of the spine, pelvis, and ribs, obscuring architecture of these bones
- Skull and appendicular bones not sclerotic

- Appendicular manifestations include periosteal thickening, ligamentous calcifications, and well-formed bone spurs at entheses

GAUCHER'S DISEASE

Clinical

- Rare, inherited enzyme deficiency (acid beta-glucosidase) results in accumulation of cerebroside lipid in macrophages (Gaucher's cells) in bone marrow, liver, spleen, lymph nodes, brain, and lungs
- Tissue infiltration by Gaucher's cells most pronounced in spleen and lymph nodes
- Most common among Ashkenazi Jews
- Type 1 ("adult") disease, the most common form, manifests in childhood but becomes most problematic in the second and third decades, with hepatosplenomegaly, anemia, fever, pneumonia, and skeletal findings that include osteonecrosis and fracture; no neurologic symptoms occur
- Type 2 disease is marked by severe neurologic findings and death in infancy
- Type 3 ("juvenile") is a rare neuronogenic form that presents earlier than type 1 disease and has the additional manifestation of chronic seizures
- Current treatment is macrophage-targeted enzyme therapy

Imaging

- Skeletal manifestations reflect marrow infiltration by Gaucher's cells
- Radiographs show diffuse expansion of the marrow space in the axial and appendicular skeleton, with generalized osteopenia, coarsened trabecular pattern, Erlenmeyer flask deformities of the femora, pathologic fractures, osteolytic lesions, and multifocal osteonecrosis
- Step-like deformities of the vertebral end plates (H vertebrae) resemble those seen in sickle cell anemia
- Patients are at increased risk of osteomyelitis
- Radiographic bone changes not commonly reversible despite otherwise effective enzyme therapy
- Gaucher's shows rapid T_2 relaxation on MRI

GIANT CELL TUMOR

Clinical

- Usually benign and solitary but may be multicentric or malignant (10%)
- Vast majority present after skeletal maturity, usually in second and third decades
- Pain is the most common presenting symptom
- Aggressive lesions may break through the cortex, invade local soft tissues, and recur after surgical resection
- Lesions in the distal radius are often aggressive

Imaging

- Purely lytic lesion, with sharply defined but nonsclerotic margins, eccentrically positioned in subarticular medullary bone
- In contrast to chondroblastoma, the physis is usually closed
- Aggressive lesions may break through cortex

GOUT

Clinical

- Asymmetric polyarthritis caused by deposition of monosodium urate crystals in articular cartilage, synovium, subchondral bone, and periarticular tissues
- Most commonly idiopathic, but also associated with various conditions (e.g., myeloproliferative diseases, chronic renal failure)
- Acute gout most commonly affects the lower extremity joints, especially the first metatarsophalangeal joint (70%), with excruciating pain and swelling

- Negatively birefringent, needle-shaped crystals in synovial fluid are diagnostic
- Chronic arthritis develops in less than 50% of cases that are recurrent

Imaging

- Asymmetric, nodular deposits of calcium urate (tophi) in periarticular tissues
- Calcification of tophi is uncommon
- Intraarticular and periarticular erosions show sclerotic margins and often have elevated "overhanging edges" extending over tophaceous nodules
- Joint space is preserved until late disease
- Periarticular osteopenia is not a prominent feature unless joint is in disuse

HEMANGIOMA

Clinical

- Benign, vascular neoplasm of bone and soft tissues seen in all ages but most commonly in middle-aged women
- May be associated with overgrowth of affected limb

Imaging

- Predilection for vertebrae, where they are very common and incidental; classically have a "corduroy" or "honeycomb" appearance in vertebrae
- Presence of fat within a vertebral body lesion on MRI is virtually diagnostic
- In the skull, lesions usually involve the facial bones (usually the mandible)
- Involvement of tubular bones is uncommon; intracortical and periosteal lesions are rare
- Phleboliths are diagnostic of soft tissue hemangiomas but not always present

HEMOCHROMATOSIS

Clinical

- Excessive iron accumulation in a variety of tissues as the result of either a primary disturbance in gastrointestinal iron absorption (primary hemochromatosis) or an increased iron load from multiple transfusions, alcoholic cirrhosis, or direct ingestion (secondary hemochromatosis)
- Diagnosis is based on increased serum iron concentration, increased transferrin saturation, and liver biopsy
- Most common in men aged 40 to 60 years
- Clinical triad: cirrhosis, skin pigmentation, diabetes
- Can lead to ascites and heart failure
- Noninflammatory arthritis initially affects the small joints of the hands but eventually can involve large joints
- Hemosiderin deposition in synovium but generally not in cartilage, whereas calcium pyrophosphate dihydrate deposition can be seen in both synovium and cartilage

Imaging

- Diffuse osteopenia is common and may be associated with biconcave vertebral deformities
- Associated with degenerative-like arthritis; indistinguishable from that seen with idiopathic calcium pyrophosphate dihydrate deposition
- Articular changes include chondrocalcinosis (40%); joint-space narrowing (often symmetric); subchondral sclerosis, collapse, and cyst formation; and osteophytosis (often distinctive, e.g., beak-like osteophytes of metacarpal heads)
- Distribution of joint involvement unusual for degenerative joint disease, i.e., metacarpophalangeal joints (most common site), radiocarpal and midcarpal joints of wrist, elbow, and shoulder

- Progression of arthritis typically slower than that associated with calcium pyrophosphate dihydrate deposition disease

HEMOPHILIA

Clinical

- X-linked recessive deficiency of factor VIII (classical hemophilia) or factor IX (Christmas disease)
- Incidence is 1 in 10,000 males
- Hemarthrosis in weight-bearing joints occurs in the vast majority of hemophiliacs

Imaging

- Radiographic features include epiphyseal overgrowth, osteopenia, dense effusions, secondary osteoarthritis with subchondral cysts, pseudotumors (intraosseous hemorrhages), and osteonecrosis
- In the knee, a wide intercondylar notch and "square" patella (erosion of inferior pole) may be present
- The ankle may show tibiotalar tilting
- Radiographic findings are usually indistinguishable from those of juvenile chronic arthritis

HYDROXYAPATITE DEPOSITION

Clinical

- Recurrent, painful deposits of calcium hydroxyapatite in periarticular tissues
- Also called *calcific tendinitis*
- Usually monoarticular but can be polyarticular
- Most common site is the shoulder
- Typical age of patients is 40 to 70 years

Imaging

- Initially thin or cloud-like periarticular calcifications usually become well-defined, amorphous collections
- Small calcific deposits may mimic fracture fragments or ossicles
- Calcifications may change or disappear over time

HYPERPARATHYROIDISM

Clinical

- Overproduction of parathormone results in excessive bone resorption and hypercalcemia by direct stimulation of osteoclasts; in the presence of intact renal function, excess parathormone also causes hypophosphatemia via phosphaturic effect on the kidneys
- Primary hyperparathyroidism is most commonly caused by adenoma of one gland or diffuse hyperplasia; parathyroid carcinoma and ectopic secretion of parathormone (e.g., from bronchogenic carcinoma) are rare causes
- Secondary hyperparathyroidism results from chronic hypocalcemic stimulation of the parathyroid glands, usually because of phosphate retention in renal failure (renal osteodystrophy), but occasionally because of intestinal malabsorption
- Tertiary hyperparathyroidism is the development of autonomous parathyroid function after long-standing secondary hyperparathyroidism
- *Pseudohyperparathyroidism* refers to hypercalcemia of malignancy resulting from secretion of parathormone-like substance by a neoplasm (e.g., from breast carcinoma)
- Laboratory abnormalities include elevated parathormone concentration (except in pseudohyperparathyroidism), hypercalcemia, hypophosphatemia (primary hyperparathyroidism, secondary hyperparathyroidism caused by malabsorption), or hyperphosphatasia (secondary hyperparathyroidism caused by renal failure)

- Initial clinical presentation usually is attributable to urinary calculi, peptic ulcer disease, or pancreatitis

Imaging

- Radiographic changes in primary hyperparathyroidism are related primarily to excessive bone resorption
- Subperiosteal bone resorption is a specific but insensitive sign that is usually seen along the radial side of middle phalanx of index and middle fingers but also can involve the phalangeal tufts; medial aspects of proximal tibia, humerus, and femur; the ribs; and lamina dura
- Other manifestations of osteoclastic resorption include intracortical tunneling, endosteal scalloping, and diffuse osteopenia resulting from trabecular bone resorption
- Enthetic bone resorption occurs at tendinous and ligamentous attachments, especially the femoral trochanters, ischial tuberosity, humeral tuberosities, calcaneus, and inferior clavicle
- Subchondral bone resorption and collapse results in widening of sacroiliac and acromioclavicular joints, symphysis pubis, and appendicular joints
- Other articular manifestations include chondrocalcinosis and marginal erosions but not joint-space narrowing
- Brown tumors are well-defined, lytic lesions of fibrous tissue and giant cells that are most common in primary hyperparathyroidism; intralesional hemorrhage produces brown appearance on gross inspection
- With renal failure (i.e., renal osteodystrophy), additional changes occur associated with concomitant vitamin D deficiency and hyperphosphatasia, including vascular calcifications, vertebral end plate sclerosis (rugger-jersey spine), mild rickets, and occasionally diffuse osteosclerosis

HYPERTROPHIC OSTEOARTHROPATHY

Clinical

- Occurs secondary to numerous benign and malignant pulmonary diseases, including lung carcinoma, pleural mesothelioma, abscess, bronchiectasis, emphysema, cystic fibrosis, Hodgkin's disease, and metastasis
- Also associated with cyanotic congenital heart disease, inflammatory bowel disease, and biliary atresia
- Digital clubbing with soft tissue swelling may be present
- Usually accompanied by periarticular pain
- The cause is unknown
- Thoracotomy often results in rapid remission
- Also called *secondary hypertrophic osteoarthropathy* to distinguish it from pachydermoperiostosis (primary hypertrophic osteoarthropathy)

Imaging

- Periostitis that spares the epiphyses
- Scintigraphy more sensitive than radiography and shows diffuse symmetric "double stripe" along diaphyses and metaphyses of tubular bones

JUVENILE CHRONIC ARTHRITIS

Clinical

- Several subgroups, as follows:
  Pauciarticular or *monoarticular disease:* very common form, shows a female predominance, most commonly affects large joints, and may be complicated by blindness from iridocyclitis
  Polyarticular disease: symmetric appendicular involvement, cervical spine is only axial site, systemic manifestations (rash, fever, splenomegaly, lymphadenopathy)

Classic systemic disease: very young patients (age under 5 years), severe systemic manifestations, only mild articular manifestations

Juvenile-onset adult type (seropositive) rheumatoid arthritis: fewer than 10% of cases, patients usually older than 10 years, shows a female predominance

Imaging

- Unlike rheumatoid arthritis, erosions, joint-space narrowing, and osteopenia are not prominent features
- Periostitis and intraarticular ankylosis are common
- Often accompanied by epiphyseal compression, joint subluxation, and growth disturbances, including epiphyseal ballooning and bone overgrowth or undergrowth
- Leg-length discrepancies are common
- Hypoplasia of fused cervical vertebral bodies and micrognathia are characteristic features

LEUKEMIA

Clinical

- Acute leukemia affects children (lymphoblastic) and adults (myeloid)
- Chronic leukemia is usually granulocytic or lymphocytic and affects adults
- Childhood leukemia is associated with lymphadenopathy, splenomegaly, and arthralgias
- Leukemia in adults usually shows milder clinical and radiographic findings

Imaging

- Common findings include osteopenia, radiolucent and radiodense metaphyseal bands, osteolytic lesions, and periostitis
- Metaphyseal osteosclerosis may be seen in rare instances
- Changes are less frequent and less severe in adults

LYMPHOMA

Clinical

- A variety of malignant lymphoreticular neoplasms (Hodgkin's disease, non-Hodgkin's lymphoma, Burkitt's lymphoma, and mycosis fungoides) affecting all ages
- May be disseminated or arise as a primary process in bone
- Primary lymphoma is uncommon but associated with a relatively good prognosis
- Burkitt's lymphoma is the most common malignancy of children in tropical Africa and typically involves the facial bones

Imaging

- Skeletal lesions most common in Hodgkin's disease
- Moth-eaten or permeative lesions may be lucent, sclerotic, or mixed
- Osteosclerotic lesions (e.g., "ivory vertebra") and periostitis are more common in Hodgkin's disease than in non-Hodgkin's lymphoma
- Primary lymphoma typically affects the distal femur and presents as a local mass before secondary symptoms become evident

MALIGNANT FIBROUS HISTIOCYTOMA

Clinical

- Malignant fibrous neoplasm occurring at any age but most commonly in fifth to seventh decades of life
- More common in men

Imaging

- Purely lytic, aggressive appearance, with moth-eaten or permeative pattern
- Most commonly in metaphysis of long bone
- Radiographically similar to fibrosarcoma
- May have sequestrum

MELORHEOSTOSIS

Clinical

- Rare, sclerosing dysplasia typically presenting after early childhood
- Symptoms include pain, swelling, and restricted range of motion
- May cause considerable deformity and disability

Imaging

- Wavy cortical hyperostosis resembling dripping candle wax is the classic appearance
- May coexist with osteopoikilosis and osteopathia striata ("overlap syndrome," mixed sclerosing dysplasias)

METASTASIS

Clinical

- Up to 15% are solitary
- Most frequent site of skeletal metastasis is the spine
- Infrequent sites include the mandible, patella, and bones distal to the elbow and knee

Imaging

- Lung cancer is most common cause of cortical metastasis and metastasis to the hand or foot
- Prostate and breast cancer are the most common sources of osteoblastic metastasis, although breast metastases are usually lytic or mixed lytic-sclerotic
- Diffuse osteoblastic metastasis is a rare cause of generalized osteosclerosis
- Renal and thyroid metastases are purely osteolytic and may have sharply corticated margins mimicking benign lesions of bone
- Bone scintigraphy is more sensitive but less specific than radiography
- MRI is the most sensitive imaging modality

MULTICENTRIC RETICULOHISTIOCYTOSIS

Clinical

- Also called *lipoid dermatoarthritis*
- Uncommon systemic disease characterized by proliferation of histiocytes in skin, mucosa, synovium, bone, and periosteum
- Cause is unknown
- Presents in adulthood, more commonly in women
- Polyarthritis resembling rheumatoid arthritis is usually the earliest manifestation, followed by development of nodular skin lesions
- Associated with carcinoma of colon, lung, breast, and cervix

Imaging

- Bilaterally symmetric erosive polyarthritis with predilection for joints of hand and wrist
- Erosions are sharply marginated as in gout
- No juxtaarticular osteopenia or periostitis
- Uncalcified cutaneous, subcutaneous, and peritendinous nodules

- 50% develop arthritis mutilans
- Severe atlantoaxial subluxation can develop early

MULTIPLE MYELOMA

Clinical

- Malignant medullary neoplasm of plasma cells
- Usually presents in patients older than 40 years of age
- Diagnosis usually made by urinary and plasma electrophoresis or bone biopsy

Imaging

- Multiple lesions are most common; solitary lesions are termed *plasmacytomas*
- Wide spectrum of radiographic appearances, including moth-eaten and permeative lesions; rib lesions are often well defined and expansive
- Axial skeletal usually involved first
- Mandible involvement, which is rare with metastasis, is present in 33% of cases
- Sclerotic lesions rare (less than 2%, associated with POEMS [polyneuropathy, organomegaly, endocrinopathy, M protein, and skin changes] syndrome)
- Hyperviscosity may result in bone infarctions
- Bone scintigraphy may be falsely negative

NEUROFIBROMATOSIS

Clinical

- This idiopathic entity (which is one of the phakomatoses) has an incidence of 1 in 3000 births
- Autosomal dominant transmission, although 50% are spontaneous
- Type I (peripheral) and type II (central) subdivisions

Imaging

- Skeletal features include scoliosis/kyphoscoliosis, ribbon ribs, vertebral deformities, posterior vertebral scalloping, pseudarthrosis (especially distal tibia and fibula), bone whittling, neural foraminal widening (caused by lateral meningocele or nerve sheath neoplasms), and bone overgrowth
- One cause of hemihypertrophy of limbs

NEUROPATHIC ARTHROPATHY

Clinical

- "Charcot joint"
- Neural deprivation of joint leads to highly destructive arthropathy, probably because of severe biomechanical derangement
- Causes include congenital insensitivity to pain, syphilis (lower extremities), syringomyelia (upper extremities), meningomyelocele, multiple sclerosis, diabetes (metatarsophalangeal and intertarsal), alcoholism, excess steroids, and various neurologic disorders

Imaging

- Radiographic changes similar to those of osteoarthritis but with greater sclerosis and fragmentation of the articular bones, abundant intraarticular debris, and marked joint distention and subluxation
- Ankylosis is uncommon

NONOSSIFYING FIBROMA

Clinical

- Benign, fibroosseous lesion termed *fibrous cortical defect* if less than 2 cm
- Highly prevalent in children (up to 30% incidence)
- Involutes in late adolescence
- Painless unless fractured

Imaging

- Lesions are subcortical and lytic with thin, lobular, sclerotic borders
- Occasionally mildly expansive
- Usually metaphyseal
- No periosteal reaction unless fractured

OCHRONOSIS

Clinical

- Also called *alkaptonuria*
- Hereditary absence of homogentisic acid oxidase results in accumulation of homogentisic acid and dark pigmentation of various connective tissues
- Urine turns dark when left in open air
- Ochronotic arthropathy results from skeletal deposition of pigment
- Arthropathy presents in fourth decade

Imaging

- Calcification of the intervertebral discs (usually lumbar) with severe disc narrowing and vacuum phenomenon but only small osteophytes
- May lead to "bamboo spine" appearance, simulating that of ankylosing spondylitis
- Vertebral osteopenia
- Arthropathy of sacroiliac joints, symphysis pubis, and large appendicular joints resembles degenerative joint disease but often with more severe sclerosis, collapse and fragmentation, multiple intraarticular bodies, and only small osteophytes
- Tendons occasionally calcified

OSTEOARTHRITIS

Clinical

- Degenerative joint disease associated with pain, swelling, stiffness, and crepitation
- Affects 14% of population
- Severity and distribution of articular changes represent balance between systemic predisposition and local biomechanical factors
- Old age is most important risk factor, but acute trauma and overuse also are important causes
- Distal interphalangeal joints are most commonly affected, but knee and hip disease cause most disability

Imaging

- Joint-space narrowing is typically eccentric, with most severe narrowing at sites of greatest joint loading
- Subchondral sclerosis, cyst formation, and osteophytosis are additional features
- Loose intraarticular bodies may develop osteochondroma

OSTEOBLASTOMA

Clinical

- Benign primary bone neoplasm characterized by osteoid and woven bone production

- Usually seen in patients under 30 years of age
- Male predominance
- Most commonly in long bones or posterior elements of spine

Imaging

- Variable radiographic appearance, including well-marginated lytic lesion, expansive (posterior vertebral elements) or aggressive; may resemble a giant osteoid osteoma or be associated with a soft tissue mass
- Nidus may calcify or be associated with sclerosis of neighboring bone

OSTEOGENESIS IMPERFECTA

Clinical

- Inherited disorder of collagen synthesis affecting bones, ligaments, sclera, skin, and dentin
- Diagnostic criteria include osteoporosis and abnormal bone fragility, blue sclerae, otosclerosis, and dentinogenesis imperfecta
- Other clinical features include joint laxity, easy bruising, premature vascular calcifications, constipation, and hypertrophic scarring
- Originally subclassified into congenita and tarda forms; the congenita form (10%) was usually sporadic and showed severe bone fragility and high infant mortality, whereas the more common tarda form (90%) showed autosomal dominant inheritance, was clinically milder, and was associated with a normal life expectancy

Imaging

- Diffuse osteopenia of variable severity involving both the axial and appendicular skeleton
- Appendicular bones are most commonly thin and gracile (tarda); short, thick bones are seen in congenita form; rarely, bones have a cystic appearance
- Bones are often bowed and fracture frequently with exuberant callus formation
- Skull radiography shows enlarged sinuses, Wormian bones, and platybasia
- Severe kyphoscoliosis and biconcave or wedge-shaped deformity of the vertebrae often occur
- Radiographic changes may be indistinguishable from those of Cushing's disease
- Prenatal ultrasonography may reveal short or fractured femora, poorly defined calvarium, and narrow thorax in fetuses with congenita or severe tarda

OSTEOID OSTEOMA

Clinical

- Benign osteoblastic lesion consisting of a central vascular osteoid tissue nidus and peripheral sclerosis
- Most often affects those aged between 7 and 25 years
- Presents with pain, which classically is worse at night and relieved by aspirin
- Lesions near articulations may be associated with lymphoproliferative synovitis

Imaging

- CT is the modality of choice for nidus localization
- Lucent nidus is less than 15 cm in size
- The lucent nidus may be calcified and appear as a "pseudosequestrum"
- Cortical lesions may have extensive surrounding reactive sclerosis
- Medullary lesions often associated with less sclerosis

OSTEOMA

Clinical

- Asymptomatic nodule of normal bone in periosteum
- Most common among men 30 to 50 years of age

- Multiple lesions associated with Gardner's syndrome

Imaging

- Small, homogeneously dense periosteal nodule with smooth or lobular margins
- Most commonly involve skull, paranasal sinuses, and mandible
- Can potentially obstruct a paranasal sinus to cause a mucocele

OSTEOMALACIA/RICKETS

Clinical

- Group of skeletal disorders associated with abnormal development and mineralization of the growth plate (rickets) or undermineralization of trabecular and cortical osteoid (osteomalacia)
- Most common cause is vitamin D deficiency resulting from dietary deficiency, intestinal malabsorption, or inadequate synthesis because of insufficient sun exposure (impaired conversion of 7-dehydrocholesterol to D_3 in skin), liver disease (impaired 25 hydroxylation of D_3), renal tubular disease (impaired 1 hydroxylation of 25-OH-D_3), anticonvulsant therapy (mechanism unclear), or, rarely, congenital hydroxylase deficiencies or target-tissue unresponsiveness
- Skeletal changes in vitamin D deficiency primarily related to disturbed blood mineral homeostasis and secondary hyperparathyroidism rather than direct effects of vitamin D on bone
- Other causes of disturbed blood mineral homeostasis, such as acquired or congenital phosphate-loosing nephropathy (Fanconi's syndrome, X-linked hypophosphatemia) and hypophosphatasia, can produce severe osteomalacia or rickets

Imaging

- Generalized osteopenia and insufficiency fractures associated with osteomalacia are nonspecific, but unmineralized osteoid lining the trabeculae may produce a subtle "smudged" appearance to spongy bone
- Pseudofractures are specific for osteomalacia but relatively uncommon; they appear as bilaterally symmetric linear lucencies perpendicular to the cortex, occasionally with sclerotic margins ("Looser's zones"), often arising in scapula, ribs, pubic rami, and proximal femora
- In the immature skeleton (rickets) additional radiographic changes include widening of the growth plate, irregularity of the zone of provisional calcification, metaphyseal fraying, and cupping; bone softening and epiphyseal displacement by asymmetric musculotendinous pull results in bowing deformities of long bones, scoliosis, basilar invagination, and triradiate pelvis

OSTEOMYELITIS

Clinical

- Presents with pain, tenderness, soft tissue swelling, and fever
- Hematogenous infection usually associated with metaphyseal localization

Imaging

- Radiographic findings require approximately 2 weeks to develop; radiography thus is not sensitive for early infection
- Usually does not cross open physis unless patient is less than 1 year of age
- Extension to adjacent joint is most common cause of pyogenic arthritis in children; therefore, associated joint effusion should be sought

OSTEOPETROSIS

Clinical

- Group of diseases characterized by defective bone resorption associated with decreased osteoclastic activity

- Results in dense fragile bones, cranial nerve compressions, anemia, and growth disturbance
- Several forms exist, with varying severity of findings, ranging from severe anemia and death in the first decade to asymptomatic individuals
- One form is associated with renal tubular acidosis and periventricular and basal ganglionic calcifications

Imaging

- Generalized osteosclerosis, especially base of skull
- Narrowing of medullary space with loss of corticomedullary distinctness
- Disturbed bone modeling may give rachitic appearance and show undertubulation
- Occasionally presents characteristic "bone-within-a-bone" appearance
- Pathologic fractures often occur

OSTEOSARCOMA

Clinical

- Malignant osteoblastic neoplasm
- Peak incidence in patients aged 10 to 30 years
- Presents with local pain, swelling, and warmth

Imaging

- Ill-defined or permeative appearance, usually with osteoid-matrix calcification
- Commonly associated with a soft tissue mass
- Most commonly metaphyseal about the knee
- Satellite lesions occasionally found in parent bone
- Rare multifocal form (osteosarcomatosis) presents with multiple isochronous skeletal lesions

PACHYDERMOPERIOSTOSIS

Clinical

- Also known as *primary hypertrophic osteoarthropathy*
- About 20-fold less common than secondary hypertrophic osteoarthropathy
- Autosomal dominant with variable penetrance
- Most common in black men
- Typically manifests in adolescence
- Clinical features include enlarged hands and feet, digital clubbing, coarsening of the skin of the face and scalp, excessive sweating, and nonspecific musculoskeletal pain
- Significant disability may occur such as kyphosis, limited range of motion, and neurologic symptoms
- In general, the disease process progresses for about 10 years before it is spontaneously arrested

Imaging

- Diffuse symmetric periostitis, primarily involving long bones
- In contrast to secondary hypertrophic osteoarthropathy, periostitis may involve epiphyses
- Bone scintigraphy is very sensitive and appears similar to that in secondary hypertrophic osteoarthropathy

PAGET'S DISEASE

Clinical

- Idiopathic condition of excessive and abnormal turnover of individual bones in middle-aged and elderly patients

- Prevalence is 3% in population over 40 years old and 10% among those older than 80 years
- Associated with local pain and deformity, pathologic fractures, nerve impingement, osteoarthritis, and rarely (1%) sarcomatous transformation
- Elevated urinary hydroxyproline and serum alkaline phosphatase reflect increased bone resorption and synthesis, respectively
- Usually patients have five to six lesions
- Pelvis is the most common site, followed by the spine and femur, but any bone can be involved
- Diagnosis usually incidental on radiography
- Treatment includes suppression of abnormal resorption with calcitonin and bisphosphonates

Imaging

- Radiography is usually diagnostic; changes can be purely lytic, mixed lytic and sclerotic, or predominantly sclerotic
- Initial lytic phase always begins at one end of a long bone and shows a sharply marginated V-shaped leading edge resembling a flame or blade of grass; additional resorptive changes include osteolytic cortical clefts
- Lytic Paget's disease in the skull (osteoporosis circumscripta) usually affects the frontal and occipital bones
- Proliferative changes include bone enlargement, cortical thickening, trabecular thickening and coarsening, and loss of corticomedullary distinctiveness
- Characteristic radiographic appearances include picture-frame vertebra and cotton-wool calvarium
- New pagetic bone is woven, not lamellar, and therefore relatively weak, leading to bowing of long bones and pathologic fractures

PAROSTEAL OSTEOSARCOMA

Clinical

- Subtype of osteosarcoma arising on the bone surface
- Most common between the ages of 25 and 40 years
- Presents with pain, swelling, and often a large palpable mass

Imaging

- Parosteal mass shows typical osteoid-matrix calcification
- Most common site is the posterior aspect of the distal femoral metaphysis
- In contrast to myositis ossificans, which shows peripheral calcification, neoplastic calcification of osteosarcoma is central
- MRI is useful for evaluating marrow involvement

PSORIATIC SPONDYLOARTHROPATHY

Clinical

- Inflammatory arthritis and enthesitis affecting a minority of patients with psoriasis of the skin
- Skin lesions almost always develop first
- Distribution of arthritis is classically asymmetric but can be symmetric or monoarticular

Imaging

- Synovitis and cartilage loss result in concentric joint space narrowing and bone erosions, as in rheumatoid arthritis
- Unlike rheumatoid arthritis, however, the distal interphalangeal joints are frequently involved; bone erosions show proliferative "whiskered" or "fuzzy" mar-

gins; periostitis and intraarticular ankylosis are seen; osteopenia is not a prominent feature
- Other findings include tuft erosion and joint malalignment
- Bilaterally asymmetric sacroiliitis is common
- Large, asymmetric, bulky paravertebral excrescences typically affect the thoracolumbar spine

REFLEX SYMPATHETIC DYSTROPHY SYNDROME

Clinical

- Often called *Sudeck's atrophy, causalgia, algodystrophy,* or *shoulder-hand syndrome*
- Presents with extremity pain, stiffness, weakness, and swelling with vasomotor instability and hyperesthesia in association with a wide variety of clinical situations, including posttraumatic, postsurgical, and postinfectious states; calcific tendinitis; cervical degenerative disc disease; cerebrovascular disease; or myocardial infarction
- Pathogenesis unknown, but an abnormal neurovascular reflex mechanism is postulated
- Most commonly affects an entire upper extremity, but any site can be affected
- Process is bilateral but typilily asymmetric
- Duration of the condition varies, but it may persist for years or become irreversible

Imaging

- Radiographic findings include soft tissue swelling associated with rapidly developing regional osteoporosis and cortical tunneling, endosteal resorption, and occasionally subperiosteal bone resorption
- Periarticular osteopenia can mimic arthritis but without significant articular erosion or joint space narrowing
- Bone scintigraphy shows regionally increased uptake caused by local hyperemia; scintigraphic changes may precede clinical or radiographic findings

REITER'S SYNDROME

Clinical

- Uncommon arthritic disorder
- Mostly affects men aged between 15 and 35 years
- Believed to be transmitted sexually or in association with epidemic dysentery
- Primarily a clinical diagnosis
- Classic triad: urethritis, conjunctivitis, and arthritis
- Other clinical findings include circinate balanitis (penile lesion), keratoderma blenorrhagicum (characteristic skin lesion, usually of soles and palms), fever, and weight loss
- Arthritis usually asymmetric and most commonly affects the lower extremities
- 75% of patients are HLA-B27 positive

Imaging

- Radiographic findings may be indistinguishable from those of psoriatic spondyloarthropathy
- Synovitis and cartilage loss result in concentric joint-space narrowing and bone erosions
- As with other seronegative arthritides, bone erosions and entheses show proliferative "whiskered" or "fuzzy" margins, and periostitis may be seen along the shafts of small bones in the foot and hand
- Intraarticular ankylosis is less common than in psoriatic spondyloarthropathy or ankylosing spondylitis, and osteopenia is not a prominent feature
- Bilaterally asymmetric sacroiliitis is common
- Asymmetric paravertebral ossifications may develop but occur less often than in psoriatic spondyloarthropathy or ankylosing spondylitis

RENAL OSTEODYSTROPHY (see *Hyperparathyroidism*)

RHEUMATOID ARTHRITIS

Clinical

- Multisystem disorder associated with symmetric polyarthritis
- Affects 2 to 4% of the population; affects females more often than males
- Any synovial joint can be involved, but most common in metacarpophalangeal and interphalangeal joints of hands
- Cartilaginous joints less commonly affected
- Arthritis has insidious onset, usually beginning in one joint first, then becoming polyarticular and symmetric
- Clinical findings include joint pain, swelling, and morning joint stiffness
- Other findings include subcutaneous nodules (25%), muscular weakness, and vascular lesions (e.g., Raynaud's phenomenon, pulmonary hypertension)

Imaging

- Arthritis characterized by concentric joint-space narrowing, nonproliferative bone erosion, juxtaarticular osteopenia, and joint malalignment
- Osteophytes and other proliferative changes do not occur unless secondary degenerative disease also present

SCLERODERMA

Clinical

- Multisystem disorder of connective tissue associated with fibrosis and small vessel disease
- Most common in adult women
- Raynaud's phenomenon is usually present and associated with sclerosis of skin over face and fingers
- Skin sclerosis can become diffuse
- The majority of patients eventually develop arthritis that may resemble rheumatoid arthritis clinically
- Additional clinical findings include subcutaneous calcinosis and those related to gastrointestinal, pulmonary, cardiac, or renal involvement

Imaging

- Tuft resorption is associated with atrophy of overlying soft tissues and subcutaneous calcifications
- Synovium may calcify and "tumoral" periarticular calcific deposits may develop
- Joint space narrowing, marginal and central bone erosions, osteophyte formation, and intraarticular ankylosis may involve the distal interphalangeal joints and resemble psoriatic arthritis

SOLITARY BONE CYST

Clinical

- Benign central medullary cyst seen almost exclusively in patients younger than 20 years of age
- High incidence of pathologic fracture
- Most common skeletal sites include the proximal humerus, proximal femur, and calcaneus

Imaging

- First arises in metaphysis, but may be seen in diaphysis as physis migrates away from lesion with skeletal growth
- Usually unicompartmental (thus the synonym *unicameral bone cyst*); however, ridges along gently lobulated surface may mimic septations when viewed en face

- Presence of a dependent fragment of bone within the lesion after pathologic fracture ("fallen-fragment" sign) is virtually pathognomonic

SPONDYLOLYSIS

Clinical

- Discontinuity at the pars interarticularis, which bridges the superior and inferior facet of a vertebra
- Believed to be an acquired condition because it is rarely seen in infants and children
- Bilateral pars defects usually result in anterior subluxation of the vertebral body with the proximal spinal column and posterior displacement of the spinous process with the distal spinal column; the spinal canal is actually widened
- L5–S1 and L4–L5 are the two most common locations

Imaging

- Radiographic diagnosis depends on oblique views but sometimes visible on lateral views
- CT is most sensitive, but MRI has almost equivalent diagnostic power and can evaluate associated disc protrusions and neural impingement
- MRI can also visualize osteochondral overgrowth at the pars defect that can narrow the lateral recess and impinge the descending nerve root

SYNOVIAL OSTEOCHONDROMATOSIS

Clinical

- Idiopathic nodular chondroid metaplasia of synovium (synovial chondromatosis)
- Usually monoarticular, but can involve more than one joint
- Large joints most commonly affected
- Chondral bodies can detach, become loose bodies nourished by synovial fluid, and ultimately calcify or ossify
- Undergoes malignant transformation in rare instances

Imaging

- Uncalcified synovial chondromatosis appears as a diffuse, nodular, high-signal intensity mass within the joint on MR images; however, only juxtaarticular erosions and joint-space widening are visible on radiographs
- Calcified or ossified osteochondral bodies are directly visible on radiographs

SYSTEMIC LUPUS ERYTHEMATOSUS

Clinical

- Common multiple organ connective tissue disorder
- Most common in black women, usually younger than 45 years of age
- Symmetric polyarthritis (hands, wrists, knees, shoulders) develops in vast majority of patients

Imaging

- Soft tissue swelling and periarticular osteopenia resemble changes of early rheumatoid arthritis
- Unlike rheumatoid arthritis, erosions and joint-space narrowing are unusual
- Jaccoud-like, deforming, nonerosive arthropathy is present in many patients with long-standing lupus, and characterized by reversible, nondisabling joint deformity without erosions or joint-space narrowing
- Osteonecrosis often complicates steroid treatment but occasionally develops spontaneously
- Soft tissue calcifications may be seen

• Increased risk of osteomyelitis

TELANGIECTATIC OSTEOSARCOMA

Clinical

• Highly aggressive, vascular subtype of the usually osteoblastic malignant neoplasm

Imaging

• Purely lytic, aggressive appearance
• May have fluid-fluid levels due to hemorrhage

THALASSEMIA

Clinical

• Group of hereditary disorders characterized by deficient globin synthesis: alpha-thalassemia (deficient alpha globin chain synthesis) and beta-thalassemia (deficient beta globin chain synthesis)
• Common among but not exclusive to patients of Italian or Greek origin ("Mediterranean anemia")
• Alpha-thalassemia, usually seen in Southeast Asia, can manifest in utero with hydrops fetalis and death
• Homozygous beta-thalassemia (thalassemia major) presents in infancy with severe anemia and hepatosplenomegaly; usually death occurs in childhood
• Heterozygous beta-thalassemia (thalassemia minor) associated with only mild clinical features
• Thalassemia intermedia is a poorly defined form with intermediate clinical findings

Imaging

• Radiographic changes relate to pronounced hematopoietic marrow hyperplasia; changes are more severe in thalassemia major than in thalassemia minor
• Initially, both appendicular and axial skeleton affected, but appendicular involvement diminishes at puberty as marrow regresses from peripheral skeleton
• In the skull, the diploic space expands with thinning of the outer table and "hair-on-end" striations; facial bones show obliteration of paranasal sinuses, hypertelorism, and malocclusion of teeth, producing characteristic "rodent" facies not usually seen in other anemias
• The spine shows severe osteoporosis and biconcave vertebral deformities
• Appendicular bones and ribs show medullary expansion, osteoporosis, cortical thinning, and coarse trabecular pattern
• Severe osteoporosis leads to insufficiency fractures
• Growth disturbances, including Erlenmeyer flask deformity and premature physeal fusion, may be seen in the extremities
• Numerous transfusions can lead to secondary hemochromatosis with arthritis and chondrocalcinosis, as seen in primary hemochromatosis
• Hyperuricemia and gouty arthritis may also be seen
• Excess iron deposition from several transfusions can cause reduced skeletal uptake of radiotracer on bone scintigraphy and decreased signal intensity in marrow on MRI

TUMORAL CALCINOSIS

Clinical

• Large, periarticular soft tissue calcifications arising in the setting of hypercalcemic states (e.g., milk-alkali syndrome, hypervitaminosis D, hyperparathyroidism, chronic renal failure, sarcoidosis)
• Rare idiopathic form occurs most frequently in black boys and adolescents and shows a familial tendency
• Masses are painless and flocculent

Imaging

- Well-demarcated extracapsular calcified mass up to 20 cm in diameter most commonly adjacent to large joints
- May contain fluid levels

THYROTOXICOSIS

Clinical

- Most common causes are toxic diffuse goiter (Graves' disease) and toxic nodular goiter (single or multiple adenomas)
- Clinical findings include fatigue, nervousness, hypersensitivity to heat, weight loss, tachycardia, palpitations, visual disturbance, and diarrhea
- Musculoskeletal abnormalities include osteoporosis, fracture, and myopathy; they are more common in men
- Thyroid acropachy, which occurs in less than 1% of patients (usually after treatment), has the following clinical findings: exophthalmos, pretibial myxedema, painless soft tissue swelling of the digits, and clubbing of the fingers; its cause is unknown

Imaging

- Radiography shows changes of high-turnover osteoporosis: osteopenia and insufficiency fractures, but more specifically cortical tunneling; in contrast to postmenopausal osteoporosis, effects are more pronounced in cortical bone than in trabecular bone
- Skeletal changes involve the spine, pelvis, skull, hands, and feet
- Accelerated skeletal maturation and premature craniosynostosis may be seen in children
- Thyroid acropachy shows characteristic radiographic features: feathery periosteal bone formation along the shafts of the tubular bones in the hands and feet associated with local soft tissue swelling

4

Alimentary Tract Imaging

■ **Maitray D. Patel,** M.D.

4

OVERVIEW

The mainstay of radiologic evaluation of the alimentary tract is the barium contrast examination, using either single-contrast or double-contrast technique. Double-contrast techniques are preferable because they provide greater mucosal detail. Single-contrast techniques are suitable for all patients who are considered too ill to undergo double-contrast maneuvers; they are also adequate in those patients in whom a nonmucosal condition is suspected. If bowel perforation is suspected, water-soluble contrast agents *only* should be administered, at least until frank perforation has been excluded. For the hypopharynx, esophagus, stomach, and proximal duodenum, double-contrast technique is achieved by using an effervescent agent that contains sodium bicarbonate, which releases carbon dioxide when mixed with liquids; the concomitant use of simethicone helps disperse bubbles rapidly. For the terminal ileum, colon, and rectum, double contrast is achieved by retrograde infusion of air using air insufflation. Barium usually is also instilled in retrograde fashion for these studies, but can be administered perorally for evaluation of the terminal ileum. The small bowel double-contrast examination (enteroclysis) relies on initial barium coating that is administered through a tube (tip in distal duodenum or proximal jejunum), followed rapidly by infusion of methylcellulose.

In general, there are a limited number of alterations in the contrast-examination appearance of any segment of bowel being evaluated, caused by a much larger list of individual diseases and pathologic processes. The broad categories of alteration are (1) caliber, (2) contour, (3) content, (4) mucosa/folds, (5) course, (6) coating, and (7) motility. Thus, when a contrast-examination study of any segment of the alimentary tract is performed or evaluated, each of the seven categories of possible alteration should be assessed. Once an abnormality is perceived, the radiologist determines the size, location, and distribution of the abnormality. The radiologist who aspires to be board certified is required to recognize alterations and be familiar with the appropriate differential diagnosis. The paragraphs that follow outline the specific differential diagnoses that are covered in section 2 of this chapter (listed in italic type).

Caliber and contour changes of the esophagus include *narrowing, ulceration, diverticula*, and *extrinsic impressions*. Other differential gamuts for the esophagus include *pharyngeal mass* and esophageal *filling defects* (alteration of content), *nodules* (alteration of filling and of mucosa/folds), *fistulas* (alteration of course), and *abnormal motility/contractions. Surgical procedures* commonly performed for the esophagus result in alteration of contour.

An important caliber change of the stomach is the *linitis plastica* appearance, in which the stomach is narrowed and poorly distensible. *Obstruction* of the stomach leads to gastric dilatation. The most common pathologic alteration of gastric contour is *outpouching/ulceration. Gas in the stomach wall* and *barium filling defects* represent changes of gastric content. Abnormality of gastric mucosa/folds may manifest as *erosions* or *fold thickening*. One of the most common surgical procedures of the stomach is some variation of the Billroth procedure (alteration in course), which has classically associated *complications* that lead to additional alterations of content or mucosa, or both.

With respect to manifestations of the broad categories of alteration in the duodenum, the board-certified radiologist should be especially familiar with causes of *obstruction* (alteration of caliber), *postbulbar ulceration* (alteration of contour), *filling defects* (alteration of content), *fold abnormality* (alteration of mucosa), and *widened sweep* (alteration of course). Most diseases that cause small bowel alterations have limited manifestations, grouped into the following differentials: *dilatation with normal folds, terminal ileal narrowing, filling defects*, and *fold abnormalities*.

Pathologic alterations of the colon and appendix predominately affect caliber, contour, content, and mucosa. The most common caliber changes manifest as global *dilatation* or *segmental narrowing*. Diffuse narrowing of the colon, also known as microcolon, results from congenital processes not discussed in this chapter (*See* **Pediatric Imaging**). A classic contour alteration for which differential considerations should be well known is the *coned cecum. Ulcers* and *thumbprinting* are other manifestations of contour change. Thumbprinting could also be classified as a mucosal/fold alteration, although the pathogenesis of thumbprinting involves the submucosal layer. Effacement of colonic folds, also known as the *smooth (ahaustral) colon*, is clearly an alteration of the mucosa. Pathologic processes that result in filling defects of the colon can be subdivided based on whether a *solitary colonic filling defect* is identified or whether there are *multiple colonic polyps*.

ALIMENTARY TRACT DIFFERENTIAL DIAGNOSES

Esophagus
    Extrinsic impressions on cervical esophagus
    Extrinsic thoracic impression
    Discrete filling defect
    Fistula
    Abnormal motility and tertiary contractions
    Narrowing
    Nodules
    Ulceration
    Diverticula
    Surgical procedures
Pharynx mass/mass effect
Stomach
    Erosions
    Complications in Billroth procedure
    Filling defect(s) in stomach
    Fold thickening
    Gas in wall of stomach
    Linitis plastica pattern
    Obstruction
    Outpouching/Ulceration
Duodenum

4

ESOPHAGUS

EXTRINSIC IMPRESSIONS ON CERVICAL ESOPHAGUS

What causes extrinsic impressions on the pharynx/cervical esophagus?

Cricopharyngeus muscle
Postcricoid impression
Thyroid or parathyroid enlargement
Lymphoid hyperplasia
Soft tissue lesion
    Abscess
    Hematoma
Related to spine
    Anterior marginal osteophyte
    Anterior herniation of intervertebral disc
    Neoplasm
    Inflammation

Cricopharyngeus muscle

Is cricopharyngeal prominence posterior or anterior?

- Posterior impression
- Prominence can be result of achalasia versus total laryngectomy
- Clinical significance of isolated cricopharyngeal achalasia unknown; present in up to 5% of asymptomatic adults
- Myotomy produces relief in over 66% of patients with significant dysphagia
- Radiographic appearance of cricopharyngeal achalasia: hemispheric or horizontal, shelf-like, posterior protrusion into barium column at C5–C6 level

FIGURES   Gore: 232, 286

Postcricoid impression

Where does the postcricoid defect occur?
What distinguishes it from true pathology?

- Anterior impression, undulating or plaque-like in shape
- Be sure that the region changes size and shape during study

FIGURE   Gore: 214

In what settings is lymphoid hyperplasia of lingual tonsil usually seen?

Lymphoid hyperplasia

- Frequently occurs after puberty, as response to allergy or repeated infection, and as result of tonsillectomy

FIGURE Gore: 253

Soft tissue lesion

- Consider abscess or hematoma (ask about relevant history)

Related to spine

Name three spinal disease processes leading to an extrinsic cervical esophageal impression.

- Consider three major categories:
    ¶ Disc and disc space: marginal osteophyte, anterior disc herniation
    ¶ Vertebral body neoplasm
    ¶ Spinal osteomyelitis

FIGURE Gore: 297

EXTRINSIC THORACIC IMPRESSION

List basic causes of extrinsic thoracic compression of the esophagus.

Normal structures
Aortic structures
Nonaortic vascular structures
Cardiac/pericardial structures
Mediastinal mass
Pulmonary mass

Normal structures

- Aortic arch
- Left mainstem bronchus
- Left inferior pulmonary vein
    ¶ Seen in about 10% of patients
    ¶ Produces indentation on anterior left wall of esophagus about 4 to 5 cm below carina

FIGURE Gore: 297

Aortic structures

- Right aortic arch
- Cervical aortic arch (rare)
- Double aortic arch
    ¶ Right usually larger and higher than left
    ¶ Barium swallow produces characteristic reverse S-shaped indentation on esophagus (seen in all vascular rings)
- Coarctation of aorta
    ¶ On plain films, "figure 3" sign seen
    ¶ "Reverse figure 3" seen on barium swallow study
- Aortic aneurysm/tortuosity

FIGURES Gore: 527, 1428

Nonaortic vascular structures

- Aberrant right subclavian artery: causes posterior esophageal indentation
- Aberrant left pulmonary artery: indents anterior esophagus and posterior trachea
- Total anomalous pulmonary venous return (TAPVR), type 3: pro-

4

4

duces anterior indentation on lower portion of esophagus, slightly below expected site of left atrial indentation
- Truncus arteriosis, type 4: dilated bronchial vessels produce discrete indentations on posterior wall of esophagus

Cardiac/paracardial structures

- Cardiac: left atrium, left ventricle
- Pericardial lesion: effusion, tumor, cyst

Mediastinal mass

- Tumor
- Lymph node enlargement
- Duplication cyst: most segmental, involving lower posterior mediastinum
- Neurenteric cysts: associated with vertebral anomalies, particularly hemivertebra, spina bifida, and scoliosis

FIGURES   Gore: 454, 483

DISCRETE FILLING DEFECT

Outline the causes of a discrete filling defect of the esophagus.

Neoplastic (benign much less common than malignant)
      Benign tumors
         Leiomyoma
         Fibrovascular polyp
         Papilloma
         Inflammatory esophagogastric polyp
         Adenoma
      Malignant tumors
         Squamous cell carcinoma
         Adenocarcinoma
         Lymphoma
         Spindle-cell sarcoma
         Gastric carcinoma with upward extension
      Metastatic disease
Other
      Varices
      Foreign bodies

Leiomyoma

What features are characteristic of leiomyoma? What features are diagnostic?

- Smooth, rounded; result of submucosal location
- Look for calcification: presence of amorphous calcification in retrocardiac esophageal mass diagnostic of leiomyoma

FIGURE   Gore: 436

Fibrovascular polyp

Are fibrovascular polyps of the esophagus typically large or small? True or false: the surface of a fibrovascular polyp usually is nodular.

- Large intraluminal filling defect
- Oval-shaped or elongated with smooth or mildly lobulated surface
- Barium can be observed to completely surround tumor

FIGURES   Gore: 438, 439

Papilloma

- Small, sessile, smooth, or slightly lobulated

FIGURE   Gore: 432

Inflammatory esophagogastric polyp

What is the cause of this lesion? How does that help in the differential diagnosis when it is seen?

- Look for inflamed prominent fold leading up to it from gastric fundus
- This lesion frequently straddles a hiatal hernia and may be associated with other findings of reflux (thought to be sequela of reflux esophagitis)

FIGURE   Gore: 434

Adenoma

What other esophageal lesion mimics adenoma? What features argue for adenoma?

- Most arise from Barrett's mucosa
- Located distal in esophagus, near gastroesophageal (GE) junction
- Can be mistaken for inflammatory esophagogastric polyp; features suggesting adenoma include large size, nodularity, and lobulation

FIGURE   Gore: 433

Squamous cell carcinoma

True or false: esophageal squamous cell carcinoma always looks ugly (more than 90% of the time).

- Appearances:
    ¶ Fungating (60%)
    ¶ Ulcerative (25%)
    ¶ Intramural, presenting as benign stricture (15%)
- Rare presentation: varicoid carcinoma; looks like varix, but does not collapse, differentiating it from varices
- Remember to look at celiac chain of nodes

FIGURES   Gore: 450–457

Adenocarcinoma

Where in the esophagus does adenocarcinoma occur?

- Usually involves GE junction or gastric fundus
- Develops in the setting of Barrett's syndrome (accounts for 20% of adenocarcinomas of esophagus)
- May give achalasia-like picture; distinguishing features include age of patient (older with cancer), duration of symptoms (shorter with cancer), and weight loss (occurs with cancer)
- Calcification unusual in esophageal carcinoma, but may rarely occur with this type (consider leiomyoma if presented with esophageal mass with amorphous calcification)

FIGURES   Gore: 459–461, 486, 487

Lymphoma

- Look for contiguous nodular involvement of both distal esophagus and stomach
- If grows inward toward lumen, can appear as filling defect
- If remains confined to submucosa, can resemble varices

FIGURES   Gore: 489–491

Spindle-cell sarcoma

- Also known as carcinosarcoma or pseudosarcoma
- Often bulky intraluminal mass

Where in the esophagus do spindle-cell sarcomas usually occur? Are these tumors difficult to image?

- Tends not to ulcerate and constrict as squamous cell does
- More often in middle of esophagus, less often distal

FIGURE   Gore: 492

Gastric carcinoma with upward extension

- Can be difficult to differentiate from adenocarcinoma of esophagus
- Look carefully at gastric cardia for associated abnormalities

FIGURE   Gore: 482

Metastatic disease

- With respect to hematogenous or lymphatic metastases, most common primary site is breast or lung
- When esophagus is directly invaded by adjacent neoplasm, usually result of larynx or thyroid primary site

FIGURES   Gore: 483–485

Varices

How are varices distinguished from varicoid tumor?

- Serpentine filling defects
- Some esophageal carcinomas may produce varicoid appearance
    - ¶ Distinguishable at fluoroscopy; variability of size and shape should be sought
    - ¶ Abrupt demarcation favors tumor

FIGURES   Gore: 501, 502

Foreign bodies

Where do foreign bodies usually get stuck in the esophagus?

- In thoracic esophagus, usually result of unchewed meat bolus
- Site of obstruction: GE junction most common, less common at aortic arch or left main bronchus
- Clinical history allows for correct diagnosis
- After impaction is relieved, possible underlying pathologic process should be sought

FIGURES   Gore: 520–522

FISTULA

List the basic causes of an esophageal fistula.

Congenital fistula
    Malignancy
        Esophageal carcinoma
        Carcinoma of lung
Perforation
    Iatrogenic
    Spontaneous
    Foreign body
Corrosive esophagitis
Inflammatory disease
    Histoplasmosis
    Tuberculosis (TB)
    Actinomycosis
    Crohn's disease

Describe the various types of congenital tracheoesophageal fistulas and their frequency.

What extraesophageal findings might be present to indicate a fistula resulting from carcinoma?

4

Congenital fistula

- Presents in neonatal period

FIGURES Gore: 1399, 1401

Esophageal carcinoma

- Tends to occur after radiation therapy, as tumor necrosis leads to fistula formation

FIGURES Gore: 456, 523

Perforation

- Left pleural effusion with pneumomediastinum classic for Boerhaave syndrome
- Can also occur after tracheoesophageal fistula repair in neonates

FIGURE Gore: 1400

TB

- Fistula extends into mediastinum or tracheobronchial tree
- Look for lymphadenopathy

FIGURE Gore: 399

Crohn's disease

- Intramural tracks can simulate fistula

FIGURE Gore: 415

ABNORMAL MOTILITY AND TERTIARY CONTRACTIONS

List five causes of abnormal esophageal motility.

Abnormal motility
    Esophagitis
    Neuropathy
    Achalasia
    Chagas disease
    Scleroderma
    Connective tissue disorders
    Associated with malignancy
    Striated muscle disorders
    Presbyesophagus
Tertiary contractions
    Presbyesophagus
    Diffuse esophageal spasm
    Esophagitis
    Early stage of achalasia
    Neuromuscular disorders
    Normal variant in older patients

Normal motility

- Three phases occur
- Primary peristalsis: "major stripping wave"; upper end of barium column assumes an inverted V-shaped configuration
- Secondary peristalsis

¶ Stripping waves similar to primary peristalsis but elicited by distention or irritation anywhere along esophagus

¶ Has radiographic appearance similar to that of primary peristalsis, but originates in body of esophagus

- Tertiary contractions:
  ¶ Uncoordinated, nonpropulsive, segmental contractions
  ¶ Function unknown
  ¶ Seen as annular or segmental contractions simultaneously displacing barium both orally and aborally from site of contraction
  ¶ Repetitive tertiary contractions not seen in normal young adults but can be seen in about 10% of normal adults in the fourth to sixth decade of life

4

Esophagitis

When in the course of esophagitis does esophageal motility become abnormal?

- Whatever the cause, earliest finding is disordered motility, with failure of stripping wave to progress past area of irritation

Neuropathy

List some neuropathic causes of disordered esophageal motility.

- Several causes
  ¶ Cerebrovascular accident (CVA)
  ¶ Postvagotomy syndrome: typically occurs with solid foods on postoperative day 7 to 14; usually disappears spontaneously and completely within 2 months
  ¶ Diabetes
  ¶ Chronic idiopathic intestinal pseudoobstruction
  ¶ Amyloidosis
  ¶ Alcoholism: selective deterioration of esophageal peristalsis most pronounced in distal portion, with preservation of sphincter function

FIGURE Gore: 356

Achalasia

Achalasia tends to manifest in what age group?

How is this useful when radiographic findings suggesting achalasia are discovered?

- Usually seen in young patients (20 to 40 years of age)
- Because achalasia is a disease of young adults, neoplasm should be suspected in the older patient with radiographic appearance of achalasia
- Distinguished from scleroderma by fact that complete emptying of esophagus does not occur, even in erect position

FIGURES Gore: 350, 351

Chagas disease

- Megacolon, ureteral dilatation, and acute or chronic myocarditis also can be seen
- Looks like achalasia radiographically

Scleroderma

What distinguishes esophageal scleroderma from achalasia?

- In contrast to achalasia, barium flows rapidly through lower esophageal sphincter (LES) when patient is upright
- Dilated esophagus with wide open LES

FIGURE Gore: 356

Connective tissue disorders

- Various types: systemtic lupus erythematosus (SLE), rheumatoid arthritis (RA), polymyositis, dermatomyositis
- Almost all have Raynaud's phenomenon

Striated muscle disorders

- Myasthenia gravis
    - ¶ Breaking of primary wave in proximal esophagus, with normal propagation through distal esophagus (affects striated muscle, not smooth muscle)
    - ¶ Improves after administration of cholinergic drugs
- Anticholinergic medications

Presbyesophagus

When should the term "presbyesophagus" be used?

- Nowadays, more broadly referred to as *nonspecific esophageal motility disorder* (NEMD)
- Refers to symptomatic patients

FIGURE   Gore: 355

Diffuse esophageal spasm (DES)

Where in the course of the esophagus does the dysmotility begin with DES?

What are the classic clinical features of DES?

- Normal peristaltic wave to level of aortic arch
- Corkscrew radiographic appearance of transient sacculations or pseudodiverticula ("rosary bead" esophagus) can be seen
- Characterized by chest pain and intermittent dysphagia; repetitive contractions on manometry; segmental contraction on barium swallow; and esophageal wall thickening

FIGURE   Gore: 353

NARROWING

List a broad differential for esophageal narrowing, with a few examples in each category.

Congenital conditions
    Esophageal web
    Lower esophageal ring/Schatzki ring
Infection
Inflammation
    Reflux esophagitis
    Corrosive esophagitis
    Barrett's esophagus
    Crohn's disease
    Eosinophilic esophagitis
Neoplastic lesions
    Carcinoma of esophagus
    Carcinoma of stomach
    Metastases
    Lymphoma
Iatrogenic causes
    Postsurgical stricture
    Postnasogastric intubation strictures
    Radiation injury
Dermatologic causes
    Epidermolysis bullosa
    Bullous pemphigoid
Intramural esophageal pseudodiverticulosis

Esophageal web

What is Plummer-Vinson syndrome?

- Usually thin; can be masslike
- Never appears on posterior wall
- Consider manifestation of Plummer-Vinson syndrome: dysphagia, anemia, atrophic glossitis, mucosal abnormalities

Lower esophageal ring/Schatzki ring

What is the difference between a lower esophageal ring and a Schatzki ring?

- Concentric narrowing several centimeters above the diaphragm, marking the junction between esophageal and gastric mucosa
- If luminal opening is greater than 13 mm, obstructive symptoms are unlikely
- Should be called Schatzki ring only if diameter is less than 13 mm (size of barium tablet)

FIGURES   Gore: 534, 535

Infection

- Discrete mucosal plaques strongly suggest candidiasis, which is most common infection

FIGURE   Gore: 389

Reflux esophagitis

Do all strictures need endoscopic evaluation?

- Classic appearance pathognomonic: smooth, tapered area of concentric narrowing in distal esophagus above a sliding hiatal hernia
- Benign cannot always be distinguished from malignant, so endoscopy is important whenever radiographic findings are equivocal

FIGURES   Gore: 371, 374

Corrosive esophagitis

What drugs most commonly cause corrosive esophagitis?

- Strictures can occur as soon as 2 weeks after ingestion
- Drugs can cause this condition; tetracycline and potassium chloride are the most common
- Increased incidence of carcinomas developing at site of stricture

FIGURES   Gore: 413, 457

Barrett's esophagus

What is Barrett's esophagus?

What is the classic appearance of a stricture caused by Barrett's esophagus?

- Classic findings are high stricture and esophageal ulceration, but most patients do not have classic picture
- More patients with Barrett's esophagus have distal esophageal strictures

FIGURES   Gore: 378–381

Crohn's disease

Can one exclude Crohn's disease from consideration if a patient has no other gastrointestinal manifestations of Crohn's disease?

- Most patients have advanced Crohn's disease of lower gastrointestinal tract; this possibility should not be considered unless other gastrointestinal involvement is present

FIGURE   Gore: 415

How are strictures caused by eosinophilic esophagitis distinguished from reflux esophagitis?

4

What radiographic features of a stricture suggest malignancy?

Eosinophilic esophagitis

- About half of patients have history of allergies
- Almost all patients have peripheral eosinophilia
- Strictures occur in upper thoracic esophagus, at level of aortic arch

FIGURE Gore: 421

Carcinoma of esophagus

- Features of malignancy include discrete, irregular, fixed strictures, often with sharply demarcated filling defects with overhanging edges bulging toward the lumen
- Associated ulceration frequently is seen

FIGURE Gore: 474

Carcinoma of stomach

- About 12% of adenocarcinomas of stomach arising near cardia invade lower esophagus

FIGURES Gore: 482, 486, 487

Metastases

- Direct invasion (as in lung carcinoma), involvement by mediastinal lymph nodes (breast and lung most common), or hematogenous metastases (most commonly from breast cancer)

FIGURES Gore: 480–485

Lymphoma

What clinical features distinguish lymphoma of the esophagus from other causes of stricture?

- Rarely presents with dysphagia as initial manifestation of disease; usually widespread

FIGURES Gore: 489–491

Iatrogenic causes

- Postsurgical stricture
- Postnasogastric intubation strictures: long area of narrowing
- Radiation injury

FIGURES Gore: 419, 545

Dermatologic causes

Where in the esophagus do epidermolysis bullosa and bullous pemphigoid tend to cause strictures?

- Tend to be located in upper thoracic esophagus

FIGURES Gore: 417, 418

Intramural esophageal pseudodiverticulosis

- Stricture found in about 90% of cases
- Located in upper third of esophagus in 66% of cases (above pseudodiverticula)
- Presence of characteristic pseudodiverticula makes the diagnosis

FIGURES Gore: 425–427

NODULES

List a differential diagnosis for entities that lead to nodular-appearing esophageal mucosa. Which are common?

Common
    Candidiasis
    Reflux esophagitis
    Glycogenic acanthosis
Uncommon
    Superficial spreading esophageal carcinoma
    Esophageal papillomatosis
    Acanthosis nigricans
    Cowden's disease
    Leukoplakia

Candidiasis

- Discrete plaques
- Ask about history of acquired immunodeficiency syndrome (AIDS), odynophagia
- Often spares distal most esophagus (in comparison with reflux, which does not)

What features help distinguish candidiasis from reflux esophagitis?

FIGURES Gore: 386, 387

Reflux esophagitis

- Distal third or half of esophagus
- Esophagus involved continuously from GE junction
- Granular mucosa (nodules poorly defined)
- Other associated findings should be sought: hiatal hernia, reflux

FIGURES Gore: 390

Glycogenic acanthosis

At what age does glycogenic acanthosis occur?

What is the treatment?

- Asymptomatic incidental finding
- Age-related phenomenon; first appears in fifth to sixth decade

FIGURE Gore: 435

Superficial spreading esophageal carcinoma

True or false: the absence of symptoms makes superficial spreading esophageal carcinoma unlikely.

- Poorly defined nodules and plaques
- May be asymptomatic

FIGURE Gore: 451

Esophageal papillomatosis

How do patients with esophageal papillomatosis present?

What is the characteristic appearance of this entity?

- Multiple discrete excrescences
- Diffuse; appears like a cobblestone surface
- Asymptomatic

FIGURE Gore: 433

Acanthosis nigricans

- When it involves esophagus, multiple verrucous proliferations throughout mucosa similar to skin changes produce radiographic appearance
- Involvement of esophagus rare; thus, diagnosis should be suggested only for patients with known skin involvement

When should acanthosis nigricans be considered as a possible diagnosis for nodular esophageal mucosa?

Leukoplakia

- Tiny nodules
- Most commonly located in middle third of esophagus
- Rare

ULCERATION

List three basic causes of esophageal ulceration, with examples of each type.

Inflammation
    Reflux esophagitis
    Barrett's esophagus
    Corrosive esophagitis
    Drug-induced esophagitis
    Radiation esophagitis
Infectious/granulomatous disorders
    Candidiasis
    Herpes
    Cytomegalovirus (CMV)
    Human immunodeficiency virus (HIV)
    TB
    Crohn's disease
Malignant lesions
    Carcinoma
    Lymphoma
Mimics of ulceration
    Intramural pseudodiverticulosis
    Mallory-Weiss tear

Reflux esophagitis

- Shallow, punctate, or linear ulcers
- Deep ulcers not as common
- If present, always involve distal esophagus (not so in infectious ulceration)
- Associated hiatal hernia should be sought

How do ulcerations from reflux differ from infectious ulcerations?

FIGURE   Gore: 395

Barrett's esophagus

- Ulceration tends to be deep and penetrating, identical to peptic gastric ulceration, as opposed to shallow ulcerations of reflux
- Accompanied by stricture
- Location higher than that typical for reflux

How do ulcerations of Barrett's esophagus differ from those seen in reflux?

FIGURE   Gore: 379

Corrosive esophagitis

- Superficial or deep ulcers
- Relevant history helps make diagnosis

FIGURE   Gore: 412

Drug-induced esophagitis

- Several drugs can cause mucosal damage, including potassium chloride tablets, tetracycline, quinidine, ascorbic acid
- Sometimes, ulceration has shape of tablet (i.e., square edges), which can be helpful in suggesting the diagnosis
- Location typically in mid-esophagus, at aortic arch or left main bronchus

Which drugs most commonly cause esophageal ulceration?

What is the classic location for drug-induced esophageal ulcers?

FIGURES   Gore: 395, 405, 406

Radiation esophagitis

- Appears similar to candidiasis
- Relevant history helps make diagnosis
- Area of abnormality confined to radiation portal

FIGURE Gore: 409

Candidiasis

- Raised plaques and pseudomembrane formation lead to "shaggy" appearance
- Immunosuppressed patients
- Deep ulcerations and sloughing
- Mucosa diffusely abnormal, which helps differentiate candidiasis from herpes and CMV, which typically cause discrete ulcers on otherwise normal appearing mucosa

FIGURE Gore: 388

How is the distinction made between candidiasis and herpes involvement of the esophagus?

Herpes

- Although herpes ulceration can be indistinguishable from candidiasis, herpes typically causes discrete ulceration on otherwise normal mucosa, whereas mucosal abnormality tends to be more diffuse with candidiasis
- Ulcers smaller than those seen with CMV
- Can be seen in non–HIV-infected patients

FIGURES Gore: 393, 394

What distinguishes the ulceration of herpes from that of CMV?

CMV

- Ulcers tend to be deep and giant, seen especially in distal third of esophagus
- HIV patients
- Often enlarges despite therapy

FIGURES Gore: 396, 397

HIV

- Ulcers appear as giant, relatively flat, ovoid or irregular barium collections in middle or, less frequently, distal esophagus
- Small satellite ulcers may be seen nearby in some cases

FIGURE Gore: 398

TB

- Rare
- When TB involves esophagus, usually it does so through direct extension from infected mediastinal lymph nodes
- Most common manifestation in esophagus: single or multiple ulcers
- Intense fibrotic response causes narrowing of esophageal lumen
- Sinuses and fistulous tracts common
- HIV patients have been shown to develop TB ulcers, which tend to be deeper than HIV ulcers and may have associated sinus tracts

FIGURES Gore: 399, 400

Crohn's disease

- Aphthous ulcers
- Long intramural tracks and fistulas may be seen in advanced cases
- Diagnosis not suggested unless patient has other gastrointestinal involvement of Crohn's disease

FIGURE   Gore: 415

Carcinoma

- Ulceration occurs with necrosis of bulky mass

FIGURE   Gore: 453

Lymphoma

- Ulceration occurs with necrosis of bulky mass
- Can be indistinguishable from esophageal carcinoma

FIGURE   Gore: 490

Intramural pseudodiverticulosis

- Characteristic appearance pathognomonic

FIGURES   Gore: 425–427

Mallory-Weiss tear

True or false: Mallory-Weiss tears are seldom diagnosed radiographically.

- Often hard to demonstrate radiographically
- 95% diagnosed endoscopically
- Linear collection of barium near GE junction

FIGURE   Gore: 513

DIVERTICULA

What are the major types of diverticula seen in the esophagus?

Pharyngeal
    Cervical
        Zenker's diverticulum (pulsion)
Midesophageal
        Traction
Distal esophageal
        Epiphrenic (pulsion)

General comments

- Walls of traction diverticula contain all esophageal layers, whereas walls of pulsion diverticula are composed only of mucosa and submucosa herniating though muscularis
- Although traction and pulsion diverticula can occur anywhere in esophagus, only the most common types are discussed here

Pharyngeal diverticula

What are three types of pharyngeal diverticula?

- True lateral pharyngeal diverticula are rare

FIGURE   Gore: 246

- Anterolateral pharyngeal diverticula result from weak area in thyrohyoid membrane, through which passes internal laryngeal nerve

¶ Referred to by several names, including *hypopharyngeal pouches*, *hypopharyngeal ears*, and *pharyngoceles*

FIGURE Gore: 245

· Laryngocele: abnormal saccular dilatation of appendix of laryngeal ventricle

FIGURE Gore: 247

Zenker's diverticulum

What is the purported pathogenesis of a Zenker's diverticulum?

· Development apparently related to premature contraction or other motor incoordination of cricopharyngeus muscle
· Occurs through defect between oblique and transverse bundles of cricopharyngeus muscle (Killian dehiscence)
· Most surgeons perform cricopharyngeal myotomy

FIGURE Gore: 249

Midesophageal diverticulum

Where do traction diverticula typically occur?

· Primarily found opposite carina
· Usually a traction diverticulum that develops in response to pull of fibrous adhesions after infection of mediastinal lymph nodes
· Calcified mediastinal node from healed granulomatous disease adjacent to diverticulum may be seen
· Tented or triangular configuration

FIGURE Gore: 527

Epiphrenic diverticulum

How does the appearance of a traction diverticulum differ from that of a pulsion diverticulum?

· Usually of pulsion type; occurs in distal 10 cm of esophagus; probably related to incoordination of esophageal peristalsis and sphincter relaxation
· Rarely symptomatic
· Tends to have a broad, short neck with rounded contour
· Usually occurs on right anterolateral esophageal surface immediately above GE junction

FIGURE Gore: 525

SURGICAL PROCEDURES

Esophageal reconstruction
Antireflux procedures
Antivarices procedure
Procedures for motility

Esophageal reconstruction

· Gastric pull through: GE reflux can occur
· Colonic interposition: through either anterior mediastinum or esophageal hiatus
· Direct anastomosis (for atresia): characteristic radiographic findings years after repair include aperistaltic esophagus distal to anastomosis and web at site of repair

FIGURE Gore: 552

Antireflux procedures

- Nissen fundoplication
- Belsey Mark IV fundoplication
- Angelchik prosthesis:
    - ¶ Silastic prosthesis around abdominal segment of distal esophagus
    - ¶ Simpler than fundoplication
    - ¶ Can migrate into thorax or erode into stomach

FIGURES   Gore: 544, 545, 547

Antivarices procedure

- Esophageal resection and reanastomosis, accompanied by splenectomy, vagotomy, and pyloroplasty
- Operative mortality high

Procedures for motility

- Cricopharyngeal myotomy
- Heller myotomy: usually accompanied by antireflux procedure (generally a Belsey 270-degree fundoplication rather than a Nissen, to avoid increasing resistance to esophageal emptying)
- Pneumatic dilatation

PHARYNX MASS/MASS EFFECT

List causes of mass effect in pharynx.

Malignancy
Mucus retention cyst
Laryngocele
Postoperative appearance from total laryngectomy
Postradiation therapy

Malignancy

- Can appear as intraluminal mass, area of mucosal irregularity, or loss of normal distensibility
- Cross-sectional imaging (CT, MR) used to determine spread of tumor

FIGURES   Gore: 260–268

Mucus retention cyst

- Smooth, spherical, submucosal filling defects

FIGURE   Gore: 255

Laryngocele

- Results from obstruction of laryngeal ventricle with subsequent enlargement of its appendix
- Most contain air, but may also contain fluid, particularly when infected

FIGURE   Gore: 247

Postoperative appearance from total laryngectomy

- Cricopharyngeus and inferior constrictor severed from their anterior attachments, so they bunch posteriorly and indent "neo-pharynx" to some extent
- Weakest area in closure is at base of tongue, where pseudodiverticula often form

FIGURE   Gore: 286

Post radiation therapy

What are the characteristic features of "mass effect" caused by radiation of the pharynx?

- Radiation edema generally subsides 6 to 8 weeks after course of radiation
- Smooth, symmetrical swelling of arytenoid, cricoid, and epiglottic mucosa is characteristic
- Ulceration is unusual and should raise the possibility of persistent tumor
- Aspiration is the rule

FIGURE   Gore: 273

STOMACH

EROSIONS

What are common causes of erosive gastritis?

Alcohol
Antiinflammatory agents
    Nonsteroidal antiinflammatory drugs (NSAIDs)
    Steroids
Crohn's disease
Viral/fungal infection
Barium precipitates (not true erosion)

What do erosions look like?

General comments

- Erosions do not penetrate beyond muscularis mucosae
- Best seen with air-contrast studies
- Appear as a tiny fleck of barium surrounded by a radiolucent halo
- Often multiple

FIGURES   Gore: 599–601

Antiinflammatory drugs

What is a distinctive finding of the erosive gastritis caused by aspirin and other antiinflammatory drugs?

- May produce distinctive linear or serpiginous erosions that tend to be clustered in body of stomach

FIGURE   Gore: 601

Crohn's disease

- Patients almost always also have Crohn's disease involving small and/or large bowel

FIGURE   Gore: 609

Viral/fungal infection

- CMV or *Candida*
- History of immunocompromise

Barium precipitate

How can one distinguish barium precipitates from erosive gastritis?

- Does not have radiolucent halo
- Does not project beyond gastric contour in profile

FIGURE Gore: 602

COMPLICATIONS OF BILLROTH PROCEDURE

List the major complications of a Billroth procedure.

Marginal ulcers
Carcinoma in gastric stump
Retained gastric antrum
Jejunogastric intussusception
Bezoars

Marginal ulcers

Do marginal ulcers occur proximal or distal to the anastomosis?

- Usually occur distal to anastomosis
- More frequently occur on efferent segment
- 10% incidence

FIGURE Gore: 756

Carcinoma in gastric stump

How is recurrent tumor differentiated from gastric stump carcinoma?

What are the radiographic features of gastric stump carcinoma?

- Incidence of carcinoma in stump is two to six times higher than in intact stomach, probably related to bile reflux
- Can present as ulceration occurring proximal to anastomosis, as opposed to marginal ulcers, typically seen on jejunal side and invariably after duodenal ulcer surgery, not gastric ulcer surgery
- Can present as decrease in size of gastric remnant secondary to infiltration
- Has to occur more than 5 years after the original surgery
- Original resection must have been for benign disease
- If these criteria are not met, it is considered recurrent tumor

FIGURE Gore: 753

Retained gastric antrum

- Retained antrum at the very end of afferent loop
- Patient has increased gastrin levels
- Diagnosis can be made with barium or technetium (Tc) study
- Perforation not common

Jejunogastric intussusception

Do gastrojejunal intussusceptions have any clinical significance?

- More commonly efferent loop (afferent loop tied down by ligament of Treitz)
- Potentially lethal complication of Billroth II
- Appears as spheroid or oval intraluminal filling defect, with contrast outlining jejunal folds
- Gastrojejunal intussusception is much more common but usually is of no significance

Bezoars

- Occur as result of stasis
- Often composed of fibrous material from fruits and vegetables
- Have mottled appearance
- Tend to float like an iceberg in barium

FIGURE Gore: 754

FILLING DEFECT(S) IN STOMACH

Organize the causes of gastric filling defects into categories based on location and etiology.

Intraluminal
    Bezoar
    Foreign body
Mucosal/mural
    Benign tumors
        Leiomyomas
        Other intramural tumors
            Lipomas
            Neurofibromas
        Polyp
            Hyperplastic polyp
            Adenomatous polyp
            Hamartoma
    Malignant tumors
        Adenocarcinoma
        Carcinoid
        Lymphoma
        Leiomyosarcoma
        Metastatic disease
    Ectopic pancreas
    Thickened folds simulating nodules
        Ménétrier's disease
        Varices
        Inflammatory or infectious gastritis
    Peptic ulcer (surrounding edematous mass; incisura)
    Eosinophilic granuloma (inflammatory fibroid polyp)
Extrinsic
    Extrinsic cystic or inflammatory masses
    Duplication cyst

Bezoar

- May have characteristic mottled or streaked appearance because of contrast medium entering interstices of bezoar
- Freely movable

FIGURE   Gore: 734

Leiomyomas

- Characteristic submucosal appearance
- May have central ulceration
- Stippled calcification may be present

FIGURES   Gore: 641–643

Other intramural tumors

- Includes lipomas and neurofibromas
- Not common; lipomas account for only 3% of benign gastric tumors
- Usually small and asymptomatic

FIGURE   Gore: 646

Hyperplastic polyp

How does the appearance of hyperplastic polyps differ from that of adenomatous polyps?

Which are more common in the stomach?

- Far more common than adenomatous polyps in stomach
- Small (5 to 10 mm)
- Sharply defined
- Possibility of Cronkhite-Canada syndrome should be considered if multiple polyps are seen

FIGURE   Gore: 630

4

Which is more likely to be symptomatic when it occurs in the stomach: hyperplastic polyp or adenomatous polyp?

Adenomatous polyp

- Usually larger than hyperplastic polyp; therefore, more likely to be symptomatic
- Irregular surface, with contrast in deep fissures and furrows
- Usually single, seen most commonly in antrum

FIGURE Gore: 632

Hamartoma

In what syndromes are gastric hamartomas found?

- Consider as part of larger syndrome
    - ¶ Peutz-Jeghers: multiple gastric and small bowel hamartomas
    - ¶ Cowden's disease, or multiple hamartoma syndrome: hamartomas of stomach and other parts of GI tract, with characteristic circumoral papillomatosis and nodular gingival hyperplasia

FIGURE Gore: 638

Adenocarcinoma

- Polypoid mass
- Ulceration common
- Usually advanced at time of presentation

FIGURES Gore: 664–666

Carcinoid

What is the classic appearance of gastric carcinoid?

- Multiple submucosal masses or bull's-eye lesions

FIGURE Gore: 712

Lymphoma

Does ulceration commonly occur in lymphoma?

- One or more submucosal masses
- Ulceration or cavitation common
- Bull's-eye lesions of similar sizes
- Does not obstruct GI tract (unless it is Hodgkin's lymphoma, which most are not)

FIGURE Gore: 699

Leiomyosarcoma

- Intramural, bulky, often with huge ulcerations; not infiltrative, as is adenocarcinoma
- Better prognosis than carcinoma

FIGURES Gore: 705–707

Metastatic disease

- None really common
- Melanoma: bull's-eye appearance typical
- Lymphoma
- Kaposi's sarcoma: target lesions typical
- Breast: can be infiltrative and give linitis plastica pattern

FIGURES Gore: 674, 685–687, 709

Ectopic pancreas

- Most common on distal greater curvature of gastric antrum within 3 to 6 cm of pylorus (but can occur anywhere in GI tract)
- Often has central dimple or umbilication representing orifice of associated duct
- Usually asymptomatic

FIGURE   Gore: 650

Eosinophilic granuloma

- Also called *inflammatory fibroid polyp*
- Most commonly located in gastric antrum; not associated with peripheral eosinophilia

FIGURE   Gore: 649

Duplication cyst

What fluoroscopic finding can be helpful in suggesting duplication cyst as a cause of a filling defect?

- Found along greater curvature
- Appears as intramural or extrinsic mass lesion
- Communication with gastric lumen occurs in 15%
- Usually symptomatic in first year of life
- Manual compression or peristalsis can make these lesions change in size and shape at fluoroscopy

FIGURE   Gore: 654

FOLD THICKENING

List a broad differential diagnosis of fold thickening.

Normal variant
Gastritis
    Acute gastritis
        Ingested agents
        Corrosive agents
        Chemotherapy
        Infection
    Chronic erosive gastritis
    Granulomatous gastritis
      Crohn's disease
      Chronic granulomatous disease of childhood
      TB
Ménétrier's disease
Infiltrative process
      Eosinophilic gastroenteritis
      Amyloidosis
Ulcer disease
      Peptic ulcer disease
      Zollinger-Ellison syndrome
Neoplasm
      Lymphoma
      Carcinoma
Varices
Adjacent inflammation
      Pancreatic disease
Pseudolymphoma

General comments

- Antral folds more than 5 mm in width are abnormal
- When stomach partially empty or contracted, folds appear thicker; thus, normal variant is a possibility

What associated finding might suggest aspirin ingestion as a cause of fold thickening?

Ingested agents

- Alcohol, aspirin, or other medications
- Distinctive linear erosions may be seen in body of stomach with aspirin and other drug ingestion

FIGURE   Gore: 601

Corrosive agents

- Acid or alkali
- Leads to strictures
- Antral narrowing most common resultant deformity

FIGURES   Gore: 619, 620

Chemotherapy

- Infusion into hepatic artery

FIGURE   Gore: 621

Infection

- Phlegmonous
    ¶ Bacterial invasion causes thickening of wall of stomach
    ¶ Duodenum and esophagus usually spared
    ¶ Usually caused by alpha-hemolytic streptococci
    ¶ Other organisms: staphylococci, *Escherichia coli*, *Clostridium perfringens*, pneumococci, and *Proteus* spp
    ¶ Fulminating and usually fatal
    ¶ Bubbles of gas may be seen in wall of stomach, a poor prognostic sign
- Candidal infection in immunocompromised patients
- Unusual infectious cause is anisakiasis, caused by *Anisakis* worm
    ¶ Causes generalized coarse, broad gastric folds
    ¶ Threadlike filling defect can be demonstrated about 30 mm in length, representing larva itself

What is the name of the worm that can infect the stomach?

Chronic erosive gastritis

- Single or multiple punctate erosions surrounded by elevated rim of mucosa

FIGURE   Gore: 600

Crohn's disease

- Tendency to have pyloroantral and duodenal involvement
- Upper GI involvement at presenting site rare

FIGURE   Gore: 609

Chronic granulomatous disease of childhood

- Usually affects boys
- Classically involves gastric antrum

FIGURE   Gore: 1457

What part of the stomach typically is involved in children with chronic granulomatous disease?

TB

- Rare in the United States

Ménétrier's disease

Should antral involvement dissuade one from considering Ménétrier's disease as a cause of marked fold thickening of the stomach?

- Thickened gastric rugae contort in convolutional pattern suggestive of gyri and sulci of brain
- In children, folds are thickened throughout stomach
- In adults, generally limited to fundus and body, but antrum can be involved
- Fold thickening greatest along greater curvature
- Stomach remains pliable and distensible (not so with gastric carcinoma)

FIGURE Gore: 605

Eosinophilic gastroenteritis

Which part of the stomach is most likely involved with eosinophilic gastroenteritis? How does this compare with Ménétrier's disease?

- Nodular pattern similar to that seen in small bowel
- Antral narrowing and rigidity

FIGURE Gore: 608

Amyloidosis

- Involves antrum
- Patient has systemic manifestations

Peptic ulcer disease

- Look for ulceration
- Thick folds radiate to ulcer

FIGURE Gore: 575

Zollinger-Ellison syndrome

Besides fold thickening, what other features suggest Zollinger-Ellison syndrome?

What test should be ordered if Zollinger-Ellison syndrome is suspected?

- Simultaneous presence of increased fluid in upper gastrointestinal tract and one or more ulcers in unusual locations strongly suggests this diagnosis
- Assessment of fasting serum gastrin level facilitates diagnosis

FIGURE Gore: 594

Lymphoma

How are thickened folds from lymphoma distinguished from those caused by Ménétrier's disease?

- Differentiation from Ménétrier's disease:
    ¶ Lymphoma suggested if enlarged folds predominantly involve distal portion of stomach, some loss of pliability, enlarged regional lymph nodes, or enlarged spleen
    ¶ Ménétrier's disease is suggested if process stops at incisura, spares lesser curvature, no ulceration or true rigidity, excess mucus shown

FIGURE Gore: 699

Carcinoma

What associated features suggest that fold thickening is caused by gastric carcinoma?

- Look for associated loss of pliability, distensibility
- Look for associated malignant-appearing ulceration

FIGURES Gore: 670, 671

Varices

What are the differentiating features of gastric varices?

- Usually in fundus and associated with esophageal varices
- If no esophageal varices, think of isolated splenic vein thrombosis
- Differentiating features:
  - ¶ Changeability of size and shape (eliminates neoplastic process)
  - ¶ Extension along lesser curvature (makes Ménétrier's disease less likely)

FIGURE Gore: 718

Pancreatic disease

- Acute pancreatitis: selective prominence of folds on posterior wall and lesser curvature (normally rugae of fundus and greater curvature are more prominent)

Pseudolymphoma

What radiographic features suggest pseudolymphoma as a cause of fold thickening?

- No characteristic features
- Indistinguishable from gastric carcinoma or lymphoma

GAS IN WALL OF STOMACH

List some causes of intramural gas in the stomach. Which are of clinical concern?

Severe gastritis
    Infectious
    Corrosive
Ischemia
Peptic ulcer with intramural perforation
Gastric outlet obstruction
Iatrogenic causes
    Gastroscopy or esophagoscopy
    Recent gastroduodenal surgery
Gastric pneumatosis
Bulla ruptured into esophageal wall

Severe gastritis

Characterize the appearance of emphysematous gastritis.

- Coliforms, hemolytic streptococci, and *Clostridium* spp have propensity to cause emphysematous gastritis
- Characterized by bubbly or mottled collections of intramural gas, not long linear collections seen with gastric emphysema
- Patients are very sick

FIGURE Gore: 618

Ischemia

- Ischemia of stomach is unusual because of abundant collateral supply, but can occur, especially in the setting of previous surgery

Peptic ulcer with intramural perforation

- Focal collection of intramural air

Gastric outlet obstruction

What is the appearance of benign gastric emphysema?

- Overdistended stomach
- Gas pattern is finely linear and sharply defined, rather than the usual, irregularly mottled pattern

Iatrogenic causes

- Gas collection is linear, circumferential
- Patients tend to be asymptomatic

LINITIS PLASTICA PATTERN

List five causes of linitis plastica.

Malignant neoplasm
    Carcinoma
    Lymphoma
    Metastases
Gastric ulcer disease
Gastritis
    Acute forms
    Granulomatous forms
Infiltrative process
    Eosinophilic gastritis
    Amyloidosis
Polyarteritis nodosa
Gastroplasty (for weight reduction)

Carcinoma

- Most common cause, called *scirrhous carcinoma of the stomach*
- Usually begins near pylorus and progresses slowly upward, fundus being least involved
- Can affect only part of the stomach
- Diffuse infiltrating gastric carcinoma causing linitis plastica may exhibit enhancement after intravenous (IV) contrast on CT

FIGURE Gore: 669

Lymphoma

What type of lymphoma incites a desmoplastic response that can be indistinguishable from gastric carcinoma?

- Residual peristalsis and flexibility of stomach are often preserved in non-Hodgkin's lymphoma (compared with carcinoma and Hodgkin's lymphoma, where usually these are lost)

Metastases

Which metastatic process is most likely to result in a linitis plastica appearance of the stomach?

- Most commonly from breast cancer

FIGURE Gore: 674

Gastric ulcer disease

- Appearance can be caused by intense spasm
- Should not persist
- "Geriatric ulcer": ulcer arising high on posterior wall of stomach (elderly patients particularly prone to this location), which results in "hourglass" deformity of stomach with healing

Acute gastritis

- Iron intoxication: iron has corrosive action on gastric mucosa
- Caustic agents can result in scarred stomach

FIGURE Gore: 620

Granulomatous infiltration

• Sarcoid, TB, Crohn's disease

FIGURES   Gore: 610, 614

Eosinophilic gastritis

• Clinical history helps suggest correct diagnosis
• Small bowel may also be involved (follow barium into small bowel to look for abnormalities)

FIGURE   Gore: 608

Amyloidosis

• Patient has systemic findings

Polyarteritis nodosa

• Narrowing of antrum can occur secondary to ischemia and inflammation

OBSTRUCTION

Outline the causes of gastric obstruction using broad categories with at least one example of each category.

Peptic ulcer disease (PUD)
Malignant tumor
     Antral or pyloric channel carcinoma
     Carcinoma of head of pancreas
     Lymphoma
Benign tumor
     Prolapsed antral polyp
Inflammatory disorders
     Crohn's disease
     Pancreatitis
     Cholecystitis
     Corrosive stricture
Congenital disorders
     Antral mucosal diaphragm
     Gastric duplication
Miscellaneous disorders
     Gastric volvulus
     Hypertrophic pyloric stenosis
     Gastric bezoar
Mimics
     Gastroparesis

Peptic ulcer disease (PUD)

• Most common cause (60 to 65%)
• Patients usually have long history of PUD
• Presence of distortion and scarring of bulb with formation of pseudodiverticula makes PUD more likely
• Conversely, a normal bulb suggests malignant disease as the cause of gastric outlet obstruction

What features are helpful in differentiating gastric outlet obstruction caused by ulcer disease from that caused by antral malignancy?

FIGURES   Gore: 576, 587

Antral carcinoma

Do antral carcinomas commonly cause gastric outlet obstruction?

• Second most common cause (30 to 35%)
• Primary scirrhous carcinoma of pyloric channel

¶ Elongated, symmetrically smooth pylorus, often with gradual tapering of proximal margin
¶ Distinguished from healed ulcer by presence of ulceration and duodenal deformity in patients with peptic disease

Carcinoma of head of pancreas

- Extrinsic compression
- Obstruction usually at duodenal level

FIGURE   Gore: 691

Lymphoma

- Involvement of both stomach and duodenum in up to one third of cases

FIGURE   Gore: 703

Prolapsed antral polyp

- Filling defect in duodenal bulb

FIGURE   Gore: 631

Inflammatory disorders

- If severe, can incite inflammatory spasm of proximal duodenum

Corrosive stricture

- History of caustic ingestion

FIGURE   Gore: 1458

Antral mucosal diaphragm

- Thin, membranous septa within 3 cm of pyloric canal
- Congenital, but may not produce symptoms until adulthood (if ever)
- Radiologically, sharply defined, bandlike defect seen in barium column, 2 to 3 cm wide, arising at right angles to gastric wall

FIGURES   Gore: 722, 1444

Gastric duplication

- CT or ultrasound can help confirm cystic nature of obstructing mass

FIGURE   Gore: 654

Gastric volvulus

- Characteristic findings:
    ¶ Double air-fluid level
    ¶ Inversion of stomach
    ¶ Cardia at same position as pylorus
    ¶ Downward pointing of pylorus and duodenum

FIGURE   Gore: 735

Hypertrophic pyloric stenosis

- Characteristic appearance on ultrasound
- Barium findings: string sign, teat sign, or shoulder sign

FIGURES Gore: 1452, 1453

Gastric bezoar

- Mottled filling defect

FIGURE Gore: 1454

Gastroparesis

What clinical history is often found in patients with gastroparesis?

- Flaccid stomach with decreased or absent peristalsis
- History of diabetes

OUTPOUCHING/ULCERATION

List a differential diagnosis for barium collecting in a cavity in the stomach.

Benign
    Peptic ulcer disease
    Gastritis
    Granulomatous disease
    Leiomyoma
    Radiation-induced ulcer
    Pseudolymphoma
    Diverticula
Malignant
    Carcinoma
    Lymphoma
    Leiomyosarcoma
    Metastases

General comments about benign-appearing ulcers

What features define a benign-appearing ulceration?

- Penetration: projection of ulcer outside normal barium-filled gastric lumen
- Hampton line, ulcer collar, ulcer mound
    - ¶ Represents overhanging resistant mucosal layer
    - ¶ Most reliable sign of benign ulcer is Hampton line; ulcer collar and mound are less so (these are thicker)
    - ¶ In mound, benign state suggested by central ulcer location; smooth, sharply delineated, gently sloping and symmetrically convex tissue around ulcer; and smooth obtuse angle of margin of mound with adjacent normal gastric wall
- Crescent sign: trapped barium in benign ulcer with occluding overhanging mucosa
- Radiation of mucosal folds to edge of crater: smooth, slender, appear to extend into edge of crater
- Size and contour of base have no relationship to malignancy or benignancy
- Location not significant except in fundus above level of cardia, where all ulcers should be considered malignant
- Caveat regarding greater curvature
    - ¶ Benign ulcers along greater curvature do not show same characteristic radiographic features of benignancy seen in the more common lesser curvature ulcers because they may cause spasm in the abundant musculature and therefore appear intraluminal
- Ellipse sign

¶ Used to determine if collection of barium represents acute ulceration or nonulcerating deformity
¶ If long axis of collection is parallel to lumen, then an ulcer is considered present
¶ Otherwise, collection is considered manifestation of nonulcerating deformity
- Other points
  ¶ Benign gastric ulcer usually heals without deformity
  ¶ Deeply penetrating ulcer may show persistent pit where mucosa has healed over crater; barium may collect in pit and mimic active ulcer

4

General comments about malignant-appearing ulcers

What features of an ulceration suggest malignancy?

- Carman's meniscus sign (also known as *Carman-Kirklin complex*)
  ¶ Semicircular meniscoid configuration seen in profile, convex to lumen
  ¶ What one sees in the meniscus is not all ulcer; rather, with compression the two sides of the tumor are opposed and the central ulcer-like area collects barium
- Base (outer margin) of barium collection located where normal gastric wall would be expected (represents intraluminal mass with ulceration, i.e., malignant)
- Abrupt transition of normal mucosa and abnormal tissue
- Nodular surrounding tissue

Peptic ulcer disease

Where in the stomach do peptic ulcers usually occur?

- Overwhelming majority
- Usually on lesser curvature or posterior wall of antrum or body

FIGURES   Gore: 566–575

Gastritis

Are the ulcers associated with gastritis large or small?

- Variable appearance
- Ulcers tend to be small, erosive type

FIGURES   Gore: 599–601

Granulomatous disease

- Small aphthoid ulcers seen with Crohn's disease

FIGURE   Gore: 609

Leiomyoma

- Ulceration occurs with necrosis of mass

FIGURE   Gore: 642

Radiation-induced ulcer

True or false: radiation-induced ulcers are less likely to perforate because of fibrosis.

- Dose more than 4500 rads
- Can occur any time between 1 month and 6 years after treatment (mean: 5 months)
- High incidence of perforation and hemorrhage
- Heals poorly

Pseudolymphoma

- Looks malignant

Diverticula

Where do gastric diverticula occur?

- Not common; if present, usually at cardia
- 75% occur on posterior wall
- Second most common location is prepyloric region; about 15% of these occur along greater curvature (85% along lesser curvature)

FIGURE   Gore: 719

Carcinoma

- *See* **General comments about malignant-appearing ulcers**

FIGURE   Gore: 667

Lymphoma

- Presence of several malignant ulcers suggests lymphoma
- Aneurysmal appearance of single, huge ulcer is characteristic

FIGURE   Gore: 699

Leiomyosarcoma

When should the possibility of leiomyosarcoma rather than just leiomyoma be considered?

- Consider if submucosal mass is larger than 2 cm

FIGURE   Gore: 706

Metastases

- Often cause "bull's-eye" lesions, with central large ulcerations
- Melanoma, lung, breast, Kaposi's sarcoma

FIGURE   Gore: 687

DUODENUM

FILLING DEFECTS

Pseudotumors
    Flexural pseudolesion
    Acute ulcer mound
    Foreign body
Non-neoplastic masses
    Ectopic pancreas
    Prolapsed antral mucosa
    Brunner's gland hyperplasia
    Benign lymphoid hyperplasia
    Heterotopic gastric mucosa
    Enlarged papilla
    Choledochocele
    Duplication cyst
    Duodenal varices or mesenteric arterial collaterals
    Intramural hematoma
Benign tumors
    Adenomatous polyp
    Leiomyoma
    Lipoma

Prolapsed/intussuscepted antral polyp
Tumors with variable malignant potential
Villous adenoma
Carcinoid
Malignant tumors
Adenocarcinoma
Ampullary carcinoma
Leiomyosarcoma
Lymphoma
Kaposi's sarcoma
Metastases

Flexural pseudolesion

Where does the duodenal pseudolesion occur?

- Characteristic location along inner aspect of superior duodenal flexure between first and second portions of duodenum
- Changeable appearance at fluoroscopy

FIGURE   Gore: 300

Ectopic pancreas

What are the characteristic features of ectopic pancreas?

- Occur most frequently in distal stomach, but can present in proximal second portion of duodenum
- Characteristic sign: fleck of barium in rudimentary central canal ("bull's-eye" appearance)
- Although other lesions have "bull's-eye" appearance (metastases, lymphoma, Kaposi's sarcoma), patients with those conditions have multiple lesions, whereas ectopic pancreas is a solitary lesion

FIGURE   Gore: 650

Prolapsed antral mucosa

Where is the characteristic location of prolapsed antral mucosa?

- Characteristic location at base of duodenal bulb
- Mushroom-shaped defect

FIGURE   Gore: 634

Brunner's gland hyperplasia

Can Brunner's gland hyperplasia present as a single filling defect?

What is the cause of the hyperplasia?

- Multiple, small, rounded polypoid elevations

FIGURE   Gore: 652

Benign lymphoid hyperplasia

Is benign lymphoid hyperplasia limited to the duodenal bulb?

- Innumerable tiny nodular defects evenly scattered throughout the duodenum
- Usually not limited to bulb

FIGURE   Gore: 653

Heterotopic gastric mucosa

How does heterotopic gastric mucosa differ in appearance from benign lymphoid hyperplasia?

- Finely nodular pattern formed by abruptly marginated, angular filling defects ranging from 1 to 6 mm
- Generally restricted to bulb (which differentiates it from benign lymphoid hyperplasia)
- Smaller and more numerous than those in Brunner's gland hyperplasia

FIGURES   Gore: 300, 624, 653

Enlarged papilla

- Usually measures 1.5 cm or less; normal can be up to 3 cm

FIGURE   Gore: 301

Choledochocele

- Smooth, extrinsic mass

FIGURE   Gore: 1632

Duplication cyst

- Usually detected early in life
- Radiologically has two patterns: well defined oval filling defect or, more commonly, sharply defined intramural defect

FIGURE   Gore: 655

Duodenal varices or mesenteric arterial collaterals

- Serpiginous
- Usually multiple, can be single

FIGURE   Gore: 719

Intramural hematoma

Where do duodenal hematomas occur?

- Occur in second or third portion of duodenum (fixed retroperitoneal portions)
- Well-defined margins
- Some degree of stenosis and obstruction
- Search for appropriate history (child abuse, motor vehicle accident)

FIGURES   Gore: 734, 1454

Adenomatous polyp

- Usually small (1 cm), smooth or lobulated, intraluminal

FIGURES   Gore: 634, 637

Leiomyoma

What barium features of a filling defect suggest a submucosal or mural origin of a mass?

- Produces fairly sharp angle at junction of defect and normal duodenal wall
- Stretched but intact mucosal folds visualized over its surface
- Central, punched-out ulcerations common

Lipoma

- Soft consistency allows them to have an elliptical appearance, conforming to lumen of bowel

FIGURE   Gore: 312

Hamartoma

- Especially with history of Peutz-Jeghers syndrome
- Polyp-like lesion

FIGURE   Gore: 638

Prolapsed/intussuscepted antral polyp

- Located at base of duodenum

FIGURE   Gore: 631

Villous adenoma

Describe the characteristic appearance of a villous adenoma.

- Ampullary region most common location
- "Soap bubble" appearance with feathery margins result of trapped barium in interstices of frond-like projections of tumor

FIGURE   Gore: 636

Carcinoid

Do duodenal carcinoids occur in proximal or distal duodenum?

- Duodenal bulb or proximal descending duodenum
- May appear submucosal or polypoid
- Single or multiple

Adenocarcinoma

Where in the duodenum is adenocarcinoma more likely to occur?

- Annular lesion; shelf-like borders
- Majority occur in third and fourth portions of duodenum
- Ask about history of Gardner's or Peutz-Jeghers syndrome

FIGURE   Gore: 679

Ampullary carcinoma

- A type of duodenal adenocarcinoma
- Important to distinguish from pancreatic carcinoma, because ampullary carcinoma has better prognosis

FIGURE   Gore: 680

Leiomyosarcoma

- Rare duodenal location
- Lobulated intramural filling defects, often with central ulceration

FIGURE   Gore: 708

Lymphoma

- Rare in duodenum as primary
- Can present as a polypoid mass or as multiple small nodules that produce a cobblestone appearance

FIGURE   Gore: 704

Kaposi's sarcoma

- Multiple submucosal masses that may have central ulceration

FIGURE   Gore: 710

Metastases

FIGURES   Gore: 685, 691, 695

OBSTRUCTION

List causes of duodenal obstruction.

Congenital obstruction

4

Duodenal atresia
Annular pancreas
Duodenal diaphragm
Intraluminal diverticulum
Midgut volvulus
Extrinsic bands (Ladd's bands)
Duodenal duplication cyst
Inflammatory disorders of duodenum
Postbulbar ulcer
Crohn's disease
TB
Strongyloidiasis
Nontropical sprue
Inflammatory disorders of pancreas
Acute pancreatitis
Chronic pancreatitis
Pseudocyst of pancreas
Malignancies
Primary pancreatic tumor
Primary duodenal tumor
Metastatic
Intramural duodenal hematoma
Superior mesenteric artery syndrome

Duodenal atresia

- Usually (80%) occurs distal to ampulla of Vater
- Higher incidence in patients with Down syndrome
- Imaging: classic double-bubble sign

Annular pancreas

- Other congenital anomalies of GI tract frequently coexist
- Down syndrome in 30%
- Imaging: results in incomplete obstruction (versus complete obstruction in duodenal atresia)

Duodenal diaphragm

- Most occur in second portion of duodenum near ampulla of Vater

Primary pancreatic tumor

- 70% arise in head, 20% in body, 10% in tail of pancreas

SMA syndrome

- Thin patient
- Relief of obstruction in prone or left decubitus position

POSTBULBAR ULCERATION

What disease processes lead to ulcers in the postbulbar region of the duodenum?

PUD
Zollinger-Ellison syndrome
Benign tumors
Malignant tumors
Primary duodenal malignancy
Metastatic malignancy
Contiguous invasion (pancreas, right colon, right kidney, gallbladder)
Invasion from lymph node metastases

Hematogenous metastases
Crohn's disease
TB
Aortoduodenal fistula
Lesions simulating ulceration
    Ectopic pancreas
    Duodenal diverticulum

General comments

- Mnemonic GUTED: granulomatous disease (TB, Crohn's disease), ulcer disease (PUD, Zollinger-Ellison syndrome), tumor (benign, malignant, metastatic), ectopic pancreas, diverticulum

Malignant tumors

- Most often duodenal adenocarcinoma, but ulcerating lymphomas and sarcomas also occur
- Most frequent cause of nonpeptic postbulbar ulceration
- Metastases, especially from melanoma, can result in ulceration

WIDENED SWEEP

List causes of a widened duodenal sweep.

Normal variant
Pancreatic lesion
    Pancreatitis
    Pancreatic pseudocyst
    Pancreatic cancer
    Metastatic replacement of pancreas
    Cystadenoma/cystadenocarcinoma
Lymph node enlargement
    Metastases
    Lymphoma
    Inflammation
Cystic lymphangioma of the mesentery
Mesenteric arterial collaterals
Retroperitoneal masses (tumors, cysts)
Aortic aneurysm
Choledochal cyst

Cystic lymphangioma of the mesentery

- Benign, unilocular or multilocular cystic structures containing serous or chylous fluid

ABNORMAL FOLDS

Name broad categories of disease that result in duodenal fold thickening, with a few examples of each type.

Inflammatory disorders
    PUD
    Brunner's gland hyperplasia
    Zollinger-Ellison syndrome
    Pancreatitis
    Cholecystitis
    Uremia (chronic dialysis)
    Crohn's disease
    TB
    Parasitic infestation
        Giardiasis
        Strongyloidiasis
    Nontropical sprue

4

Neoplastic disorders
    Lymphoma
    Metastases to peripancreatic lymph nodes
Diffuse infiltrative disorders
    Whipple's disease
    Amyloidosis
    Mastocytosis
    Eosinophilic enteritis
    Intestinal lymphangiectasis
Vascular disorders
    Duodenal varices
    Mesenteric arterial collaterals
    Intramural hemorrhage
    Chronic duodenal congestion
    Ischemia
Cystic fibrosis
Edema

General comments

- Abnormal folds can manifest in many ways:
  - ¶ Thickened folds (highly subjective)
  - ¶ Shortening and straightening of folds
  - ¶ Bulbous rounding of crest of fold
  - ¶ Fold thickening in abnormal locations for PUD (i.e., beyond second portion of duodenum)
  - ¶ Punctate erosions

PUD

- Coarse folds can be obliterated by compression

Brunner's gland hyperplasia

- Filling defects not obliterated by compression

Uremia (chronic dialysis)

- Not related to hyperacidity or PUD

Giardiasis

- Involves both duodenum and jejunum

Strongyloidiasis

- If duodenum involved, jejunum also abnormal

Diffuse infiltrative disorders

- Usually do not affect duodenum alone; also involve small bowel

Mastocytosis

- Dense bones
- May have coexisting gastric polyps

Eosinophilic enteritis

- Gastric antrum commonly involved
- Almost always affects jejunum if it involves duodenum
- Peripheral eosinophilia

Duodenal varices

- Four major radiographic appearances
    - ¶ Collateral flow in dilated superior pancreaticoduodenal vein can cause vertical compression defect on duodenal bulb about 1 cm distal to pylorus
    - ¶ Small varices produce diffuse polypoid mucosal pattern in duodenum, difficult to distinguish from Brunner's gland hyperplasia
    - ¶ Serpiginous filling defects are the result of larger, dilated submucosal veins
    - ¶ Occasionally, isolated varix presents as discrete filling defect on medial aspect of descending duodenum

Mesenteric arterial collaterals

- Dilated pancreaticoduodenal arcade secondary to atherosclerotic disease affecting proximal celiac axis or SMA

Chronic duodenal congestion

- From portal hypertension or congestive heart failure (CHF)

Ischemia

- Secondary to radiation therapy, collagen vascular diseases, and Henoch-Schönlein purpura

Edema

- Numerous causes: hypoproteinemia, venous obstruction, lymphatic obstruction, and angioneurotic edema

SMALL BOWEL

GENERAL COMMENTS ABOUT IMAGING

Outline an approach to evaluation of the small bowel on barium studies.

Approach to analysis

- Determine if small bowel dilated: should not exceed 3 cm in diameter
- Analyze fold thickness
    - ¶ Normal folds are smooth, regular, less than 3 mm thick
    - ¶ Determine whether fold thickening is regular, irregular, or nodular
- Analyze distribution of abnormality
    - ¶ Diffuse or localized?
    - ¶ In duodenum, jejunum, ileum, or terminal ileum?
    - ¶ Is stomach also involved?
    - ¶ Is cecum abnormal?
- Look for contour abnormalities
    - ¶ Extrinsic impression
    - ¶ Ulceration
    - ¶ Response to desmoplastic process
- Look carefully for filling defects

DILATED SMALL BOWEL WITH NORMAL FOLDS

What is the differential diagnosis for dilated small bowel with normal folds?

Obstruction
Postvagotomy

Ileus
Scleroderma
Sprue
    Celiac/nontropical
    Tropical

Obstruction

- Suspect obstruction if you see more than two air-fluid levels
- Relative paucity of air in colon

FIGURES   Gore: 938, 940, 941

Ileus

- Usually, there is a preponderance of gas in colon
- Focal ileus may be the result of adjacent inflammation, as in pancreatitis

Scleroderma

What characteristics are seen in the small bowel with scleroderma?

- Usually affects duodenum with dilatation
- Decrease in distance between valvulae conniventes ("hidebound" appearance) differentiates it from other causes of dilatation such as obstruction or sprue
- Pseudosacculation of small bowel may occur (intermittent fibrosis leading to outpouching)

FIGURE   Gore: 868

Celiac/nontropical sprue

Where does celiac disease usually manifest in the small bowel?

Characterize its appearance on barium studies.

- Usually middle and distal jejunum
- Variability in fold pattern
  - ¶ In jejunum, folds of normal thickness but number decreased
  - ¶ In some cases, folds prominent, particularly in duodenum
  - ¶ In ileum, prominent folds create "jejunization" appearance
  - ¶ Occasionally, folds diminished; rarely, folds lost, creating "moulage" sign (develops when increased secretions obscure mucosal folds)
- Can exhibit transient intussusception ("coiled spring" appearance)

FIGURES   Gore: 873, 874

Tropical sprue

- Radiologic findings similar to those in celiac disease

FOLD ABNORMALITIES

List the causes of small bowel dilatation with thick folds.

Dilated small bowel with thick folds
    Ischemia
    Hemorrhage
    Radiation therapy
    Crohn's disease
    Zollinger-Ellison syndrome
    Lymphoma
    Whipple's disease

Amyloid
Abetalipoproteinemia

List causes of normal caliber small bowel with thick folds.

Normal caliber small bowel with thick folds
    Vascular (tend to be regular, localized, or diffuse)
        Ischemia
        Hemorrhage
        Radiation therapy
    Inflammatory (tend to be irregular, localized, or diffuse)
        Crohn's disease
        Zollinger-Ellison syndrome
    Infiltrative (tend to be irregular, except abetalipoproteinemia, diffuse)
        Eosinophilic enteritis
        Amyloid
        Whipple's disease
        Mastocytosis
        Abetalipoproteinemia
    Infective (tend to be irregular, localized)
        TB
        Yersinia spp
        Typhoid fever
        Giardiasis
        Strongyloidiasis
        Cryptosporidiosis
        Infections in immunosuppressed patients
        Histoplasmosis
    Neoplastic (tend to be irregular, localized)
        Lymphoma
        Metastases
        Carcinoid: in ileum
    Edema (tend to be regular, diffuse)
        Hypoproteinemia
        Venous obstruction
        Lymphatic obstruction
        Angioneurotic edema
        Lymphangiectasia
    Other
        Cystic fibrosis
        Graft-versus-host disease

Nodules on folds (mnemonic: WHILMA)
    Whipple's disease
    Histoplasmosis
    Lymphoma, lymphangiectasia, lymphoid hyperplasia
    Macroglobulinemia and mastocytosis
    Amyloid and abetalipoproteinemia

Gastric and small bowel thickening (mnemonic: MALEZ)
    Ménétrier's disease
    Amyloid
    Lymphoma
    Eosinophilic enteritis
    Zollinger-Ellison syndrome

General comments

- List of differential diagnoses is large, and some entities look nothing like the others
- Easiest approach: memorize entire list; then, when going through the differential, go through list systematically but do not mention entities that do not even remotely resemble the case at hand

Which diseases tend to affect the duodenum and jejunum? Jejunum and ileum? Terminal ileum?

- Generalized (definitely not absolute) lists of pattern of involvement
  A. Predominantly duodenal and/or jejunal involvement
     1. Cystic fibrosis
     2. Whipple's disease
     3. Giardiasis
     4. Strongyloidiasis
  B. Predominantly jejunal and/or ileal involvement
     1. Amyloid
     2. Lymphoma
     3. Graft-versus-host disease
  C. Predominantly terminal ileal involvement
     1. Crohn's disease
     2. TB
     3. *Yersinia* spp
     4. Typhoid fever
  D. Other patterns
     1. Sprue: duodenal and ileal
     2. Eosinophilic enteritis: stomach, all small bowel

Ischemia

What "buzz words" are used to describe the changes resulting from acute ischemia of small bowel?

- Rigid, narrowed, thickened loops of small bowel
- "Stacked-coin" appearance of symmetrically thickened valvulae conniventes
- "Thumbprinting": occurs as edema progresses
- Spasm and hypermotility favorable signs; dilatation and stasis imply transmural infarction
- Localized perforations form "pneumatosis intestinalis"

FIGURES Gore: 969, 970

Hemorrhage

Why is the duodenum prone to hemorrhage in blunt trauma?

- In blunt trauma, think of duodenum (fixed position)
- Uniform, regular thickening of folds in symmetric, spike-like configuration (classic buzz word is "stack of coins")

FIGURE Gore: 976

Radiation therapy

Describe changes caused by radiation therapy.

- Edema from progressive vasculitis leads to straight, thickened folds and a spiked contour of bowel lumen; bowel loops separated by thick walls; abrupt angulations caused by fibrosis

FIGURES Gore: 938, 974, 975

Crohn's disease

- Begins by showing aphthous ulcers, mucosal fold thickening, and mucosal fold distortion; then progresses to deep linear ulceration, nodular cobblestone pattern, and eventual stenosis
- Fistulas and sinus tracts occur
- Separation of bowel loops by wall thickening and induration of mesentery
- Scattered islands of mucosa are pseudopolyps

How is spasm distinguished from fibrosis in the setting of Crohn's disease?

- Fixed narrowing of fibrosis distinguished from spastic narrowing of Crohn's disease by lack of proximal bowel dilatation in latter

FIGURES Gore: 827–831

Zollinger-Ellison syndrome

· Proximal involvement (duodenum and jejunum)
· Increased fluid

FIGURE Gore: 883

Eosinophilic enteritis

Are folds regular or irregular in eosinophilic enteritis?

· Initially, regular symmetric thickening of folds when mucosa and lamina propria are involved
· Later, extensive transmural involvement causes irregular fold thickening, angulation, and saw-toothed contour of small bowel

FIGURE Gore: 881

Amyloid

What changes in the ileum are suggestive of amyloidosis?

Is the bowel caliber normal?

· Characterized by sharply demarcated thickening of folds throughout small bowel (occasionally, involvement is patchy and uneven)
· Folds can be symmetric or irregular
· Appearance of prominent ileal folds resembling valvulae conniventes of jejunum (jejunization) suggests amyloidosis
· Caliber of bowel normal (mild dilatation as disease progresses)

FIGURE Gore: 870

Whipple's disease

· Mucosal fold thickening and irregular fold distortion
· Predominantly duodenal and jejunal involvement
· Focal extrinsic mass effect can be noted along mesentery secondary to adenopathy
· Lumen may be normal or slightly dilated

Is small bowel involvement proximal or distal in Whipple's disease?

· Intestinal lymphangiectasia may simulate findings in Whipple's disease, except for its distribution; Whipple's disease affects proximal small bowel, whereas intestinal lymphangiectasia involvement is diffuse

FIGURE Gore: 886

Mastocytosis

What non-GI finding helps diagnose mastocytosis?

· Look for dense bones

FIGURE Gore: 885

Abetalipoproteinemia

· Small bowel dilatation with mild to moderate fold thickening
· Typically regular, diffuse

FIGURE Gore: 885

TB

· Can be almost impossible to distinguish from Crohn's disease
· Potentially distinguishing features include

What are possible distinguishing features of TB compared with Crohn's disease?

    ¶ Ulcers in TB are annular, whereas those in Crohn's disease are linear
    ¶ More involvement of cecum in TB, with widely patent ileocecal valve

FIGURE Gore: 849

Yersinia spp

How do patients with Yersinia spp infection present?

- Terminal ileum is the most commonly involved site, but can affect entire small bowel and colon in severe cases
- Clinical symptoms mimic appendicitis
- At early stage looks like early Crohn's disease (irregular thickened folds, aphthous ulcerations, cobblestone appearance of mucosa), but it is transient, with complete resolution of symptoms and lesions within a few weeks

FIGURE   Gore: 850

Typhoid fever

Is the cecum involved in typhoid fever?

- Limited to terminal ileum
- Proliferation of organisms in Peyer's patches of terminal ileum produces raised plaques, giving the appearance of thickened mucosal folds
- No skip areas, no fistulas, and positive splenomegaly differentiate from Crohn's disease

Giardiasis

Is involvement proximal or distal with giardiasis?

- Present with diarrhea
- Fold pathology most apparent in duodenum and jejunum
- Folds have distinctively nodular appearance when seen on end
- Also seen: spasm and irritability; hypermotility; with or without hypersecretion

FIGURE   Gore: 848

Strongyloidiasis

Is involvement proximal or distal in strongyloidiasis?

- Most prominent in jejunum and duodenum, with thick folds
- In severe cases, ulceration, paralytic dilatation
- In chronic disease, narrow, rigid jejunal loops with absent mucosal folds

FIGURES   Gore: 847, 848

Infections in immunosuppressed patients

What small bowel infections affect immunocompromised patients?

- Cryptosporidiosis: proximal small bowel more often affected than distal; thick folds; mucosal atrophy (long standing); increased secretions
- CMV: thickened folds; can lead to ulceration and perforation
- *Mycobacterium avium intracellulare*

FIGURES   Gore: 854, 855

Histoplasmosis

- Can affect small bowel; diffuse, fine, nodular thickening of folds

Lymphoma

Discuss the spectrum of findings seen with small bowel lymphoma.

- Spectrum of radiologic findings includes:
  - ¶ Mesenteric mass: results in mass effect along mesenteric border of small intestine, with spiculation and tethering of small bowel loops; thickened nodular folds in region of tethering indicate areas of tumor invasion
  - ¶ Mantle of enlarged lymph nodes: "sandwich sign"
  - ¶ Bowel wall thickening, occasionally constricting napkin-

ring lesion; usually fairly long segment as opposed to adenocarcinoma; does not tend to obstruct
¶ Aneurysmal dilatation of bowel (after necrosis and cavitation)

FIGURES   Gore: 822, 902

Metastases

Which metastases most commonly affect the small bowel?

- From melanoma or tumors of breast, ovary, GI tract

Carcinoid

What type of reaction does carcinoid incite in surrounding tissues? Why?

- Characteristic CT appearance of soft tissue mass with radiating stellate pattern of linear densities caused by local release of serotonin
- CT findings can be simulated by other neoplastic or inflammatory disorders such as metastases, retractile mesenteritis, and Crohn's disease
- Liver metastases almost always hypervascular

FIGURE   Gore: 905

Hypoproteinemia

- Causes include nephrosis, cirrhosis, and protein-losing enteropathy

FIGURE   Gore: 872

Lymphangiectasia

Compare findings seen with lymphangiectasia with those of Whipple's disease.

- Diffuse, thickened folds with fine nodularity
- Increased secretions
- Has diffuse enteric involvement in comparison with more proximal involvement of Whipple's disease

FIGURE   Gore: 888

Cystic fibrosis

Which part of the small bowel is most affected by cystic fibrosis?

- Can lead to coarse nodular thickening of mucosa, particularly in duodenum and proximal jejunum

FIGURE   Gore: 884

Graft-versus-host disease

- Not uncommon to find changes in small bowel, colon, and esophagus after allogeneic bone marrow transplants
- Changes include crypt cell necrosis, ulcerations, vascular dilatation, and edema; occurs throughout GI tract, especially in ileum, where it can look like Crohn's disease (ulceration, nodularity, fold effacement)

FIGURE   Gore: 859

Macroglobulinemia

- Gamma globulin deficiency states can affect small bowel, manifested as nodular lymphoid hyperplasia (this can also be seen in giardiasis)
- Waldenström's macroglobulinemia results in fine granular pattern along small bowel folds

FIGURE   Gore: 821

TERMINAL ILEUM NARROWED WITH ABNORMAL CECUM

List the differential diagnosis for terminal ileum narrowed with abnormal cecum.

TB
Crohn's disease
Lymphoma
Carcinoid
Postradiation therapy
Ischemia

TB

See entry under Fold Abnormalities

Crohn's disease

What is the characteristic appearance of Crohn's disease?

- Longitudinal ulcers predominate
- Terminal ileum more affected than cecum
- Cobblestone pattern is characteristic

FIGURES   Gore: 834, 835, 839

FILLING DEFECT

List the differential diagnosis for a filling defect in the small bowel.

Benign tumors
    Adenoma
    Leiomyoma
    Lipoma
    Hemangioma
    Hamartomatous polyp
Malignant tumor
    Carcinoid
    Lymphoma
    Leiomyosarcoma
    Adenocarcinoma
Metastases
Intussusception

Adenoma

- Usually small (1 to 3 cm)
- Sessile or pedunculated
- Usually asymptomatic

FIGURE   Gore: 893

Leiomyoma

Why is a small bowel leiomyoma more likely to be detected than a small bowel adenoma?

- Bleeding is a common presentation as the tumor ulcerates
- Hypervascular, so enhances uniformly on CT, unless necrotic
- May show calcification

FIGURE   Gore: 894

Lipoma

What features of a filling defect suggest lipoma?

- Sharply demarcated
- Often pedunculated

- Configuration of tumor may change during compression or peristalsis

FIGURE   Gore: 896

Hemangioma

What syndromes are associated with small bowel hemangiomas?

- Generally not big enough to be seen on barium studies
- Consider tuberous sclerosis and Turner's, Osler-Weber-Rendu, and blue rubber bleb nevus syndromes
- Phleboliths sometimes present
- Over 80% symptomatic, with bleeding the usual presenting symptom

FIGURE   Gore: 896

Hamartomatous polyp

List the syndromes that result in hamartomatous polyps of the small bowel.

- Seen with Peutz-Jeghers syndrome and Cowden's disease

FIGURE   Gore: 897

Carcinoid

Where do small bowel carcinoids occur?

Are carcinoid tumors easily distinguishable from other small bowel tumors?

- Far more common in ileum than jejunum (10:1)
- May seem mucosal or submucosal in origin, so not easily differentiated from other lesions
- Presence of one or two additional polyps of similar appearance strengthens suspicion for carcinoid

FIGURE   Gore: 904

Lymphoma

- Tends to originate at multiple sites

Leiomyosarcoma

Describe the typical appearance of a small bowel leiomyosarcoma.

- Bulky
- Appears as extrinsic mass displacing adjacent bowel loops
- Like leiomyomas, these ulcerate and bleed

FIGURE   Gore: 913

Adenocarcinoma

What part of the small bowel is typically affected by adenocarcinoma?

Name three conditions that predispose patients to small bowel adenocarcinoma.

- Rare; less common than leiomyosarcoma
- Tends to occur in duodenum (50%) and proximal small bowel, whereas lymphoma is more common distally
- Precancerous conditions: celiac disease, Crohn's disease, Peutz-Jeghers syndrome

FIGURES   Gore: 843, 908–910

Metastases

What are the mechanisms of metastatic involvement of the small bowel?

- Mechanisms of involvement include:
    - ¶ Hematogenous: breast, lung, kidney, melanoma, Kaposi's sarcoma
    - ¶ Direct spread from contiguous tumor (renal, adrenal, pancreatic)
    - ¶ Intraperitoneal seeding (ovarian, appendix, colon)

What type of metastasis is prone to develop intussusception? Why?

- Melanoma metastases prone to develop intussusception because of submucosal location

4

FIGURES Gore: 924–926, 961

Intussusception

- Narrow, tapered, barium-filled channel outlines intussusceptum (advancing proximal segment)
- Coiled-spring appearance occurs when barium refluxes into lumen of intussuscipiens

FIGURES Gore: 961–963

What is the name for the segment of bowel that surrounds the intussuscepted segment of bowel?

COLON AND APPENDIX

CONED CECUM

List the differential diagnosis for a coned cecum.

Crohn's disease
Infection
      Amebiasis
      TB
      Actinomycosis
      Yersinia spp
      Typhlitis
Inflammation
      Appendicitis
      Diverticulitis
Adenocarcinoma
Lymphoma
Ulcerative colitis

Crohn's disease

Can the terminal ileum be normal in a patient with Crohn's disease?
What other clues may be present on a radiograph to suggest Crohn's disease?

- Look for concomitant involvement of terminal ileum (although isolated colonic involvement found in up to 20% of patients)
- Look for other clues that are associated with Crohn's disease or its treatment
    - ¶ Nephrolithiasis
    - ¶ Gallstones
    - ¶ Ankylosing spondylitis
    - ¶ Sacroiliitis
    - ¶ Avascular necrosis of femoral heads

FIGURES Gore: 837, 1135

Amebiasis

Would you expect the terminal ileum to be abnormal in a patient with amebiasis?

- Skip lesions common in acute disease
- Terminal ileum invariably spared

FIGURES Gore: 1148, 1149

TB

- Features closely resemble those of Crohn's disease
- Exuberant mural thickening present that tends to be greater than that in Crohn's disease
- In contrast to Crohn's disease, fistulas and sinus tracts rare

True or false: fistula formation is not uncommon with TB.

Is it common with actinomycosis?

FIGURES Gore: 1147, 1148

Actinomycosis

Why does actinomycosis result in disease if it is a part of the normal gut flora?

- Consider whenever thinking about Crohn's disease or TB
- Ask about recent penetrating trauma or surgery

Yersinia spp

What feature of cecal disease would argue against Yersinia?

- Stenosis not a common feature

FIGURE   Gore: 1146

Typhlitis

When should typhlitis be considered in the differential diagnosis?

- Consider in appropriate clinical setting

FIGURE   Gore: 1152

Appendicitis

- Presence of an appendicolith makes this diagnosis quite likely

FIGURES   Gore: 1318, 1475

Diverticulitis

Because both appendicitis and cecal diverticulitis can be clinically similar, what barium finding would help distinguish between them?

- Look for diverticula in other parts of colon
- Mucosal folds should be preserved
- Look for gradual zone of transition
- Usually, major competing clinical diagnosis is appendicitis; thus, finding normal-appearing appendix on CT makes this diagnosis more likely

FIGURES   Gore: 1079–1083

Adenocarcinoma

Could you reasonably expect the mucosa overlying a lesion to be normal if the lesion is caused by adenocarcinoma?

- Unless superimposed infection is present, significant inflammatory changes are not seen on CT
- Abrupt transition
- Destruction of mucosa
- "Apple-core" configuration

FIGURES   Gore: 1170–1183, 1277, 1278

Lymphoma

What feature of a large cecal mass would support the diagnosis of lymphoma?

- Can extend into terminal ileum from cecum
- Tends not to obstruct
- Mucosal surface smooth, indicating submucosal infiltration rather than mucosal ulceration

FIGURE   Gore: 1201

Ulcerative colitis

True or false: the key to excluding ulcerative colitis is the demonstration of an abnormal terminal ileum, indicating a disease process that is not confined to the colon.

- No skip lesions; thus, would have to involve whole colon in order to affect cecum
- Look for changes of backwash ileitis in terminal ileum

FIGURES   Gore: 1113, 1114

4

MULTIPLE COLONIC POLYPS

Name three general categories of diseases that lead to multiple polypoid lesions in the colon. Give specific examples of each category.

Any of the polyposis syndromes
    Familial adenomatous polyposis syndrome (encompasses familial polyposis and Gardner's syndrome)
    Peutz-Jeghers syndrome
    Turcot's syndrome
    Cronkhite-Canada syndrome
    Juvenile polyposis
    Cowden syndrome
Related to colitis (postinflammatory pseudopolyps)
    Ulcerative colitis/Crohn's disease
    Pseudomembranous colitis
Neoplasm
    Lymphoma
    Kaposi's sarcoma
Other
    Lymphoid follicles
    Colitis cystica profunda
    Pneumatosis cystoides intestinalis

Familial adenomatous polyposis syndrome

Describe the major extracolonic manifestations of familial adenomatous polyposis syndrome.

- Numerous extracolonic manifestations

FIGURES   Gore: 1229–1232

Peutz-Jeghers syndrome

True or false: Peutz-Jeghers syndrome leads to innumerable colonic polyps.

- When polyps occur in colon, there are fewer there than in small bowel (1 to 10 in colon versus too numerous to count in small bowel)

FIGURES   Gore: 1234–1236

Turcot's syndrome

Is the type of polyp seen in Turcot's syndrome premalignant (adenomatous rather than hyperplastic)? Is colectomy an important part of the management of patients with Turcot's syndrome?

- Associated with intracerebral tumors (usually glioblastomas)
- Patients usually die of their brain tumor before colon becomes a clinical issue

Cronkhite-Canada syndrome

What is the typical clinical setting of Cronkhite-Canada syndrome?

- Innumerable small to moderate-sized polyps
- Older adults with alopecia, skin pigmentation, and atrophy of fingernails and toenails
- No malignant potential

FIGURE   Gore: 1239

Juvenile polyposis of the colon

What is the difference between juvenile polyposis of the colon and an isolated juvenile polyp?

- Increased risk of malignancy

FIGURES   Gore: 1240, 1241

Cowden syndrome

- Inquire about breast and thyroid disease

FIGURE   Gore: 1238

Ulcerative colitis and Crohn's disease

Do polyps form during the active phase or healing phase of inflammatory bowel disease?

- Postinflammatory pseudopolyps occur when denuded mucosa is overgrown
- Polyps may be small and rounded, long and filiform, or proliferate into something resembling villous adenoma

FIGURES Gore: 1111, 1112

Pseudomembranous colitis

- "Lesions" irregular, numerous
- Mucosa not normal in appearance

FIGURES Gore: 1156, 1157

Kaposi's sarcoma

What clinical features must exist before the diagnosis of GI Kaposi's sarcoma is strongly entertained?

How do lymph nodes involved with Kaposi's sarcoma behave on CT?

- Patient must have AIDS and, in general, demonstrate skin lesions of Kaposi's sarcoma
- Submucosal location results in smooth nodular appearance
- May have central umbilication

FIGURE Gore: 2685

Lymphoid follicles

- Uniformly sized; mucosa otherwise normal

FIGURE Gore: 1034

Colitis cystica profunda

- Submucosal appearing

FIGURE Gore: 1297

Pneumatosis cystoides coli

- Usually in left colon
- Lucent

ULCERS

What diseases cause ulcers of the colon?

Crohn's disease
Ulcerative colitis
Other colitis
    Amebiasis
    TB
    Shigellosis
    Yersinia spp infection
    CMV infection
Behçet's syndrome

Crohn's disease

Are colonic ulcers caused by Crohn's disease deep or superficial?

- Ulcers are superficial (aphthoid)
- Look for concomitant small bowel involvement (though 20% of patients have only colonic disease)

FIGURES Gore: 1133, 1134

Distinguish between ulcerative colitis and Crohn's disease.

Ulcerative colitis

- Mucosa appears granular in early stages, with loss of markings seen in late stages
- Ulcers described as "collar button"
- No skip areas

FIGURE   Gore: 1109

Amebiasis

- Right colon and rectal involvement, with skip areas
- Acute stages characterized by ulceration
- Chronic stages characterized by contraction of bowel; also by ameboma formation
- Generally spares ileum

Is the ileum involved in amebiasis?

TB

- Features mimic those of Crohn's disease
- Some findings more suggestive of TB than other entities
    - ¶ Oval or circumferential transverse ulcers
    - ¶ Loss of anatomic demarcation between ileum and right colon (Stierlin's sign)
    - ¶ Right-angle intersection between ileum and cecum, with marked hypertrophy of ileocecal valve (Fleischner's sign)

What are some of the classic signs of TB colitis?

Shigellosis

- Predominantly left-sided involvement

FIGURE   Gore: 1145

Which side of the colon is more commonly involved with shigellosis?

Yersinia spp infection

- Stenosis not a feature
- Involvement more extensive in small bowel than in colon

FIGURE   Gore: 1146

CMV infection

- Consider if patient has AIDS
- Usually right-sided involvement

Which patients get CMV colitis?

Behçet's syndrome

- Mimics Crohn's disease

THUMBPRINTING

Vascular causes
    Ischemia
    Intramural hemorrhage (coagulopathy)
    Traumatic hematoma
    Hemolytic-uremic syndrome
Advanced colitis (any cause)
    Ulcerative colitis
    Crohn's disease
    Amebiasis
    CMV infection
    Pseudomembranous colitis

Tumor
 Lymphoma
 Metastases
Miscellaneous
 Pneumatosis cystoides coli
 Amyloidosis

Ischemia

- Thumbprinting is classic plain film and barium enema finding of ischemia
- Usually caused by low flow states or small vessel disease rather than by occlusive arterial disease; thus, often a diffuse process
- Occurs in older patients
- Next step in work-up is colonoscopy, not angiography

Would an angiogram be useful in diagnosis of colonic ischemia?

FIGURES   Gore: 2702, 2703

4

Intramural hemorrhage

- Can be caused by any cause of coagulopathy

Traumatic hematoma

- Focal
- May be iatrogenic (i.e., caused by colonoscopy)
- Look for other signs of trauma, such as broken bones or free intraperitoneal fluid

FIGURES   Gore: 2593, 2594

Hemolytic-uremic syndrome

- Pediatric patients

Advanced colitis (any cause)

- Tends to be diffuse abnormality

FIGURES   Gore: 1157, 1294

Pneumatosis cystoides coli

- Look for lucency along wall of colon
- More common on left side of colon
- Obstructive lung disease is a "risk factor"

FIGURE   Gore: 186

Amyloidosis

- Tends to be sharply demarcated

FIGURE   Gore: 1022

SOLITARY COLONIC FILLING DEFECT

Using broad categories, give a differential diagnosis for a solitary colonic filling defect.

Benign tumor
 Adenoma
 Hyperplastic polyp
 Lipoma
 Hemangioma

Malignant tumor
    Adenocarcinoma
    Carcinoid
    Lymphoma
    Cloacogenic carcinoma
Infection
    Ameboma
    Diverticular abscess
Miscellaneous
    Intussusception
    Related to appendix

4

Adenoma

What feature makes a polyp more likely to be benign?

• Polyp very likely benign if stalk longer than 2 cm

FIGURES   Gore: 1162, 1164, 1167, 1168

Hyperplastic polyp

• Indistinguishable from adenoma
• Diagnosis made by the pathologist, not radiologist

Lipoma

What features of a mass favor lipoma?

• Soft, pliable, may change appearance with change in position or with compression

FIGURES   Gore: 1209–1211

Hemangioma

The presence of clustered round calcifications associated with a filling defect suggests what entity?

• Phleboliths may be found
• Usually located in rectum or sigmoid colon
• Polypoid forms smooth, broad-based, sessile lesions

Adenocarcinoma

• Polyp more likely to be malignant with increasing size

FIGURES   Gore: 1170–1172

Carcinoid

Are carcinoids small or large when they are discovered?

• In rectum, usually appear as sessile polyps
• Elsewhere in colon, usually in right colon and bulky in size

FIGURE   Gore: 1207

Lymphoma

True or false: lymphomas are large tumors and therefore likely to result in bowel obstruction.

• Wide spectrum of appearances
    ¶ Multiple nodules
    ¶ Large polypoid intraluminal mass
    ¶ Less common appearances include focal stricturing, aneurysmal dilatation, large ulcerating mass with multiple fistulas
• Tend not to obstruct despite large size

Cloacogenic carcinoma

What is characteristic of cloacogenic carcinoma?

- Highly suggestive radiographic appearance: plaque-like filling defect with well-defined proximal and distal margins at anorectal junction

Ameboma

- Usually annular constricting rather than polypoid appearance

FIGURE   Gore: 1149

Diverticular abscess

What are some features that distinguish diverticular abscess from adenocarcinoma, in terms of the finding of a filling defect in the colon?

- Look for presence of other diverticula
- Clinical setting helps to differentiate, but carcinoma can present with infection
- Other features that help differentiate from cancer: gradual zone of transition, preserved mucosal folds
- Specific diagnosis made only when there is extravasation of contrast from diverticulum

FIGURE   Gore: 1081

Intussusception

- Search for coiled-spring appearance
- CT shows pathognomonic appearance of intussuscepted mesenteric fat

FIGURES   Gore: 1255, 1256

Related to appendix

- Inverted stump
- Mucocele
- Characteristic location and appearance

FIGURES   Gore: 1335, 1337

SEGMENTAL COLONIC NARROWING

List a broad differential diagnosis for segmental colonic narrowing with a few examples of each entity.

Malignant disorders
    Adenocarcinoma
    Metastases
    Lymphoma
    Carcinoid
    Direct spread from adjacent tumor
Inflammatory/infectious disorders
    Crohn's disease
    Ulcerative colitis
    Diverticulitis
    Ameboma
    Lymphogranuloma venereum (LGV)
Vascular disorders
    Ischemia
    Radiation colitis
Miscellaneous
    Endometriosis
    Hemangioma

Adenocarcinoma

What radiographic and clinical features of a segmental colonic process favor neoplasm?

- Features that favor adenocarcinoma include abrupt transition at site of obstruction, rigid and narrowed lumen, mucosal destruction, and apple-core configuration with overhanging margins
- Look for polyps/lesions elsewhere in the colon because synchronous lesions are found in 5% of cases
- Evidence of chronic gastrointestinal blood loss makes this diagnosis more likely than other causes of segmental narrowing

FIGURES   Gore: 1054, 1171, 1174

Metastases

Describe the mechanisms by which metastases can involve the colon.

- Direct invasion by contiguous cancers arising in cervix, prostate, ovary, gallbladder, uterus, and kidney
- Direct invasion by noncontiguous cancers arising in pancreas (via transverse mesocolon) or stomach (via gastrocolic ligament)
- Intraperitoneal seeding: think of ovarian cancer in women
- Hematogenous spread: melanoma, lung, breast

FIGURES   Gore: 1214–1216, 1218–1225

Lymphoma

Does lymphoma cause segmental narrowing?

- Focal stricture a less common presentation but possible
- Generally, lymphoma does not cause obstruction
- Overlying mucosa smooth because disease process is submucosal

FIGURES   Gore: 1201, 1202

Carcinoid

True or false: colonic carcinoids are aggressive tumors with poor prognosis.

- Rectal carcinoids are more common than colonic carcinoids; their behavior is less aggressive
- When in colon, carcinoids are more aggressive and larger; tend to occur in right colon
- May demonstrate desmoplastic response, so look for tethering of adjacent bowel loops

FIGURE   Gore: 1207

Crohn's disease

What extraintestinal findings might help implicate Crohn's disease?

- Look for other sites of abnormality (skip lesions)
- Search for fistulas, aphthoid lesions, ulcers
- Extraintestinal clues: nephrolithiasis, gallstones, ankylosing spondylitis, sacroiliitis, and avascular necrosis of femoral heads

FIGURES   Gore: 1129, 1135

Ulcerative colitis

Could ulcerative colitis cause focal narrowing of the hepatic flexure? How?

- Strictures occur in 10% of patients
- Benign strictures caused by ulcerative colitis usually in distal colon and may be reversible
- Nonreversible strictures located in more proximal portion of colon may be neoplastic

FIGURE   Gore: 1115

Diverticulitis

What features suggest diverticulitis rather than carcinoma as the cause of an area of segmental narrowing?

What features suggest diverticulitis rather than carcinoma as the cause of an area of segmental narrowing?

- Features that favor diverticulitis as cause of stricture
    - ¶ Gradual zone of transition
    - ¶ Only partial obstruction
    - ¶ Preserved mucosal folds (oftentimes not present, however)
    - ¶ Presence of other diverticula
- Site of involvement usually sigmoid colon

Where does diverticulitis typically occur? How can CT help if diverticulitis is suspected?

- CT is the examination of choice if diverticulitis suspected; in general, adjacent inflammatory changes are more extensive than those seen with neoplasm (unless superimposed perforation present)
- Evidence of diverticula should be sought elsewhere
- Clinical evidence of chronic gastrointestinal blood loss makes this diagnosis less likely than malignancy

FIGURES Gore: 1079–1083, 1086

4

Ameboma

- Short regions of involvement with marked granulation (ameboma) occur in 10% of patients
- Skip lesions typically seen, so other areas of disease should be sought
- More common in right colon

FIGURE Gore: 1149

Lymphogranuloma venereum (LGV)

- Involvement limited to rectum
- Barium enema findings mimic those of Crohn's disease

FIGURE Gore: 1295

Ischemia

True or false: sacculation of the stricture wall argues against ischemia as the cause. Where do ischemic strictures occur?

- Strictures occur after insult, as quickly as 3 weeks
- Usually not obstructive
- May be smooth and tapered or eccentric with sacculations
- Because colonic ischemia usually is caused by low flow states, strictures that result from ischemia tend to occur at watershed zones of arterial supply

FIGURE Gore: 2704

Radiation colitis

- History is key
- Narrowing caused by radiation can be acute (as result of spasm, edema) or chronic (as result of effect of radiation on microvascularity)

What features of a stricture favor radiation as a possible cause?

- Narrowing typically has tapered margins and symmetrical appearance, with preserved mucosal pattern
- Other clues of radiation in the area should be sought (for example, bony changes)

FIGURE Gore: 2712

Endometriosis

Where does endometriosis usually affect the colon?

- Crenulated pattern, usually located along anterior wall of rectum or inferior wall of sigmoid

FIGURES Gore: 1221, 1301, 1302

The presence of clustered round calcifications associated with a filling defect suggests what entity?

Hemangioma

- Phleboliths may be found
- Usually located in rectum or sigmoid colon
- Circumferential lesion with scalloped contours and nodular mucosal surface pattern

FIGURE   Gore: 1205

DILATED COLON

List the main considerations when the colon appears abnormally dilated. Which is the most common? List five causes of colonic obstruction.

Obstruction
    Carcinoma
    Diverticulitis
    Volvulus
    Intussusception
    Adhesions
    Hernia
Toxic megacolon
Ischemia
Ileus

Carcinoma

Is colon cancer a common cause of obstruction?

What is the mechanism of obstruction in colon cancer?

Characterize the clinical symptoms of colon carcinoma.

- Most common cause of obstruction in adults in the United States
- Can cause obstruction as result of luminal narrowing, intussusception, or perforation and abscess formation
- Sigmoid colon the most common site of obstruction; rectum is not because of its distensibility
- Symptoms usually subacute or chronic

FIGURE   Gore: 1173

Diverticulitis

If diverticulitis is suspected clinically, which imaging test is usually most helpful to further evaluate?

- Site of obstruction usually the sigmoid colon
- CT the examination of choice if diverticulitis suspected
- Evidence of diverticula should be sought elsewhere

FIGURES   Gore: 1079–1088, 1090–1095, 1251, 1252

Volvulus

- More common in sigmoid colon or cecum; not common in transverse colon
- Beak sign seen on barium enema examination
- If sigmoid volvulus suspected, prone film should be tried to see if air moves to rectum; if so, there is no sigmoid volvulus

FIGURES   Gore: 176, 177, 1253, 1254

Intussusception

What is the classic plain film finding that suggests intussusception?

What does intussusception look like on CT or ultrasound?

- Look for crescent sign on plain films, coiled spring appearance on barium enema, or target appearance on CT or ultrasound
- In adults, always has a pathologic lead point

FIGURES   Gore: 1254–1256

Adhesions

- More commonly affects small bowel than colon
- When adhesions occur in colon, usually involve mobile, redundant portions such as cecum or sigmoid colon
- Bowel loops become angulated, tethered

Hernia

- Less likely to affect colon than small bowel

FIGURE Gore: 1257

4

Toxic megacolon

What disease most commonly leads to toxic megacolon?

True or false: barium studies are important in the diagnosis of toxic megacolon.

- Most commonly occurs in setting of ulcerative colitis
- Barium study contraindicated if toxic megacolon suspected, because of risk of perforation (colonic wall is pathologically very thin in this condition, although it appears thickened radiographically)

FIGURES Gore: 1102, 1119

Ischemia

- Patients usually older
- Thumbprinting the classic finding
- Usually relates to low flow states or small vessel disease rather than occlusion or embolus; thus, angiography not of much use

FIGURES Gore: 2702–2705

Ileus

- Often has metabolic basis
- May be result of drugs
- Usually, small bowel also dilated

FIGURE Gore: 2631

SMOOTH (AHAUSTRAL) COLON

List four entities that lead to a featureless colon.

Cathartic abuse
Ulcerative colitis
Radiation colitis (late)
Ischemic colitis (late)

Cathartic abuse

What distinguishes cathartic colon from other causes of a featureless colon?

- Typically right colonic involvement
- Colon dilated or normal in caliber, as opposed to relative narrowing seen in other conditions leading to ahaustral appearance

Ulcerative colitis

- Haustra lost with chronic disease because colon foreshortened

FIGURES Gore: 1113, 1114

Radiation colitis, ischemic colitis

- Colon becomes featureless years after incident
- Lumen somewhat narrowed

Figure References

Gore RM, Levine MS, Laufer I: Textbook of Gastrointestinal Radiology. Philadelphia: WB Saunders, 1994.

4 ALIMENTARY TRACT DISEASE ENTITIES

ABETALIPOPROTEINEMIA

Clinical

- Rare; autosomal recessive inheritance
- Biopsy results in detection of foamy lipid material in cytoplasm of intestinal epithelial cell; this is pathognomonic
- Malabsorption of fat, progressive neurologic deterioration, and retinitis pigmentosa
- Acanthocytosis (thorny appearance of red blood cells) is characteristic

Imaging

- Small bowel dilatation with mild to moderate fold thickening
- Typically regular, diffuse

ACHALASIA

Clinical

- Two pathophysiologic features:
    Hypertonic lower esophageal sphincter (LES)
    Lack of peristalsis in body of esophagus (where smooth muscle starts), although classically, primary peristalsis is absent throughout entire esophagus
- Pathologically: decrease in neural elements, especially ganglionic cells of myenteric plexus at LES
- Disease of the young (20 to 40 years)
- Increased incidence of carcinoma in patients with achalasia
- Treatment: hydrostatic pneumatic dilatation initially; if unsuccessful, Heller myotomy

Imaging

- Plain films: retained food and fluid in esophagus; widened mediastinum with air-fluid level, primarily on right, secondary to dilated and tortuous esophagus
- Barium studies
    "Rat-tail" or "beak" sign: smooth, conical narrowing of distal esophageal segment extending 1 to 3 cm
    To distinguish from stricture, stand patient up: in achalasia, weight of barium column opens LES; in stricture, LES does not open
    Barium retention above LES for longer than 2.5 seconds after swallowing
- Differentiated from scleroderma in that complete emptying of esophagus does not occur even in erect position
- Because achalasia is a disease of young adults, neoplasm should be suspected in an older patient with the radiographic appearance of achalasia

ACTINOMYCOSIS

Clinical

- Part of normal flora of bowel; pathologic process ensues only when contact occurs with tissues not normally exposed, as in penetrating trauma, surgery (often in setting of antecedent appendectomy), in presence of long-standing intrauterine device (IUD)
- Predilection for fistula formation in right lower quadrant

Imaging

- Inflammatory mass and fistula
- Consider whenever thinking about Crohn's disease or TB

ADENOCARCINOMA, OF COLON

Clinical

- Most common cancer in the United States population
- Second most common cause of cancer mortality
- About 50% of colonic cancers occur in the rectum and sigmoid
- Risk factors: age, personal or family history of colorectal polyps or cancer, chronic ulcerative colitis
- About 5% of patients with colon carcinoma have synchronous carcinomas elsewhere in colon
- Most important complications of colorectal cancer: bleeding, bowel obstruction, perforation

Imaging

- Features of polyps that suggest possible malignancy:
    Size greater than 2 cm
    Serial growth
    Short, thick stalk (long, thin stalk generally a sign of benign polyp)
    Irregular or lobulated head of polyp
- Advanced cancers: majority of patients; generally annular or large polypoid tumors
- CT
    Limitations of CT imaging for staging:
        CT poor means of determining depth of spread of tumor in bowel wall
        CT not good at detecting intraperitoneal spread of neoplasm
        Spread to lymph nodes also problematic; using 15 mm as upper size limit, sensitivity is only 26%
    CT reserved for patients suspected of having locally extensive or widespread disease
    CT good for detecting recurrence after abdominoperineal resection (barium enema, endoscopy not good)

ADENOCARCINOMA, OF DUODENUM

Clinical

- Majority occur in third and fourth portions of duodenum
- Increased incidence in patients with Gardner's or Peutz-Jeghers syndrome

ADENOCARCINOMA, OF ESOPHAGUS

Clinical

- Develops in setting of Barrett's esophagus (accounts for 20% of adenocarcinomas of esophagus)
- Most found in distal esophagus, tending to involve gastric cardia; may ultimately be classified as gastric in origin; about 90% of all carcinomas arising at GE junction are adenocarcinomas

• May give achalasia-like picture; distinguishing features include age of patient (older with cancer), duration of symptoms (shorter with cancer), and weight loss (occurs with cancer)

Imaging

• Calcification extremely unusual in esophageal carcinoma but rarely may occur with this type (think of leiomyoma if presented with esophageal mass with amorphous calcification)

ADENOCARCINOMA, OF STOMACH

Clinical

• Decreasing incidence throughout the world, including United States
• Higher prevalence in Japan, Chile, Iceland
• Risk factors: gastric atrophy, achlorhydria, hypochlorhydria, pernicious anemia
  Related to nitrates in stomach
  Achlorhydria promotes bacterial overgrowth in stomach, leading to increased nitrates
• Route of spread:
  (1) Hematogenous to liver and lungs
  (2) Direct extension along ligamentous attachments
  (3) Regional nodal dissemination
  (4) Diffuse spread throughout peritoneal surfaces of abdominal cavity

Imaging

• Radiographic appearance of adenocarcinoma varies: polypoid, infiltrative, hyperrugosity, ulceration
• Occasionally, punctate calcifications seen within thickened wall are essentially diagnostic of colloid carcinoma or mucinous adenocarcinoma (represent psammoma bodies)

ADENOMA, OF COLON

Clinical

• Sessile polyps have greater risk of malignancy than pedunculated lesions
• 5% incidence of malignancy; incidence rises with increasing size of adenoma
• Another important indicator of malignancy: presence or absence of stalk; polyps with stalk more than 2 cm long almost never associated with malignant invasion

Imaging

• Detection rate by barium enema: 85% for double-contrast studies versus 60% for single-contrast studies
• Because colorectal adenomas grow slowly, reexamination every 3 years is sufficient

ADENOMATOUS POLYP, OF STOMACH AND DUODENUM

Clinical

• Constitute less than 20% of all gastric polyps
• Premalignant, but less so than colonic adenomas
• Found in stomach of patients with pernicious anemia and chronic atrophic gastritis

Imaging

• Most frequently seen in antrum as solitary lesions
• No special features; these look like polyps in the colon

AMEBIASIS

Clinical

- Rare in United States
- Infestation of colon can lead to spread to liver and lungs, resulting in abscesses
- Two stages: acute ulcerative stage and chronic fibrotic stage

Imaging

Acute stage
- Shallow ulceration
- More severe disease associated with irritability, spasm, loss of haustra
- Most commonly involves cecum, ascending colon, or rectum, but any part of colon can be affected
- Skip lesions

Chronic stage
- Shortening and contraction of bowel, most marked in cecum (results in cone-shaped cecum)
- Amebomas: polypoid masses or annular constricting lesions
- Invariably spares terminal ileum

AMYLOID

Clinical

- Can involve all areas of GI tract
- Segmental involvement in 70% of cases
- No evidence of hypersecretion
- Arteriolar compression can lead to ischemic disease

Imaging

- Characterized by sharply demarcated thickening of folds throughout small bowel (occasionally, involvement is patchy and uneven)
- Folds can be symmetric or irregular
- Appearance of prominent ileal folds resembling valvulae conniventes of jejunum (jejunization) suggests amyloidosis
- Caliber of bowel normal (mild dilatation as disease progresses)

ANNULAR PANCREAS

Clinical

- Other congenital anomalies of GI tract frequently coexist
- Down syndrome in 30%

Imaging

- Results in incomplete obstruction (versus complete obstruction in duodenal atresia)

ANTRAL MUCOSAL DIAPHRAGM

Clinical

- Thin, membranous septa within 3 cm of pyloric canal
- Congenital, but may not produce symptoms until adulthood (if ever)

Imaging

- Sharply defined, 2 to 3 cm wide, bandlike defect in barium column, arising at right angles to gastric wall

APPENDICITIS

Clinical

- Pathogenesis related to luminal obstruction, usually as result of fecal residue (fecaliths)
- Characteristic clinical presentation of pain at McBurney's point (2 inches medial to the right anterior superior iliac spine) not always present; wide variety of atypical presentations; radiographic procedures become useful in atypical cases

Imaging

- CT:
    Most accurate imaging modality for detection of appendicitis
- Ultrasound:
    Can be useful but CT has higher sensitivity
    Technique uses graded compression of right lower quadrant with linear 5-MHz transducer; normal appendix may be visualized as having a thickness of 6 mm or less; more than 6 mm is considered evidence of appendicitis; demonstration of a fecalith or fluid collection also indicative of appendicitis
    Diagnosis can be made with confidence when abnormal appendix is identified or when appendicolithiasis present in right lower quadrant

BARRETT'S ESOPHAGUS

Clinical

- Replacement of normal stratified squamous lining of lower esophagus with columnar epithelium
- Ulceration tends to be deep and penetrating, identical to peptic gastric ulceration, as opposed to shallow ulcerations of reflux
- Accompanied by stricture
- Increased incidence of adenocarcinoma (10%)

Imaging

- Classic findings: high stricture and esophageal ulceration; however, most patients do not have the classic picture
- Fine reticular or granular pattern on double-contrast esophagrams more sensitive but less specific

BEHÇET'S SYNDROME

Clinical

- Rare condition with buccal and genital ulcerations as well as skin and ocular manifestations
- In GI tract, Behçet's syndrome usually involves colon, producing localized or diffuse form of colitis in 20% of patients
- Hemorrhage and perforation frequent complications

Imaging

- Tends to mimic Crohn's disease more than ulcerative colitis, although ulcers in Behçet's are larger than in those in Crohn's disease

BENIGN LYMPHOID HYPERPLASIA

Clinical

- Usually pathologically insignificant
- Can be seen with hypogammaglobulinemia and giardiasis

Imaging

- Most commonly presents as innumerable tiny nodular defects evenly scattered throughout duodenum
- Resembles that seen in terminal ileum
- Multiple small, round filling defects usually not limited to bulb

BEZOAR, GASTRIC

Clinical

- Types:
  1. Trichobezoar: hair
  2. Phytobezoar: vegetable matter; occurs postgastrectomy (i.e., Billroth procedure)
  3. Concretion bezoar: ingested material such as paints, resins, etc.
- May pass into small bowel and obstruct at terminal ileum (happens with Billroth procedures)

Imaging

- Irregular filling defect
- May float
- On fluoroscopy, cannot be broken into smaller pieces with manual manipulation (food clumps that mimic bezoar can be broken)

BRUNNER'S GLAND HYPERPLASIA

Clinical

- Submucosal glands that produce mucus-like substance to protect duodenum from gastric acid
- Finding hyperplasia of these glands suggests hyperacidity

Imaging

- Multiple, small, rounded polypoid elevations

CARCINOID, OF COLON

Clinical

- Represents 15% of carcinoid tumors
- When located in colon, majority lie in rectum; these rectal carcinoids rarely metastasize
- Colonic carcinoids much more aggressive than rectal carcinoids and frequently located in cecum or right colon
- 5-year survival of patients with large bowel carcinoid tumors:
  - Rectal   83%
  - Colonic   50%

Imaging

- Right colonic carcinoids have two general appearances:
  - Bulky, larger than 5 cm, sessile and fungating intraluminal masses
  - Irregular annular lesions
- Rectal carcinoids appear as sessile polyp

CARCINOID, OF SMALL BOWEL

Clinical

- Most common primary small bowel tumor
- Arises from cells deep in crypts of Lieberkühn

- Malignancy related to size; lesions larger than 2 cm consistently demonstrate metastases (to lymph nodes and liver)

Imaging

- Characteristic CT appearance of soft tissue mass with radiating stellate pattern of linear densitites caused by local release of serotonin
- CT findings can be simulated by other neoplastic or inflammatory disorders such as metastases, retractile mesenteritis, and Crohn's disease
- Liver metastases almost always hypervascular

CATHARTIC ABUSE

Imaging

- Haustrations of colon obliterated, resulting in featureless colon and terminal ileum
- Usually involves right colon more than left
- Colon usually dilated or normal caliber
- Does not ulcerate (mucosal surface remains normal)

CHAGAS DISEASE

Clinical

- Infection caused by *Trypanosoma cruzi*
- Also can see megacolon, ureteral dilatation, acute or chronic myocarditis

Imaging

- Looks like achalasia

CLOACOGENIC CARCINOMA

Clinical

- Arises from remnants of cloacal membrane located at anorectal junction

Imaging

- Highly suggestive radiographic appearance: plaque-like filling defect with well-defined proximal and distal margins at anorectal junction

COLITIS, CMV

Clinical

- Generally involves right side of colon, sometimes extending to distal ileum (small bowel otherwise spared)
- Early disease characterized by nodular lymphoid hyperplasia
- Moderate disease results in discrete multifocal ulceration, scattered on a background of normal mucosa
- Advanced disease leads to deeper ulcers, mucosal edema, and thickened bowel wall
- Hemorrhagic CMV colitis can be fatal in patients with AIDS

Imaging

- Bowel wall typically hypodense on CT but may be hyperdense, reflecting hemorrhagic component of the disease

COLITIS, RADIATION

Clinical

- Usually doses in excess of 4500 rads needed to produce complications (which occur in only approximately 10% of patients)
- Acute effects: edema, spasm, ulceration, and fistulas possible; perforation rare
- Chronic effects: need 6 to 24 months to occur; primarily manifest as decreased bowel caliber; with more severe damage, smooth, symmetrical strictures may be seen

COLITIS, TB

Clinical

- Primary disease acquired by drinking nonpasteurized milk
- Secondary disease usually results from ingestion of infected sputum
- Only approximately 50% of patients with intestinal TB have radiographically evident pulmonary disease
- Affects ileocolic region in 80 to 90% of patients

Imaging

- Features closely resemble those of Crohn's disease: edema and ulceration; contracted, cone-shaped cecum; narrowed terminal ileum; ileocecal valve may be fixed in gaping position
- Certain abnormalities considered more characteristic of TB than of other entities:
    Oval or circumferential transverse ulcers
    Loss of anatomic demarcation between ileum and right colon (Stierlin's sign)
    Right-angle intersection between ileum and cecum with marked hypertrophy of ileocecal valve (Fleischner's sign)
- Other suggestive features: extremely short segments of involvement of ileum or cecum; lymphadenopathy, especially with low-density centers on CT; ascites

COLITIS CYSTICA PROFUNDA

Clinical

- Postinflammatory condition (typically after severe case of bacillary dysentery); usually presents as multiple submucosal filling defects in rectum, but can be single; can affect other segments
- Islands of regenerating epithelium result in mucous cysts, which rise to the surface and empty; thus, characterized by mucous cysts in muscularis mucosa
- Most often seen in young adults

Imaging

- Cysts may produce intraluminal filling defects
- Segmental proliferative changes usually present in rectum or sigmoid should not be mistaken for adenocarcinoma

COWDEN DISEASE

Clinical

- Multiple hamartomas
- Mucocutaneous papules
- Breast and thyroid disease

CRICOPHARYNGEUS MUSCLE

Clinical

- Posterior impression
- Prominence can be caused by achalasia and by total laryngectomy

- Clinical significance of isolated cricopharyngeal achalasia is unknown; present in up to 5% of asymptomatic adults
- Myotomy produces relief in over 33% of patients with significant dysphagia

Imaging

- Radiographic appearance of cricopharyngeal achalasia: hemispherical or horizontal, shelf-like posterior protrusion into barium column at C5 to C6 level

CROHN'S DISEASE, OF COLON

Clinical

- Approximately 20% have disease limited to colon; 40% have disease limited to small bowel; 40% have disease in both small and large bowel
- Rectum often spared, but anal disease not uncommon (up to 80% in one study)
- Risk of colon carcinoma increased, but only 25% that of ulcerative colitis

Imaging

- Barium enema
    - Aphthous ulcers one of the early manifestations
    - Ulcers increase in number and size and become coalescent to form irregular longitudinal or transverse ulcers (leads to cobblestone pattern)
    - Fibrosis leads to strictures
    - Fistulas
    - Skip areas
    - Pseudopolyps
- CT
    - Thickened bowel wall
    - "Double-halo" appearance: inner, low-density ring with attenuation near water surrounded by higher density ring of muscularis propria and serosa (not specific for Crohn's disease)
    - Fistulas and abscesses
    - "Creeping fat": fibrofatty proliferation of the mesentery
    - Enlarged mesenteric nodes
- Extraintestinal imaging findings: nephrolithiasis, gallstones, ankylosing spondylitis, sacroiliitis, and AVN of femoral heads

Distinguishing from ulcerative colitis (UC)

- UC a contiguous confluent process starting from the rectum; Crohn's disease characterized by skip areas, asymmetric involvement
- UC may lead to shallow ulcerations that are not discrete; ulcers in Crohn's disease discrete and deep, commonly with fistula
- Granular mucosa common in UC and uncommon in Crohn's disease
- Severe anal/perianal disease exceptionally rare in UC but characteristic of Crohn's disease
- Spontaneous fistula and sinus tracts not seen in UC but characteristic of Crohn's disease

CROHN'S DISEASE, OF SMALL BOWEL

Clinical

- Involvement usually begins in terminal ileum
- Can affect almost any part of GI tract (usually spares rectum)
- Most common pattern (55%) is involvement of both colon and ileum; Crohn's colitis alone seen in 15%
- Characterized by ulcerations, rigid thickening of bowel wall that produces pipelike narrowing, loss of mucosal pattern, skip lesions, and creeping fat
- Peak incidence between 20 and 40 years of age, but 20% diagnosed in pediatric age group
- Frequent recurrence after surgery, usually at site of anastomosis

- Increased incidence of adenocarcinoma
- Complications: fistula to other organs/bowel loops, abscess, partial small bowel obstruction more common than total obstruction

Imaging

- Begins by showing aphthous ulcers, mucosal fold thickening, and mucosal fold distortion; progresses to deep linear ulceration, nodular cobblestone pattern, and eventual stenosis
- Fistulas and sinus tracts occur
- Separation of bowel loops by wall thickening and induration of mesentery
- Scattered islands of mucosa are pseudopolyps
- Fixed narrowing of fibrosis distinguished from spastic narrowing of Crohn's disease by lack of proximal bowel dilatation in the latter

CROHN'S DISEASE, OF STOMACH

Clinical

- Tendency to have pyloroantral and duodenal involvement
- Can occur without disease in jejunum
- Presentation with upper GI symptoms as first manifestation of Crohn's disease is rare
- Combined gastroduodenal disease occurs in 2 to 20% of patients with Crohn's disease

CRONKHITE-CANADA SYNDROME

Clinical

- Gastrointestinal polyposis, alopecia, skin pigmentation, and atrophy of fingernails and toenails
- Middle-aged women commonly affected; patients die from malnourishment
- Polyps occur in stomach and colon of all affected patients, where they are too numerous to count; occur in small bowel in 50% of patients
- These polyps have no malignant potential

DIFFUSE ESOPHAGEAL SPASM

Clinical

- Normal peristaltic wave to level of aortic arch
- Characterized by chest pain and intermittent dysphagia; repetitive contractions on manometry; segmental contraction on barium swallow; esophageal wall thickening

Imaging

- Corkscrew radiographic appearance of transient sacculations or pseudodiverticula ("rosary bead" esophagus) can be seen

DIVERTICULA, OF DUODENUM

Clinical

- 1 to 5% incidence on UGI examination; 20% at autopsy
- Most contain only mucous membrane layer
- Not congenital; congenital diverticulum more accurately called *duplication cyst*
- Usually asymptomatic
- If perforated, does not lead to pneumoperitoneum because usually retroperitoneal (usually off medial aspect of second portion of duodenum, which is retroperitoneal); extravasated air is contained in anterior pararenal space

DIVERTICULA, GASTRIC

Clinical

- Not common; if present, usually at cardia
- 75% occur on posterior wall
- Second most common location is prepyloric region, with about 15% of these occurring along greater curvature (85% along lesser curvature)

DIVERTICULITIS, OF COLON

Clinical

- Colonic diverticula are acquired herniations of the mucosa and portions of the submucosa through the muscularis propria
- Wall of diverticulum eroded, resulting in perforation
- Inflammatory process usually localized; free perforation into peritoneal cavity uncommon

Imaging

- CT is imaging study of choice in severe diverticulitis
- Barium study:
  Defer for 2 to 3 days to allow perforation to wall off
  Do a single-contrast study
  Most common finding is eccentric narrowing of lumen caused by pericolic or intramural inflammatory mass
  Spasm will be seen
  Most direct evidence of diverticulitis is demonstration of extraluminal collection of contrast material
- When considering this diagnosis, look for evidence of other diverticula elsewhere in colon; if none evident, then less likely to be diverticulitis

DUODENAL ATRESIA

Clinical

- Usually (80%) occurs distal to ampulla of Vater
- Higher incidence in those with Down syndrome

Imaging

- Classic double-bubble sign

DUPLICATION CYST, OF ESOPHAGUS

Clinical

- Also known as *gastroenteric cyst*
- Lined by esophageal, gastric, or small intestinal mucosa
- Also called *esophageal duplication*
- Rare lesion; presents as a round or oval posterior mediastinal mass
- Most are segmental, involving lower posterior mediastinum
- Both spherical and tubular duplications can be seen; spherical type generally does not communicate with esophageal lumen

Imaging

- Sometimes can localize with Tc^{99} pertechnetate (gastric mucosa)

ECTOPIC PANCREAS

Imaging

- Usually single
- Occur most frequently in distal stomach but can present in proximal second portion of duodenum

- Characteristic sign: fleck of barium in rudimentary central canal

ENDOMETRIOSIS

Clinical

- 15 to 20% of cases involve large bowel

Imaging

- Most frequent finding: single extramucosal mass associated with crenulated mucosal pattern
- Usually located along anterior wall of rectum or inferior wall of sigmoid

ENTERITIS, EOSINOPHILIC

Clinical

- Most commonly affects stomach and small bowel (jejunum mostly, although duodenum and proximal ileum may also be affected)
- Rarely involves colon
- Peripheral eosinophilia with infiltration of intestines with eosinophils and edema
- History of food allergy in about 66% of patients
- More common in young patients
- Responds to steroids

Imaging

- Initially, regular, symmetric thickening of folds when involving mucosa and lamina propria
- Later, extensive transmural involvement causes irregular fold thickening, angulation, and saw-toothed contour of small bowel

ENTERITIS, GIARDIAL

Clinical

- Present with diarrhea
- Spasm, irritability, hypermotility, and hypersecretion are other manifestations
- Fold pathology most apparent in duodenum and jejunum
- Folds have distinctively nodular appearance when seen on end

ENTERITIS, IN IMMUNOSUPPRESSED PATIENT

Clinical

- Cryptosporidiosis: proximal small bowel affected more often than distal; thick folds; mucosal atrophy (long standing); increased secretions
- CMV: thickened folds; can lead to ulceration and perforation

ENTERITIS, RADIATION

Clinical

- Minimum dose of 4200 to 4500 rads needed over 4-week period; usually seen when more than 6000 rads given
- Most develop within 6 months to 2 years after radiotherapy (although acute radiation enteritis is a clinical entity)
- Previous surgery increases risk of radiation enteritis, because small bowel loops often are fixed

Imaging

- Edema from progressive vasculitis leads to straight, thickened folds and spiked contour of bowel lumen; bowel loops separated by thick walls; abrupt angulations caused by fibrosis

ENTERITIS, *STRONGYLOIDES* SPP

Clinical

- May affect duodenum, but jejunum invariably also involved
- Most prominent in jejunum and duodenum with thick folds
- In severe cases, ulceration, paralytic dilatation
- In chronic disease, narrow, rigid jejunal loops with no mucosal folds

Imaging

- Findings in chronic disease: "lead pipe" appearance
- Findings in acute disease: nonspecific fold thickening

ENTERITIS, TB

Clinical

- Most common cause of inflammatory bowel disease in underdeveloped countries
- Predisposition for ileum and proximal colon
- Less than 50% of patients with intestinal involvement have lung disease
- Almost impossible to distinguish from Crohn's disease (but some say ulcers in TB are annular, whereas they are linear in Crohn's disease)

ENTERITIS, TYPHOID FEVER

Clinical

- Limited to terminal ileum

Imaging

- Proliferation of organisms in Peyer's patches of terminal ileum produces raised plaques, giving appearance of thickened mucosal folds
- No skip areas, no fistulas, and positive splenomegaly differentiate this entity from Crohn's disease

ENTERITIS, *YERSINIA* SPP

Clinical

- Terminal ileum most commonly involved site, but can affect entire small bowel and colon in severe cases
- Results in lymphoid hyperplasia, with subsequent smooth nodular terminal ileal lesions that can extend into ascending colon (more small bowel involvement than colonic involvement)
- Symptoms in children mimic appendicitis; may be more protracted in adults
- No proven effective therapy

Imaging

- Scattered small nodules, discrete punctate aphthous or larger ulcers may be seen
- Simulates Crohn's disease, but stenosis not a common feature
- Involvement of colon typically right sided, but left side can be involved
- Looks like Crohn's disease early in its course (irregular thickened folds, aphthous ulcerations, cobblestone appearance of mucosa), but it is transient; symptoms and lesions resolve completely within a few weeks

EOSINOPHILIC GASTROENTERITIS

Clinical

- Infiltration of GI tract by eosinophils
- Affects primarily the antrum (when it involves the stomach)
- Peripheral eosinophilia
- Pain, diarrhea, weight loss improved by steroids

Imaging

- Nodular pattern similar to that seen in small bowel
- Antral narrowing and rigidity

ESOPHAGITIS, CANDIDAL

Clinical

- Raised plaques and pseudomembrane formation
- Immunosuppressed patients

Imaging

- Spectrum of findings:
  - (1) Initially, abnormal motility seen
  - (2) Subsequently, small marginal filling defects with fine serrations
  - (3) Later, irregular cobblestone pattern
  - (4) Classic pattern: shaggy marginal contour caused by deep ulcerations and sloughing
- Mucosa diffusely abnormal, which helps differentiate candidiasis from infection with herpes and CMV, which typically give discrete ulcers on otherwise normal appearing mucosa

ESOPHAGITIS, CMV

Clinical

- Mimics herpes infection
- Initially, vesicles seen; these progress to ulcers
- Ulcers tend to be deep, seen especially in distal third of esophagus
- HIV patients
- Often enlarges despite therapy

ESOPHAGITIS, CORROSIVE

Clinical

- Strictures can occur as soon as 2 weeks after ingestion
- Causes changes most commonly seen in lower 66% of esophagus; alkali more damaging than acid in the esophagus (penetrates into deeper layers, whereas acid produces coagulative necrosis, inhibiting further penetration)
- Drugs can cause: tetracycline, potassium chloride most common, especially in patients with mitral valve disease and subsequent left atrial enlargement
- Increased incidence of carcinoma developing at site of stricture

ESOPHAGITIS, DRUG INDUCED

Clinical

- Ulcers tend to occur at places where tablets might temporarily lodge (proximal or middle esophagus) because of obstruction by a prominent aortic arch or ingestion immediately before retiring to sleep
- Several drugs can cause mucosal damage, including potassium chloride tablets, tetracycline, quinidine, and ascorbic acid

4

Imaging

- Ulceration sometimes has shape of tablet (i.e., square edges), which can be helpful in suggesting the diagnosis

ESOPHAGITIS, HERPETIC

Clinical

- Normal mucosal surface between discrete ulcers
- Site of infection may relate to area of previous trauma (i.e., nasogastric tube)
- Immunosuppressed patients
- Patients often do not have oral lesions

Imaging

- Typically multiple ulcers
- Although herpes ulceration can be indistinguishable from candidiasis, herpes typically causes discrete ulceration on otherwise normal mucosa, whereas mucosal abnormality tends to be more diffuse with candidiasis

ESOPHAGITIS, HIV

Clinical

- Electron microscopy shows cells infected with HIV (similar to HIV encephalitis)
- Recently described syndrome of odynophagia and giant esophageal ulcers
- May develop during acute HIV infection (immediately after seroconversion) but usually seen in patients who have had HIV for an extended period
- Some patients have characteristic distinctive maculopapular rash involving face, trunk, and upper extremities
- Once diagnosis is established (by negative cultures for other organisms on brushings, etc.), treatment is unclear; some advocate no treatment (self-limited), others suggest steroids or zidovudine (AZT)

Imaging

- Appear as giant, relatively flat, ovoid or irregular barium collections in middle or, less frequently, distal esophagus; small satellite ulcers may be seen nearby in some cases

ESOPHAGITIS, REFLUX

Clinical

- Associations:
  - Hiatal hernia
  - Zollinger-Ellison syndrome: increased acid in stomach; duodenal ulcers inhibit gastric emptying
  - Vomiting
  - Chalasia of infancy: lower esophageal sphincter fails to remain normally closed between swallows; found in immediate postnatal period
  - Pregnancy
  - Scleroderma
  - Medication
  - Surgery
- Complications: Barrett's esophagus, stricture, intramural pseudodiverticulosis

Imaging

- Single-contrast findings: hazy, serrated border; shallow, irregular protrusions; strictures
- Air-contrast findings

Mucosal granularity

Superficial erosions: longitudinal collection of barium surrounded by radiolucent halo

Ulcers

Strictures

"Wrinkled" mucosa secondary to transient contraction of longitudinal muscles results in fine transverse lines, known as *cat waves*; this finding associated with reflux; is a transient phenomenon

Caveats: air-producing granules attach to esophageal lumen and can produce false-positive studies

• May find inflammatory polyp associated with thick gastric fold

ESOPHAGITIS, TB

Clinical

• Rare
• When esophagus involved, usually through direct extension from infected mediastinal lymph nodes
• Most common manifestation in esophagus is single or multiple ulcers
• Intense fibrotic response causes narrowing of esophageal lumen
• Sinuses and fistulous tracts common
• HIV patients have been shown to develop TB ulcers, which tend to be deeper than HIV ulcers and may have associated sinus tracts

FAMILIAL ADENOMATOUS POLYPOSIS SYNDROME

Clinical

• Thought to represent a spectrum of the same disease; called *Gardner's syndrome* when associated osteomas and soft tissue lesions (epidermoid cysts most common) are present
• Autosomal dominant gene; 33% of cases arise from mutation, 66% inherited
• Cancer risk: 10% every 10 years (100% will get cancer by age 100 years)
• Polyps present by age 15 to 20 years; 2 to 5 mm in size
• Surgery performed in mid to late teens
• Numerous extracolonic manifestations, as follows

Gastric involvement
• Fundal gastric polyp; 20 to 60% of patients; not premalignant; spares antrum; can also occur in patients without polyposis syndromes, usually middle-aged women
• Gastric adenomas: more prevalent in Japan than in United States; preferentially involve antrum; premalignant, a few cases of adenocarcinoma reported
• Recommendation: follow polyps closely, no prophylactic gastrectomy

Duodenal involvement
• 60 to 100% of patients; second most common site of involvement after colon; multiple and small, hard to detect radiographically; premalignant

Periampullary involvement
• 12% of patients develop periampullary carcinoma

Jejunal and ileal involvement
• 60% incidence of polyps in Japanese literature

Mesenteric fibromatosis
• Aggressive fibrous tumor, locally invasive but without metastases; high rate of occurrence after colectomy

Skeletal/dental involvement
• Multiple osteomas; common sites: outer table skull, angle mandible, frontal sinus; may precede GI signs; long bone cortical hyperostosis

Skin and eye involvement
- Epidermal cysts in 65%

Thyroid involvement
- Increased risk of thyroid cancer (papillary type); ratio of women to men affected 4:1; ages 15 to 35 years

Imaging

GI tract
- Filling defects

Mesenteric fibromatosis
- Radiographic findings: noncalcified soft tissue mass that may displace loops; homogeneous, no necrosis (helps distinguish from lymphoma, leiomyosarcoma)
- Hyperechoic or hypoechoic on ultrasound

Skeletal/dental involvement
- Focal densities at sites of osteomas
- Long bone cortical hyperostosis

FIBROVASCULAR POLYP, OF ESOPHAGUS

Clinical

- Rare, but second most common type of solid benign tumor of esophagus

Imaging

- Large intraluminal filling defect
- Oval-shaped or elongated with smooth or mildly lobulated surface
- Barium can be observed to completely surround the tumor

GASTRITIS, CHRONIC EROSIVE

Clinical

- Also known as *varioliform* or *verrucous gastritis*
- Cause unknown; may relate to peptic acid secretion and/or food allergy
- Single or multiple punctate erosions surrounded by elevated rim of mucosa

GASTRITIS, CORROSIVE

Clinical

- Acid or alkali
- Leads to strictures
- Antral narrowing most common resultant deformity

GASTRITIS, INFECTIOUS

- Phlegmonous:
  - Bacterial invasion causes thickening of wall of stomach
  - Duodenum and esophagus usually spared
  - Usually caused by alpha hemolytic streptococci
  - Other agents include staphylococci, *Escherichia coli*, *Clostridium welchii*, pneumococci, and *Proteus* spp
  - Fulminating and usually fatal
  - Bubbles of gas may be seen in wall of stomach, a poor prognostic sign
- Candidal infection in immunocompromised patients
- Unusual infectious cause is anisakiasis, caused by *Anisakis* worm, which causes generalized coarse, broad gastric folds; can demonstrate threadlike filling defect about 30 mm in length, representing larva itself

GIARDIASIS

Clinical

- Most common infection involving duodenum
- Increased intestinal secretions and irritability

Imaging

- Causes thick folds in duodenum and jejunum

GLYCOGENIC ACANTHOSIS

Clinical

- Common benign condition; multiple white plaques seen at endoscopy, and they create a nodular appearance
- 3 to 15% incidence in the population
- Degenerative condition in which glycogen accumulates intracellularly
- Patients asymptomatic
- No malignant potential

HEMANGIOMA, OF BOWEL

Clinical

- Rare, but frequently misdiagnosed at endoscopy
- Associated with high mortality rate as result of bleeding
- Consider tuberous sclerosis, Turner's syndrome, Osler-Weber-Rendu syndrome, and blue rubber bleb nevus syndrome

Imaging

- Phleboliths may be found
- Usually located in rectum or sigmoid colon
- Suspect the diagnosis whenever plain films demonstrate phleboliths in young patient with GI bleeding or when phleboliths occur in clusters along expected course of rectosigmoid colon
- Generally not big enough to be seen on barium studies
- Barium enema can show circumferential lesion with scalloped contours and nodular mucosal pattern

HENOCH-SCHÖNLEIN PURPURA

Clinical

- Affects children and young to middle-aged adults
- Affects skin, joints, kidneys, and GI tract
- Classic clinical triad: palpable purpura (nonthrombocytopenic), arthritis, and abdominal pain
- Cause unknown; presumed related to allergic vasculitis
- Edematous mucosa with features of congestion and hemorrhage on barium studies
- Intussusceptions can occur in childhood form, but unusual in adults

Imaging

- Straightened and thickened folds on barium studies
- Lumen usually widened
- Tends to involve small bowel

HERNIA, GASTROESOPHAGEAL

Clinical

Hiatal hernia
- Gastroesophageal junction above diaphragmatic hiatus
- "Lines" to remember:
  - B ring demarcates stomach from esophagus and should lie at diaphragm (if higher, hiatal hernia present)
  - A ring marks beginning of esophageal ampulla
  - Z line demarcates transition from squamous cell epithelium to columnar epithelium

Paraesophageal hernia
- Gastroesophageal junction in normal location, but portion of fundus of stomach lies above hiatus
- Distal esophagus usually displaced posteriorly and to right
- Unusual type of paraesophageal hernia: fundus herniates through separate congenital defect in diaphragm; exceedingly rare

HETEROTOPIC GASTRIC MUCOSA

Imaging

- Finely nodular pattern formed by abruptly marginated, angular filling defects ranging from 1 to 6 mm
- Generally restricted to bulb (differentiates it from benign lymphoid hyperplasia)
- Filling defects smaller and more numerous than those seen with Brunner's gland hyperplasia

HYPERPLASTIC POLYP, OF COLON

Clinical

- Represents degenerative changes in mucosa
- Because radiographic findings are nonspecific, diagnosis made only by pathologist

Imaging

- Indistinguishable from sessile adenomas
- Usually less than 5 mm in size but can be larger with about 10% larger than 1 cm
- Minority of lesions are pedunculated

HYPERPLASTIC POLYP, OF STOMACH

Clinical

- Accounts for 75 to 90% of all gastric polyps
- Not premalignant
- Probably represents excessive regenerative hyperplasia in areas of chronic gastritis
- Majority less than 1 cm

Imaging

- Smooth, sessile, round or oval lesions
- Range in size from 5 to 10 mm
- Tend to be clustered in gastric fundus or body
- Be careful not to mistake an anterior wall polyp with a hanging droplet of barium for a central ulceration on a posterior wall polyp

INTUSSUSCEPTION, IN ADULTS

Clinical

- Uncommon
- Colonic intussusception usually caused by colon cancer

- Small bowel intussusception usually related to benign tumor or metastatic lesion
- Often chronic and relapsing in adults, so history often reflects recurrent episodes of subacute obstruction

Imaging

- Plain film:
    "Crescent" sign is virtually pathognomonic and may be seen
- Barium studies:
    Coiled spring appearance of contrast trapped between intussusceptum and intussuscipiens
    Hydrostatic or pneumatic reduction usually contraindicated in adults because of high incidence of malignant cause that will require laparatomy anyway
- Ultrasound:
    Target-like lesion, resulting from hypoechoic rim caused by mesentery and edematous wall of intussuscipiens and hyperechoic center produced by compressed mucosal, submucosal, and serosal interfaces
- CT:
    Target sign (analogous to that described for ultrasound); sausage-shaped mass with alternating layers of high and low attenuation; reniform mass

ISCHEMIA, OF COLON

Clinical

- Usually related to decreased blood flow (low-flow states) or small vessel disease; occlusion of large vessels rare
- Patients usually older than 50 years

Imaging

- Thumbprinting classic plain film and barium enema finding of actively ischemic bowel
- Other findings include transverse ridging, spasm, and ulceration
- In late stages, barium enema demonstrates strictures
- Barium enema should not be done if gangrene or perforation is suspected or if diffuse peritoneal signs are present
- Because pathogenesis usually relates to low-flow states rather than occlusion, angiography often not of great value and generally not indicated; rather, colonoscopy can be helpful to establish the diagnosis and to exclude other causes

ISCHEMIA, OF SMALL BOWEL

Clinical

- Acute occlusive ischemia most often caused by thrombosis, usually involving proximal segment of SMA, resulting in extensive infarction
- Acute segmental ischemia may occur from occlusion of small arteries (emboli) but is usually nonocclusive in origin, resulting from severe vasoconstriction of intramural arterioles, which occurs with sudden decreased cardiac output or occasionally with digitalis ingestion

Imaging

- Plain films:
    Rigid, narrowed, thickened loops of small bowel
    "Stacked coin" appearance of symmetrically thickened valvulae conniventes
    Thumbprinting: occurs as edema progresses
    Spasm and hypermotility favorable signs; dilatation and stasis imply transmural infarction
    Localized perforations form "pneumatosis intestinalis"
- Angiography:
    Thrombus may be seen; these patients may benefit from low-dose streptokinase

Mesenteric vasoconstriction may be seen; intraarterial infusion of vasodilators such as tolazoline and papaverine may reverse the vasoconstrictive changes
- CT

Often done first because of nonspecific presentation

Pneumatosis intestinalis and portal venous gas are late findings

Excludes other processes

Thrombosis of SMA, pneumoperitoneum, bowel dilatation, bowel wall thickening

Unremarkable CT does not exclude the diagnosis
- Sequelae of ischemia: fistulas, sinus tracts can occur; healing can lead to strictures, pseudodiverticula

ISLET CELL TUMOR

Clinical

- 10% located in duodenal wall
- Hypervascular

Imaging

- *See Imaging of Abdominal Viscera*

JUVENILE POLYPOSIS

Clinical

- Two main categories: isolated juvenile polyp of childhood and juvenile polyposis of colon or entire GI tract

Juvenile polyp
- Hamartoma with low risk of malignant change
- Although often solitary, can be multiple with 25% of patients having more than four polyps
- Often located in rectum, but more than half are not
- Present with painless bleeding
- Spontaneous autoamputation common

Juvenile polyposis of colon or GI tract
- Diagnostic criteria include the presence of six or more juvenile polyps in colon or rectum, juvenile polyps throughout GI tract, and/or juvenile polyps in patients with family history of juvenile polyposis
- Patients have increased risk of developing malignancy
- About 25% of cases transmitted genetically as autosomal dominant trait

KAPOSI'S SARCOMA

Clinical

- AIDS-related neoplasm
- Occurs more frequently in homosexual and bisexual men with AIDS than in intravenous drug users
- Skin lesions generally antedate GI involvement
- Characteristic appearance on endoscopy

Imaging

- Barium studies:

Typically 1 to 2 cm, well defined, smooth and nodular, reflecting submucosal origin

Central umbilication may be noted, resulting in "bull's eye" or "target" appearance, but not seen in most lesions
- CT:

Isolated area of nodular mural thickening highly suggestive of Kaposi's sarcoma in patients with AIDS; other causes of bowel wall thickening in AIDS patients either more diffuse (infections) or bulky (lymphoma)

Mild or absent lymphadenopathy (compared with common presence of lymphadenopathy in lymphoma)

Involved lymph nodes may show striking enhancement

LARYNGOCELE

Clinical

- Result from obstruction of laryngeal ventricle with subsequent enlargement of its appendix
- Most contain air, but may contain fluid, particularly when infected

LEIOMYOMA, OF ESOPHAGUS

Clinical

- Most common benign tumor of esophagus (51% of benign tumors)
- Intramural mass
- Unlike gastric leiomyomas, rarely bleed or ulcerate
- Most frequently found in lower third of esophagus
- Most asymptomatic, found incidentally

Imaging

- Smooth, rounded
- No evidence of infiltration, ulceration
- May have large extramural component
- Rarely, may contain enough calcium to be visible radiographically; presence of amorphous calcification in retrocardiac esophageal mass diagnostic of leiomyoma

LEIOMYOMA, OF STOMACH

Clinical

- Most common benign tumor of stomach (40%)
- Usually single, 1 to 2% multiple
- Can be very large
- Tend to bleed
- 5% demonstrate coarse calcification
- Can be intraluminal, intramural, or extramural

Imaging

- Usually presents as discrete submucosal mass, but exophytic lesions exist; these tent gastric wall because of traction by base or pedicle of the mass
- May have punctate, granular, or finely stippled calcification

LEIOMYOSARCOMA

Clinical

- Intramural, bulky, often with huge ulcerations; not infiltrative like adenocarcinoma
- Rarely spread to lymph nodes; rather, invade and spread hematogenously to liver, less commonly to lung
- Extensive neovascularity

Imaging

- Present as lobulated intramural filling defects, often with central ulceration
- Hypervascular by angiography
- Both hypoechoic and echogenic appearances by ultrasound have been described

4

LEUKOPLAKIA, OF ESOPHAGUS
Clinical

- Small, round foci of epithelial hyperplasia
- No impairment of peristalsis
- Most commonly located in middle third of esophagus

LIPOMA
Clinical

- Next most common benign neoplasm of colon after adenoma
- Right side more frequently affected, especially in cecum
- Usually asymptomatic

Imaging

- Sessile submucosal mass or polypoid lesion on broad-based pedicle
- Sharply demarcated
- Pliable; thus, may change shape with palpation or change in position
- CT allows definitive diagnosis

LYMPHANGIECTASIA
Clinical

- Bowel wall filled with dilated lymphatics
- Congenital or acquired
- Protein loss secondary to rupture of dilated lymphatics

Imaging

- Diffuse thickened folds with fine nodularity
- Increased secretions
- Has a diffuse enteric involvement in comparison to the more proximal involvement of Whipple's disease

LYMPHOGRANULOMA VENEREUM (LGV)
Clinical

- Caused by *Chlamydia trachomatis*
- Often related to anal intercourse
- Leads to proctitis
- Characterized by deep ulceration, stricturing, and rectovaginal fistulas

LYMPHOID FOLLICLES
Clinical

- Multiple, uniformly sized, round nodular elevations; 1 to 4 mm in diameter, evenly distributed on otherwise normal mucosa
- Normal feature on barium enema in younger patients
- Frequently associated with neoplasms (90%) when seen in older patients (over 40 years of age); therefore, if lymphoid follicles are seen on barium enema of older patient, look carefully for neoplasm

LYMPHOMA, OF COLON
Clinical

- Colon third most common primary site of lymphoma involving GI tract (after stomach and small bowel)
- Non-Hodgkin's lymphoma accounts for practically all colonic lymphomas

Imaging

- Wide spectrum of appearances:
    Multiple nodules
    Large polypoid intraluminal mass
    Less common appearances include focal stricturing, aneurysmal dilatation, large ulcerating mass with multiple fistulas

LYMPHOMA, OF DUODENUM

Clinical

- Rare in duodenum as primary
- More commonly, duodenum invaded by retroperitoneal lymphoma or extension of gastric lymphoma, or involved as part of generalized lymphoma

Imaging

- Presents as polypoid mass or multiple small nodules producing a cobblestone appearance

LYMPHOMA, OF ESOPHAGUS

Clinical

- Rare as primary in esophagus
- Transcardial extension of gastric lymphoma, occurs in 2 to 10%

Imaging

- Contiguous nodular involvement of both distal esophagus and stomach
- If grows inward toward lumen, can appear as filling defect
- If remains confined to submucosa, can resemble varices

LYMPHOMA, OF SMALL BOWEL

Clinical

- Distribution: localized to one segment in about 75% of patients, most frequently the ileum; may be discrete mass or nodule; multiple lesions in 10 to 20%
- Usually, non-Hodgkin's lymphoma in small bowel; if Hodgkin's, result is marked fibrosis
- 20% of primary malignant tumors in small bowel are lymphoma
- Lymphoma tends to involve ileum, whereas adenocarcinoma more common in proximal small bowel and duodenum; both can result in regional lymph node enlargement
- 25% of patients with disseminated lymphoma have small bowel involvement at autopsy, but often incidental finding
- May be complication of long-standing sprue (in which case it is T-cell lymphoma, rather than the usual B-cell type)

Imaging

- Spectrum of radiologic findings:
    Mesenteric mass
        Results in mass effect along mesenteric border of small intestine, with spiculation and tethering of small bowel loops
        Thickened nodular folds in region of tethering indicate areas of tumor invasion
    Mantle of enlarged lymph nodes: "sandwich sign"
    Bowel wall thickening, occasionally constricting napkin-ring lesion
        Usually fairly long segment as opposed to adenocarcinoma
        Does not tend to obstruct
    Aneurysmal dilatation of bowel (after necrosis and cavitation)

LYMPHOMA, OF STOMACH

Clinical

- Represents 5% of stomach tumors (95% are adenocarcinomas)
- Location of lymphoma in GI tract: stomach, 50%; small bowel, 30 to 40%; ileocecal, 12 to 15%; colon, 10%
- Size: most more than 5 cm, average about 10 cm
- Stomach most common extranodal location for lymphoma (15 to 20% of patients)
- Hodgkin's disease rare in stomach; more common cell types are diffuse histiocytic and poorly differentiated non-Hodgkin's lymphoma
- Does not obstruct GI tract (unless it is Hodgkin's disease)
- Secondary involvement of intestinal tract occurs in more than 50% of patients with non-Hodgkin's lymphoma and 10 to 20% of patients with Hodgkin's disease
- Presents in sixth decade

Imaging

- Location: no predilection for antrum (as there is in gastric adenocarcinoma)
- Patterns: no pathognomonic appearance
      Large masses, especially if nodular or with bizarre forms
      Large single ulcer or multiple ulcers
      Combination of masses and ulcers
      Rarely, manifested only by large gastric folds and some rigidity of stomach
      Linitis plastica appearance can be seen with Hodgkin's disease
- Extension
      10% into esophagus (same as adenocarcinoma)
      33% into duodenum (six times that of adenocarcinoma), but because adenocarcinoma is more common, cannot use extension as a differential point
- CT features:
      Focal gastric wall thickening with distortion of the normal rugal fold pattern is the hallmark of gastric lymphoma on CT
      Absence of obstruction
- Can be difficult to differentiate from carcinoma: more flexible gastric wall, enlarged spleen, associated prominence of regional lymph nodes all favor lymphoma

MALLORY-WEISS TEAR

Clinical

- Involves only mucosa
- Most tears gastric (76%); remainder gastroesophageal or esophageal
- Most commonly result of vomiting
- 25% of patients have multiple tears

Imaging

- Often hard to demonstrate radiographically

MASTOCYTOSIS

Clinical

- Mast cell proliferation of dermis, reticuloendothelial system, and bowel wall
- Coarse nodular thickening of small bowel folds
- Patients with mastocytosis at increased risk for developing peptic ulcer disease (PUD) (secondary to histamine release by mast cells)

Imaging

- Look for dense bones

MECKEL'S DIVERTICULUM

Clinical

- Represents persistence of omphalomesenteric duct
- Located on antimesenteric border of ileum

- Rule of 2s: occurs in 2% of population, 20% develop complications, complications usually occur before age 2 years, and usually located 2 feet from ileocecal valve
- Most frequent clinical manifestation is GI bleeding; less common complications include intestinal obstruction and inflammation; those with bleeding contain ectopic gastric mucosa (present in 25% of all patients, 50% of symptomatic patients, and over 90% of bleeding patients)
- Complications:
  Bleeding
  Inflammation
  Small bowel obstruction by ileoileal intussusception, small bowel volvulus, internal hernia, local inflammation
  Perforation
  Enterolith formation
  Formation of giant diverticulum

Imaging

- Radionuclide scanning with Tc^{99} pertechnetate can be done to detect gastric mucosa, which is found in 80 to 90% of asymptomatic pediatric patients but less than 50% of adults
- Modality of choice to detect ectopic gastric mucosa in Meckel's diverticulum: nuclear scintigraphy; false positives occur with appendicitis, peptic ulcer, hemangioma, abscess, intussusception, Crohn's disease, lymphoma of small bowel, dilated renal pelvis, and partial ureteral obstruction

MÉNÉTRIER'S DISEASE

Clinical

- Protein-losing enteropathy associated with huge gastric rugal folds secondary to marked submucosal edema of stomach
- Particularly prominent along greater curvature
- May have malignant potential
- Usually hyposecretion of acid and excessive secretion of gastric mucus occur
- Two distinct forms:
  Acute but transient form in children, in whom disease usually is benign and self-limited
  Chronic form primarily affects adults
- Symptoms include pain, vomiting, peripheral edema, GI bleeding, and weight loss
- Associated with benign gastric ulcers, even though acid production is absent or decreased (acid has little to do with gastric ulcers; it plays a role in duodenal ulcers)

Imaging

- Thickened gastric rugae contort in convolutional pattern suggestive of gyri and sulci of brain
  In children, folds are thickened throughout stomach
  In adults, generally limited to fundus and body, with little or no involvement of antrum
- Peristalsis and motility often sluggish

MOTILITY, OF ESOPHAGUS

Imaging

- Three phases, as follows

Primary peristalsis
- "Major stripping wave": upper end of barium column assumes an inverted V-shaped configuration

Secondary peristalsis
- Stripping waves similar to those in primary peristalsis but elicited by distention or irritation anywhere along esophagus

- Radiographic appearance similar to that of primary peristalsis, but originates in body of esophagus

Tertiary contractions
- Uncoordinated, nonpropulsive, segmental contractions
- Function unknown
- Seen as annular or segmental contractions simultaneously displacing barium both orally and aborally from site of contraction
- Repetitive tertiary contractions not seen in normal young adults but can be seen in about 10% of normal adults in fourth to sixth decades of life

NEURENTERIC CYSTS

Clinical

- Also known as the "split notochord" syndrome
- Results from incomplete separation of foregut from notochord
- Typically connect by stalk to meninges, often maintain attachment to esophagus
- Associated with vertebral anomalies, particularly hemivertebra, spina bifida, and scoliosis

NEUROPATHY, OF ESOPHAGUS

- Variety of causes
     (1) Cerebrovascular accident (CVA)
     (2) Postvagotomy syndrome
          Typically occurs with solid foods on postoperative days 7 to 14
          Usually disappears spontaneously and completely within 2 months
     (3) Diabetes
     (4) Chronic idiopathic intestinal pseudoobstruction
     (5) Amyloidosis
     (6) Alcoholism
          Selective deterioration of esophageal peristalsis most pronounced in distal portion, with preservation of sphincter function

OBSTRUCTION, OF COLON

Clinical

- Usually caused by cancer
- Although numerous other causes of colonic obstruction exist, most common to remember include diverticulitis, volvulus, intussusception, adhesions, hernias, strictures, and extrinsic masses

Imaging

- Plain films correctly suggest diagnosis of obstruction in 60 to 70% of patients; however, about 20% of patients have no plain film evidence of obstruction
- If obstruction is suspected, first imaging procedure generally is an enema, usually with water soluble medium so as not to preclude CT or colonoscopy (if patient has pseudoobstruction, barium remains in colon for days)
- Once the colon is cleared by enema examination, next imaging test is somewhat controversial; traditionally, upper GI with small bowel follow-through (SBFT) performed with barium, but recent studies have demonstrated utility of CT

OBSTRUCTION, OF SMALL BOWEL

- Suspect if more than two air-fluid levels seen
- Causes:
     Extrinsic bowel lesions
          (1) Adhesions: most common cause
          (2) Hernias: second most common cause, external or internal (through mesentery)
          (3) Masses

  (4) Volvulus
  (5) Congenital bands
Luminal lesions
  (1) Tumor
  (2) Gallstone
  (3) Foreign body
  (4) Bezoar
  (5) Intussusception: no leading edge pathology in 20% of adult cases and almost all pediatric cases
  (6) Meconium ileus
Bowel wall
  (1) Strictures: neoplastic, inflammatory, chemical, anastomotic, radiation therapy, amyloid
  (2) Vascular insufficiency
  (3) Congenital atresia or stenosis: triple-bubble sign of jejunal atresia

4

PAPILLOMA, OF ESOPHAGUS

Clinical

- All reported esophageal papillomas have been benign, but malignant potential remains uncertain
- Lesions very small, so diagnostic frequency may be underestimated
- Solitary lesions, usually 0.5 to 1.5 cm
- Rarely, multiple lesions present in condition called *esophageal papillomatosis*
- Most patients asymptomatic

Imaging

- Sessile, smooth, or slightly lobulated
- Can mimic early esophageal carcinoma

PEPTIC ULCER DISEASE (PUD)

Clinical

- Only 5% of benign PUD gives postbulbar ulcers

Imaging

- Shallow, flattened niche on medial aspect (rarely lateral) of upper second portion of duodenum; usually associated with an incisura, an indentation defect on opposite duodenal margin

PERFORATION, OF ESOPHAGUS

Clinical

- Causes:
 Iatrogenic most common
  (1) Endoscopy
   0.1% incidence
  (2) Pneumatic dilatation for achalasia
   4 to 5% incidence
  (3) Sengstaken-Blakemore tubes
   35% incidence
 Spontaneous (Boerhaave's syndrome)
- In adults, spontaneous perforation almost always occurs along left posterior wall of lower esophagus
- Boerhaave's syndrome usually result of repetitive forceful emesis

Imaging

- Air can reach potential space lying between parietal pleura and left crus of diaphragm, accounting for V-shaped gas collection (superomedial to stomach fundus) described by Naclerio (Naclerio's sign)
- 25% of perforations are missed when water soluble contrast used; barium is the contrast of choice after frank perforation is excluded by water soluble agent
- Boerhaave's syndrome can present as left pleural effusion with pneumomediastinum

PEUTZ-JEGHERS SYNDROME

Clinical

- Autosomal dominant
- Polyps are hamartomas in small bowel; in stomach, duodenum, and colon they can be adenomatous
- No risk of malignancy for hamartomatous polyps in small bowel
- Slightly increased risk of carcinoma in stomach, duodenum, and colon as result of adenomatous polyps

Imaging

- Polyps found predominantly in small bowel (too numerous to count)
- When polyps occur in colon, fewer present compared with small bowel (usually approximately 1:10)

PNEUMATOSIS CYSTOIDES COLI

Clinical

- Multiple gas-containing cysts in bowel wall
- Vary in size from few millimeters to centimeters
- Most commonly seen in left colon
- Cause unknown
- Some patients have chronic obstructive pulmonary disease or pyloric obstruction, possibly related to cause of this condition

POSTCRICOID IMPRESSION

Clinical

- Anterior impression
- Lax mucosal folds over submucosal pharyngeal venous plexus
- Occurs at about C6 level
- Seen in 70 to 90% of adults
- No clinical significance

PRESBYESOPHAGUS

Imaging

- Components:
    - (1) Failure of complete peristaltic wave
    - (2) Tertiary contractions
    - (3) Aperistalsis (no muscular response to swallowing)
    - (4) Absence of contraction of lower esophageal sphincter (LES) or failure of relaxation of LES

PSEUDODIVERTICULOSIS, OF ESOPHAGUS

Clinical

- Not true diverticula; rather, represent dilated submucosal glands
- These diverticula harbor *Candida* spp in 50%; fungus not believed to be causative, however, but related to reflux

- Approximately 93% associated with esophageal strictures located above level of pseudodiverticula
- Esophagitis cystica a variation in which glands become obstructed and secreted mucus forms retention cysts
- Dysphagia in 75%

Imaging

- Stricture found in approximately 90% of cases; located in upper third of esophagus in 66% of cases (above pseudodiverticulum)
- Associated stricture usually smooth
- Pseudodiverticula seen as numerous flask-shaped, pinhead-sized outpouchings

PSEUDOLYMPHOMA

Clinical

- Gastric lymphoid hyperplasia
- Thought to represent nonspecific late reaction to chronic PUD
- Has been described in small bowel

Imaging

- Characterized by large ulcer with surrounded mass and associated regional or generalized enlargement of rugal folds

PSEUDOMEMBRANOUS COLITIS

Clinical

- Often caused by *Clostridium difficile*
- Clinical setting: patient receiving antibiotics has sudden onset of watery diarrhea, often with fever, abdominal pain, and leukocytosis

Imaging

- CT may show marked, low-density mural thickening with swollen haustra and thin, intervening streaks of trapped contrast material
- Small, irregular plaques seen on mucosal surface on air-contrast barium enema; thumbprinting noted on single-contrast barium enema

SCHATZKI RING

Imaging

- Concentric narrowing several centimeters above diaphragm marking junction between esophageal and gastric mucosae; if luminal opening more than 12 to 13 mm, obstructive symptoms unlikely; should be called Schatzki ring only if diameter less than 13 mm (size of a barium tablet)

SCLERODERMA, OF DUODENUM AND SMALL BOWEL

Imaging

- Usually affects duodenum with dilatation
- Generally no increased secretions
- Most dramatic change is diminished peristaltic activity
- Decrease in distance between valvulae conniventes ("hidebound" appearance) differentiates it from other causes of dilatation such as obstruction or sprue
- Pseudosacculation of small bowel may occur (intermittent fibrosis leading to outpouching)
- Rarely, intramural pneumatosis
- Dermatomyositis can give picture identical to that of scleroderma

4

SCLERODERMA, OF ESOPHAGUS

Clinical

- Striated muscle not affected by scleroderma
- Can occur in any portion of GI tract, resulting in poor motility, dilatation, and sacculation

Imaging

- Normal stripping wave that clears upper esophagus (striated muscle not affected by scleroderma) but stops at about the level of the aortic arch will be seen
- In contrast to achalasia, barium flows rapidly through LES when patient is upright
- Dilated esophagus with wide-open LES; therefore, high incidence of reflux esophagitis and subsequent strictures
- Other connective tissue diseases that can mimic scleroderma are systemic lupus erythematosus, Raynaud's disease, rheumatoid arthritis, Sjögren's syndrome, and mixed connective tissue disease (may affect entire esophagus)

SHIGELLOSIS

Clinical

- Infection may occur in outbreaks; increased prevalence in homosexuals
- Shigella produces diarrhea-causing toxin that can be absorbed, leading to extraintestinal symptoms
- Infection usually self-limiting

Imaging

- Predominantly left-sided colitis
- Ulceration common: deep ulcers that may have collar button appearance; aphthous ulcers; flat ulcers

SMA SYNDROME

Clinical

- Term used to describe the obstruction of third portion of duodenum by overlying SMA
- Causes:
  Asthenic persons
  Congenitally small vascular angle
  Prolonged bed rest or immobilization
  Weight loss (loss of retroperitoneal fat)
  Can be seen in patients with reduced duodenal peristalsis
  Can be seen with any space-occupying process within aorticomesenteric angle (i.e., inflammatory thickening of bowel wall or mesenteric root)

Imaging

- Pronounced dilatation of first and second portions of duodenum
- To differentiate from organic obstruction, patient should assume prone or left decubitus position under fluoroscopy; with organic obstruction, little relief of obstruction should occur, whereas with SMA syndrome, there should be relief

SPRUE

Clinical

Celiac/nontropical
- Celiac and nontropical sprue basically same disease in different age groups (celiac sprue occurs in children)
- Caused by intolerance to gluten (allergic response)
- Steatorrhea

- Association with intestinal malignancy (lymphomas; carcinomas less commonly)

Tropical
- Infectious origin
- Malabsorption leads to deficiency of folic acid and vitamin B12 (uncommon in celiac disease)
- Responds to antibiotic therapy and folic acid administration
- Radiologic findings similar to those in celiac disease

Imaging

- Usually in mid and distal jejunum
- Dilatation of small bowel, typically in mid bowel; degree correlates with degree of steatorrhea
- Usually transit time slowed
- Variability in fold pattern:
    In jejunum, folds of normal thickness but decreased in number
    In some cases, prominent folds, particularly in duodenum
    In ileum, prominent folds create "jejunization" appearance
    Occasionally folds diminished and rarely lost, creating "moulage" sign (develops when increased secretions obscure mucosal folds)
- Secretions
    Flocculation of barium used to be seen secondary to secretions but no longer seen with new barium preparations
    Leads to dilution of barium
- Can exhibit transient intussusception ("coiled-spring" appearance)
- Ulceration rare

SQUAMOUS CELL CARCINOMA, OF ESOPHAGUS
Clinical

- Most common histology (90%)
- Dissemination via direct extension, lymphatic diffusion, and hematogenous spread
- Lymphatic diffusion:
    May travel to nodes quite distant from orignal tumor
    10 to 20% with cervical esophageal carcinoma will have metastases in celiac chain of subdiaphragmatic nodes
- Verrucous carcinoma: unusual subtype; locally aggressive, not invasive, rarely metastatic
- Rarely presents with bleeding, usually with dysphagia
- Overall 5-year survival, 4 to 10%
- Risk factors: tobacco, alcohol, caustic stricture, achalasia, prior head and neck cancer, Plummer-Vinson syndrome
- More proximal lesions technically more difficult to resect

Imaging

- Early radiologic finding: flat, plaquelike lesion, occasionally with central ulceration; as cancer progresses, luminal irregularities occur; advanced lesions encircle lumen completely
- Appearances: fungating (60%); ulcerative (25%); intramural, presenting as benign stricture (15%)
- Rare presentation: varicoid carcinoma (looks like varix); does not collapse, differentiating it from varices
- CT good for detecting invasion (but not into aorta)
- CT not sensitive for assessing nodal involvement because many involved nodes are not enlarged
- Remember to look at celiac chain of nodes

SQUAMOUS CELL CARCINOMA, OF OROPHARYNX
Clinical

- Spread: early to cervical lymph nodes; hematogenous metastases to lung, mediastinum, ribs, liver occur later

4

- Specific locations and behavior
  - (1) Base of tongue: exophytic irregular mass
  - (2) Supraglottic tumor: tends to remain compartmentalized; thus, may spread extensively to aryepiglottic fold, false vocal cord, preepiglottic space, and paralaryngeal space without involving true vocal cord
  - (3) Hypopharynx: most commonly arises from pyriform sinus; can extend through thyrohyoid membrane or cricothyroid articulation; tumors arising from posterior pharygeal wall or in postcricoid region anteriorly the most aggressive
- Multiple primary tumors in 15%
- Verrucous carcinoma relatively uncommon type of epidermoid cancer that spreads in plaquelike fashion rather than extending deeply into submucosa; occurs in 1 to 2% of patients

SPINDLE CELL SARCOMA, OF ESOPHAGUS

Clinical

- Also called *carcinosarcoma* or *pseudosarcoma*
- Tumor of connective tissue origin
- Metastases do not occur until late, so survival rates better than those of squamous cell carcinoma

Imaging

- Often bulky, intraluminal mass
- Tends not to ulcerate and constrict as squamous cell does

TOXIC MEGACOLON

Clinical

- Most severe complication of ulcerative colitis, potentially fatal
- Extensive inflammation leads to disintegration of normal tissue cohesion and decreased muscle tone, resulting in paper-thin, dilated colon
- Can complicate other forms of colitis, including ischemic colitis, Crohn's disease, and pseudomembranous colitis

Imaging

- Hallmark of toxic megacolon is dilatation
- Cecum should not measure more than 9 cm in diameter and transverse colon should not measure more than 6 cm in diameter
- Although colonic wall is pathologically thin in this condition, it appears thick on plain films
- Barium studies should not be performed

TURCOT'S SYNDROME

Clinical

- Intracerebral tumors (usually glioblastomas) and colon polyps (adenomatous)
- Autosomal recessive
- Occurs in patients in their teens
- Patients usually die of brain tumor before colon becomes a clinical issue

TYPHLITIS

Clinical

- Word derived from Greek *typhlon*, meaning cecum
- Refers to inflammatory changes seen in cecum of patients with agranulocytosis, usually after chemotherapy for leukemia

• These changes include inflammatory infiltration, bleeding, infection, ischemia

Imaging

• Ileocecal dilatation with air-fluid levels
• Small bowel obstruction
• Marked low-density mural thickening in right colon on CT
• Thumbprinting
• Most important differential consideration to exclude is *C. difficile* infection

ULCER, GASTRIC

Imaging

Benign-appearing ulcers
• Penetration: projection of ulcer outside normal barium-filled gastric lumen
• Hampton line, ulcer collar, ulcer mound: represent overhanging resistant mucosal layer; most reliable sign of benign ulcer is Hampton line; ulcer collar and mound are less so (these are thicker)
• In mound, benignancy suggested by:
  Central ulcer location
  Smooth, sharply delineated, gently sloping, and symmetrically convex tissue around ulcer
  Smooth, obtuse angle of margin of mound with adjacent normal gastric wall
• Crescent sign: trapped barium in benign ulcer with occluding overhanging mucosa
• Radiation of mucosal folds to edge of crater: smooth, slender, appear to extend into edge of crater
• Size and contour of base have no relationship to malignancy or benignancy
• Location: no significance except in fundus above level of cardia, where all ulcers should be considered malignant
• Caveat: benign ulcers along greater curvature do not show same characteristic radiographic features of benignancy seen in more common lesser curvature ulcers because they can cause spasm in the abundant musculature and therefore appear intraluminal
• Ellipse sign: used to determine if collection of barium represents acute ulceration or nonulcerating deformity
  If long axis of collection parallel to lumen, then ulcer
  Otherwise, collection considered manifestation of nonulcerating deformity
• Benign gastric ulcer usually heals without deformity
• Deeply penetrated ulcer may show a persisting pit where mucosa has healed over crater; barium may collect in pit and mimic active ulcer

Malignant-appearing ulcers
• Carman's meniscus sign (also called *Carman-Kirklin complex*)
  Semicircular meniscoid configuration seen in profile, convex to lumen
  What is seen in meniscus is not all ulcer; rather, with compression the two sides of the tumor are opposed and central ulcer-like area collects barium
• Base (outer margin) of barium collection located where normal gastric wall would be expected (represents intraluminal mass with ulceration; i.e., malignant)
• Abrupt transition of normal mucosa and abnormal tissue
• Nodular surrounding tissue

ULCERATIVE COLITIS (UC)

Clinical

• Disease always begins in rectum; proximal spread occurs in continuous fashion
• Terminal ileum normal in vast majority of cases; "backwash ileitis" accounts for ileal disease
• Incidence 1 per 1000
• More frequent in Jewish and white populations
• Most commonly presents in second through fourth decades
• Complications:

(1) Carcinoma
Risk starts when disease present for about 8 years; 5 to 8% at 15 years, 12% at 20 years, 25% by 25 years
If UC limited to rectum or sigmoid, no cancer predisposition
Tends to be multiple and proximal to splenic flexure
May appear as strictures (these tumors are infiltrating, spread along bowel wall)
(2) Toxic megacolon
(3) Hepatobiliary disease
Pericholangitis, fatty infiltration, chronic active hepatitis, cirrhosis, sclerosing cholangitis, and primary carcinoma of bile ducts
(4) Arthritis

Imaging

- Plain films:
  Toxic megacolon: dilatation of transverse colon (averaging 8.5 cm; normal less than 5.5 cm)
  Coarsely irregular contour to bowel margin
  Need to repeat films frequently
- Barium enema:
  Earliest finding: indistinct fine or coarse granular mucosal pattern
  With disease progression, ulcers become undermined, leading to "collar button" appearance
  Chronic findings: loss of rectal valves and colonic folds; widening of presacral space and rectal narrowing
  Acute inflammatory polyps: mucosal remnants in areas of diffuse ulceration
  Postinflammatory polyps: seen in 15 to 25%; may be filiform or sessile; filiform polyps seen as small linear filling defects, with or without branching
  Rectum can be less severely involved than other portions of colon, or even spared; disease limited to right side of colon excludes ulcerative colitis

Distinction from Crohn's disease

- UC is a contiguous confluent process starting from rectum, whereas Crohn's disease is characterized by skip areas, asymmetric involvement
- UC may lead to shallow ulcerations that are not discrete, whereas ulcers in Crohn's disease are discrete and deep, commonly with fistulas
- Granular mucosa is common in UC and uncommon in Crohn's disease
- Severe anal/perianal disease is rare in UC and characteristic of Crohn's disease
- Spontaneous fistula and sinus tracts not seen in UC but characteristic of Crohn's disease

VARICES, OF ESOPHAGUS

Clinical

Causes
- Portal hypertension: connection between left gastric (coronary) vein of portal system and azygos and hemiazygos venous system
  (1) Cirrhosis
  (2) Carcinoma of pancreas
  (3) Pancreatitis
  (4) Retroperitoneal inflammatory disease
  (5) High-viscosity, slow-flow states (e.g., polycythemia)
- Noncirrhotic liver disease
  (1) Metastatic carcinoma
  (2) Carcinoma of liver
  (3) Congestive heart failure
- Superior vena cava obstruction (termed *downhill* varices because blood flows toward abdomen)

(1) Mediastinal tumors (e.g., bronchogenic carcinoma): tend to be confined to upper esophagus

(2) Chronic fibrosing mediastinitis: can involve the entire esophagus

- 20% die within month of first bleed
- 60% who have second bleed die at that time

Imaging

- Serpentine filling defects
- Compressible
- Barium contrast technique:
    First coat with high-density barium
    Next put patient in supine oblique position and wait for 2 to 3 minutes (allows time to fill varices)
    Most commonly shown in lower third of esophagus (unless downhill variety)
    Early varices generally situated on right anterolateral wall of distal esophagus and therefore most easily identified in left anterior oblique projection

VARICES, GASTRIC

Clinical

- Usually in fundus and associated with esophageal varices
- If no esophageal varices, think of isolated splenic vein thrombosis

Imaging

- Differentiating features:
    Changeability of size and shape (eliminates neoplastic process)
    Extension along lesser curvature (makes Ménétrier's disease less likely)

VOLVULUS, GASTRIC

Clinical

- Organoaxial (around long axis): greater curvature cephalic to lesser curvature
- Mesenteroaxial: cardia to right of antrum ("axial")
- Occurs in conjunction with large esophageal or paraesophageal hernia
- Can also be secondary to eventration or paralysis of diaphragm

Imaging

- Findings: double air-fluid level, inversion of stomach, cardia at same position as pylorus, downward pointing of pylorus and duodenum
- Vascular compromise uncommon

VOLVULUS, SIGMOID

Clinical

- Accounts for 1 to 2 % of intestinal obstruction in United States
- Acute presentation

Imaging

- Classic appearance: dilated loop of sigmoid colon with inverted U configuration, with dense white line pointing to pelvis (representing apposed inner walls of sigmoid)
- Results in obstruction of more proximal colonic segments and absence of rectal air
- If suspected, try prone film: if air moves to rectum, no sigmoid volvulus present

4

WEB, OF ESOPHAGUS

Clinical

- Typical transverse web always arises from anterior wall of esophagus, never posterior wall, just below level of cricopharyngeus muscle
- Rarer circumferential web concentrically narrows esophagus
- *Ring* refers to structure thicker than 3 mm, circumferential narrowing of lumen
- Rarely symptomatic
- Plummer-Vinson syndrome:
    Esophageal webs in association with dysphagia, iron-deficiency anemia, atrophic glossitis and mucosal lesions
    Occurs predominantly in middle-aged women
    Increased incidence of pharyngeal carcinomas

Imaging

- Usually thin; can be mass-like
- Never appears on posterior wall

WHIPPLE'S DISEASE

Clinical

- Hallmark: periodic acid–Schiff-positive macrophages extensively infiltrating lamina propria of small bowel
- Fold pathology most often seen in duodenum and proximal jejunum
- Abdominal pain, diarrhea, occasionally lympadenopathy and arthritis (nonde-forming arthritis an important feature)
- Antibiotic therapy results in improvement

Imaging

- Mucosal fold thickening and irregular fold distortion
- Predominantly duodenal and jejunal involvement
- Focal extrinsic mass effect can be noted along mesentery secondary to adenopathy
- Lumen may be normal or slightly dilated
- Intestinal lymphangiectasia may simulate findings in Whipple's disease, except for its distribution: Whipple's disease affects proximal small bowel, whereas intestinal lymphangiectasia involvement is diffuse

ZOLLINGER-ELLISON SYNDROME

Clinical

- Most cases occur in bulb, but more often postbulbar than is benign PUD
- Gastrin-secreting, non-beta islet cell tumor
- Occasional ectopic location (i.e., wall of duodenum)
- Most common location of ulcer is duodenal bulb
- Clinical findings suggesting this syndrome: ulcer that will not heal, recurrent ulcer at anastomosis after partial gastrectomy, ulcers in atypical locations

Imaging

- Multiple ulcers distal to bulb, thickening of gastric and duodenal folds, evidence of hypersecretion all suggest Zollinger-Ellison syndrome

Abdominal Viscera Imaging

■ Maitray D. Patel, M.D.

OVERVIEW

Examinations and discussions of the gastrointestinal system other than the alimentary tract generally include the liver, gallbladder, biliary tract, pancreas, and spleen; collectively, these structures are referred to as the *abdominal organs* for the purposes of this discussion. Although the spleen is more properly classified functionally with the hematologic and lymphatic system, its location in the abdomen often results in its concomitant evaluation when radiographic techniques are applied to the abdomen. The goal of this chapter is to provide an overview of the imaging techniques (other than scintigraphy) applied to evaluation of abdominal organs and a framework for the evaluation of disease processes that affect these organs.

Although plain film radiographs can provide clues to the diagnosis of alimentary tract abnormalities, they usually provide little diagnostic information with regard to diseases that affect the abdominal organs. Plain films may be used to evaluate for abnormal calcifications, but even in this role, plain film radiography is limited in its conclusions. Approximately 80% of gallstones are not visible on plain film radiographs, so the absence of calcifications on a radiograph does little to distinguish between diagnostic possibilities in a patient who presents with right upper quadrant pain. Chronic pancreatitis can lead to calcifications in the pancreatic bed, but the diagnosis of chronic pancreatitis is usually well established in these patients. Certain neoplasms can calcify in different patterns, but computed tomography (CT) provides far more information than can be obtained by plain film radiographs.

Ultrasound is often chosen as the initial cross-sectional imaging modality for the evaluation of the abdominal organs, usually because it is relatively cheaper than CT and magnetic resonance (MR). The findings on ultrasound may necessitate further imaging with cholangiography (usually via endoscopic retrograde cholangiopancreatography [ERCP]), CT, or MR, when it appears that these other modalities can provide additional useful information. Ultrasound is usually bypassed as the initial imaging tool in those instances when another modality is demonstrably superior (as in staging for known malignancies, specific evaluation of the pancreas, or evaluation of generalized trauma) or when the disease process under consideration is not clearly localized to the abdominal organs (as in abscess searches). When additional cross-sectional imaging is needed or when ultrasound has significant limitations for the clinical question at hand, CT is usually performed, with MR reserved for problem solving.

Although a number of disease processes can involve the abdominal organs with numerous manifestations, there are recurring themes that present more commonly. In addition, certain manifestations have classic associations that are useful to recognize. With respect to the gallbladder and biliary tract, pathologic processes commonly result in diffuse or focal alteration of the caliber of the ducts (*see* the following topics in the **Differential Diagnosis** section of this chapter: *Dilated Bile Ducts; Narrowed or Thick-walled Ducts; Stricture*), the appearance of filling defects (*Intraluminal Filling Defect in Common Bile Duct; Gallbladder Intraluminal Filling Defect/Mass*), or changes in the appearance of the wall (*Narrowed or Thick-walled Ducts; Gallbladder Wall Abnormality*). Pneumobilia has a classic set of associated disorders that should be recognized.

In the liver, there are several disease entities to consider when one detects diffuse alterations of echogenicity, attenuation, or enhancement (*Diffuse Increased Attenuation; Diffuse Abnormality of Enhancement; Diffuse Abnormality of Echogenicity*). In the pancreas and spleen, such diffuse abnormalities usually only have one cause (inflammation for the pancreas, global vascular insult for the spleen), thereby not resulting in differential considerations. In the liver, spleen, and pancreas, the identification of calcification helps to focus the discussion toward associated disease entities. In the liver, spleen, and pancreas, the identification of masses or mass-like areas should prompt the radiologist to determine whether they are primarily cystic or solid, which helps to organize the evaluation into specific differentials (*Liver Mass, Cystic Appearing; Liver Mass, Not Primarily Cystic Appearing; Cystic Pancreatic Lesions; Pancreatic Mass/Focal Abnormality; Cystic Splenic Mass; Solid Splenic Mass*). The considerations for the cause of a solid liver mass can be further limited if a central scar is identified or if the liver abnormality appears geographic rather than mass-like. Since few disease entities lead to portal vein thrombosis, this is an important finding to observe. Other classic differential gamuts in the liver include recognition of those malignancies that lead to hypervascular-appearing metastases and those diseases that result in portal hypertension.

ABDOMINAL VISCERA DIFFERENTIAL DIAGNOSES

Biliary Tract and Gallbladder
    Dilation
    Narrowed or thick-walled ducts
    Stricture
    Intraluminal filling defect in common bile duct
    Pneumobilia
    Gallbladder intraluminal filling defect/mass
    Gallbladder wall abnormality
Liver
    Calcifications
    Mass with central scar
    Diffuse increased attenuation
    Cysts
    Mass(es), not primarily cystic appearing
    Hypervascular metastases
    Portal hypertension
    Diffuse increase in echogenicity
    Diffuse abnormality of enhancement
    Geographic lesion
    Portal vein thrombosis
    Hepatic visceral echogenic foci

Pancreas
       Cystic pancreatic lesions
       Pancreatic mass/focal abnormality
       Pancreatic calcification
Spleen
       Calcifications
       Cystic splenic mass
       Solid splenic mass

BILIARY TRACT AND GALLBLADDER

DILATION

List the differential diagnosis for dilated bile ducts.

Obstruction
Caroli's disease
Choledochal cyst
Bacterial cholangitis
Acquired immunodeficiency syndrome (AIDS) cholangitis
Sclerosing cholangitis
Clonorchiasis
Recurrent pyogenic cholangitis (RPC)

Obstruction

What is the most common cause of obstruction?

Organize the causes of obstruction of the extrahepatic bile duct based on location.

What are the sonographic features of obstruction?

What is the commonly stated upper limit of normal measurement of the common hepatic duct?

If enlargement of the duct is borderline, how can the possibility of obstruction be further evaluated noninvasively?

Does the absence of dilatation exclude obstruction?

- Dilated ducts most likely caused by intraductal stone
- Other common entities include:
  - ¶ Carcinoma (bile duct, pancreas, ampulla)
  - ¶ Strictures (iatrogenic, postinflammatory)
  - ¶ Pancreatitis
  - ¶ Periportal adenopathy
- Administration of a fatty meal is a provocative test to determine if ductal dilatation is caused by obstruction

FIGURES Putnam and Ravin: 1005–1007, 1009

Caroli's disease

Describe the pathologic changes seen with Caroli's disease.

How do patients with Caroli's disease present?

What other disease states are associated with Caroli's disease?

Describe sonographic findings with Caroli's disease.

What other organ should be scanned in a patient in whom Caroli's disease is suspected?

What complication should be carefully sought when Caroli's disease is suspected?

- Ducts appear saccular
- Associated choledochal cyst may be seen
- Look for intraductal calculi or periportal fibrosis
- Look at the kidneys on ultrasound, searching for autosomal recessive polycystic kidney disease or medullary sponge kidney
- 100-fold increase in bile duct carcinoma occurs in these patients

FIGURES Gore: 1633; Gedgaudas-McLees: 234; Putnam and Ravin: p. 1015

How does ductal dilatation differ between choledochal cysts and obstruction?

How are choledochal cysts believed to originate?

Which patients tend to get choledochal cysts? How and when do they usually present?

Choledochal cyst

- Dilatation more focal than seen with obstruction
- Involvement of extrahepatic duct more common
- More likely in pediatric patient
- Calcification of wall is extremely rare

FIGURE   Gore: 1629–1632

Bacterial cholangitis

- Small, hepatic abscesses that communicate with the ducts may be seen
- Abscesses look like irregular saccular outpouchings of the duct

FIGURE   Gore: 1738

What is the most common appearance of AIDS cholangitis?

What other clues may be present on an ultrasound scan to indicate the diagnosis?

AIDS cholangitis

- Most common pattern of disease: dilated extrahepatic and intrahepatic ducts that abruptly terminate at level of papilla
- Other patterns include dilated intrahepatic ducts and thick-walled extrahepatic ducts
- Look for markedly echogenic, normal to large-sized kidneys if given an ultrasound scan

FIGURE   Gore: 1740

Sclerosing cholangitis

- Usually more narrowing than dilatation, although dilatation is a feature

Which ducts are more affected with clonorchiasis—extrahepatic or intrahepatic?

What other feature do dilated ducts have with clonorchiasis?

Clonorchiasis

- Look for diffuse dilatation of intrahepatic ducts with relative sparing of large ducts
- Periductal changes more severe in this condition

FIGURES   Gore: 1742, 1743

To help diagnose RPC, what should be searched for?

Recurrent pyogenic cholangitis (RPC)

- Intraductal calculi
- When obstruction is caused by an intraductal stone, dilated ducts are seen proximal to the stone; with recurrent pyogenic cholangitis, dilatation is seen proximal and distal to the stone

NARROWED OR THICK-WALLED DUCTS

What entities lead to narrowed and/or thick-walled bile ducts?

Sclerosing cholangitis
AIDS cholangitis
Cholangiocarcinoma
    Bacterial cholangitis
    Clonorchiasis
    Recurrent pyogenic cholangitis (RPC)
Cirrhosis
    General
    Primary biliary cirrhosis

Sclerosing cholangitis

Should extensive ductal dilatation be expected with sclerosing cholangitis?

Describe the features of sclerosing cholangitis.

- Combined features of short strictures, "beading," "pruning," diverticula, and mural irregularities suggest the diagnosis
- Presence of diverticular outpouchings in the setting of ductal irregularity is highly suggestive of primary sclerosing cholangitis (PSC); unfortunately, only approximately 25% of patients with PSC have diverticulae
- Dilatation not a predominant feature; usually short and discontinuous in this condition

FIGURE   Gore: 1730–1733

AIDS cholangitis

What other clues may be present on an ultrasound scan to indicate AIDS cholangitis?

How is the diagnosis of AIDS cholangitis made?

- Duct may be dilated without wall thickening or may appear to be of normal caliber with wall thickening
- Diarrhea is an associated clinical finding; may be caused by coexisting cytomegalovirus (CMV) infection of bowel
- Tends to involve papilla, which is uncommon with primary sclerosing cholangitis
- Look for other clues of AIDS infection, e.g., echogenic kidneys on ultrasound examination
- Diagnosis usually made by ERCP; however, consistent ultrasound appearance in an AIDS patient with appropriate clinical and biochemical features (markedly elevated alkaline phosphatase level with nearly normal bilirubin value) is sufficient to establish the diagnosis

FIGURE   Gore: 1740

Cholangiocarcinoma

What features help distinguish cholangiocarcinoma from PSC?

- In 90% of cases, cholangiocarcinoma presents as focal stricture or polypoid mass (less common), not as diffuse narrowing of ducts; however, 10% of cases are characterized by relatively diffuse ductal abnormality
- Diverticula do not occur with cholangiocarcinoma; PSC should be considered instead
- Cholangiocarcinoma can occur in the setting of PSC
- Cholangiocarcinoma is suggested in the setting of PSC when:
    ¶ Strictures and dilatation form relatively rapidly (PSC is slowly progressing)
    ¶ Intraluminal filling defects are more than 1 cm
    ¶ Mural thickening is more than 5 mm
- If suspicion of cholangiocarcinoma is raised by cholangiogram, do CT

Bacterial cholangitis

- Look for small hepatic abscesses that communicate with biliary tree

FIGURE   Gore: 1738

Clonorchiasis

True or false: The extrahepatic ducts are spared with clonorchiasis.

- Has marked periductal changes
- Usually involves peripheral small bile ducts, sparing extrahepatic ducts

FIGURES   Gore: 1742, 1743

RPC has predilection for which part of the biliary system?

Recurrent pyogenic cholangitis (RPC)

- May affect any segment of biliary tree, but typically involves lateral segment of left lobe most extensively
- Intrahepatic ductal stones commonly found

FIGURE   Gore: 1740

Cirrhosis, general

- Corkscrew appearance of ducts
- Examine liver surface for nodularity

Primary biliary cirrhosis

What clinical and radiographic features characterize primary biliary cirrhosis?

- Much more common in females (ratio of females to males, 9:1)
- Not irregular in appearance

FIGURE   Gore: 1737

STRICTURE

List a broad differential for biliary stricture.
Iatrogenic causes
    Surgery
    Hepatic artery chemotherapy
Sequela of inflammation
    Sclerosing cholangitis
    Infectious cholangitis
    Pancreatitis
Malignant causes
    Cholangiocarcinoma
    Hepatoma
Extrinsic compression
    Periportal nodes
    Mirizzi's syndrome

Surgery, iatrogenic

- Stricture at site of cystic duct
- Look for surgical clips

FIGURES   Gore: 1755, 1770

Hepatic artery chemotherapy, iatrogenic

- Look for evidence of cancer (i.e., colostomy bag)

FIGURE   Gore: 1741

Sclerosing cholangitis

Why pay attention to a dominant stricture in a patient with sclerosing cholangitis?

- Diffuse abnormality
- About 25% of patients have a "dominant stricture," which may represent cancer

Infectious cholangitis

Where do the strictures tend to occur in patients with AIDS cholangitis?

In patients with clonorchiasis?

- Includes pyogenic cholangitis, AIDS cholangitis, recurrent pyogenic cholangitis, and clonorchiasis

Pancreatitis

- Distal stricture

FIGURES Gore: 1586, 1601

Cholangiocarcinoma

What is the work-up for suspected cholangiocarcinoma?

- Classically occurs at hilum (Klatskin's tumor)
- Diagnosis made by biopsy, usually at ERCP
- Presence of associated mass extending into liver suggests diagnosis
- May cause lobar hepatic atrophy

FIGURES Gore: 1586, 1718–1721, 1756

Hepatoma

- Look for associated mass on cross-sectional imaging study
- Although both cholangiocarcinoma and hepatoma can present as masses, hepatoma is more likely to result in portal vein thrombosis

Periportal nodes

- Diagnosis made on cross-sectional imaging study

FIGURE Gore: 1585

Mirizzi's syndrome

- Consider if patient has symptoms of cholecystitis (i.e., Murphy's sign, fever, right upper quadrant pain)

FIGURE Gore: 1596

INTRALUMINAL FILLING DEFECT IN COMMON BILE DUCT

What is the differential diagnosis of a filling defect in the common bile duct?

Choledocholithiasis
Pseudocalculus
Air bubbles
Cholangiocarcinoma
Hemobilia
Parasitic infections
Sludge ball

Choledocholithiasis

What maneuvers help to diagnose choledocholithiasis?

- May move with gravity
- Usually casts acoustic shadow on ultrasound examination
- Usually patient has concomitant gallstones

FIGURES Gore: 1589, 1653, 1654, 1662–1667

Pseudocalculus

What can be done if sphincter of Oddi spasm is suspected?

- Represents sphincter of Oddi or Boyden spasm
- Should not persist
- Glucagon administration may relieve spasm

FIGURE Gore: 1588

5

5

Air bubbles

• Will rise with gravity
• More air bubbles seen in nondependent areas of liver and biliary system

FIGURE Gore: 1596

Cholangiocarcinoma

Is it common for cholangiocarcinoma to appear as a polypoid filling defect?

• Much more likely to result in stricture rather than an intraluminal filling defect

FIGURES Gore: 1719, 1723

Hemobilia

How may the suspicion of hemobilia as the cause of a filling defect be confirmed?

• No acoustic shadowing
• Has patient had recent trauma or intervention (e.g., transjugular intrahepatic portosystemic shunt [TIPS], percutaneous transhepatic cholangiogram [PTC])?
• Does patient have bleeding disorder?
• Resolves spontaneously

Parasitic infections

• Linear filling defect

FIGURES Gore: 1741, 1742

Sludge ball

• No acoustic shadowing on ultrasound

PNEUMOBILIA

What are the common causes of pneumobilia?

Iatrogenic causes
    Surgical fistulization
    After papillotomy during ERCP
Cholecystoenteric fistula from gallstone erosion
Duodenal ulcer perforation into gallbladder
Gallbladder carcinoma perforation into gastrointestinal (GI) tract
Septic cholangitis

Iatrogenic causes

• Most common cause, usually the result of surgically created anastomosis of extrahepatic duct with bowel

FIGURE Gore: 1580

Cholecystoenteric fistula from gallstone erosion

What other radiographic signs should be sought if Bouveret's syndrome is suspected?

• Also known as *gallstone ileus*
• Refers to passage of gallstone directly from inflamed gallbladder into bowel
• Look for calcified structure on plain film, which represents gallstone in the bowel
• Classically has small bowel dilatation, but not necessarily, because gallstone can erode directly into colon
• Bouveret's syndrome refers to gastric outlet obstruction caused by a gallstone that has eroded into the stomach

FIGURE Gore: 1653

Duodenal ulcer

- Nasogastric aspirate should be positive for heme

Gallbladder carcinoma

- Usually advanced when enteric fistula occurs
- Heterogeneous mass typically seen in gallbladder fossa
- Echogenic areas may represent air or stones (which are associated with gallbladder carcinoma)

Septic cholangitis

What differentiates septic cholangitis from other causes of pneumobilia?

- Not a common cause of pneumobilia
- By definition, patients appear septic

GALLBLADDER INTRALUMINAL FILLING DEFECT/MASS

List the differential for a gallbladder filling defect.

Gallstones
Sludge
Hemobilia
Parasitic infection
Cholesterol polyp
Polypoid tumor
Sloughed mucosa

Gallstones

- Generally mobile but can be adherent
- Acoustic shadowing present; in equivocal cases:
    - ¶ Make sure focal zone of transducer is on suspected stone
    - ¶ Use highest frequency transducer possible

FIGURES   Gore: 1577, 1638–1642, 1644, 1646

Sludge

- Generally obeys gravity
- No acoustic shadowing
- Can appear tumefactive ("sludge ball"), in which case it can be adherent to the wall of the gallbladder; in these cases, sludge often has different echogenicity than the wall of the gallbladder, which helps indicate that it does not arise from the wall (like a tumor)

FIGURE   Gore: 1643

Hemobilia

- No acoustic shadowing
- Usually in specific clinical settings (trauma, bleeding disorder)

Parasitic infection

- Ascariasis
- May be mobile

Cholesterol polyp

- One form of cholesterolosis
- Nonmobile, can be multiple
- Ultrasound can be characteristic, with "ring down" artifact

Polypoid tumor

- Gallbladder carcinoma
- Metastatic melanoma
- Any of several rare benign tumors

Sloughed mucosa

- Can occur in acute cholecystitis
- Assess patient's tenderness (sonographic Murphy's sign)

GALLBLADDER WALL ABNORMALITY

List considerations for focal or diffuse gallbladder wall abnormality.

Cholecystitis
    Acute
    Emphysematous
    Acalculous
    Chronic
Hyperplastic cholecystoses
Cholesterolosis
Adenomyomatosis
Gallbladder carcinoma
Porcelain gallbladder
Gallbladder varices
Metastatic melanoma
Nonspecific causes of thickened wall

Acute cholecystitis

What are the sonographic features of early acute cholecystitis? What features occur as inflammation progresses?

- Look for stones and evaluate for sonographic Murphy's sign
- Findings with advanced inflammation include associated gallbladder wall thickening, strandlike debris within gallbladder lumen, and pericholecystic fluid

FIGURES   Gore: 1648, 1649

Emphysematous cholecystitis

- Hyperechoic foci in wall with dirty acoustic shadowing
- Can be confused with adenomyomatosis

FIGURE   Gore: 1650

Acalculous cholecystitis

- Suspect if gallbladder is tensely dilated (i.e., more than 6 cm in transverse diameter) without visualization of stones

Chronic cholecystitis

How is acute cholecystitis differentiated from chronic cholecystitis?

- Patients generally do not have sonographic Murphy's sign and are not acutely ill
- Functional imaging with nuclear medicine may help diagnose this condition
- Gallstones invariably are present

Cholesterolosis

- Diffuse form of cholesterolosis (which leads to "strawberry gallbladder") generally is not radiographically visible
- More focal forms result in cholesterol polyps and plaques, which can be multiple and visible by imaging

FIGURE Gore: 1710

Adenomyomatosis

What other entity should be considered and excluded when the sonographic diagnosis of adenomyomatosis is considered?

- Characteristic appearance on cholecystography
- Look for ring down artifact from hyperechoic foci in wall of gallbladder
- Consider the possibility that hyperechoic foci in gallbladder wall is caused by air (emphysematous cholecystitis)

FIGURES Gore: 1622, 1645, 1707, 1708

Gallbladder carcinoma

How may a gallbladder wall tumor be distinguished from tumefactive sludge?

- Can present as diffuse or focal wall thickening, but usually as an invasive mass
- Apply color Doppler to the wall thickening to determine whether neovascularity is detectable

FIGURES Gore: 1713–1716

Porcelain gallbladder

- Characteristic plain film
- Ultrasound can be somewhat confusing, mimicking appearance of a gallbladder packed with stones

FIGURE Gore: 1656

Gallbladder varices

- Turn on color Doppler
- Evaluate portal vein (gallbladder varices occur in the setting of portal vein thrombosis)

Nonspecific causes of thickened wall

- List of causes of gallbladder wall thickening is too long to memorize
- Think principally of any disorder that leads to imbalance in oncotic pressure of intravascular system (i.e., liver disease, renal failure, heart failure)
- Many AIDS patients have thick gallbladder walls, a nonspecific feature and not necessarily associated with AIDS cholangitis

LIVER

CALCIFICATIONS

Name five causes of hepatic calcification.

Infections
    Echinococcus spp
    Disseminated granulomas: tuberculosis (TB), histoplasmosis
    Pneumocystis carinii pneumonia (PCP)
Tumors
    Cysts
    Fibrolamellar hepatoma

5

Hepatoblastoma
Intrahepatic cholangiocarcinoma
Metastases
Other causes
Intrahepatic choledocholithiasis
Hepatic artery aneurysm
Phleboliths/calcified thrombus
Capsular calcification

Echinococcus spp

Describe the type of calcification seen with echinococcus.

What does calcification of an echinococcal cyst indicate?

- Peripheral curvilinear calcification visible on plain films in 20 to 30%
- Calcification of the cyst wall indicates death of organism

FIGURE Gore: 1957

Disseminated granulomas: TB, histoplasmosis

What is the most common cause of focal hepatic calcification?

- Probably most common cause of calcification of liver

PCP

Are numerous or few calcifications found with PCP?

- Punctate calcifications; may coalesce to form dense clumps
- Calcifications in kidneys, spleen, pancreas, and lymph nodes also may be seen
- Findings not specific for PCP; also reported with *Mycobacterium avium intracellulare* (MAI) and CMV, but less commonly

FIGURE Gore: 1964

Cysts

- Usually do not have calcification

Fibrolamellar hepatoma

Where does the calcification occur in fibrolamellar hepatoma?

- Stellate calcification can occur in central scar

FIGURE Gore: 1913

Hepatoblastoma

What clinical features help to determine that a calcified liver mass is hepatoblastoma?

- Large mass in a child
- Presents in first 3 years of life
- If calcifications are present, they tend to be multifocal and punctate

FIGURE Gore: 1916

Intrahepatic cholangiocarcinoma

Is calcification common with cholangiocarcinoma?

Are calcifications caused by ductal stones in this case?

- Usually large at presentation
- Calcification frequently seen
- Not associated with choledocholithiasis

FIGURES Gore: 1919, 1920

Metastases

What types of hepatic metastasis show calcification?

- From mucinous adenocarcinoma of lung, colon, ovary, or stomach
- Also from melanoma, insulinoma, neuroblastoma

True or false: Recurrent pyogenic cholangitis typically shows intrahepatic calcifications associated with small masses caused by fibrosis.

Intrahepatic choledocholithiasis

- No associated mass
- Consider recurrent pyogenic cholangitis, especially in patients from the Pacific Rim

FIGURE   Gore: 1739

What shape of calcification suggests the diagnosis of hepatic artery aneurysm?

Hepatic artery aneurysm

- Curvilinear calcification

True or false: Phleboliths are commonly found in hepatic hemangiomas.

Phleboliths/calcified thrombus

- Phleboliths may be seen infrequently in hemangiomas

What disease processes lead to hepatic capsular calcification?

Capsular calcification

- Results from hematoma, infection, or meconium peritonitis

MASS WITH CENTRAL SCAR

- Fibrolamellar hepatocellular carcinoma
- Focal nodular hyperplasia
- Hemangioma

General comments

- Two types of central scar described on MRI:
    ¶ Collagenous: low signal on T2; occurs in hemangiomas, hepatomas, and focal nodular hyperplasia (FNH)
    ¶ Inflammatory: high signal on T2; occurs most commonly in FNH, generally not in fibrolamellar carcinoma, and not at all in hemangioma

Describe the MRI features of a central scar that assist in predicting the correct diagnosis.

Fibrolamellar hepatocellular carcinoma

- Central scar calcification makes fibrolamellar hepatoma a more likely diagnosis than FNH

FIGURE   Gore: 1914

What feature of a central scar suggests hepatoma rather than FNH?

Focal nodular hyperplasia

- Central scar does not calcify

FIGURE   Gore: 1872

Hemangioma

- Central scar seen with giant hemagiomas represents areas of fibrosis

FIGURE   Gore: 1867

What type of hemangiomas develop central fibrosis?

DIFFUSE INCREASED ATTENUATION

Name five causes of a dense liver on CT.

Thorotrast
Hemochromatosis
Amiodarone therapy
Gold therapy
Wilson's disease
Glycogen storage disease

Hemochromatosis

What other structures can help confirm the suspicion of hemochromatosis as a cause of a dense liver?

- Primary hemochromatosis is tenfold more common in men
- Increased attenuation of lymph nodes, pancreas, and adrenal cortex also may be seen, so these areas should be examined

Wilson's disease

How old are patients who present with Wilson's disease?

- Excess copper deposition in liver, kidneys, brain, and cornea
- Presents between the ages of 6 and 20 years

CYSTS

List five broad categories of disease that can lead to hepatic cysts.

Cystic neoplasm
    Metastases
    Adenoma/hepatoma with hemorrhage
    Biliary cystadenoma
    Biliary cystadenocarcinoma
    Mesenchymal hamartoma
Infection
    Pyogenic abscess
    Amebic abscess
    Echinococcal cyst
Posttraumatic: hematoma or biloma
Developmental
    Congenital cyst
    Caroli's disease
    Choledochal cyst
Vascular
    Pseudoaneurysm/arteriovenous malformation (AVM)
Peliosis hepatis

General comments

How common are cysts in the liver: less than 1%, 1 to 10%, 10 to 50%, or over 50%?

- Affects 2 to 7% of population
- Congenital (failure of involution of intrahepatic biliary ductules) more common than acquired (trauma, inflammation, parasitic disease)

Congenital cyst

True or false: The presence of septation or slight wall irregularity makes congenital hepatic cyst unlikely?
Where else might one look for evidence that cysts in the liver are congenital hepatic cysts?

- Multiple cysts associated with polycystic kidney disease; seen in at least one third of patients with adult polycystic renal disease
- May be septated or show slight wall irregularity, usually because of previous hemorrage

Necrotic metastases

How do metastases become cystic appearing?
Is it reasonable to include metastasis on the differential diagnosis for a thin-walled cyst?
What types of metastases are more likely to be cystic?

- Caused by necrosis of rapidly growing metastases: thus, one should see thick-walled margins and internal debris when seriously considering this possibility
- Types of primary neoplasms to consider: choriocarcinoma, mucinous pancreatic carcinoma, leiomyosarcoma, small cell carcinoma
- Ovarian carcinoma studs outside of liver with cystic implants; rarely causes intrahepatic lesions

Adenoma/hepatoma with hemorrhage

True or false: Hemorrhage into a neoplasm can make the neoplasm appear entirely cystic.

- Pathologic mass evident, with irregular cystic component

Biliary cystadenoma/cystadenocarcinoma

Biliary cystadenomas tend to be found in what type of patient?

- Generally affects middle-aged women
- Rare
- Usually large, ranging from 3 to 25 cm
- Cystadenoma may be indistinguishable from congenital hepatic cyst

Mesenchymal hamartoma

In what age group are mesenchymal hamartomas found?

What are the major competing diagnoses in this age group? How is mesenchymal hamartoma differentiated?

- Discovered in first 3 years of life
- Large, multicompartmental mass, often 15 cm or more in diameter
- Differentiated from hepatoblastoma and infantile hemangioendothelioma by its prominent cystic components

Pyogenic abscess

What finding would strongly suggest pyogenic abscess?

- When solitary, usually multilocular
- May appear as a cluster of smaller, irregular cysts (so-called "cluster sign")
- Presence of gas helps to confirm pyogenic nature

Amebic abscess

Where are hepatic amebic abscesses typically located?

- Most amebic liver abscesses are solitary, often located in right lobe of the liver adjacent to the liver capsule
- Pleuroperitoneal involvement in 10 to 20%

Echinococcal cyst

What imaging feature strongly suggests echinococcal disease as the cause of a cyst?

- Daughter cysts seen as secondary cysts or septated regions within the large cyst strongly suggest diagnosis
- With time, may appear nearly solid on ultrasound, as cyst fills with material
- About 50% calcify
- Aspiration may lead to anaphylaxis

Hematoma

- Internal septations and fibrinous strands are a common feature as hematoma liquefies

Biloma

- Internal debris uncommon

Caroli's disease

What feature of intrahepatic cysts suggests Caroli's disease?

- Intrahepatic cystic spaces communicate with biliary tree

5

Choledochal cyst

- Located in porta hepatis
- Presents in childhood

Pseudoaneurysm/AVM

What maneuver is essential when vascular origin of a cystic mass is a consideration?

- Doppler interrogation is the key to diagnosis
- Should be considered in the patient with a history of previous liver biopsy or other injury

Peliosis hepatis

How large are the cystic areas seen with peliosis hepatis?

- Rare; multiple, blood-filled cystic spaces in liver (ranging from 1 to 5 mm)
- Asymptomatic, incidental finding at autopsy; seen in patients with chronic diseases such as TB, cancer, and hematologic disorders

MASS(ES), NOT PRIMARILY CYSTIC APPEARING

Name four nonneoplastic causes of a liver mass.

Nonneoplastic
    Pyogenic abscess
    Parasitic abscess
    Hematoma
    Regenerating nodule
    Focal fatty infiltration
    Focal fatty sparing
    Hepatic infarct

Name two benign hepatic tumors.

Benign tumor
    Cavernous hemangioma
    Adenoma
    Focal nodular hyperplasia

Name four malignant tumors found in the liver.

Malignant tumor
    Hepatoma
    Lymphoma
    Metastasis
    Cholangiocarcinoma
    Angiosarcoma

Pyogenic abscess

What is the best clue to suggest that a mass is a pyogenic abscess?

- Can be difficult to differentiate from neoplasm on basis of imaging; clinical history important
- Often has irregular borders
- Look for gas
- May be of variable echogenicity on ultrasound

Parasitic abscess

Describe imaging features of parasitic abscesses.

- Smooth borders
- Often with uniform low level echoes on ultrasound
- Internal daughter cysts may be seen (echinococcal)
- History of travel in endemic area

Hematoma

Examination of what region of the liver may assist in determining that an intrahepatic mass is a hematoma?

- History of trauma
- Look for associated subcapsular blood

Focal fatty infiltration or sparing

Describe features associated with focal fatty infiltration or sparing.

- Geographic or regional in appearance
- One or more of the borders may be straight, especially where they abut a vessel that is not displaced

Hepatic infarct

What clinical history is usually present when the diagnosis of hepatic infarct is considered?

- Peripheral, wedge shaped
- Seen especially in setting of liver transplant

Cavernous hemangioma

Describe the imaging features of a cavernous hemangioma.

- Often found incidentally
- Globular peripheral enhancement implicates the diagnosis on CT
- Increased through-sound transmission on ultrasound may be difficult to demonstrate
- Often peripherally located

Hepatic adenoma

What is the classic history of hepatic adenoma?

Which nuclear medicine test may be helpful? Why?

- Classic history: oral contraceptive use
- May bleed
- Usually large before becoming symptomatic
- Sulfur-colloid nuclear medicine study shows lack of uptake (no Kupffer cells)

Focal nodular hyperplasia

Describe imaging features that suggest focal nodular hyperplasia.

- Many have Kupffer cells and thus are scintigraphically active
- Lack peripheral enhancement
- Central scar
- Arterial supply radiates in a spoke-wheel fashion

Hepatoma

Distinguish multifocal hepatoma from multiple metastases.

What finding implicates hepatoma as the cause of a liver mass?

- When multifocal, usually one dominant mass exists with surrounding smaller masses
- Portal vein invasion most commonly seen with hepatoma

Lymphoma

Is lymphoma in the differential diagnosis for an echogenic mass?

- Usually diffuse involvement of liver in immunocompetent persons
- In those with AIDS, focal hepatic lesions more common
- Hypovascular
- Very low echogenicity is common; can appear almost cystic on ultrasound examination

Metastasis

Distinguish the typical imaging finding of metastatic disease from that of hepatoma.

- Tends not to cause portal vein thrombosis
- Often distinguished from multifocal hepatoma by absence of dominant mass

Cholangiocarcinoma

What feature of the surface of the liver near a cholangiocarcinoma may help in suggesting this diagnosis? What causes this feature?

- May result in local hepatic atrophy, such that surface of the liver adjacent to the tumor is slightly concave
- Dilated ducts peripheral to lesion

Angiosarcoma

What clinical history is suggestive of angiosarcoma?

- Associated with Thorotrast exposure
- These lesions are quite vascular

HYPERVASCULAR METASTASES

Which metastases tend to be hypervascular? What does this mean in terms of imaging?

Choriocarcinoma
Renal cell carcinoma
Carcinoid
Islet cell tumors
Thyroid carcinoma

General comments

- To remember this list, think of tumors that have endocrine origin or that can elaborate hormone-like substances (renal cell carcinoma can produce erythropoietin, choriocarcinoma produces βhCG, etc.)
- Hypervascularity results in increased echogenicity on ultrasound, bright enhancement on CT, and hyperintensity on MRI
- MRI not useful in patients with vascular primary tumors to distinguish hepatic metastases from hemangiomas: both very bright on T2-weighted images

PORTAL HYPERTENSION

Give an organized differential diagnosis for portal hypertension based on the site of impedance to flow.

Extrahepatic presinusoidal
    Portal vein/splenic vein occlusion
    Arterioportal fistula
Intrahepatic presinusoidal
    Congenital hepatic fibrosis
    Primary biliary cirrhosis
    Schistosomiasis
Intrahepatic sinusoidal
    Cirrhosis
    Sclerosing cholangitis
Posthepatic postsinusoidal
    Budd-Chiari syndrome
    Polycythemia
    Inferior vena cava obstruction (IVC)

Portal vein/splenic vein occlusion

Name diseases to consider when portal vein or splenic vein occlusion is identified.

- Considerations: pancreatitis, hepatoma, trauma, infection
- When caused by infection, site of infection usually is the appendix; organism is *Bacteroides* spp

Arterioportal fistula

Name two causes of arterioportal fistula.

- Causes include trauma and hepatoma

Primary biliary cirrhosis

Who gets primary biliary cirrhosis?

- Occurs in middle-aged women

Cirrhosis

List causes of cirrhosis.

Which is the most common cause in the United States?

- Causes of cirrhosis in United States:
    - ¶ Alcohol abuse: 30 to 60%
    - ¶ Postnecrotic: 10 to 30%
    - ¶ Biliary cirrhosis: 10 to 20%
    - ¶ Pigment cirrhosis: 2 to 5% (hemochromatosis, Wilson's disease)

Sclerosing cholangitis

Sclerosing cholangitis is associated most commonly with what disease?

- Most commonly associated with ulcerative colitis

Budd-Chiari syndrome

What are the clinical features of Budd-Chiari syndrome?

- Clinical triad: hepatomegaly, right upper quadrant pain, ascites

DIFFUSE INCREASE IN ECHOGENICITY

Fatty infiltration
Cirrhosis
Hepatic fibrosis
Gaucher's disease
Hemochromatosis

Fatty infiltration

What finding confirms the diagnosis of diffuse fatty infiltration of the liver?

- Most common cause of echogenic liver
- Identifying areas of focal sparing confirms diagnosis
- Poor sound penetration

Cirrhosis

What finding helps to diagnose cirrhosis?

- Look for nodular liver surface

DIFFUSE ABNORMALITY OF ENHANCEMENT

Budd-Chiari syndrome
Hepatic venoocclusive disease
Cirrhosis
Right-sided venous congestion

Budd-Chiari syndrome

Describe the features of Budd-Chiari syndrome on CT, nuclear medicine, angiography, and MRI.

- CT findings:
    - ¶ Fan-shaped appearance of abnormality in liver with central sparing (contrast trying to drain peripherally gives fan-shaped appearance)
    - ¶ Caudate lobe spared (drains independently directly into IVC)
    - ¶ No visualization of hepatic veins
    - ¶ Prominent retroperitoneal collaterals
    - ¶ Prolonged, nonhomogeneous parenchymal opacification
    - ¶ Compressed intrahepatic cava often seen secondary to swollen liver

- Nuclear medicine finding: may see "hot spot" on technetium-sulfur colloid study because caudate is the only normal liver present
- Angiography: "spider web" network of veins
- MRI: serpiginous collateral vessels (flow voids); also seen in some normal individuals

Hepatic venoocclusive disease

How does the imaging of hepatic venoocclusive disease differ from that of classic Budd-Chiari syndrome?

- Variant of Budd-Chiari syndrome in which small hepatic venules are diffusely occluded
- Occurs in patients with bone marrow transplant and those with hepatic radiation therapy
- Findings similar to those of Budd-Chiari syndrome except that hepatic veins may be visualized on CT and ultrasound scans
- Hepatic venography (retrograde injection into hepatic vein) shows "spider web" appearance of collaterals

Cirrhosis

What findings help to identify patients with cirrhosis?

- Look for secondary signs of cirrhosis: varices, splenomegaly, ascites
- Nodular liver surface

Right-sided venous congestion

What findings suggest venous congestion as a cause of abnormal liver enhancement?

- Causes include heart failure or restrictive pericarditis
- Enlarged IVC and hepatic veins

GEOGRAPHIC LESION

Infarct
Focal fatty infiltration
Focal fatty sparing
Radiation change

Definition

- An area of focal abnormal echotexture, attenuation, or enhancement without mass effect

Infarct

Describe typical location and clinical setting for hepatic infarction.

- Not common secondary to dual hepatic blood supply
- Clinical setting: shock, severe biliary disease, anesthesia, liver transplantation
- CT: wedge-shaped, low-density area extending to periphery; look also for splenic or renal infarcts; intrahepatic bilomas also have been described

Focal fatty infiltration

What is the common location for focal fatty infiltration?

- Tends to occur around porta hepatis
- No mass effect

Focal fatty sparing

What are the common locations for fatty sparing?

- Rest of liver must demonstrate features of fatty infiltration (increased echogenicity or decreased attenuation)
- Commonly found near falciform ligament, adjacent to gallbladder, or in porta hepatis
- No mass effect

Radiation change

Does hepatic radiation result in long-term CT abnormalities?

- Causes fatty infiltration and extensive fibrosis
- Onset 2 to 6 weeks after therapy; need at least 3500 rads
- Liver usually returns to normal in 3 to 5 months
- CT: sharply defined region of low attenuation

PORTAL VEIN THROMBOSIS

Name four causes of portal vein thrombosis.

Idiopathic
Secondary
    Tumor
    Intraabdominal sepsis
    Clotting disorder
    Trauma

Tumor

What maneuver can be diagnostic of tumor thrombus?

- Thrombosis is caused by invasion or compression
- Presence of arterial signal on Doppler within the thrombus makes hepatoma very likely

Intraabdominal sepsis

What is the usual cause of septic thrombosis of the portal vein?

- Not lethal
- Infection with *Bacteroides* spp predisposes patient to this condition because it elaborates clotting enzymes; appendix often primary site
- Can also develop from pancreatitis
- Microabscesses develop in liver

Clotting disorder

- Clinical diagnosis; no helpful imaging features

Trauma

What additional findings suggest a traumatic cause of portal vein thrombosis?

- Look for other findings suggesting trauma, such as lacerations, hemoperitoneum, or rib fractures

HEPATIC VISCERAL ECHOGENIC FOCI

What is the differential for echogenic foci within the abdominal viscera?

Prior infection
Intrahepatic ductal stones
Pneumobilia
Portal venous gas
Hepatitis

Prior infection

What infectious agents are responsible for echogenic foci in the spleen in patients with AIDS?

- TB and histoplasmosis may demonstrate 2- to 3-mm echogenic foci, seen within the spleen and liver
- Tiny echogenic foci may be seen in the spleen, liver, and kidneys in patients with AIDS, secondary to disseminated pneumocystis, mycobacteria, or CMV

FIGURES   Rumack: 95 (granulomatous disease), 61 (PCP), 101 (MAI)

Intrahepatic ductal stones

What is the usual cause of intrahepatic ductal stones?

- Usually secondary to recurrent pyogenic cholangitis
- Shadowing medium-echogenicity foci are seen within the intrahepatic and extrahepatic ducts

FIGURE Rumack: 128

Pneumobilia

What features of hepatic echogenic foci suggest pneumobilia?

- Can be secondary to incompetent sphincter of Oddi, surgery, or erosion into the common bile duct of a stone or ulcer
- Echogenic foci are linear, and more are seen in the left lobe of the liver in supine patient (nondependent)

FIGURE Rumack: 129

Portal venous gas

What characteristic finding is seen on pulse-wave Doppler examination of the portal venous system in cases of portal venous gas?

- Usually secondary to pneumatosis intestinalis
- Look for evidence of bowel ischemia (thick-walled bowel, echogenic foci within bowel wall), and echogenic foci within the liver
- Unlike pneumobilia, no left-sided preference
- May see high-amplitude spikes on Doppler examination of the portal venous system

Hepatitis

True or false: The liver is normally slightly echogenic relative to renal cortex.

True or false: Diffuse gallbladder wall thickening is fairly specific for an intrahepatic process, such as hepatitis.

- Liver parenchyma may have decreased echogenicity, accentuating the portal triads, which appear bright
- The liver is hypoechoic relative to renal cortex (usually iso- to slightly hyperechoic)
- Gallbladder wall thickening is a nonspecific finding that is often associated

FIGURE Rumack: 55

PANCREAS

CYSTIC PANCREATIC LESIONS

List the differential diagnosis for cystic pancreatic lesions.

Pseudocyst
Simple cyst
Abscess
Neoplasm
      Necrotic adenocarcinoma
      Cystic neoplasms
      Cystic metastases
      Lymphangioma
Mimics
      Splenic artery aneurysm

Pseudocyst

What other sonographic features might one find in cases of pancreatic pseudocyst?

- Communication with duct (rare in cystadenoma/adenocarcinoma)
- Look for signs of chronic pancreatitis: calcifications, ectatic duct

FIGURES Gore: 2142, 2156

Simple cyst

What conditions are associated with simple pancreatic cysts?

- No septations or enhancement
- Seen in polycystic kidney disease, cystic fibrosis, von Hippel-Lindau disease

Abscess

- Patient septic

FIGURE Gore: 2150

Necrotic adenocarcinoma

- Thick, irregular wall

Cystic neoplasms

Which is more likely to be malignant: serous or mucinous adenoma?

- Microcystic/serous adenoma (benign)
- Macrocystic/mucinous adenoma
- Adenocarcinoma
- Solid and papillary epithelial neoplasm

FIGURES Gore: 2175, 2176, 2178

Cystic metastases

- Lung, ovary, melanoma

Lymphangioma

What anatomic feature separates lymphangioma from other cystic pancreatic masses?

- May cross fascial boundaries

Splenic artery aneurysm

- May mimic cystic lesion on ultrasound; use color Doppler to rule this out

FIGURE Gore: 2152

PANCREATIC MASS/FOCAL ABNORMALITY

What are the main considerations when a focal mass is identified in the pancreas?

Neoplasm
    Epithelial
        Ductal adenocarcinoma
        Serous cystadenoma
        Mucinous cystadenoma/carcinoma
        Solid and cystic papillary neoplasm
    Acinar cell carcinoma
        Pancreatoblastoma
    Islet cell
        Insulinoma
        Gastrinoma
        Somatostatinoma
        Glucagonoma
        VIPoma (i.e., tumor that secretes vasoactive intestinal peptide)
    Metastases
Inflammatory
    Acute pancreatitis
    Pseudocyst
    Abscess

Ductal adenocarcinoma

- Obliteration of fat surrounding celiac axis and superior mesenteric artery (SMA) has long been considered a characteristic of pancreatic carcinoma, but nonpancreatic tumors also can do this
- Dilated ducts usually present

FIGURES   Gore: 2165, 2166

Serous cystadenoma

- Cysts less than 2 cm; more than six cysts
- Calcification rarely occurs within tumor (20%); when present, it is stellate and central

FIGURE   Gore: 2175

Mucinous cystadenoma

- Cysts more than 2 cm; fewer than six cysts
- 40% calcify; can have stellate appearance but calcification is classically peripheral (as opposed to central calcifications of serous tumors)

FIGURE   Gore: 2176

Solid papillary epithelial neoplasm

- Usually in tail of pancreas
- Occurs in young women (mean age, 24 years)

FIGURE   Gore: 2178

Acinar cell carcinoma

- Large (2 to 12 cm)
- Greater tendency to be centrally necrotic

Pancreatoblastoma

- Large and echogenic on ultrasound
- Inhomogeneous solid mass on CT

Insulinoma

- Tumors manifest when quite small because of powerful effect of insulin

FIGURE   Gore: 2181

Gastrinoma

- Zollinger-Ellison syndrome
- 60% multiple, 60% malignant with metastases

Somatostatinoma

- Diabetes, gallstones, weight loss

Glucagonoma

- Symptoms: rash (thigh, buttocks), glucose intolerance, weight loss, anemia, venous thrombosis

VIPoma

- Symptoms: watery diarrhea, hypokalemia, achlorhydria

Metastases

- From melanoma; cancer of breast, lung, kidney, GI tract, prostate

Acute pancreatitis

- Look for signs of inflammation: fat stranding, retroperitoneal fluid

Pseudocyst

- Chronic sequela of pancreatitis
- Look for other features of chronic pancreatitis: calcification, dilated pancreatic duct, thickening of retroperitoneal fascial planes

Abscess

- Patient septic

PANCREATIC CALCIFICATION

What disease entities should be considered when pancreatic calcifications are detected?

Chronic pancreatitis
    Any cause, but especially hereditary
    Pseudocyst
Neoplasm
    Serous cystadenoma
    Mucinous cystadenoma/carcinoma
    Islet cell
Vascular calcification
    Splenic artery
    Splenic artery aneurysm

Chronic pancreatitis

- Identification of a dilated duct is helpful

Neoplasm

- Serous cystadenomas show central calcifications compared with peripheral calcifications seen with mucinous cystadenomas
- Islet cell tumors can calcify as they get bigger

Vascular calcification

- Splenic artery aneurysm is a complication of pancreatitis

SPLEEN

CALCIFICATIONS

Outline a differential diagnosis for splenic calcification.

Disseminated infection
    Granulomatous disease (TB, histoplasmosis)
    Pneumocystis carinii

Vascular
    Infarcts
    Splenic artery (with or without aneurysm)
    Hemangioma (phleboliths)
Calcified cyst
    Echinococcal disease
    Old hematoma
Metastases that calcify
    Colon
    Ovarian

Granulomatous disease

Can active granulomatous splenic infections be calcified?

• Calcification indicates that focus of disease is old

Pneumocystis carinii

• Immunocompromised patient
• Look for additional calcifications in liver, kidneys, and lymph nodes
• Calcifications in spleen tend to be coalescent compared with punctate calcifications in liver
• May also result in low-attenuation lesions in liver and spleen
• Presence of calcification does not mean infection is quiescent or healed

Can active disseminated Pneumocystis *infections be calcified?*

FIGURE Gore: 2257

Splenic infarct

What underlying diseases should be considered if one identifies splenic infarction?

• Numerous causes
• May be due to underlying sickle cell disease or bacterial endocarditis

FIGURE Gore: 2261

Echinococcal disease

True or false: Calcification of echinococcal disease in the spleen is usually detectable on plain films.

• Uncommon
• Calcification usually subtle, not seen on plain films

Metastases

Which metastases calcify?

• Metastases that tend to ossify or calcify can be recalled using the mnemonic CHOMP:
    CH: chondrosarcoma
      O: osteosarcoma
     M: mucinous adenocarcinomas (ovary, gastrointestinal tract)
      P: papillary thyroid carcinoma

CYSTIC SPLENIC MASS

List the differential diagnosis for cystic splenic mass.

Epidermoid cyst
Sequela of trauma
    Hematoma
    Traumatic cyst
    Degenerated infarct

FIGURE Gore: 2259

Infection
    Splenic abscess
    Echinococcal cyst
Inflammation
    Pancreatic pseudocyst
Cystic neoplasm

Epidermoid cyst

- Congenital; increases slowly in size with time
- True cyst (has epithelial lining)

FIGURE   Gore: 2267

Trauma

- Remote history

Splenic abscess

- May have reactive left pleural effusion

FIGURE   Gore: 2252

Echinococcal cyst

- Daughter cysts
- Wall calcification

Pancreatic pseudocyst

- Look for other findings of pancreatitis

FIGURE   Gore: 2269

Cystic neoplasm

- Metastatic tumors to spleen can be cystic (think of melanoma)

FIGURE   Gore: 2268

SOLID SPLENIC MASS

List common entities to consider for a solid splenic mass.

Sarcoma
Lymphoma
Metastases
Hemangioma

Sarcoma

- Most frequent primary malignancy of spleen
- Occurs in middle-aged to older adults

FIGURES   Gore: 2277, 2278

Lymphoma

- Approximately 50% of patients with lymphoma have splenic involvement
- Splenic involvement usually is microscopic and is manifested as splenomegaly without discrete mass
- On CT, look for contour abnormalities, because 70% of lymphomatous involvement of spleen is subcapsular

- Solitary or multifocal mass also in spectrum of possibilities
- Sonographically hypoechoic (may mimic cyst)

FIGURES   Gore: 2279–2282

Metastases

- From cancer of breast, lung, ovary; melanoma

FIGURE   Gore: 2284

Hemangioma

- Most common benign tumor of spleen
- May be part of generalized angiomatosis (Klippel-Trénaunay-Weber syndrome)
- Calcifications may be seen on CT

FIGURES   Gore: 2271, 2272

Figure References

Gedgaudas-McClees RK: Handbook of Gastrointestinal Imaging. New York: Churchill Livingstone, 1987.

Gore RM, Levine MS, Laufer I: Textbook of Gastrointestinal Radiology. Philadelphia: WB Saunders, 1994.

Putnam CE, Ravin CE: Textbook of Diagnostic Imaging, 2nd ed. Philadelphia: WB Saunders, 1994.

Rumack CM, Wilson SR, Charboneau JW: Diagnostic Ultrasound. St. Louis: Mosby Year Book, 1991.

GASTROINTESTINAL VISCERA DISEASE ENTITIES

ABSCESS, OF LIVER

Clinical

- Usually related to ascending biliary infection; thus, organism usually gram negative
- Before antibiotic era, was usually caused by diverticulitis, perforated viscus, or inflammatory bowel disease (IBD)
- Can be caused by systemic bacteremia
- Treatment of choice is percutaneous drainage

Imaging

- Ultrasound:
    Irregular, encapsulated cavity of variable internal echoes depending on gas, debris, etc.; need to differentiate from necrotic neoplasm, hematoma, complicated cysts, and amebic abscess; with treatment, the echo amplitude of the lesion increases; may end up with residual area of increased echogenicity
- CT:
    Varies from smoothly marginated, fluid-filled cavity to higher density mass indistinguishable from neoplasm; often with irregular borders

ACINAR CELL CARCINOMA

Clinical

- Large (2 to 12 cm); can arise anywhere in the pancreas
- Metastasizes to nodes, liver, lung
- Males affected more often than females
- Release lipase: subcutaneous fat necrosis, polyarthralgia, eosinophilia, lytic bone lesions

ADENOCARCINOMA, OF PANCREAS

Clinical

- 3% of all cancers in United States
- Metastases: liver (hematogenous) most common followed by nodes (posterior pancreatic), peritoneum, and lungs (via lymphatics)
- 70% in head; 45% near common bile duct (CBD)
- Weight loss, fatigue
- Obstructive jaundice
- Poor long-term survival (1% 5-year survival)

Imaging

- CT:
    Focal mass
    Dilated CBD and pancreatic duct (PD) (sensitive, not specific)
    Rounded uncinate
    Obliteration of fat surrounding celiac axis and SMA has long been considered characteristic of pancreatic carcinoma, but nonpancreatic tumors can also do this, such as metastases (consider esophageal squamous cell carcinoma), lymphoma (uncommon for lymphoma to do this, however), primary small bowel adenocarcinoma (rare tumor, unusual location), and diffuse retroperitoneal endocrine tumor
    Obliteration of fat surrounding celiac axis has also been described in chronic pancreatitis
- Ultrasound:
    Hypoechoic mass; dilated ducts; can be identified as focal change in texture on ultrasound scan without glandular enlargement
- Angiography:
    Hypovascular (islet cells are hypervascular)
- ERCP:
    Double duct sign (narrowing of both CBD and PD) can be caused by pancreatitis; stricture of PD permits presumptive diagnosis of cancer 90% of the time

ADENOMA, OF LIVER

Clinical

- Composed of hepatocytes only; no Kupffer cells
- Malignant degeneration infrequently described
- Associated with oral contraceptive use; occasionally seen in men, often with history of androgen use for anemia
- Tends to be large before it is symptomatic
- May present with acute abdomen from spontaneous hemorrhage
- Management: stop birth control pills; if no regression, excise

Imaging

- Nuclear medicine:
    Does not take up technetium-sulfur colloid because does not contain Kupffer cells; however, there is a study demonstrating 13 hepatic adenomas that did have Kupffer cells; uptake occurred in three cases
- Angiography:
    No specific features, but 50% of adenomas are hypovascular (compare with FNH)
- Sonography:
    No specific features to differentiate from other neoplasms, but sonolucent areas within mass, indicative of necrosis or hemorrhage, tend to suggest adenoma
- CT:
    Adenomas show variable enhancement, may have foci of hemorrhage
- MRI:
    Without hemorrhage, has iso- to hypointense T1 signal and iso- to hyperintense T2 signal; with hemorrhage, has increased signal on T1 and T2

ANGIOSARCOMA, OF LIVER

Clinical

- Most common primary malignant sarcoma of liver
- Associated with Thorotrast exposure; Thorotrast emits alpha particles; delay time of 20 to 30 years; other tumors associated with Thorotrast include hepatomas and cholangiocarcinomas
- These lesions are quite vascular

BUDD-CHIARI SYNDROME

Clinical

- Characterized by narrowing or occlusion of hepatic veins
- Several causes:
    Hypercoagulability (polycythemia, oral contraceptives)
    Congenital webs or membranes of IVC or hepatic veins
    Compression or direct invasion by tumors (hepatoma, renal cell carcinoma, adrenal or pancreatic carcinoma)
- Clinical triad: hepatomegaly, right upper quadrant pain, ascites

Imaging

- CT:
    Fan-shaped appearance of abnormality in liver with central sparing (contrast trying to drain peripherally gives fan-shaped appearance)
    Caudate lobe spared (drains independently directly into IVC); caudate lobe appears relatively large; not seen in caval forms, in which IVC is affected
    No visualization of hepatic veins
    Prominent retroperitoneal collaterals
    Prolonged, nonhomogeneous parenchymal opacification
    Compressed intrahepatic cava often seen secondary to swollen liver
- Nuclear medicine:
    May see "hot spot" on technetium-sulfur colloid study because caudate is the only normal liver present
- Angiography:
    "Spider web" network of veins
- MRI:
    Serpiginous collateral vessels (flow voids); also seen in some normal individuals

CARCINOMA, OF GALLBLADDER

Clinical

- Cholelithiasis found in almost all cases; in contrast, cholangiocarcinoma has no association with gallstones
- Calcification of gallbladder wall in about 25% of cases; in patients who have calcified or porcelain gallbladder, frequency of gallbladder carcinoma is as high as 60%
- Modes of spread:
    Invasion, especially to liver, but also to duodenum, stomach, etc.
    Lymphatic dissemination to porta nodes, cystic nodes, pericholedochal nodes, and superior and posterior pancreaticoduodenal and periaortic nodes
    Vascular spread uncommon
    Intraperitoneal spread common
    Neural spread occurs relatively frequently and is associated with more aggressive tumors
    Intraductal spread least common but most frequently seen in cases of papillary adenocarcinoma of gallbladder
- Most primary carcinomas are adenocarcinomas, either mucinous or nonmucinous;

less commonly, adenosquamous and squamous cell carcinomas occur; malignant melanoma is the most common metastasis to gallbladder
- Usually in women over the age of 65 years; peak incidence: 6th and 7th decades; ratio of women to men affected, 4:1
- If tumor is confined to the gallbladder, can be resected easily; unfortunately, usually not detected until late; 5-year survival less than 5%

Imaging

- CT and ultrasound findings:
    Variable; can have relatively normal gallbladder with stones to large, invasive mass
    Three patterns described:
        Polypoid mass projecting into lumen
        Focal or diffuse wall thickening
        Generalized mass invading into liver (most common)
    Other findings reflect biliary obstruction, nodal involvement, and hematogenous metastases

CAROLI'S DISEASE

Clinical

- Condition characterized by segmental saccular dilatation of intrahepatic bile ducts
- Also known as *communicating cavernous ectasia of the intrahepatic biliary system*
- Propensity for developing biliary calculi and recurrent attacks of cholangitis
- Associations: may arise de novo, infantile polycystic kidney disease (IPKD), congenital hepatic fibrosis, medullary sponge kidney

Imaging

- Ultrasound:
    Intrahepatic biliary duct saccules and nonobstructing intrahepatic calculi
    Can develop periportal fibrosis, which is an alternative presentation (associated with congenital hepatic fibrosis)
    Ductal ectasia may result in portal vein within portal triad being completely surrounded by dilated biliary duct; this is known as *intraluminal portal vein sign*
    May coexist with choledochal cyst
    Examine kidneys for IPKD or medullary sponge kidney

CHOLANGIOCARCINOMA

Clinical

- No association with choledocholithiasis; gallstones can be present, but no particular association (as there is with gallbladder carcinoma)
- Men slightly more commonly affected than women; ratio approximately 2 or 3 to 1
- Increased frequency with the following:
    Primary sclerosing cholangitis
    Ulcerative colitis
    Clonorchiasis (in Asians)
    Biliary atresia
    Chronic cholangitis with or without hepatolithiasis
    Thorotrast exposure
    Hemochromatosis
    Choledochal cysts

Imaging

- Imaging features depend on location; in general, three types seen, as outlined below

Intrahepatic
- In this location, tumors usually exophytic, intrahepatic masses indistinguishable from other hepatic malignancies
- Possible focal or segmental biliary dilatation
- Cholangiocarcinoma tends to cause hepatic atrophy, so that dilated ducts are seen with hepatic parenchymal atrophy; this atrophy not always seen with cholangiocarcinoma, does not occur with hepatomas or metastases
- Abundant mucin secretion, which can calcify, sometimes occurs

Hilar
- When tumor occurs at bifurcation of right and left hepatic ducts, called *Klatskin's tumor*
- Ultrasound:
    Isolation of right and left bile duct segments
    Mass or bile duct wall thickening at hilus
    Because this tumor is scirrhous in nature, ultrasound may not detect a mass; if mass is seen, usually poorly defined
    Portal vein thrombosis can occur but not as frequently as in hepatoma
- CT:
    Better demonstrates mass, which is usually hypodense (precontrast and postcontrast)
    Lobar hepatic atrophy in combination with biliary dilatation can be seen and should strongly suggest cholangiocarcinoma
- Cholangiography:
    Irregular narrowing or obstruction
    Necessary to completely evaluate proximal extent of hilar cholangiocarcinoma
    Differentiation from:
    Hilar lymphadenopathy: compresses and displaces ducts rather than invading them
    Benign strictures: generally short and cause symmetric narrowing

Distal duct
- Usually small
- Cholangiography:
    Shows short stricture
    Polypoid mass less commonly seen
- Tumors at this level often more easily detected with ultrasound than with CT

Other Points
- Features that suggest malignancy in a patient with sclerosing cholangitis: progression of strictures, marked biliary dilatation above a dominant stricture, polypoid ductal mass 1 cm or more in diameter

CHOLANGITIS, AIDS

Clinical

- Thought to be caused by CMV, *Cryptosporidium* spp, and/or *Microsporidia*
- Appearance similar to that of sclerosing cholangitis, except AIDS cholangitis affects ampulla with stenosis, but sclerosing cholangitis typically does not
- In addition to biliary tract signs and symptoms, patients can have severe abdominal pain and diarrhea from related cryptosporidial enteritis
- Papillotomy can provide symptomatic relief, but bile duct inflammation progresses

Imaging

- Ultrasound:
    Dilated ducts, classically with abrupt termination at papilla; "hyperechoic nodule" may be seen at papilla; duct wall thickening
- Cholangiograms:
    Typically show intrahepatic and extrahepatic bile duct irregularities and strictures; papillary stenosis can occur in isolation or associated with more proximal duct strictures

CHOLANGITIS, BACTERIAL

Clinical

- Bacterial cholangitis nearly always is associated with biliary obstruction
- Underlying cause of obstruction more likely to be benign than malignant
- *Escherichia coli* the most common infecting organism

Imaging

- Ultrasound: purulent bile may be identified as echogenic material within involved ducts
- Cholangiography:
    Irregular tubular filling defects
    Multiple small hepatic abscesses that communicate with the biliary tree commonly seen
    Care must be taken not to inject too much contrast into an obstructed, infected system because of the risk of septicemia
    Chronic bouts of cholangitis lead to stricture formation

CHOLANGITIS, RECURRENT PYOGENIC

Clinical

- Formerly known as *Oriental cholangiohepatitis*
- Characterized by intrahepatic formation of pigmented stones with recurrent exacerbation and remission of abdominal pain frequently associated with jaundice, chills, and fever
- Stones are bilirubin stones (not cholesterol stones, which are passed from the gallbladder and can result in ascending cholangitis seen in Westerners)
- Two theories of pathogenesis:
    (1) Chronic infestation (i.e., clonorchiasis, ascariasis) leads to ductal injury/strictures resulting in areas of bile stasis; stagnation is a set-up for bacterial infestation, at which time the chronic infesting organism is killed; the killed larvae/ova then act as nuclei for formation of intrahepatic stones
    (2) Poor hygiene leads to portal septicemia; infection is excreted into bile, resulting in cholangitis when obstruction is present because of ductal injury/strictures from chronic infestations, stones, tumor
- Recurrent attacks of fever, chills, abdominal pain, jaundice
- Increased risk of cholangiocarcinoma

Imaging

- Intrahepatic and extrahepatic duct stones seen in 80% of patients
- Disproportionate dilatation of extrahepatic ducts and major intrahepatic ducts; peripheral intrahepatic ducts normal to small; this occurs because of peribiliary fibrosis that characterizes this disease
- Cholangiography: focal strictures, acute peripheral tapering, straightening, rigidity, decreased arborization, increased branching angle
- Prominent periportal echogenicity representing pericholangitis and periportal fibrous thickening
- In chronic stages can lead to parenchymal loss and segmental atrophy; atrophy may correlate with degree of portal vein obstruction
- When involvement is segmental, it tends to involve left lateral segment first, followed by posterior segment on right lobe
- Cases have been described that show complete obstruction of portal vein; this does not necessarily mean associated malignancy

Differential diagnosis

- Gallstone passed into bile duct: dilated ducts are seen proximal to the stone, whereas with recurrent pyogenic cholangitis, dilatation is seen proximal and distal to the stone

- Clonorchiasis: causes diffuse dilatation of intrahepatic ducts with relative sparing of large ducts; periductal changes are more severe with clonorchiasis
- Sclerosing cholangitis: may show duct dilatation and thickening, but dilatation is focal and discontinuous, with beaded or serpiginous course
- Caroli's disease: differentiation possible by presence of dilated saccules in intrahepatic ducts

CHOLECYSTITIS, ACUTE

Clinical

- In 90 to 95% of patients, caused by impacted calculus in cystic duct
- Right upper quadrant pain, fever
- Murphy's sign: palpation of gallbladder causes inspiratory arrest

Imaging

- General considerations:
  - Positive sonogram more reliable than negative sonogram
  - Negative HIDA scan more reliable than positive HIDA scan
- Ultrasound:
  - Evaluates presence of gallstones, focal tenderness (sonographic Murphy's sign), wall thickening, and pericholecystic fluid
  - Presence of stones in setting of right upper quadrant pain and fever has 90% positive predictive value for cholecystitis; if positive sonographic Murphy's sign also is present, positive predictive value goes up to 99% for pain relieved by cholecystectomy
  - Important points about sonographic Murphy's sign:
    - Either positive or negative; an equivocal sign is negative
    - Pain has to be focal and repeatable
    - If sonographic Murphy's sign is positive and stones are not seen in a patient in whom cholecystitis is suspected, perform HIDA scan
  - Ways to differentiate acute from chronic cholecystitis by ultrasound:
    - (1) Sonographic Murphy's sign
    - (2) Visualization of impacted stone in cystic duct
    - (3) Perigallbladder fluid: specific, not sensitive for acute cholecystitis
    - (4) Increased gallbladder wall thickness seen in both, thus is nonspecific; also seen in several other settings, including AIDS, ascites, alcoholic liver disease, hepatitis, heart failure, renal disease, multiple myeloma, and gallbladder carcinoma
- Biliary scintigraphy: *See* **Nuclear Medicine** chapter for details
  - Highly accurate (95%)
  - Diagnosis relies on nonvisualization of gallbladder; need to have delayed images (4 hours) to help exclude chronic cholecystitis
  - Rim of increased activity (caused by pericholecystic hyperemia) may be seen

CHOLECYSTITIS, ACALCULOUS

Clinical

- Approximately 5 to 10% of cases of acute cholecystitis occur in the absence of gallstones
- When it occurs, usually it is in the setting of a patient with multiple system abnormalities (e.g., intensive care unit patients)

Imaging

- HIDA scans can be falsely normal in these patients
- Diagnosis should be suspected in anyone with markedly distended gallbladder (more than 6 cm in transverse dimension)
- When diagnosis suspected in intensive care unit patient, a reasonable approach is to place a cholecystotomy tube to decompress the gallbladder, with the idea that

it is better to place a tube in a patient without acalculous cholecystitis than to miss the diagnosis in a patient who has the condition, given its high morbidity and mortality

CHOLECYSTITIS, CHRONIC

Clinical

- No clearly defined histologic criteria; pathologic findings include variable amount of inflammation of gallbladder wall and varying degrees of transmural thickening and fibrosis
- Preoperative clinical diagnosis of chronic cholystitis is based on presence of calculi in patients with symptoms suggesting gallbladder disease (chronic or episodic right upper abdominal pain, fatty food intolerance)

Imaging

- Quantification of contractile and symptomatic response to cholecystokinin being investigated as diagnostic scintigraphic test

CHOLECYSTITIS, EMPHYSEMATOUS

Clinical

- Infection with gas-forming bacteria causes gas to accumulate in the gallbladder wall and surrounding soft tissues
- Cholelithiasis not a major pathogenetic factor
- Three times more common in men
- 20 to 30% of cases occur in diabetics

Imaging

- Ultrasound:
    Look carefully for echogenic focus in wall of gallbladder with dirty acoustic shadowing
- Mural air is more obvious on CT; can be seen on plain film

CHOLECYSTOSES, HYPERPLASTIC

- Generic term to describe diverse group of benign, nonneoplastic, noninflammatory abnormalities of the gallbladder
- Two conditions have emerged as reasonably well-defined pathologic entities, namely cholesterolosis and adenomyomatosis

Clinical

Cholesterolosis
- Also called *strawberry gallbladder* (whitish cholesterol deposits on hyperemic mucosa)
- Abnormal accumulation of cholesterol precursors in macrophages, epithelium, and stroma of gallbladder wall
- Two forms:
    Planar variety most common: inner surface of gallbladder looks like fine reticular carpet
    Polypoid form: consists of discrete excrescences that grow to about 1 cm
- Often asymptomatic
- Neoplastic transformation does not occur

Adenomyomatosis
- Characterized by hyperplastic changes, including mucosal proliferation, muscular wall thickening, and intramural diverticulae (Rokitansky-Aschoff sinuses)
- Types: focal or diffuse, circumferential, fundal; more commonly segmental than diffuse
- Can get microcalculi in sinuses
- Often asymptomatic

Imaging

Cholesterolosis
- Planar form not radiographically appreciated; thus, discussion is limited to cholesterol polyps, the second form of cholesterolosis
- Ultrasound:
    Single or multiple fixed, nonshadowing echogenic foci that project into lumen; characteristic ring down artifact suggestive of cholesterol composition may be seen

Adenomyomatosis
- Oral cholecystography: contrast within sinuses (look like diverticulae); gallbladder can have hourglass or segmented appearance
- Ultrasound:
    Thickening of wall with identification of intramural diverticula
    Bile in sinuses produces anechoic spaces within wall
    Those containing stones or sludge appear echogenic
    Can have ring-down artifact
- Can simulate a mass in fundus in that there is hyperplasia without formation of Rokitansky-Aschoff sinuses
- Gallbladder can become compartmentalized

CHOLEDOCHAL CYST

Clinical

- Classification (Todani modification of the Alonso-Lej classification)
            (1) Fusiform dilation of entire common duct, common hepatic duct, or both
            (2) Localized, eccentric, cystic diverticulum off common duct
            (3) Dilation of distal intramural portion of common bile duct (choledochocele)
            (4) Any combination of cysts that may include intrahepatic cystic dilatation
            (5) Pure intrahepatic variant of Caroli's disease
- Abnormal dynamics believed to create cyst, caused by common bile duct joining pancreatic duct abnormally at right angles
- Uncommon (incidence approximately 0.2 to 0.5 per 1,000,000)
- Increased incidence in females (4:1) and Asians
- 33% of patients have jaundice in first year of life; approximately 70% diagnosed by age 16 years
- Triad of intermittent jaundice, pain, and abdominal mass characteristic in older patients, but present in only 25% of pediatric patients with choledochal cyst
- Increased incidence of cholangiocarcinoma
- Patients prone to develop bile duct carcinoma
- Patients predisposed to cholangitis (caused by stasis)

Imaging

- Plain films:
    Mass displacing bowel gas may be seen; calcification of wall is rare
- Barium study:
    Displacement of gastric antrum anteriorly, inferiorly, to left; choledochocele shows rounded filling defect in duodenum near ampulla of Vater
- Ultrasound:
    Cystic mass in porta hepatis, fluid filled and separate from gallbladder; can demonstrate connection of cyst with biliary system
- Tc^{99m}-labeled iminodiacetic acid (IDA):
- Accumulation and stasis of tracer within choledochal cyst

Differential diagnosis

- Other fluid-filled masses in the area:
    Hepatic cyst
    Pancreatic pseudocyst
    Ovarian cyst

Omental cyst
Mesenteric cyst
Enteric duplication
Hepatic artery aneurysm
Spontaneous perforation of an extrahepatic bile duct

CHOLEDOCHOLITHIASIS

Clinical

- Majority of stones in bile ducts originate in gallbladder and migrate to common duct
- Approximately 10 to 15% of patients undergoing cholecystectomy for cholelithiasis have concomitant choledocholithiasis
- In the United States, only 5% are primary duct stones
- Nearly 50% of patients have no symptoms
- Most commonly used treatment options include extraction through T-tube tract and endoscopic removal

Imaging

- Operative and T-tube cholangiography:
    Has high accuracy for detection of common duct stones (about 80 to 99%)
    All patients undergoing cholecystectomy should have operative cholangiography
    Postoperative T-tube cholangiography should detect any residual calculi left at the time of operation; these calculi usually can be extracted percutaneously
- ERCP:
    Indicated when CT and ultrasound fail to reveal a stone in the face of compelling clinical suspicion
- Transhepatic cholangiography:
    Used when ERCP fails or when there has been previous biliary-enteric surgery
- Ultrasound:
    Common bile duct stones can be seen in 75 to 80% of patients
    Technical maneuvers that can help visualize distal common bile duct include patient positioning (semierect position, slightly right posterior oblique) and having patient drink water
    10% of stones do not cast acoustic shadow
- CT:
    Routinely used when patients have obstructive jaundice and ultrasound fails to show cause; look for "target" or "crescent" sign

CHOLELITHIASIS

Clinical

- Causes:
    Nonhemolytic
        Positive family history
        Obesity
        Diabetes
        Pregnancy
        Estrogen therapy
        Cystic fibrosis
        Enteric causes (chronic GI infection, diet, interruption of enterohepatic circulation of bile salts)
    Hemolytic causes (result of hemolytic anemia causing pigment stones)
        Congenital spherocytosis
        Sickle cell anemia
        Thalassemia
        Other causes of accelerated red blood cell destruction
- Occurs in 10 to 20% of the population in United States
- Women affected twice as often as men

Imaging

- Plain films:

    About 10 to 15% of gallstones contain enough calcium to be visualized on plain films

    Shrinkage of cholesterol crystals as a stone becomes dehydrated can lead to dendritic cracks containing nitrogen gas, resulting in Mercedes-Benz sign

- Ultrasound:

    Procedure of choice

    Accuracy in detection exceeds 95%

    Diagnosis made by demonstration of nonfixed echogenic foci within gallbladder lumen with acoustic shadowing

    Small stones may not show acoustic shadowing (which depends on diameter of sonic beam in relation to diameter of stone); differential diagnosis for this nonfixed foci without shadowing includes sludge, pus, mucin, or blood

- Oral cholecystography: once the gold standard, now reserved for cases in which ultrasound examination is equivocal or when compelling clinical symptoms suggest gallbladder disease and ultrasound is normal

CIRRHOSIS

Clinical

- Generic term: refers to chronic destruction and distortion of normal hepatic architecture with replacement by fibrosis and regenerating nodules
- Causes of cirrhosis in United States:

Alcohol abuse	30 to 60%
Postnecrosis	10 to 30%
Biliary cirrhosis	10 to 20%
Pigment cirrhosis	2 to 5% (hemochromatosis, Wilson's disease)

Imaging

- Overall liver size decreases and caudate lobe hypertrophies; some say that ratio of caudate to right lobe of more than 0.6 indicates cirrhosis
- Ultrasound:

    Parenchymal heterogeneity with decreased penetration caused by fibrosis

    This appearance also seen with fatty infiltration, but secondary signs of cirrhosis (varices, splenomegaly, ascites: occur with development of portal hypertension) help to distinguish the two

    Look for recanalized umbilical vein, which occurs in up to 20% (now thought to be caused by dilated veins adjacent to irrevocably scarred umbilical vein)

CLONORCHIASIS

Clinical

- Parasitology: fluke lays eggs in biliary system of host; eggs excreted, then eaten by snails; metamorphosis occurs; flukes escape to penetrate scales of fish, then encyst in muscles of fish; fish eaten by host; cyst freed by action of gastric juice; adults migrate from duodenum into biliary system and reside in intrahepatic ducts
- Factors in pathogenesis: mechanical obstruction of biliary tract by fluke, congestion of bile, and effects of metabolites on surrounding tissues, leading to fibrosis
- Epithelium of bile duct undergoes edema and desquamation; later metaplasia
- Endemic in Southeast Asia, from Japan to Vietnam
- Flukes live for decades, so can be recognized in emigrants
- Minimal clinical symptoms
- Increased risk of developing cholangiocarcinoma

Imaging

- Cholangiography:

    Filling defects: round, linear, filamentous, rice-like, and oval; 2 to 10 mm

Dilatation of peripheral small intrahepatic ducts; extrahepatic bile ducts not dilated

The heavier the infestation, the more likely that filling defects of extrahepatic ducts and gallbladder will be seen

- Ultrasound: thickening of bile ducts

Differential diagnosis

- Cancer along bile ducts: obstructing lesion usually visualized; entire biliary tree proximal to obstruction is dilated, not just peripheral small bile ducts
- Choledocholithiasis with recurrent pyogenic cholangitis: intrahepatic bile ducts not dilated or dilated minimally; extrahepatic ducts much more dilated
- Sclerosing cholangitis: ducts much more irregular and serpiginous, appear to be discontinuous rather than diffusely dilated; extrahepatic ducts also involved (not seen with clonorchiasis)
- Caroli's disease: saccular dilatation rather than diffuse dilatation

ECHINOCOCCAL CYST

Clinical

Echinococcus granulosus
- Sheep and cattle
- Seen in Australia, New Zealand, parts of Africa, Middle East, South America, and Central Europe
- Produces well-defined expansile cystic lesions
- Classic teaching: aspiration contraindicated, can lead to anaphylaxis

Echinococcus alveolaris (multilocularis)
- Rodents
- Seen in Russia, Central Europe, Canada, Alaska, and Japan
- Produces infiltrating lesions with irregular margins that resemble slow-growing hepatic tumors rather than cysts

Imaging

Echinococcus granulosus
- CT:

Cysts, calcification of cyst wall (indicates death of cyst), daughter cysts (indicate active cyst), membrane detachments

ENDOCRINE TUMORS OF PANCREAS

- Slow growing, hypervascular, rare vascular encasement
- Insulinoma benign; all others malignant to varying degrees
- 20% show calcification (coarse) versus 2% with calcification in ductal adenocarcinoma
- Necrosis rare because blood supply good (hypervascular)
- Insulinoma, gastrinoma present when small; glucagonoma, VIPoma, somatostatinoma present when large
- Nonfunctioning islet cell tumors: present when large, with central necrosis, enhancement, coarse calcification; periaortic adenopathy more common than retropancreatic aortocaval extension

Insulinoma
- Benign; 10% multiple

Gastrinoma
- Zollinger-Ellison syndrome
- 60% multiple; 60% malignant with metastases

Somatostatinoma
- Diabetes mellitus, gallstones, weight loss; very slow growing

Glucagonoma
- Symptoms: rash (thigh, buttocks), glucose intolerance, weight loss, anemia, venous thrombosis

VIPoma
- Symptoms: watery diarrhea, hypokalemia, achlorhydria (WDHA)

FOCAL NODULAR HYPERPLASIA (FNH)

Clinical

- Usually up to 5 to 6 cm in diameter, nonencapsulated, composed of hepatocytes, bile ducts, and variable complement of Kupffer cells
- Central fibrous stellate scar in many
- Hemorrhage rare
- Multiple in 20%
- Usually incidental finding
- Predominantly affects women (4:1)
- No definite association with oral contraceptives has been shown

Imaging

- Nuclear medicine: FNH has variable scintigraphic uptake because amount of Kupffer cells variable; about 40% have increased uptake
- Ultrasound: no distinguishing sonographic features, can be hyperechoic or hypoechoic
- CT:

    Appears as well-circumscribed lesion with central, stellate fibrous scar, lacks peripheral enhancement

    With contrast, transient hyperdensity seen, followed by isodensity

    Presence of transiently increased attenuation of central focus on dynamic images suggests FNH (blood supply often radiates from center, causing spoke-wheel appearance on angiography)

- Arteriography:

    Well-circumscribed, hypervascular mass with dense blush in capillary and portal venous phase

    Numerous tortuous vascular channels present, representing hypertrophied normal vasculature

    Classically, arterial supply radiates in spoke-wheel fashion

    In parenchymal phase, fine granular appearance and lucent septa seen

- MRI:

    Many isointense on all sequences; some slightly hypo T1 and hyper T2

    Central scar common, often inflammatory (hyper T2 signal)

    Response to gadolinium: rapid enhancement and rapid washout, just as with hepatoma and vascular metastases

HEMANGIOMA, OF LIVER

Clinical

- Common: autopsy series shows about 5% incidence
- Multiple in 10 to 20%
- Usually subcapsular or marginal in location
- Calcifications uncommon
- 4.5 to 9 times more common in women
- No increase in complications (versus other types of tumors) when biopsied with a needle smaller than 18 gauge

Imaging

- CT:

    (1) Fills in from periphery, eccentrically; 85% of lesions larger than 2 cm in diameter show this pattern; small lesions (less than 15 mm) often do not have this pattern

    (2) Dynamic scanning: pick level; inject about 150 mL contrast; scan

at 30 seconds, 1 minute, 2 minutes, etc., up to about 20 minutes; some recommend delayed scans (i.e., 6 hours) to assist in diagnosis
(3) Typical findings: peripheral location; homogenous after enhancement; sharply defined; brightly enhanced nodular or corrugated borders as enhancement progresses; early in examination, border usually does not form continuous rim but appears as bright papillary projections pointing toward center of lesion; central focus or cleft of low density representing fibrosis often seen in large hemangiomas

- Nuclear medicine
     (1) Increased blood pool activity with a discordant (decreased) flow pattern noted; no such mismatch of flow and blood pool activity (both increased) with hepatomas
     (2) Because these tumors do not have hepatocytes, decreased activity on technetium-sulfur colloid study
     (3) Problems
     A. Size less than 2 cm, not enough signal: planar images detect 12% of lesions less than 2 cm and (single photon emission computed tomography) brings this up to 22%
     B. Location near major vessel
     (4) Mimics: hepatic angiosarcoma and hepatoma, both of which tend to be hyperperfused on immediate images, whereas hemangiomas appear hypoperfused unless small

- Angiography:
     (1) Feeding vessels large
     (2) Arteries displaced by mass
     (3) Lakes of contrast late in arterial phase which, unlike those of other vascular tumors, persist during and past capillary and venous phases for up to 30 seconds
     (4) Neovascularity, draining veins, or arterial-portal venous shunting never seen except in rare pediatric patient with giant cavernous hemangioma

- Ultrasound:
     (1) Usually strongly echogenic masses, but may be relatively echopenic
     (2) Other lesions with similar pattern: FHN, hepatic adenoma, hepatocellular carcinoma, solitary hepatic metastasis
     (3) Flow not seen on Doppler because flow is too slow
     (4) May have increased through-sound transmission
     (5) Atypical hemangioma suggested by solid hepatic tumor with well-defined echogenic border and inhomogeneous internal echo pattern with hypoechoic components

- MRI:
     (1) Increased signal on T2
     (2) Sharply defined, often lobulated
     (3) Peripheral, homogeneous, no rim or halo
     (4) In more than 50%, central low signal scar (collagenous)
     (5) Accuracy of MRI less than 100% because vascular metastases also have prolonged T2, resulting in increased signal on T2
     (6) Response to gadolinium: same as in CT, fills in from periphery

HEMOCHROMATOSIS

Clinical

- Two forms:
     Primary: abnormal iron absorption
     Secondary: more common; iron overload (transfusions)
- Present with liver failure, diabetes, skin pigmentation, arthropathies, cardiac disease, and hypogonadism
- Primary form: tenfold more common in men; symptoms occur between ages 40 and 60 years

Imaging

- Increased density of liver on CT
- Increased attenuation of lymph nodes, pancreas, adrenal cortex may also be seen on CT

HEPATITIS

Imaging

- Ultrasound: in acute hepatitis there can be increased echogenicity of portal vein walls and decreased echogenicity of edematous liver cells
- Scintigraphy: decreased uptake of colloid relative to spleen; differentiates between biliary atresia and neonatal hepatitis: in biliary atresia, good liver extraction with no excretion; in hepatitis, poor extraction and poor excretion
- CT: may see no abnormality; gallbladder wall may be thickened, but this is a nonspecific finding that occurs in a number of conditions

HEPATOMA

Clinical

- Also called hepatocellular carcinoma (HCC)
- Alpha fetoprotein (AFP) level elevated in 80 to 95% (vast majority)
- Modes of spread:
    Extrahepatic tumor spread most often occurs via local extension or regional lymph node involvement
    Distant metastases: regional lymph nodes, lungs, and brain; also bone and spleen
- Associated with hemochromatosis, schistosomiasis, aflatoxin, hepatitis B, cirrhosis, and previous Thorotrast administration
- Uncommon before age 40 years except for distinct subtype called *fibrolamellar hepatocarcinoma,* which occurs in noncirrhotic livers of adolescents and adults under age 35 years; equal incidence in males and females; small central calcification occur in approximately 33% of these patients; better prognosis

Imaging

- CT/general:
    Three forms:
        (1) Solitary mass (30%); common in Japan
        (2) Dominant mass with one or more smaller "satellite" lesions (65%); common in United States
        (3) Diffuse (5%)
    Calcification in 10 to 25%: discrete, dense, or stippled
    Portal vein invasion: occurs in approximately 33% of cases; much more likely caused by hepatoma than other liver tumor or metastases; invasion of IVC and hepatic arteries and veins also common (these tumors invade vessels much more readily than do metastases); best assessed by CT arterioportography
    Flow patterns may be altered because of arterioportal shunts through tumor; this can also be seen in trauma and cirrhosis; congestive hepatomegaly from cardiac disease and hepatic venoocclusive disease also lead to unusual flow patterns
- Angiography:
    Dilated hepatic arteries and feeding vessels with bizarre neovascularity; thrombus in portal vein; arteriovenous shunting
- MRI:
    Low-intensity peripheral rim, corresponding to fibrous pseudocapsule, has been seen on T1 and T2 images
    Low T1 signal, high T2 signal
    Central heterogeneous fat may have increased T1 signal
    Can have inflammatory (hyperintense T2) or collagenous (hypointense T2) central scar

Invasion of vessels with tumor thrombus; increased signal in vessel with enlargement of vein

Response of hepatoma to gadolinium:

Rapid increase in signal, followed by rapid washout

Not a specific pattern, also seen with vascular metastases, FNH

This pattern is not seen in hemangiomas

- Nuclear medicine:

Combination of decreased Tc^{99m}-sulfur colloid accumulation and normal or increased Ga^{67} citrate activity

Hepatic abscesses and, less commonly, metastatic tumors to liver may have similar appearance

- Ultrasound:

Spectrum of findings; no classic picture; use color Doppler to look for portal vein invasion

- Multifocal HCC can be distinguished from metastases as follows:

No dominant mass favors metastases; HCC usually has one large mass and much smaller satellite lesions

Calcification: favors metastases

Marginal enhancement: metastases

Lack of protrusion from liver surface: metastases

ISLET CELL TUMOR

Clinical

- Can secrete hormones normally found in adult pancreas (insulin, glucagon, somatostatin), hormones normally found in fetal pancreas or other glands or tissues (gastrin, vasoactive intestinal polypeptide, serotonin, cortisol), or a combination of different peptides
- Majority found in pancreas, but 10% located in duodenal wall
- Hormonally active tumors usually quite small at time of clinical presentation

Imaging

- Diagnosis of functional islet cell tumor made on clinical grounds and confirmed on laboratory tests
- Role of imaging is to confirm presence of suspected tumor and localize for surgery
- Ultrasound:

(1) Hypoechoic compared with rest of pancreas, well demarcated, round or oval

(2) Anechoic regions correspond to necrosis, and shadowing hyperechoic regions correspond to calcification, both of which are seen in larger tumors (which tend to be malignant)

(3) Intraoperative ultrasound is the most sensitive imaging test, detecting 85 to 100% of tumors

- CT:

(1) To visualize small tumors, need bolus, contrast-enhanced, thin-section dynamic technique; even then, the smallest tumors will not be seen

(2) May identify calcification and areas of necrosis in larger tumors

- Arteriography

(1) Used occasionally for identification of gastrinomas and insulinomas (other islet cell tumors larger and rarely require arteriography)

(2) Characteristic feature is dense, homogeneous, circumscribed parenchymal blush

(3) When all else has failed, one can try transhepatic portal venous sampling for localizing gastrinomas and insulinomas

- MRI:

(1) With present techniques, not as sensitive as CT or ultrasound

(2) When visible, these tumors are generally brighter on T2-weighted images than pancreatic adenocarcinoma

5

LYMPHOMA

Clinical

Liver
- Usually diffuse involvement of liver, but multiple focal nodules can be seen
- In AIDS, multiple focal hepatic lesions more common
- Liver usually involved late rather than early
- Lymphoma is hypovascular

Spleen
- Approximately 50% of patients with lymphoma have splenic involvement
- Spleen always is involved when liver is involved
- Usually, splenic involvement is microscopic

Imaging

Spleen
- CT:
    Look for contour abnormalities, because 70% of lymphomatous involvement of spleen is subcapsular

METASTASIS, TO LIVER

Clinical

- Wide variety of primary neoplasms can metastasize to liver
- Diffuse pattern of involvement often seen with carcinoma of breast
- Lesions less than 1.5 cm discovered in work-up for metastases (AJR 158:535–539, 1992)
    Single lesion: 65% benign, 5% malignant, 30% indeterminate
    Two to four lesions: 60% benign, 20% malignant, 20% indeterminate
    Conclusion: many lesions discovered in patients with known primary cancer are not metastases; if therapy is going to be altered, further work-up needed to be sure these are metastases before patient is discharged

Imaging

- Ultrasound:
    Metastases from GI tract usually are hyperechoic; however, other types of metastases can also be hyperechoic, and not all GI metastases are hyperechoic
- CT versus CT arterioportography (CTAP) versus MRI:
- Research is continuing, but CTAP appears to be most sensitive technique for identifying liver metastases
- Intraoperative ultrasound even more sensitive than CTAP for identifying metastases

MIRIZZI'S SYNDROME

- Unusual cause of common bile duct obstruction
- Consists of impacted stone in cystic duct that lies near and parallel to common bile duct
- The mass of the stone and surrounding inflammation result in partial obstruction of common bile duct
- In such cases, cystic duct typically has a low insertion into common bile duct, resulting in its parallel course with common bile duct

MUCINOUS CYSTADENOMA, OF PANCREAS

Clinical

- Also called *macrocystic adenoma*
- 80% in body and tail
- Malignant potential (as opposed to microcystic variety); thus, needs resection
- Ratio of males to females affected, 6:1

Imaging

- CT: focal low attenuation, cysts often visible
- In general, but not always, cysts are larger than 2 cm and fewer than 6 cysts are present
- 40% calcify; can have stellate appearance, but calcification is classically peripheral (as opposed to central calcifications of serous tumors)

OBSTRUCTION, OF BILIARY TRACT

Clinical

- Differential diagnosis based on site of obstruction
    - (1) Periportal
        Cholangiocarcinoma
        Carcinoma of gallbladder
        Metastatic disease (lymph node enlargement): colon, breast, lung, lymphoma
        Hepatoma invading bile duct
    - (2) Mid-common duct
        Pancreatic cancer
        Cholangiocarcinoma
        Iatrogenic stricture (post cholecystectomy)
        Metastatic disease
        Sclerosing cholangitis
        Chronic pancreatitis
        Common duct stone
        Mirizzi's syndrome
    - (3) Periampullary
        Pancreatic cancer
        Ampullary cancer
        Common duct stone
        Ampullary stenosis
        Choledochal cyst/choledochocele
        Villous adenoma of duodenum
        Duodenal diverticulum

Imaging

- Ultrasound:
    Commonly used to assess presence or absence of bile duct obstruction
    Common hepatic duct (the duct just as it becomes extrahepatic) almost always visualized sonographically and should be less than 6 mm in diameter; if more than 6 mm, it is dilated; however, after the age of 60 years, 1 mm per decade can be added to range of normal (thus, 7 mm normal for 70-year-old)
    7 to 11 mm is a gray zone; ducts in this range may be large normal ducts, ducts enlarged as result of previous biliary tract disease, or large ducts secondary to obstruction
    Intrahepatic ductal dilatation seen as "double ducts" throughout hepatic parenchyma, representing dilated duct adjacent to portal vessel
- Obstruction can occur without dilatation:
    Is a cause of false-negative ultrasound scan
    Most commonly results from choledocholithiasis, with small stones that transiently obstruct
    Other causes: sclerosing cholangitis, pancreatitis, ampullary stenosis, and even malignant entities such as pancreatic carcinoma or cholangiocarcinoma
- Provocative tests:
    In equivocal cases (i.e., duct measures 7 to 11 mm), fatty meal can be given
    Fatty meal should decrease duct caliber from 0 to 3 mm; increase in duct caliber implies benign fibrosis or spasm at sphincter of Oddi, choledocholithiasis, or small tumor

5

• Limitation of ultrasound:
   Low success rate in determining site and cause of obstruction (27 to 50%); CT more successful than ultrasound in establishing site and cause of obstruction but is more expensive
   Other techniques to evaluate patency of bile ducts are ERCP and transhepatic cholangiography

PANCREATITIS, ACUTE

Clinical

• Mild forms lead to edema and leukocytic infiltration only
• Severe forms can progress to necrotization, hemorrhage, suppuration
• Raised pancreatic amylase, lipase levels in blood and urine
• Conditions in which pancreatitis occurs:
   Biliary tract disease
   Alcoholism
   Hyperparathyroidism
   Trauma
      Blunt/penetrating injury
      Surgery
      Penetrating ulcer
   Infection
      Mumps
      Parasites
   Hereditary (autosomal dominant)
   Hyperlipidemia
   Drugs
   Pregnancy
   Idiopathic in about 20% of patients
• Complications:
   Hemorrhagic pancreatitis: hyperdense areas on CT
   Pseudocyst formation
   Abscess: most commonly caused by *E. coli*; occurs 2 to 4 weeks after acute insult
   Pseudoaneurysm of splenic artery (might suggest when focus of hyperintensity is seen in midst of pancreas on CT study)
   Splenic vein thrombosis

Imaging

• All studies may be normal
• Plain films:
   Colon cut-off sign: dilated transverse colon, with abrupt change to gasless descending colon
   Sentinel loop: localized ileus of adjacent bowel (usually duodenum)
   Left-sided pleural effusion
• Upper GI study:
   Poppel's sign: edematous swelling of papilla
• Cholangiography:
   Gently tapered narrowing of common bile duct
• Ultrasound:
   Hypoechoic enlarged pancreas; peripancreatic fluid collection; fluid in pararenal space; generally pancreas will not image well because of ileus
• CT:
   Increased size with edema (low density); loss of peripancreatic fat planes; nonenhancement of variable portions of the pancreas may have prognostic value; thickening of anterior pararenal fascia

PANCREATITIS, CHRONIC

Imaging

• Plain films:
   Numerous calcifications

- ERCP:
    Dilated tortuous duct; clubbed side branches; beading, chain of lakes, string of pearls
- CT:
    Findings reflect atrophy of gland with calcifications, ductal dilatation
- Ultrasound:
    In a large percentage, echogenicity is normal; identification of dilated duct helpful; calcifications may be detected, but none will be seen by CT

PANCREATOBLASTOMA

Clinical

- Occurs in head/uncinate of pancreas
- 4 to 17 cm, cystic degeneration, hemorrhage, necrosis
- Occurs before age of 7 years
- Usually metastases at diagnosis

Imaging

- Large and echogenic on ultrasound; solid mass on CT

PELIOSIS HEPATIS

Clinical

- Rare; multiple, blood-filled cystic spaces in liver (ranging from 1 to 5 mm)
- Asymptomatic, incidental finding at autopsy; seen in patients with chronically debilitating diseases such as TB, cancer, hematologic disorders

PNEUMOCYSTIS CARINII INFECTION, EXTRAPULMONARY

Clinical

- Extrapulmonary *P. carinii* infection in patients with AIDS can result in punctate calcifications in liver, spleen, kidneys, adrenal glands, and lymph nodes
- May also result in low-attenuation lesions in liver and spleen
- Presence of calcification does not mean that infection is quiescent or healed
- This pattern is of more historical importance than practical relevance because aerosolized pentamidine, which is thought to predispose AIDS patients to develop extrapulmonary PCP, is no longer used for PCP prophylaxis

PNEUMOBILIA

Imaging

- Plain films:
    Linear lucencies seen over right upper quadrant, with central pattern (as opposed to peripheral pattern that may be seen with portal venous gas)
- Ultrasound:
    Linear echogenic areas in liver with dirty shadowing; in supine patient, more of these echogenic lines seen in left lobe of liver because of its nondependent position

PORCELAIN GALLBLADDER

Clinical

- Exact cause not known; possibly result of elevation of intraluminal and mural calcium carbonate levels in the setting of chronic cholecystitis
- Symptoms suggestive of biliary disease often absent
- Patients usually aged more than 45 years
- Ratio of females to males affected, 5:1
- Virtually all patients with porcelain gallbladder have gallstones

- Cholecystectomy the appropriate therapy because of increased incidence of gallbladder carcinoma (12 to 61%)

Imaging

- Calcification of gallbladder wall
- May be confused on ultrasound as multiple gallstones filling gallbladder lumen

PRIMARY BILIARY CIRRHOSIS (PBC)

Clinical

- Idiopathic destructive disorder of interlobar and septal bile ducts leading to cirrhosis
- Generally occurs in middle-aged women (90% of patients with PBC are women)
- Cholelithiasis associated
- Alteration in cell-based immunity an important feature of PBC
- Serum marker: antimitochondrial antibodies
- Variably characterized by pruritus, hyperpigmentation, xanthelasma/xanthoma formation
- Poor survival once diagnosed

Imaging

- Early in the disease, cholangiograms normal
- Important differences compared with primary sclerosing cholangitis: bile duct deformities much less severe; diverticular outpouchings and mural irregularities typically not seen
- As cirrhosis progresses, intrahepatic ducts become attenuated

SCLEROSING CHOLANGITIS (SC)

Clinical

- Idiopathic disorder consisting of periductal inflammation predominantly involving extrahepatic bile ducts, but can involve intrahepatic bile ducts also; about 25% have normal extrahepatic ducts
- Chronic/intermittent obstructive jaundice and/or fever
- Associations: most commonly associated with ulcerative colitis (25% of cases); other reported associations (not important to memorize): retroperitoneal fibrosis, mediastinal fibrosis, orbital pseudotumor, Riedel's thyroiditis
- Propensity to develop bile duct carcinoma

Imaging

- Cholangiography:
    Irregular, multisegmented narrowing of both extrahepatic and intrahepatic ducts
    Nodular beaded appearance of duct is characteristic
    Saccular or segmental dilatation of ducts can be seen, but dilatation rarely marked
    Biliary diverticula and webs are well-documented cholangiographic features of SC but not specific

Differential Diagnosis

- Cholangiocarcinoma:
    Difficult to distinguish SC from carcinoma histologically; moreover, SC can lead to cholangiocarcinoma
    Cholangiocarcinoma and SC can be focal; if abnormality diffuse, SC more likely
    Helpful radiographic finding: little diverticulae off wall of biliary tract suggestive of SC

SC does not cause ductal dilatation; if biliary tree dilated in SC, consider superimposed neoplastic obstruction
- Primary biliary cirrhosis: smooth narrowing of entire intrahepatic system; does not involve extrahepatic system
- Cirrhosis: ducts crowded; corkscrew, twisted appearance
- Healing of acute cholangitis
- AIDS cholangitis
- FUDR (chemotherapeutic agent)-induced cholangitis

SEROUS CYSTADENOMA, OF PANCREAS

Clinical

- Also called *microcystic adenoma*
- No malignant potential
- Affects males and females with equal frequency; more common in elderly patients

Imaging

- Appears as focus of low attenuation on CT (microcysts not visible); centrally hypervascular
- Criteria: cysts less than 2 cm; more than six cysts
- Cysts do not communicate with ductal system
- Calcification uncommon within tumor (20%); when present, is stellate and central

SOLID PAPILLARY EPITHELIAL NEOPLASM OF PANCREAS

Clinical

- Rare, low-grade malignancy
- Occurs in tail of pancreas
- Malignant potential exists but is low; a slow-growing tumor
- Occurs in young women (mean age, 24 years)

VARICES, GALLBLADDER

Clinical

- Unusual manifestation of portal hypertension
- Often associated with portal vein thrombosis

Imaging

- Difficult to visualize with angiography; readily demonstrable with ultrasound, CT, and MRI
- Ultrasound:
    Thickened gallbladder wall with anechoic areas, which tend to be more serpentine than those seen with acute cholecystitis and which fill with color when color Doppler is applied; need to confirm venous nature with duplex Doppler because increased arterial flow in gallbladder wall can be seen in acute cholecystitis
- CT:
    Nodular enhancement of gallbladder wall caused by vessels crossing perpendicular to scan plane; enhancing small vessels in pericholecystic fat may also be seen
- MRI:
    Varices visible with flow-sensitive techniques

VENOOCCLUSIVE DISEASE, HEPATIC

Clinical

- Variant of Budd-Chiari syndrome, in which small hepatic venules are diffusely occluded

- Occurs in patients with bone marrow transplant and those who undergo hepatic radiation therapy

Imaging

- Findings similar to those in Budd-Chiari syndrome, except that hepatic veins may be visualized on CT and ultrasound
- Hepatic venography (retrograde injection into hepatic vein) shows "spider web" appearance of collaterals

WILSON'S DISEASE

Clinical

- Rare, autosomal recessive condition
- Excess copper deposition in liver, kidneys, brain, and cornea
- Leads to cirrhosis, renal tubular acidosis, basal ganglia dysfunction, and Kayser-Fleischer rings
- Presents between ages of 6 and 20 years

5

Genitourinary Tract Imaging

- ## Carl L. Kalbhen, M.D.
- ## Steven D. Frankel, M.D.

OVERVIEW

The genitourinary system includes the kidneys, renal collecting systems, ureters, urinary bladder, urethra, adrenal glands, and male and female genital tracts. These structures can be affected by a wide variety of disease processes, and many imaging methods are available for assessment. This chapter describes the pathologic entities that can involve the adult genitourinary system; diseases that are exclusive to children can be found in the pediatric imaging chapter, and obstetrical conditions are discussed in the ultrasound chapter.

THE KIDNEYS

Plain film radiography has a limited role in the assessment of renal pathology. Its main use is to evaluate for abnormal calcifications, and it can also assess renal size and identify large mass lesions. Intravenous urography (IVU) involves obtaining serial radiographs after the intravenous administration of iodinated contrast media; it is a simple and inexpensive examination that can assess renal size, shape, position, contour, and function. IVU also has a limited role in detecting and characterizing renal masses.

Renal ultrasound may be performed to assess renal size and location and to detect parenchymal calcifications and mass lesions. Function can be indirectly determined by evaluation of cortical thickness and echogenicity. Ultrasound is of particular use in confirming the cystic or solid nature of a focal mass. With the use of both gray-scale and Doppler techniques, ultrasound also may be used to characterize masses and to evaluate the renal vasculature directly. Ultrasound is commonly performed on renal allografts to assess for rejection, functional complications, and fluid collections. Ultrasound is also used to guide percutaneous biopsy.

Computed tomography (CT) of the kidneys should be performed both with and without the intravenous administration of iodinated contrast media. The precontrast images are useful to evaluate for subtle calcifications and to measure the attenuation values of focal lesions (e.g., fat in an angiomyolipoma, fluid in a cyst). Postcontrast

CT is the examination of choice in the evaluation of renal trauma and to identify and characterize focal renal masses. It also obtains the same functional information available from IVU. CT angiography using spiral (helical) equipment can be useful in the evaluation of the renal vasculature. Spiral CT also can be performed to obtain multiplanar and three-dimensional reconstructions of renal masses. Although no additional diagnostic information is obtained by these reconstructions, the display of anatomic relationships on these images is useful to surgeons preoperatively.

Magnetic resonance imaging (MRI) is, in general, only slightly inferior to contrast-enhanced CT in the evaluation of renal parenchymal pathology. MRI is not as sensitive as CT in the detection of small lesions, and MRI cannot reliably identify calcifications. It is, however, of particular use in the evaluation of patients who cannot undergo contrast-enhanced CT (e.g., those with renal failure, allergy). Noncontrast MR images are more sensitive than noncontrast CT images in the evaluation of focal lesions, and many patients who are not candidates for iodinated CT contrast media are able to receive MR contrast agents (gadolinium chelates). Additionally, MR angiography can be performed to obtain vascular information without the need for intravenous contrast media.

Nuclear medicine techniques are extremely useful to evaluate functional abnormalities, and they also may detect mass lesions. Intravenously injected radiopharmaceuticals can evaluate renal blood flow, and specific agents are available that assess glomerular filtration (DTPA) and tubular function (hippuran, MAG3). As with ultrasound, nuclear medicine is of particular use in the evaluation of renal transplant patients.

Renal angiography is an invasive procedure, and its role in the evaluation of renal parenchymal pathology has diminished with the advent of cross-sectional (ultrasound, CT, and MRI) techniques. Certain lesions do, however, have characteristic findings on angiography (e.g., oncocytoma). Despite the development of CT and MR angiography, conventional angiography remains the gold standard in the assessment of vascular pathology, and it also can be used for therapeutic embolization (e.g., in trauma and vascular tumors).

THE RENAL COLLECTING SYSTEMS AND URETERS

Cross-sectional imaging has a limited role in the evaluation of the renal collecting system and ureters. Ultrasound, CT, and MRI are all applicable when dilatation is present, but their usefulness is limited in the assessment of collecting systems and ureters with normal caliber. The exception is that noncontrast CT can detect nearly all collecting system and ureteral calculi, even those not visible on radiographs.

IVU is the examination of choice to detect and evaluate calculi, obstruction, urothelial lesions, and abnormalities of position and caliber. When ureteral opacification on IVU is not optimal, cystoscopic retrograde ureteral catheterization and injection of contrast (retrograde) can be performed; it is an even more sensitive examination. Nuclear medicine is not specifically performed to evaluate the collecting system and ureters, but obstruction and abnormalities of position and caliber are easily detected. Angiography has no definite role in the evaluation of collecting system and ureteral pathology, although a urothelial neoplasm typically appears less vascular than a parenchymal renal adenocarcinoma.

THE URINARY BLADDER

Cystoscopic evaluation by a urologist is the method of choice to assess most pathologic processes in the bladder; biopsy and therapeutic intervention also may be performed during the diagnostic examination. Imaging of bladder, however, is useful in many instances. Radiographs can identify bladder calculi and calcifications in the bladder wall. Voiding cystourethrography (VCUG) and its nuclear medicine counterpart are the best methods to evaluate for vesicoureteral reflux. Direct injection of contrast into the bladder during cystography and bladder opacification during IVU are useful techniques to assess mucosal contour and integrity and abnormalities of size, shape, and position.

In addition to detecting mucosal abnormalities visible by other techniques, ultrasound, CT, and MRI of the bladder may detect intramural and extrinsic lesions that otherwise would go unnoticed. Angiography has no real role in the diagnostic evaluation of the bladder, although it can be used to embolize bleeding lesions (e.g., in severe hemorrhagic cystitis).

THE MALE URETHRA

VCUG, retrograde urethrography (RUG), and sonourethrography are the best methods for assessment of urethral pathology. VCUG is better for assessing the posterior portion, and RUG and sonourethrography are better for assessing the anterior portion. RUG should always be performed before placement of a Foley catheter in cases of suspected urethral injury. MRI is useful to differentiate simple urethral strictures from narrowing caused by a mass lesion. CT is rarely used to assess the urethra, and nuclear medicine and angiography have no defined role in its evaluation.

THE ADRENAL GLANDS

Radiographs can identify adrenal calcifications and large masses. Ultrasound can detect many adrenal masses but is of limited usefulness in further characterization. CT and MRI are sensitive for the detection of adrenal lesions, and both can be used for characterization, particularly in differentiating definitely benign lesions (i.e., presence of fat) from potentially malignant lesions. Nuclear medicine radiopharmaceuticals are available that can detect and characterize masses in the cortex (NP-59) and medulla (MIBG). Angiography can be used to detect very small and vascular lesions, and adrenal venous sampling can lateralize hormone-producing tumors.

THE FEMALE GENITAL TRACT

Radiographs are useful only to identify large or calcified lesions of the female genital tract. Hysterosalpingography (HSG) can assess focal and diffuse abnormalities of the endometrial cavity and fallopian tubes. It is most commonly obtained as part of the work-up for infertility, and the "flushing of the fallopian tubes" during the procedure is believed to make it possible for many patients to become pregnant shortly after the examination. HSG can be performed with either water soluble or oil-based contrast media: the former is somewhat safer (i.e., if intravasation occurs) and the latter has a slightly higher likelihood of subsequent pregnancy.

Ultrasound is generally the initial examination in the evaluation of known or suspected female genital tract pathology. Both transabdominal and endovaginal images can be obtained, and no ionizing radiation is required. Ultrasound is performed at some point during most pregnancies, and it is the best technique to assess the cystic or solid nature of a mass. MRI offers better lesion characterization than ultrasound but is more expensive and time consuming. CT is infrequently performed to evaluate the female genital tract, but it can be used to identify and characterize masses. Nuclear medicine and angiography are not specifically performed in the evaluation of the female genital tract.

THE SCROTUM AND PROSTATE

Radiographs can detect prostate masses and calcifications, but they have no real role in the evaluation of scrotal pathology. Similarly, IVU is not used to assess the scrotum but often indirectly identifies prostate enlargement as extrinsic compression on the bladder base. Scrotal ultrasound and transrectal ultrasound (TRUS) of the prostate are the initial and often only diagnostic examinations of these structures. Scrotal ultrasound can detect and characterize most testicular and extratesticular lesions, with Doppler as a powerful adjunct. TRUS can be used to identify and characterize prostate lesions and to guide prostate biopsies. MRI can be used to further characterize scrotal lesions and to detect and stage prostate carcinoma. Nuclear medicine is useful for differentiating testicular inflammation from torsion. Angiography can be used to embolize varicoceles, but it has no defined diagnostic use in either the scrotum or prostate.

GENITOURINARY IMAGING DIFFERENTIAL DIAGNOSES

Renal parenchyma
    Small kidney(s)
    Large kidney(s)
    Absent, delayed, or persistent nephrogram
    Solitary cystic renal mass
    Multiple bilateral renal cysts (macroscopic)
    Complex renal mass
    Solid renal mass
    Renal cortical calcification
    Renal medullary calcification
Renal collecting system and ureter
    Filling defect(s)
    Dilatation
    Narrowing
    Medial ureteral deviation
    Lateral ureteral deviation
Urinary bladder
    Bladder filling defect(s)
    Small capacity bladder (with or without wall calcification)
Male urethra
    Urethral narrowing
Adrenal gland
    Adrenal enlargement
    Adrenal calcification
Uterus
    Uterine enlargement or mass
    Intrauterine filling defect(s)
Adnexa
    Cystic adnexal mass
    Solid adnexal mass
Scrotum
    Intratesticular mass
    Extratesticular mass

RENAL PARENCHYMA

SMALL KIDNEY(S)

List the main diagnostic considerations when one or both kidneys are small.

Which causes tend to be unilateral and which tend to be bilateral?

List two congenital processes that may result in a small kidney.

List two forms of nephropathy that may result in a small kidney.

Congenital
    Hypoplasia
    Multicystic dysplastic kidney (adult)
Nephropathy
    Obstructive
    Reflux
Radiation nephritis
Renal infarction/ischemia
End-stage renal disease
Amyloidosis

Hypoplasia

What causes must be excluded before it is concluded that a small kidney is congenitally hypoplastic?

How many calyces does a normal kidney have?

- Unilateral small but functional kidney secondary to incomplete development
- No prior history of infection, radiation, hypertension, obstruction, reflux, resection, etc.
- Normal number of calyces is 6 to 14

FIGURES Barbaric: 73; Dunnick: 18

Multicystic dysplastic kidney (adult)

How does the size of a multicystic dysplastic kidney usually change over time?

Are calcifications common in multicystic dysplastic kidneys?

- Unilateral congenitally nonfunctioning kidney is large in utero or at birth
- Majority decrease in size with age and often are not detectable in older children and adults (many patients followed with serial ultrasound)
- 30% of adults have curvilinear calcifications in the renal bed

FIGURES Barbaric: 73, 74; Dunnick: 125, 126

Obstructive nephropathy

Under what conditions does obstructive nephropathy result in a small kidney?

- Unilateral or bilateral renal parenchymal loss secondary to chronic obstruction
- Kidneys usually large because of hydronephrosis; can be small if parenchymal loss predominates or if obstruction is corrected

Reflux nephropathy

Is reflux nephropathy a common cause of parenchymal scarring?

Which renal pole is usually affected by reflux nephropathy?

Where in relation to the calyx does the parenchymal scarring of reflux nephropathy typically occur?

- Unilateral or bilateral parenchymal loss secondary to chronic reflux
- Most common cause of parenchymal scarring
- Upper pole usually affected
- Parenchymal thinning adjacent to clubbed calyx (differential diagnosis (ddx) to renal infarction/ischemia)
- Reflux may no longer be present (surgery or spontaneous resolution)

FIGURES Barbaric: 139; Dunnick: 182, 295

Radiation nephritis

What size is an acutely radiated kidney?

What is the typical threshold dose to induce radiation nephritis?

- Unilateral or bilateral, depending on port
- Kidneys initially normal in size or enlarged, become small with time
- Typical threshold dose: 2000 to 2500 rads over 5 weeks; may occur after only 1000 rads

Renal infarction/ischemia

What size is an acutely infarcted or ischemic kidney?

Where in relation to the calyx is there relative parenchymal sparing in chronic ischemia?

- Unilateral or bilateral atrophic kidney(s) resulting from chronically reduced blood supply
- Acutely infarcted/ischemic kidney normal or enlarged
- Focal or diffuse parenchymal loss seen chronically with relative sparing adjacent to collecting system (ddx to reflux nephropathy)

FIGURES Dunnick: 197, 198

End-stage renal disease

What are the complications of end-stage renal disease? How are they best evaluated?

- Bilateral small kidneys secondary to several causes
- CT most important test to evaluate for complications of acquired renal cystic disease of uremia and renal adenocarcinoma (dialysis patients usually able to receive intravenous contrast)

FIGURES Barbaric: 199; Dunnick: 227

Amyloidosis

How does the size of kidneys affected by amyloidosis usually change over time?

- Kidneys bilaterally affected
- Kidneys normal in size or enlarged in early stages
- Kidneys small in late stages and collecting system often attenuated

LARGE KIDNEY(S)

List the main diagnostic considerations when one or both kidneys are large.

Which causes tend to be unilateral and which tend to be bilateral?

Compensatory hypertrophy
Renal vein thrombosis
Ureteral duplication
Trauma
Hydronephrosis
Renal infarction/ischemia
Pyelonephritis
Infiltrative malignancies
Amyloidosis
Hereditary renal cystic disease
    Autosomal dominant polycystic kidney disease
    Autosomal recessive polycystic kidney disease
Acquired immunodeficiency syndrome (AIDS) nephropathy
Acute tubular necrosis (ATN)

Compensatory hypertrophy

- Any cause of unilateral small or absent kidney can cause hypertrophy of contralateral kidney

Renal vein thrombosis

How does the size of a kidney affected by renal vein thrombosis change over time?

- Usually unilateral process
- Kidney enlarged in acute renal vein thrombosis
- Kidney normal in size or small in chronic renal vein thrombosis
- Thrombus should be sought directly with ultrasound/CT/MRI/angiography

FIGURES Barbaric: 245–247; Dunnick: 202, 203

Ureteral duplication

What is the "drooping lily" sign?

What may occur at the insertion of the upper pole moiety ureter in a duplicated system?

- Unilateral process more common than bilateral process
- Ipsilateral kidney of duplicated system usually enlarged
- If upper pole moiety is obstructed, cystic upper pole mass seen on ultrasound/CT/MRI and "drooping lily" sign (inferior displacement of lower pole moiety by poorly functioning hydronephrotic upper pole moiety) seen on IVU
- Ectopic ureter/ureterocele from upper pole moiety (Weigert-Meyer rule) should be sought

FIGURES Barbaric: 74, 75; Dunnick: 29–32

Trauma

What is the best examination to evaluate for renal trauma?

Does a normal, "one-shot IVU" exclude significant renal injury?

- Unilateral or bilateral depending on mechanism and extent of trauma
- Hemorrhage (subcapsular, intraparenchymal) causes renal outline to be enlarged
- Contrast CT is the examination of choice
- IVU, particularly "one-shot IVU," may miss significant injury
- Evidence of other visceral injury, intraperitoneal/retroperitoneal hemorrhage, and fractures should be sought

FIGURES Barbaric: 318–327; Dunnick: 300–308

Hydronephrosis

Under what conditions is a hydronephrotic kidney normal in size or small?

- Unilateral or bilateral renal enlargement because of collecting system/pelvis dilatation

- Seen with reflux, obstruction, and nonobstructive causes (meg-aureter, residual hydronephrosis after correction of reflux or obstruction)
- Kidneys may be normal in size or small in chronic reflux/obstruction if parenchymal loss secondary to nephropathy predominates over hydronephrosis

FIGURES   Barbaric: 111–117, 139; Dunnick: 23, 24, 360–362, 366, 367

Renal infarction/ischemia

How does the size of a chronically ischemic or infarcted kidney change over time?

What is the cortical rim sign?

- Unilateral or bilateral process
- Acutely ischemic/infarcted kidney normal in size or enlarged
- Chronically ischemic/infarcted kidneys are small
- Look for cortical rim sign (1- to 2-mm, thin, enhancing rim of peripheral parenchyma supplied by capsular arteries) on IVU/CT/angiography

Pyelonephritis

Why is an infected kidney typically enlarged?

Which patients are predisposed to emphysematous pyelonephritis?

- Unilateral or bilateral process
- Infection causes edema, microabscesses, and tubular obstruction by purulent material, which can result in renal enlargement
- Foci of gas imply emphysematous pyelonephritis and suggest underlying diabetes
- Focal fluid or gas (or both) collections seen with abscesses

FIGURES   Barbaric: 129–137; Dunnick: 166–168, 170, 171

Infiltrative malignancies

Which malignancies may diffusely infiltrate the kidneys without causing a focal mass?

Is the renal disease in these patients ever asymptomatic?

Should patients with multiple myeloma undergo examinations that require intravenous iodinated contrast media?

- Kidneys usually affected bilaterally
- Infiltrative renal malignancies (no focal mass) include leukemia, myeloma, and diffuse forms of lymphoma and metastases
- Renal involvement often asymptomatic
- Kidneys usually heterogeneous and poorly functioning
- Look for evidence of disease and previous treatment (surgery, radiation) elsewhere
- Use of intravenous iodinated contrast media controversial in myeloma patients: may induce precipitation of Bence Jones proteins in renal tubules and cause or worsen renal failure

FIGURES   Barbaric: 173–175; Dunnick: 155, 156, 231

Amyloidosis

- Kidneys affected bilaterally
- Kidneys normal in size or enlarged in early stages
- Kidneys small in late stages and collecting system often attenuated

FIGURE   Dunnick: 232

Autosomal dominant polycystic kidney disease

At what age do patients with autosomal dominant polycystic kidney disease typically present?

Do all of the cysts in these patients qualify as simple?

What nonrenal manifestations occur in patients with autosomal dominant polycystic kidney disease?

- Bilateral renal enlargement caused by numerous macroscopic cysts of varying sizes
- Typically a disease of adults but can present at any age (even in neonates)
- Cysts often complicated by hemorrhage and may have calcifications
- Associated with cerebral aneurysms and evidence of cysts in liver and pancreas; cysts less commonly seen in thyroid, testes, seminal vesicles, and ovaries

FIGURES   Barbaric: 87–88; Dunnick: 124

Do the kidneys appear echogenic in autosomal recessive polycystic kidney disease?

Are individual cysts identifiable?

What is the relationship between the severity of renal and hepatic disease in these patients?

What is found histologically in kidneys affected by AIDS nephropathy?

Is acute tubular necrosis reversible?

Should patients with ATN undergo examinations that require intravenous iodinated contrast media?

List the main diagnostic considerations when the nephrogram is absent, delayed, or persistent. Which causes are vascular? Which causes are parenchymal?

Autosomal recessive polycystic kidney disease

- Bilateral renal enlargement caused by small saccular enlargement of medullary collecting ducts
- Numerous interfaces between cysts make kidneys appear echogenic on ultrasound
- Cysts generally too small to be individually visualized (may be identified with high-resolution ultrasound equipment)
- Evidence of associated hepatic fibrosis/cysts, portal hypertension, and varices should be sought
- Renal disease more severe than hepatic disease in infants
- Hepatic disease more severe than renal disease in older children

FIGURE Dunnick: 123

AIDS nephropathy

- Kidneys bilaterally normal in size or enlarged
- Histologic abnormalities include interstitial infiltrates/fibrosis, focal/segmental glomerulosclerosis, microcystic dilatation of tubules, and intratubular casts

FIGURE Dunnick: 234

Acute tubular necrosis (ATN)

- Bilateral enlarged kidneys or allograft with persistently and increasingly dense nephrograms
- Reversible oliguric or nonoliguric renal failure
- Several chemical and ischemic causes
- Iodinated contrast media (in addition to being a potential cause of ATN) may worsen renal failure and are contraindicated

FIGURES Barbaric: 254; Dunnick: 226, 229

ABSENT, DELAYED, OR PERSISTENT NEPHROGRAM

Vascular
    Renal ischemia/infarction
    Renal vein thrombosis
Hypotension/contrast reaction
Parenchymal
    Acute tubular necrosis (ATN)
    Glomerulonephritis
    Pyelonephritis
Obstruction
Agenesis

Renal ischemia/infarction

- Unilateral or bilateral process
- Ischemic kidney demonstrates delayed, persistent nephrogram
- Infarcted kidney demonstrates nearly absent nephrogram
- Cortical rim sign should be sought on IVU/CT/angiography

FIGURE Dunnick: 304

Renal vein thrombosis

- Usually unilateral process
- Delayed, persistent nephrogram seen on IVU/CT/angiography in acute thrombosis

- Thrombus should be sought directly with ultrasound/CT/MRI/angiography

FIGURES Barbaric: 245–247; Dunnick: 202, 203

Hypotension/contrast reaction

Why is the nephrogram delayed and persistent in cases of hypotension and contrast reactions?

What should the radiologist supervising IVU do if the early films show absent or decreased function?

- Bilateral delayed/persistent nephrogram secondary to underlying cardiac disease, trauma, or severe contrast reaction
- Decreased glomerular filtration caused by the renal arterial vasoconstriction in response to systemic hypotension
- Patient whose early films show absent/decreased function should always be evaluated

FIGURES Barbaric: 65; Dunnick: 226

Acute tubular necrosis

- Persistently and increasingly dense nephrogram in enlarged native kidneys or transplant allograft
- Reversible oliguric or nonoliguric renal failure
- Several chemical and ischemic causes
- Iodinated contrast media (in addition to being a potential cause of ATN) may worsen renal failure and are contraindicated

FIGURES Barbaric: 254; Dunnick: 226, 229

Glomerulonephritis

List three causes of glomerulonephritis.

- Bilateral delayed, persistent nephrograms seen acutely
- Chronically small, smooth kidneys, uncommonly with cortical calcifications
- Typically autoimmune (e.g., poststreptococcal, IgA nephropathy, Goodpasture's syndrome)

Pyelonephritis

Why is the nephrogram diminished in pyelonephritis?

- Unilateral or bilateral, focal or multifocal
- Diminished function caused by edema, tubular obstruction, and impaired blood flow
- Excretion and concentration of contrast decreased or absent
- Nephrogram often striated on IVU/CT

FIGURES Barbaric: 129–136; Dunnick: 166, 167, 170, 176–178

Obstruction

Why does the nephrogram become hyperdense over time in obstruction?

- Delayed and persistently hyperdense nephrogram seen in acute obstruction
- Postulated causes of hyperdensity: tubular distention during obstruction allows for increased volume of contrast media; sodium and water resorption from tubules increases during obstruction and causes concentration of contrast media

FIGURES Barbaric: 108; Dunnick: 360, 366

Agenesis

Is bilateral renal agenesis uncommon clinically? Why or why not?

Which renal and nonrenal anomalies are associated with unilateral renal agenesis?

- Unilateral complete congenital renal absence; bilateral agenesis rare and incompatible with life
- Compensatory hypertrophy of contralateral kidney
- Associated findings include ipsilateral adrenal agenesis (8 to 10%), contralateral renal anomalies (incidence increased twofold), and ipsilateral genital anomalies

FIGURES Barbaric: 72; Dunnick: 18

6

SOLITARY CYSTIC RENAL MASS

List the main diagnostic considerations for a solitary cystic renal mass.

List the two types of simple renal cysts.

Simple cyst
  Cortical
  Sinus
Calyceal diverticulum
Papillary necrosis cavity

Renal cortical cyst

- Cyst originating from and located within or adjacent to renal cortex

What are the ultrasound and CT criteria for a simple cyst?

- Ultrasound criteria: anechoic; uniformly thin, smooth wall (can have thin internal septation); posterior acoustic enhancement
- Caveat:
- Gain needs to be optimized; noise can artificially be made to appear as internal echoes, and true internal echoes in a solid mass can be artificially eliminated
- CT criteria:
- Water density (0 to 20 HU), uniformly thin, smooth wall (can have thin internal septation); no enhancement

What causes the "claw" or "beak" sign on IVU?

- "Claw" or "beak" sign should be sought on IVU secondary to smooth, sharp margin of displaced cortex

FIGURES Barbaric: 185–187; Dunnick: 117, 118

Renal sinus cyst

How can a renal sinus cyst be differentiated from a dilated renal pelvis?

- Cyst located within renal sinus (can originate from sinus structures or adjacent cortex)
- Imaging criteria same as for renal cortical cyst
- Can be confused with hydronephrosis or dilated pelvis on ultrasound
- Collecting system or pelvis (or both) likely to be displaced or attenuated on IVU/CT, but neither accumulates contrast (differential diagnosis to hydronephrosis)

FIGURES Barbaric: 197, 198; Dunnick: 132, 133

Calyceal diverticulum

How can a calyceal diverticulum be differentiated from a cyst?

How can a calyceal diverticulum be differentiated from a papillary necrosis cavity?

- Indistinguishable from cyst on ultrasound and nonenhanced CT
- Accumulates contrast on IVU and enhanced CT (differential diagnosis to cyst)
- Extends eccentrically from affected calyx (differential diagnosis to papillary necrosis cavity)
- Actual communicating channel usually not directly visualized (differential diagnosis to papillary necrosis cavity)

FIGURES Barbaric: 83, 84; Dunnick: 131, 286, 287

Papillary necrosis cavity

- Focal or multifocal loss of papilla leads to widening or clubbing of calyx
- Accumulates contrast on IVU and enhanced CT (differential diagnosis to cyst)
- Extends centrally from affected calyx (differential diagnosis to calyceal diverticulum)
- Communicating channel usually obvious (differential diagnosis to calyceal diverticulum)

FIGURES Barbaric: 260–264; Dunnick: 283–285

MULTIPLE BILATERAL RENAL CYSTS (MACROSCOPIC)

List the main diagnostic considerations for multiple macroscopic bilateral renal cysts.

Autosomal dominant polycystic kidney disease
Von Hippel-Lindau disease
Tuberous sclerosis
Acquired cystic disease of uremia

Autosomal dominant polycystic kidney disease

How do the renal and cyst sizes vary between autosomal dominant polycystic kidney disease and von Hippel-Lindau disease?

- Numerous cysts of varying sizes in enlarged kidneys (kidneys and cysts larger than in von Hippel-Lindau disease)
- Cysts often complicated by hemorrhage and may have calcifications
- Associated with cerebral aneurysms and evidence of cysts in liver, pancreas, and, less commonly, thyroid, testes, seminal vesicles, and ovaries

FIGURES   Barbaric: 87, 88; Dunnick: 124

Von Hippel-Lindau disease

Aside from renal cysts, what renal and nonrenal findings are associated with von Hippel-Lindau disease?

- Multiple small (usually 0.5 to 3.0 cm) cysts in normal-sized or mildly enlarged kidneys (kidneys and cysts smaller than those in autosomal dominant polycystic kidney disease)
- Associated renal adenocarcinomas (40%, usually multiple), pheochromocytomas (10%), cerebellar and spinal hemangioblastomas, retinal angiomatosis, pancreatic cysts and islet cell tumors, and epididymal cystadenoma should be sought

FIGURE   Barbaric: 180

Tuberous sclerosis

Are the renal cysts in patients with tuberous sclerosis typically small or large?

Are renal cysts or angiomyolipomas more common in patients with tuberous sclerosis?

- Small (less than 3 cm) cysts in normal-sized kidneys may occur in patients with tuberous sclerosis
- Renal angiomyolipomas are more common (80%) than renal cysts; fat density renal masses should be sought

FIGURE   Dunnick: 128

Acquired renal cystic disease of uremia

- Renal cysts in small, end-stage kidneys of dialysis patients
- Cysts may be complicated by hemorrhage and contain calcifications
- Associated solid masses, which occur in 7% (1% develop adenocarcinomas), should be sought

FIGURES   Barbaric: 199; Dunnick: 130

COMPLEX RENAL MASS

List the main diagnostic considerations for a complex cystic renal mass.

Complicated cyst
Abscess
Hematoma
Cystic renal adenocarcinoma
Multilocular cystic nephroma

How does a simple renal cyst become complicated?

Can a complicated renal cyst be differentiated from a renal neoplasm?

Complicated cyst

- Cortical or sinus cyst complicated by hemorrhage, infection, or both
- Does not meet ultrasound/CT criteria for simple cyst (e.g., thick, irregular, calcified wall; internal septations; internal echoes; measures more than 20 HU)
- Contents of true complicated cyst do not enhance on CT/MRI (differential diagnosis to neoplasm)
- Further work-up often indicated to exclude malignancy

FIGURES Barbaric: 188–194; Dunnick: 119, 120, 122

How does the wall of a renal abscess differ from the wall of a cyst?

Renal abscess

- Collection of purulent material within or adjacent to renal parenchyma
- Usually contains internal echoes on ultrasound and measures more than 20 HU on CT
- Thick, irregular wall enhances with contrast on CT/MRI
- Foci of gas may be present secondary to infection by gas-forming organisms

FIGURES Barbaric: 132–137; Dunnick: 171–174

How does the ultrasound and CT appearance of a renal hematoma change over time?

What is the MRI appearance of a renal hematoma?

What must be excluded in a patient with a renal hemorrhage who has no history of trauma and no coagulation abnormalities?

Renal hematoma

- Initially hyperechoic on ultrasound and high attenuation on CT
- Becomes hypoechoic on ultrasound and low attenuation on CT over time
- MRI appearance varies; generally bright on T1- and T2-weighted images
- Lack of trauma, anticoagulation, or bleeding diathesis suggests underlying neoplasm (renal adenocarcinoma more common than angiomyolipoma)

FIGURES Barbaric: 223; Dunnick: 300, 305–308

What usually causes a renal adenocarcinoma to appear cystic?

Cystic renal adenocarcinoma

- Cystic appearance of renal adenocarcinoma is more often the result of necrosis than true cystic components
- Associated enhancing solid mass or mural nodule should be sought

FIGURES Barbaric: 167, 168, 188–191; Dunnick: 139, 145

Are adult men or women more commonly diagnosed with a multilocular cystic nephroma?

Are multilocular cystic nephromas always resected?

Multilocular cystic nephroma

- Benign cystic mass containing multiple septations that typically enhance with contrast and may have calcifications
- Typically a disease of young boys, adolescent girls, and middle-aged women
- Treated surgically because cystic renal adenocarcinoma (Wilms' tumor in children) cannot be excluded by imaging

FIGURES Barbaric: 163; Dunnick: 127

SOLID RENAL MASS

List the main diagnostic considerations when a solid renal mass is discovered.

Which causes are benign neoplasms?

Which causes are malignant neoplasms?

Benign neoplasms
    Oncocytoma
    Angiomyolipoma
Malignant neoplasms
    Renal adenocarcinoma

Urothelial carcinoma (invasive)
Lymphoma
Metastases
Inflammation/infection
Focal infection
Xanthogranulomatous pyelonephritis
Hematoma

Oncocytoma

Can an oncocytoma be reliably diagnosed by imaging? By preoperative biopsy or fine-needle aspiration?

- Benign renal neoplasm that cannot be reliably differentiated from renal adenocarcinoma at imaging
- Pathologic diagnosis requires several sections showing no clear cell carcinoma (fine-needle aspiration or core biopsy not adequate; surgical resection required)

What are the classic findings of an oncocytoma at CT? At angiography?

- Central scar on CT (30%) and "spoke-wheel" vascularity on angiography (80%) should be sought

FIGURES Barbaric: 162; Dunnick: 146

Angiomyolipoma

What is the relationship between tuberous sclerosis and angiomyolipoma?

- Benign neoplasm composed of fat, smooth muscle, and blood vessels
- 80% of patients with tuberous sclerosis have angiomyolipomas; less than 40% of patients with angiomyolipomas have tuberous sclerosis

Can any renal masses other than angiomyolipoma contain fat?

- Demonstration of fat within a renal mass is virtually diagnostic (isolated case reports of fat seen at imaging within renal adenocarcinoma and Wilms' tumor)

What is the typical appearance of an angiomyolipoma at ultrasound?

- Typically a highly echogenic mass on ultrasound
- Vascular lesion on angiography

FIGURES Barbaric: 160, 161; Dunnick: 150, 151

Renal adenocarcinoma

What percentage of renal adenocarcinomas contain calcifications at imaging?

- Most commonly appears as a heterogeneous solid mass
- Although only 8 to 18% have calcifications, 87% of nonperipherally calcified renal masses are malignant

What percentage of nonperipherally calcified renal masses are malignant?

- 30% discovered incidentally at imaging

What percentage of renal adenocarcinomas are discovered incidentally at imaging?

- 95% hypervascular at angiography (differential diagnosis to transitional cell carcinoma)

How may angiography help differentiate a parenchymal adenocarcinoma from an invasive transitional cell carcinoma?

- Important to assess for renal vein and inferior vena cava (IVC) invasion
- Contrast CT is the best method for detection of small lesions

What is the best imaging study to detect small adenocarcinomas?

- CT and MRI nearly equally useful for staging

FIGURES Barbaric: 165–171; Dunnick: 137–145

Urothelial carcinoma (invasive)

What percentage of renal pelvis transitional cell carcinomas are invasive?

- Vast majority of upper tract urothelial tumors are transitional cell carcinoma (TCC)
- 70% of renal pelvis TCCs are invasive

Are urothelial carcinomas frequently calcified?

- Calcification rare (differential diagnosis to parenchymal adenocarcinoma)
- Hypovascular at angiography (differential diagnosis to parenchymal adenocarcinoma)

How often are transitional cell carcinomas multicentric?

- Multiple TCC lesions frequent (30% of collecting system and pelvic TCCs are multifocal at discovery; 40 to 80% of patients with upper tract TCC will, at some time, develop tumor elsewhere)

FIGURES Barbaric: 177–179; Dunnick: 293–295

Lymphoma

How commonly does renal lymphoma appear as multiple masses? As a solitary mass?

Is primary renal lymphoma common?

- Various renal manifestations: 45% multiple masses, 15% solitary mass
- Enhances less than parenchyma on contrast CT, hypoechoic on ultrasound
- Look for associated adenopathy or evidence of lymphoma elsewhere (primary renal lymphoma rare)

FIGURES Barbaric: 174, 175; Dunnick: 155, 156

Metastases

Are metastases to the kidneys common at autopsy? At imaging?

Are patients with metastases to the kidneys generally symptomatic from their renal disease?

- 12 to 20% autopsy incidence in cancer patients; much lower incidence at imaging
- Renal lesions usually not symptomatic
- Look for evidence of previous surgery and primary tumor or metastases elsewhere

FIGURES Barbaric: 172, 173; Dunnick: 157

Focal infection

What associated findings suggest infection as the cause of a focal renal mass?

- Focal area of low attenuation on contrast CT
- Look for infiltration of perinephric fat
- Foci of gas imply emphysematous pyelonephritis
- Well-defined fluid and/or gas collection implies abscess

FIGURES Barbaric: 130, 131; Dunnick: 169–171, 174

Xanthogranulomatous pyelonephritis (XGP)

Is XGP usually diffuse or focal?

How frequently are staghorn calculi found in association with XGP?

- 85% diffuse, 15% focal
- Rare chronic suppurative renal infection
- Classic triad: staghorn calculus (75%), absent or diminished contrast excretion, poorly defined mass
- Can be difficult to distinguish from renal adenocarcinoma at imaging

FIGURES Barbaric: 146; Dunnick: 179, 180

Hematoma

- Initially hyperechoic on ultrasound and high attenuation on CT
- Becomes hypoechoic on ultrasound and low attenuation on CT over time
- MRI appearance varies; generally bright on T1- and T2-weighted images
- In the absence of trauma, anticoagulation, or bleeding diathesis, underlying neoplasm (renal adenocarcinoma more common than angiomyolipoma) should be suspected

FIGURES Barbaric: 223; Dunnick: 300, 305–308

RENAL CORTICAL CALCIFICATION

List the main diagnostic considerations for renal cortical calcifications.

Acute cortical necrosis
Hereditary chronic nephritis (Alport's syndrome)
Glomerulonephritis
Oxalosis

Acute cortical necrosis

What is associated with most cases of acute cortical necrosis? List three other associations.

- Tram-track calcification throughout cortex with medullary sparing secondary to ischemic necrosis
- Characteristic sparing of thin rim of outer cortex secondary to preserved capsular blood supply
- More than 66% of cases associated with pregnancy; other associations include burns, sepsis, toxins, transfusion reactions, dehydration, peritonitis

FIGURES   Barbaric: 254; Dunnick: 229, 255

Hereditary chronic nephritis (Alport's syndrome)

What are the clinical components of Alport's syndrome?

- Cortical calcifications in small, smooth kidneys
- Characteristic clinical triad: hematuria, nerve deafness, and ocular abnormalities

Glomerulonephritis

Is cortical calcification a common finding in chronic glomerulonephritis?

- Cortical calcification may occur in chronic cases but is uncommon
- Small, smooth kidneys more common in chronic cases
- Delayed, persistent nephrogram seen acutely
- Typically autoimmune (e.g., poststreptococcal infection, IgA nephropathy, Goodpasture's syndrome)

Oxalosis

What renal findings in addition to cortical calcification may be seen with oxalosis?

What small bowel abnormalities predispose to oxalosis?

- Hyperoxaluria (hereditary or enteric) results in precipitation of calcium oxalate
- Can involve cortex and medulla and lead to urolithiasis
- Predisposing conditions of inflammatory bowel disease and small bowel resection should be sought

FIGURE   Dunnick: 261

RENAL MEDULLARY CALCIFICATION

List the main diagnostic considerations for renal medullary calcification.

Hypercalcemic states
Renal tubular acidosis
Medullary sponge kidney
Oxalosis
Papillary necrosis

Hypercalcemic states

List five hypercalcemic states.

- Hypercalcemia leads to hypercalciuria, which makes possible medullary precipitation of calcium salts
- Several causes: hyperparathyroidism, paraneoplastic syndromes, sarcoidosis, milk-alkali syndrome, hypervitaminosis D, others

Renal tubular acidosis

Is medullary calcification more commonly seen with type I or type II renal tubular acidosis?

- Associated hypercalciuria and lack of citrate leads to medullary calcification and calcium phosphate stone formation
- Clinical and radiographic manifestations essentially only with type I (distal) disease
- Autosomal dominant, sporadic, and acquired causes
- 70% of patients are female

FIGURE   Dunnick: 256

Medullary sponge kidney

How can the medullary calcifications of medullary sponge kidney be differentiated from other medullary calcifications?

- Dilated tubules allow urine stasis and intratubular precipitation of calcium salts
- Calcifications become obscured by excreted contrast media on IVU/CT (differential diagnosis to extratubular medullary calcifications)

FIGURES Barbaric: 85; Dunnick: 257, 285, 286

Oxalosis

- Hyperoxaluria (hereditary or enteric) results in precipitation of calcium oxalate
- Can involve cortex and medulla and lead to urolithiasis
- Predisposing conditions of inflammatory bowel disease and small bowel resection should be sought

FIGURE Dunnick: 261

Papillary necrosis

What findings other than medullary calcification suggest papillary necrosis?

- Dystrophic calcification can involve the infarcted papilla
- Look for other evidence of papillary necrosis (e.g., dilated distorted calyces, filling defects corresponding to sloughed papilla)

FIGURES Dunnick: 283–285

RENAL COLLECTING SYSTEM AND URETER

FILLING DEFECT(S)

List the main diagnostic considerations for filling defects in the renal collecting system and ureters.

Urothelial carcinoma
Leukoplakia
Malacoplakia
Ureteritis cystica
Fungus ball
Collateral vessels
Urolithiasis
Blood clot
Papillary necrosis (sloughed papilla)

Urothelial carcinoma

List three histologic types of urothelial carcinoma. Which is the most common? Where does urothelial carcinoma most commonly occur?

Is TCC of the collecting system and ureter frequently multifocal?

What is the Bergman or "goblet" sign?

- Transitional cell carcinoma (TCC) is twice as common as squamous cell carcinoma, which is twice as common as adenocarcinoma
- Bladder most common site; collecting system and pelvis next most common site; ureter least common site
- Multiple TCC lesions frequent (30% of collecting system and pelvic TCCs are multifocal at discovery; 40 to 80% of patients with upper tract TCC will, at some time, develop tumor elsewhere)
- Ureteral dilatation distal to tumor (Bergman or "goblet" sign; differential diagnosis to calculus) may be seen

FIGURES Barbaric: 177–179, 298, 299; Dunnick: 153, 154, 293–295, 377, 378

Leukoplakia

Where does leukoplakia occur?

Is leukoplakia premalignant?

- Multiple, poorly defined filling defects
- Bladder the most common site, followed by collecting system and pelvis, then ureter
- Premalignant: may develop into squamous cell carcinoma
- Evidence of associated infection or calculi should be sought

Malacoplakia

Where does malacoplakia occur?

Which disease is associated with malacoplakia?

Is malacoplakia premalignant?

- Multiple smooth, scalloped filling defects
- Bladder most common site, followed by ureter, then collecting system and pelvis
- Associated with diabetes, not premalignant
- Look for associated inflammatory renal mass, which occurs in 16% of cases

FIGURE Dunnick: 380

Ureteritis cystica

Where does ureteritis cystica occur?

What may cause a predisposition to ureteritis cystica?

- Bladder (cystitis cystica) the most common site, followed by ureter (ureteritis cystica), then collecting system and pelvis (pyelitis cystica)
- Multiple small (2 to 4 mm), smooth round filling defects that may be larger in pelvis and bladder
- Look for associated infection, calculi, and stents

FIGURES Barbaric: 294, 295; Dunnick: 381

Fungus ball

Which patients are predisposed to developing fungus balls in the urinary collecting system, ureter, or bladder?

- Renal fungal infection may result in fungus balls within collecting system and pelvis, ureter, or bladder
- Should be suspected in patients with diabetes, altered immunity, or indwelling catheters

FIGURES Barbaric: 147; Dunnick: 186

Collateral vessels

Which conditions can cause recruitment of ureteral collateral vessels?

- In renal artery stenosis or occlusion and renal vein thrombosis or compression, enlargement of ureteral collateral vessels may cause ureteral notching

FIGURES Barbaric: 228; Dunnick: 191

Urolithiasis

Where do calculi tend to lodge?

How can a radiolucent ureteral calculus be differentiated from a carcinoma?

What percentage of urinary calculi are visible on radiographs?

- Calculi are often less dense than excreted contrast and appear as filling defects
- Tend to lodge at ureteropelvic junction, iliac vessel crossing, and ureterovesical junction
- Usually narrowing immediately distal to calculus secondary to spasm (differential diagnosis to urothelial carcinoma)
- Look for calcification on scout radiograph (92% are radiopaque)

FIGURES Barbaric: 99–101; Dunnick: 259–270

Blood clot

What normally prevents the formation of blood clots in urine?

- Blood clots in renal collecting system or pelvis, ureter, and bladder appear as filling defects on contrast examinations
- Presence of urokinase in urine normally hinders clot formation
- Search for cause of bleeding (e.g., tumor, trauma, or urolithiasis)

FIGURE Dunnick: 291

6

Papillary necrosis (sloughed papilla)

- Sloughed papilla may lodge in pelvis, ureter, or bladder and present as filling defect
- Look for dilated or distorted calyx

FIGURES Barbaric: 261; Dunnick: 285

DILATATION

List the main diagnostic considerations for dilatation of the collecting system or ureter.

Obstruction
Vesicoureteral reflux
Megaureter
Pregnancy
Residua of previous obstruction or reflux

Obstruction

List 10 causes of collecting system and ureteral obstruction.

- Dilatation occurs proximal to site of obstruction
- Several causes, including urolithiasis, urothelial carcinoma, papillary necrosis, fungus ball, blood clot, congenital malformation (ureteropelvic junction, ureterovesical junction), extrinsic mass, stricture, ureterocele, upper pole moiety of duplicated system, Fraley syndrome, endometriosis, and retroperitoneal fibrosis

FIGURES Barbaric: 108–117; Dunnick: 364–369

Vesicoureteral reflux

Why does vesicoureteral reflux usually occur during voiding?

- Degree and proximal extent of dilatation indicative of severity or grade
- Usually occurs during voiding because bladder pressure is highest then

FIGURES Barbaric: 139; Dunnick: 295, 375–377

Megaureter

What is the anatomic defect in megaureter?

Is vesicoureteral reflux associated with megaureter?

How can the degree of ureteral tortuosity help to differentiate megaureter from reflux and obstruction?

- Deficient longitudinal muscle in distal ureter leading to nonobstructive dilatation proximally
- Look for classic "beak-like" configuration at ureterovesical junction
- No reflux at VCUG
- Ureter typically not as tortuous as in obstruction or reflux

FIGURES Dunnick: 370, 371

Pregnancy

Why does pregnancy result in ureteral dilatation?

Is the right or left ureter more likely to be dilated in pregnancy?

- Cause debated: hormonal versus obstructive
- Involves proximal two thirds of ureters; the right ureter is more often involved than the left
- Usually persists several weeks postpartum

FIGURES Barbaric: 487; Dunnick: 390

Residua of previous obstruction or reflux

- Dilatation may persist indefinitely after resolution or correction of causative factor(s)

NARROWING

List the main diagnostic considerations for narrowing of the collecting system or ureter. List five extrinsic causes.

Extrinsic causes
    Endometriosis
    Renal sinus lipomatosis
    Renal sinus cyst
    Retroperitoneal fibrosis
    Retroperitoneal neoplasm/lymphadenopathy
    Stricture
Infection
    Tuberculosis (TB)
    Schistosomiasis

Endometriosis

Is ureteral involvement by endometriosis common?

- Urinary tract involvement in 1%; involves bladder more often than ureter
- May cause narrowing at site of implant and, perhaps, proximal obstruction

FIGURE Dunnick: 386

Renal sinus lipomatosis

What are the usual clinical findings in renal sinus lipomatosis?

- Narrowing or splaying of renal collecting system and pelvis secondary to prominent sinus fat
- Incidence increases with age, generalized obesity
- No obstruction or other clinical consequence
- Increased renal sinus fat should be sought on ultrasound, CT, or MRI

FIGURE Dunnick: 53

Renal sinus cyst

- Narrowing or splaying of renal collecting system and pelvis secondary to parapelvic or peripelvic cyst
- Can be confused with hydronephrosis or dilated pelvis on ultrasound
- Does not accumulate contrast on IVU or CT (differential diagnosis to hydronephrosis)

FIGURES Barbaric: 197, 198; Dunnick: 132, 133

Retroperitoneal fibrosis

What is the characteristic appearance of ureters narrowed by retroperitoneal fibrosis?

What structures may be obstructed by retroperitoneal fibrosis?

- Ureteral narrowing (characteristic "rat-tail" appearance) may result from extrinsic compression by retroperitoneal fibrous tissue
- Proximal ureters may also be medially deviated
- Ureters and IVC may become obstructed
- Look for enhancement of retroperitoneal fibrous tissue on CT or MRI

FIGURES Barbaric: 302–304; Dunnick: 388, 389

Retroperitoneal neoplasm/lymphadenopathy

- Retroperitoneal neoplasm or lymphadenopathy adjacent to ureter can cause focal narrowing, which should be apparent on CT/MRI

Stricture

List five causes of ureteral stricture.

- Can result from previous radiation, infection or inflammation, urolithiasis, trauma, and surgery or instrumentation

FIGURES Barbaric: 282, 283; Dunnick: 387

Tuberculosis

What findings other than collecting system/pelvis and ureteral narrowing are associated with renal tuberculosis?

What percentage of patients with renal tuberculosis have an abnormal chest radiograph? Active pulmonary disease?

- Multiple areas of narrowing and irregularity involve renal collecting system and pelvis (Kerr sign) and ureter
- Look for the associated findings of renal parenchymal calcification and scarring, papillary necrosis, small volume bladder, and bladder calcifications
- 30% have abnormal chest radiograph; fewer than 5% have active pulmonary disease

FIGURES Barbaric: 141–145; Dunnick: 184–185, 384

Schistosomiasis

Where does urinary schistosomiasis occur?

What is the classic radiographic finding in urinary schistosomiasis?

- Bladder most commonly affected, but ureter involved in 30% of cases
- Mucosal irregularity and varying degrees of stricture and dilatation
- Calcifications in wall of bladder and distal ureters is classic finding

FIGURES Barbaric: 145; Dunnick: 383

MEDIAL URETERAL DEVIATION

List the main diagnostic considerations for medial ureteral deviation.

Iliac lymphadenopathy
Iliac artery aneurysm
Retrocaval ureter
Pelvic lipomatosis
Pelvic surgery
Psoas hypertrophy
Retroperitoneal fibrosis

FIGURE Dunnick: 373

Iliac lymphadenopathy

- Lymphadenopathy adjacent to iliac vessels may displace distal ureters medially
- Enlarged nodes readily apparent on CT or MRI

FIGURE Dunnick: 373

Iliac artery aneurysm

- Look for aneursym of iliac artery may displace ipsilateral distal ureter medially
- Dilated vessel readily apparent on CT/MRI/angiography
- Look for atherosclerotic calcifications in aneurysm on radiograph

Retrocaval ureter

Is a retrocaval ureter right-sided, left-sided, or bilateral?

- Right ureter lies medial to vertebral pedicle at L2–L3 level
- May also cause right ureteral obstruction
- Relationship of right ureter to IVC should be sought on CT/MRI/angiography

FIGURES Barbaric: 291; Dunnick: 27

What happens to the bladder and rectosigmoid colon in pelvic lipomatosis?

Can pelvic lipomatosis obstruct the ureter or IVC?

Pelvic lipomatosis

- Medial deviation of distal ureters by abundant fat in pelvis
- Bladder narrowed and displaced cephalad ("inverted pear")
- Rectosigmoid colon may be elevated
- Rarely results in ureteral or IVC obstruction
- Look for increased pelvic fat on CT and MRI

FIGURES   Barbaric: 378; Dunnick: 412

Pelvic surgery

- Absence of pelvic organs such as uterus or rectosigmoid colon permits distal ureters to lie medial to expected locations

Psoas hypertrophy

- Enlargement of psoas muscles may cause medial deviation of distal ureters and lateral deviation of proximal ureters
- Look for psoas enlargement on radiograph, CT, and MRI

FIGURE   Dunnick: 372

Retroperitoneal fibrosis

- Proximal ureters may be medially deviated
- Ureters and IVC may be obstructed or narrowed
- Look for enhancement of retroperitoneal fibrous tissue on CT and MRI

FIGURES   Barbaric: 302–304; Dunnick: 388, 389

LATERAL URETERAL DEVIATION

List the main diagnostic considerations for lateral ureteral deviation.

Aortic aneurysm
Aortocaval lymphadenopathy
Pelvic mass
Psoas hypertrophy

Aortic aneurysm

- Aneurysm of aorta may displace proximal ureters laterally
- Dilated aorta readily apparent on CT, MRI, and angiography
- Look for atherosclerotic calcifications in aneurysm on radiograph

Aortocaval lymphadenopathy

- Lymphadenopathy adjacent to aorta and IVC may displace proximal ureters laterally
- Enlarged nodes readily apparent on CT and MRI

FIGURE   Dunnick: 373

Pelvic mass

- Mass in pelvis may displace distal ureters laterally
- Mass readily apparent on CT and MRI

FIGURES   Barbaric: 475, 476

Psoas hypertrophy

- Enlargement of psoas muscles may cause lateral deviation of proximal ureters and medial deviation of distal ureters
- Look for psoas enlargement on radiograph, CT, and MRI

URINARY BLADDER

BLADDER FILLING DEFECT(S)

List the main diagnostic considerations for filling defects in the urinary bladder.

Urothelial carcinoma
Leukoplakia
Malacoplakia
Cystitis cystica
Fungus ball
Urolithiasis
Blood clot
Papillary necrosis (sloughed papilla)
Benign prostatic hypertrophy
Ureterocele

Urothelial carcinoma

What is the most common histology for urothelial carcinoma of the bladder?

Is TCC of the bladder frequently multifocal?

Which conditions are associated with squamous cell carcinoma? With adenocarcinoma?

- Transitional cell carcinoma (TCC) more common than squamous cell carcinoma (SCC), which is more common than adenocarcinoma (ADC)
- Bladder the most common location, followed by collecting system and pelvis, then ureter
- Multiple TCC lesions frequent (more than 30% of bladder TCCs are multifocal at discovery; 3 to 5% of patients with bladder TCC will, at some time, develop upper urinary tract tumor)
- SCC associated with schistosomiasis and chronic infection and inflammation
- ADC associated with exstrophy, cystitis glandularis, urachal remnant at bladder dome (85% of urachal carcinomas are ADC)

FIGURES   Barbaric: 367–373; Dunnick: 416–418

Leukoplakia

- Multiple poorly defined filling defects
- Bladder the most common location, followed by collecting system and pelvis, then ureter
- Premalignant: may develop into squamous cell carcinoma
- Search for evidence of associated infection or calculi

Malacoplakia

- Multiple smooth, scalloped filling defects
- Bladder the most common location, followed by ureter, then collecting system and pelvis
- Associated with diabetes; not premalignant

Cystitis cystica

Where can the filling defects of ureteritis cystica become large?

- Bladder (cystitis cystica) the most common location, followed by ureter (ureteritis cystica), then collecting system and pelvis (pyelitis cystica)
- Multiple small (2 to 4 mm), smooth, round filling defects, which may be larger in pelvis and bladder
- Associated with infection, calculi, and stents

FIGURES   Barbaric: 361; Dunnick: 404

Fungus ball

- Renal fungal infection may result in fungus balls within collecting system and pelvis, ureter, or bladder
- Should be suspected in patients with diabetes, altered immunity, indwelling catheters

FIGURES   Barbaric: 148; Dunnick: 186

Urolithiasis

Which conditions predispose to bladder calculi?

Are bladder calculi usually the result of migrant renal calculi?

- Calculi are often less dense than excreted contrast and appear as filling defects
- Bladder calculi usually result from stasis (outlet obstruction, diverticuli, neurogenic disorders), infection, or foreign bodies; less commonly calculi result from migrant renal calculi

FIGURES   Barbaric: 355, 356; Dunnick: 421–424

Blood clot

- Blood clots in renal collecting system and pelvis, ureter, and bladder appear as filling defects on contrast examinations
- Presence of urokinase in urine hinders clot formation
- Search for cause of bleeding (e.g., tumor, trauma, or urolithiasis)

Papillary necrosis (sloughed papilla)

- Sloughed papilla may lodge in pelvis, ureter, or bladder and present as filling defect
- Look for dilated or distorted calyx at origin of sloughed papilla

Benign prostatic hypertrophy

What finding on IVU suggests benign prostatic hypertrophy? How does the central gland in benign prostatic hypertrophy appear at TRUS? At MRI?

- Enlarged prostate can appear as large filling defect at bladder base
- Look for elevation of bladder base and distal ureters ("J" hooking) on IVU
- Bladder outlet may be obstructed
- Prostatic calcifications may be seen on radiograph, TRUS, and CT
- Central gland enlarged and heterogeneous on TRUS and MRI

FIGURES   Barbaric: 412–414; Dunnick: 441–443

Ureterocele

List the two basic types of ureteroceles.

What does the "cobra-head" appearance associated with ureterocele represent?

Name the congenital anomaly associated with an ectopic ureterocele.

- Can be simple or ectopic
- Smooth, round filling defect in bladder represents dilated prolapsed distal ureter
- Opacifies with contrast if unobstructed on IVU ("cobra head" appearance) and CT
- Ureteral duplication is associated with ectopic ureterocele
- Early cystogram images should be examined carefully; ureterocele may become effaced by distended bladder

FIGURES   Barbaric: 288, 290; Dunnick: 31–33

SMALL CAPACITY BLADDER (WITH OR WITHOUT WALL CALCIFICATION)

List the main diagnostic considerations for small bladder capacity.

Which two causes are chronic infections?

Chronic infection
   Schistosomiasis
   Tuberculosis
   Noninfectious cystitis

Schistosomiasis

What findings other than a small bladder capacity are associated with schistosomiasis?

Is schistosomiasis a premalignant condition?

- Reduced bladder capacity common
- Calcifications in bladder and distal ureters characteristic
- Mucosal irregularity, inflammatory pseudopolyps, ureteritis cystica, ureteral dilatation and stricture, and fistulas also may be seen
- Causes predisposition to squamous cell carcinoma

FIGURES Barbaric: 145; Dunnick: 401

Tuberculosis

- Long-standing tuberculosis causes an interstitial cystitis resulting in fibrosis, decreased capacity and, in rare instances, calcifications
- Associated findings include renal parenchymal calcification and scarring, papillary necrosis, autonephrectomy, and irregularity and stenosis in collecting system/pelvis and ureter

FIGURE Dunnick: 399

Noninfectious cystitis

List three types of noninfectious cystitis.

Is bladder calcification commonly associated with noninfectious cystitis?

- Several types, including radiation (usually from treatment of bladder or cervical carcinoma) cystitis, chemical (typically cyclophosphamide) cystitis, interstitial cystitis
- Chronic inflammation results in fibrosis, decreased capacity and, rarely, calcifications
- In radiation cystitis, radiation changes in adjacent tissues and evidence of primary or metastatic tumor should be sought

FIGURES Barbaric: 362–364; Dunnick: 402

MALE URETHRA

URETHRAL NARROWING

List the main diagnostic considerations for urethral narrowing.

Trauma
Stricture
Carcinoma

Trauma

Name the three types of urethral injury.

Should a Foley catheter be placed before or after RUG in patients with a suspected urethral injury?

- Urethra stretched but intact in type 1 injuries
- Urethra ruptured above urogenital diaphragm in type 2 and below urogenital diaphragm in type 3 injuries
- Look for other evidence of trauma
- RUG should always be performed before catheterization in suspected urethral injuries

FIGURES Barbaric: 332–334; Dunnick: 318, 321

What conditions may cause a urethral stricture?

How does a congenital urethral stricture typically differ in appearance from an acquired urethral stricture?

Can urethral stricture be differentiated from carcinoma by RUG? By VCUG? By MRI?

List three histologic types of urethral carcinoma. Which is the most common? Which portion of the urethra is typically involved by squamous cell carcinoma? By transitional cell carcinoma?

List the main diagnostic considerations for adrenal enlargement.

Which causes are benign neoplasms?

Which causes are malignant neoplasms?

How does adrenal enlargement resulting from hyperplasia differ in appearance from enlargement secondary to other causes?

List five causes of adrenal hyperplasia.

Which is more common, nonhyperfunctioning or hyperfunctioning adrenocortical adenoma?

Which syndrome results from hyperadrenocorticism? Which from hyperaldosteronism?

What is the likelihood that an adrenal mass with a CT attenuation of less than 0 HU is malignant?

Are adrenal myelolipomas or adenomas more common?

Stricture

- Acquired (e.g., infection, trauma, instrumentation, indwelling catheter) more common; narrowing can be diffuse or localized
- Congenital less common; usually short and weblike
- Cannot be differentiated reliably from carcinoma at VCUG/RUG; MRI often helpful

FIGURES Barbaric: 432–434; Dunnick: 466–474

Carcinoma

- Associated with, and often indistinguishable from, stricture
- Squamous cell carcinoma (SCC) more common than transitional cell carcinoma (TCC), which is more common than adenocarcinoma (ADC)
- SCC usually involves bulbous portion; TCC usually involves posterior portion

FIGURES Dunnick: 478–480

ADRENAL GLAND

ADRENAL ENLARGEMENT

Hyperplasia
Benign neoplasms
   Adenoma
   Myelolipoma
   Pheochromocytoma
Malignant neoplasms
   Carcinoma (cortical)
   Metastases/lymphoma
Hemorrhage

Hyperplasia

- Bilateral adrenal enlargement without focal mass (adrenal shape maintained)
- Numerous causes include idiopathic, inborn error of metabolism, pituitary tumor, ectopic hormone production, exogenous hormone source
- Cushing disease: hyperadrenocorticism secondary to adrenocorticotropic hormone-producing pituitary adenoma

FIGURES Barbaric: 206; Dunnick: 333

Adenoma

- Common, benign adrenocortical tumor containing fatty elements
- Nonhyperfunctioning type more common than hyperfunctioning type (Cushing's syndrome if hyperadrenocorticism; Conn's syndrome if hyperaldosteronism)
- Homogeneous low attenuation on CT (less than 0 HU 100% specific for benignity)
- Diagnosed on MRI with fat suppression or chemical shift imaging

FIGURES Barbaric: 204, 205; Dunnick: 331, 332, 334, 343–345

Myelolipoma

- Small, rare, benign adrenal tumor containing myeloproliferative cells and fat

- Echogenic on ultrasound
- Fat attenuation on CT
- Suppresses with fat saturation on MRI and may show chemical shift artifact

FIGURES Barbaric: 214; Dunnick: 347, 348

Pheochromocytoma

What percentage of pheochromocytomas are malignant? Extraadrenal? Bilateral? Familial?

Should patients with suspected or known pheochromocytomas receive intravenous iodinated contrast media?

- 10% malignant; 10% extraadrenal (30% in children); 10% bilateral; 10% familial
- Solid mass on ultrasound and CT
- Hyperintense on MRI T2-weighted images
- Uptake of MIBG
- Iodinated contrast controversial; hypertensive reaction possible

FIGURES Barbaric: 212; Dunnick: 336, 337

Carcinoma (cortical)

Are adrenocortical carcinomas typically functional?

How often are calcifications seen in an adrenocortical carcinoma on CT?

- Uncommon
- Usually large at presentation
- 50 to 80% functional
- Generally heterogeneous masses on ultrasound, CT, and MRI
- Calcifications seen in 30% on CT

FIGURES Dunnick: 345–347

Metastases/lymphoma

- Adrenal gland is common site of metastases
- Generally heterogeneous masses on ultrasound, CT, and MRI
- Investigate for the site of primary tumor and other metastases

FIGURES Barbaric: 205; Dunnick: 351–354

Hemorrhage

How old is the typical patient with adrenal hemorrhage?

How does the appearance of adrenal hemorrhage change over time on ultrasound? On CT?

- More common in newborns than in older children and adults
- Initially hyperechoic on ultrasound, decreases in echogenicity over time
- Initially high attenuation on CT, decreases in attenuation over time
- Calcification common in later stages

FIGURE Dunnick: 349

ADRENAL CALCIFICATION

List the main diagnostic considerations for adrenal calcification.

Hemorrhage
Granulomatous disease
Neoplasms

Hemorrhage

- Calcification is common in the later stages of adrenal hemorrhage

FIGURES Barbaric: 215; Dunnick: 349

Granulomatous disease

List three granulomatous diseases that may cause adrenal calcification.

- Adrenal calcification common in tuberculosis, histoplasmosis, and blastomycosis

Neoplasms

- Calcification may occur in adenomas, carcinomas, and pheochromocytomas; it is nonspecific

UTERUS

UTERINE ENLARGEMENT OR MASS

List the main diagnostic considerations for uterine enlargement or mass.

Leiomyoma
Adenomyosis
Pregnancy
Gestational trophoblastic disease
Endometrial carcinoma
Obstruction

Leiomyoma

What is the most common location for a uterine leiomyoma?
Which location is most likely to affect fertility?

- Intramural most common (more than 95%), followed by subserosal, then submucosal, which is most likely to affect fertility
- Calcifications frequently seen on radiograph and CT
- Well-defined mass of low to intermediate signal on T1-weighted images; low-signal intensity on T2-weighted images (differential diagnosis to adenomyosis)

FIGURES Barbaric: 465–467; Callen: 604–607, 666–669

Adenomyosis

How can adenomyosis be differentiated from a leiomyoma by MRI?

Is adenomyosis associated with endometriosis?

- Ill-defined area of low-signal intensity contiguous with junctional zone on T2-weighted images (differential diagnosis to leiomyoma)
- May contain foci of high-signal intensity on T1- and T2-weighted images
- Associated with endometriosis

FIGURES Barbaric: 466; Callen: 603, 670

Pregnancy

- Endometrial cavity distended by products of conception
- Clinical history and level of human chorionic gonadotropin (hCG) should lead to diagnosis

Gestational trophoblastic disease

List the three major forms of gestational trophoblastic disease.

Which is the most malignant?

What is the typical ultrasound appearance of gestational trophoblastic disease?

- Ranges from benign to malignant; 90% hydatidiform mole, 5 to 8% invasive mole, 1 to 2% choriocarcinoma
- Large, moderately echogenic mass in endometrial cavity at ultrasound (invasive mole may infiltrate myometrium; choriocarcinoma may have distant metastases)
- Associated with very high levels of hCG and theca lutein cysts

FIGURES Callen: 616–622

Endometrial carcinoma

What is the normal width of the endometrial stripe in a woman of menstrual age? In a postmenopausal woman?

- Small lesions may not be detectable or may show only widening of endometrial stripe at ultrasound (normally less than 14 mm during menstrual years, less than 8 mm in postmenopausal years)
- Large or advanced lesions may invade myometrium or spread beyond the uterus
- Dynamic enhanced MRI useful to assess depth of invasion

FIGURES Barbaric: 470, 471; Callen: 609, 671, 672

Obstruction

List three causes of an obstructed uterus.

- Dilated, blood-filled endometrial cavity
- Several causes, including cervical tumor/stenosis, imperforate hymen, vaginal web or atresia
- Look for bright signal intensity material within uterine cavity on T1-weighted images

INTRAUTERINE FILLING DEFECT(S)

List the main diagnostic considerations for intrauterine filling defects.

Asherman's syndrome (uterine synechiae)
Endometrial polyp
Endometrial carcinoma
Submucosal uterine leiomyoma
Pregnancy
Gestational trophoblastic disease

Asherman's Syndrome (uterine synechiae)

List three causes of Asherman's syndrome.

- Irregular filling defects in endometrial cavity may partially or completely obliterate it
- Causes include surgery or instrumentation, infection, and pregnancy

FIGURE Callen: 610

Endometrial polyp

Are endometrial polyps common?

How can endometrial polyps be differentiated from endometrial carcinoma at imaging?

- Single or multiple filling defects
- Size varies: may be large enough to prolapse through cervix
- Common; found in 10% of women
- Cannot be differentiated from endometrial carcinoma by imaging techniques

FIGURE Callen: 601

Endometrial Carcinoma

- May see filling defect indistinguishable from endometrial polyp
- Small lesions may not be detectable or show only widening of endometrial stripe at ultrasound (normal stripe less than 14 mm during menstrual years, less than 8 mm in postmenopausal years)
- Large or advanced lesions may show myometrial invasion or extrauterine spread
- Dynamic enhanced MRI useful to assess depth of invasion

FIGURES Barbaric: 470, 471; Callen: 609, 671, 672

Submucosal Uterine Leiomyoma

- Submucosal leiomyoma typically appears as endometrial filling defect
- Least common type of leiomyoma but most likely to result in infertility
- Calcifications may be seen on radiograph and CT
- Well-defined mass of low to intermediate signal on T1-weighted images, low-signal intensity on T2-weighted images (differential diagnosis to adenomyosis)
- Additional leiomyomas should be sought because several usually are present

FIGURES Barbaric: 466; Callen: 605, 668

Pregnancy

- Endometrial cavity distended by products of conception
- Clinical history and hCG level should lead to diagnosis

Gestational Trophoblastic Disease

- Ranges from benign to malignant; 90% hydatidiform mole, 5 to 8% invasive mole, 1 to 2% choriocarcinoma
- Large moderately echogenic mass in endometrial cavity at ultrasound (invasive mole may infiltrate myometrium; choriocarcinoma may have distant metastases)
- Associated with very high levels of hCG and theca lutein cysts

FIGURES Callen: 616–622

ADNEXA

CYSTIC ADNEXAL MASS

See Chapter 11 (Ultrasound).

Tuboovarian abscess

What findings in addition to tuboovarian abscess may be seen in pelvic inflammatory disease?

- Complex adnexal mass on ultrasound, CT, or MRI
- Other evidence of pelvic inflammatory disease (e.g., endometrial fluid, pelvic peritoneal fluid, pyosalpinx or hydrosalpinx) should be sought

Ectopic pregnancy

Where do most ectopic pregnancies occur?

What is the likelihood of an intrauterine pregnancy coexisting with an ectopic pregnancy?

- Complex adnexal mass (97% tubal, 1% ovarian) on ultrasound, CT, or MRI
- No evidence of intrauterine pregnancy (only approximately 1:7000 intrauterine pregnancies coexist with an ectopic pregnancy)
- In indeterminate cases, patient should be followed with serial ultrasound and hCG levels

FIGURES Callen: 650–657

SOLID ADNEXAL MASS

See Chapter 11 (Ultrasound).

SCROTUM

INTRATESTICULAR MASS

List the main diagnostic considerations for an intratesticular mass.

Testicular germ cell tumor
Testicular stromal tumor
Orchitis
Trauma

Testicular germ cell tumor

Which histologic type of testicular germ cell tumor is most common?

What is its typical ultrasonographic appearance?

Which serum markers may be elevated in testicular germ cell tumors?

Can a "burned-out" germ cell tumor metastasize?

- Seminoma most common histology, typically homogeneously hypoechoic at ultrasound
- Nonseminomatous typically heterogenous mixed echogenicity at ultrasound
- "Burned-out" tumors: echogenic focus at ultrasound
- Many tumors associated with elevated levels of alpha-fetoprotein (AFP) or hCG, or both
- Retroperitoneal lymphadenopathy should be sought when an intratesticular mass is discovered ("burned-out" tumors may still metastasize)
- An intratesticular tumor should be sought when retroperitoneal lymphadenopathy is discovered in a young man

FIGURES Barbaric: 456; Dunnick: 495–497

Testicular stromal tumor

Name two histologic types of testicular stromal tumor.

Are these common lesions?

- Typically hypoechoic masses (may have associated cysts) at ultrasound
- These uncommon lesions include Leydig cell tumor, Sertoli cell tumor, gonadoblastoma

Orchitis

What extratesticular findings are associated with orchitis?

- Focal or diffuse hypoechoic areas in testis correspond to site of inflammation at ultrasound
- Associated with epididymitis
- Increased flow should be sought by Doppler ultrasound or nuclear medicine

FIGURE Dunnick: 505

Trauma

What extratesticular findings are associated with testicular trauma?

- Intratesticular hemorrhage heterogeneously hypoechoic on ultrasound
- Hematocele and scrotal hemorrhage or edema should be sought

FIGURE Dunnick: 499

EXTRATESTICULAR MASS

List the main diagnostic considerations for an extratesticular mass.

Epididymitis
Spermatocele
Epididymal cyst
Hydrocele
Trauma (hematocele)
Varicocele
Hernia

Epididymitis

- Enlargement of the head and body of epididymis
- Heterogeneous and predominantly hypoechoic at ultrasound
- Associated with orchitis
- Increased flow should be sought at Doppler ultrasound or nuclear medicine

FIGURES Barbaric: 454; Dunnick: 505

Spermatocele

- Cystic mass in epididymis at ultrasound
- May be loculated and have a few internal echoes
- Occurs only in head (differential diagnosis to epididymal cyst)

FIGURE Dunnick: 503

Epididymal cyst

How can an epididymal cyst be differentiated from a spermatocele?

- Anechoic mass in epididymis at ultrasound
- May be multiple and measure up to 2 cm
- May occur in head, body, or tail (differential diagnosis to spermatocele)

Hydrocele

What percentage of normal men have a hydrocele?

What conditions may cause a secondary hydrocele?

- Anechoic extratesticular fluid at ultrasound
- Small, idiopathic hydroceles present in more than 60% of normal men
- May also occur secondary to inflammation, tumor, trauma, torsion

FIGURES Barbaric: 452; Dunnick: 502, 503

Trauma (hematocele)

- Extratesticular fluid containing internal echoes at ultrasound
- Associated with intratesticular hemorrhage or injury and scrotal hemorrhage or edema

FIGURE Dunnick: 499

Varicocele

What size is the normal pampiniform plexus?

What percentage of normal men have an idiopathic varicocele?

What percentage of infertile men have an idiopathic varicocele?

What must be suspected when a right-sided varicocele is discovered?

- Serpiginous hypoechoic tubular structures at ultrasound
- Enlargement of pampiniform plexus (normally less than 3 mm)
- Vascular flow identifiable by Doppler ultrasound and often at gray scale
- Idiopathic: predominantly left-sided; size increases with upright position or Valsalva maneuver; occurs in 15% of normal men, 40% of infertile men
- Secondary: no side predilection, no change with position or Valsalva maneuver (intraabdominal mass causing venous compression suggested when a right-sided varicocele is discovered)

FIGURES Barbaric: 458–460; Dunnick: 504

Hernia

- Complex, echogenic, peristaltic mass at ultrasound
- Scrotal gas should be sought on radiograph or CT

Figure References

Barbaric ZL: *Principles of Genitourinary Radiology,* 2nd ed. New York: Thieme, 1994.
Callen PW: *Ultrasonography in Obstetrics and Gynecology,* 3rd ed. Philadelphia: WB Saunders, 1994.
Dunnick NR, Sandler CM, Amis ES, Newhouse JH: *Textbook of Uroradiology,* 2nd ed. Baltimore: Williams & Wilkins, 1997.

GENITOURINARY IMAGING DISEASE ENTITIES

ACQUIRED RENAL CYSTIC DISEASE OF UREMIA

Clinical

- Renal cysts in uremic patients; cause unclear
- 40% overall incidence in dialysis patients; 80 to 90% after 5 years
- Solid masses develop in up to 7% (renal adenocarcinoma in 1%)

Imaging

- Small, end-stage kidneys
- Multiple bilateral cysts, may be hemorrhagic

ACUTE CORTICAL NECROSIS

Clinical

- Rare, irreversible ischemic necrosis of cortex with characteristic sparing of medulla and thin rim of outer cortex (preserved capsular blood supply)
- More than 66% of cases associated with pregnancy; other associations include burns, sepsis, toxins, transfusion reactions, dehydration, and peritonitis

Imaging

- Early: diffusely enlarged kidneys
    IVU:
        Absent/faint opacification
    Ultrasound:
        Loss of corticomedullary differentiation
- Late: small, smooth kidneys; "tram-track" cortical calcifications

ACUTE TUBULAR NECROSIS (ATN)

Clinical

- Most common form of acute reversible renal failure
- Can be oliguric or nonoliguric
- Chemical causes: iodinated contrast media, antibiotics (especially aminoglycosides), chemotherapeutic agents, hemoglobin, myoglobin, heavy metals, and solvents
- Ischemic causes: trauma, surgery, burns, hypotension, postpartum status, renal transplantation

Imaging

- Enlarged kidneys
- IVU:
    Persistently increasingly dense nephrogram
- Ultrasound:
    Gray-scale appearance varies (often appears normal), elevated resistive indices (RIs)
- MRI:
    Loss of corticomedullary differentiation on T1-weighted images
- NM:
    Poor DTPA concentration, progressive parenchymal accumulation of hippuran/MAG3

ADDISON'S DISEASE

Clinical

- Primary adrenal insufficiency (requires more than 90% cortical loss)
- Idiopathic atrophy (usually autoimmune) most common cause in United States
- Other causes include granulomatous disease, especially tuberculosis (TB), hemorrhage, and metastases

Imaging

- Small adrenal glands
- Enlarged adrenal glands if acute inflammation, hemorrhage, or metastases

ADENOMYOSIS

Clinical

- Invasion of myometrium by endometrial glands
- Common in women of menstrual age; associated with endometriosis

Imaging

- Ultrasound:
    Poorly defined hypoechoic and heterogeneous myometrial areas may be visualized, but study must be meticulously performed and experienced sonologist must veiw in real time.
- MRI:
    Low-signal area in myometrium contiguous with junctional zone on T2-weighted images; may contain high-signal foci on T2- and T1-weighted images; lesions poorly defined and demarcated compared with leiomyomas

ADRENAL HEMORRHAGE

Clinical

- Newborns: birth trauma, hypoxia, septicemia, coagulopathies
- Older children and adults: anticoagulation, sepsis (Waterhouse-Friderichsen syndrome if secondary to meningococcemia), trauma, tumor

Imaging

- Radiograph:
    Soft tissue mass displacing kidney inferiorly; calcification is common in later stages and can develop in weeks
- Ultrasound:
    Initially hyperechoic mass that decreases in echogenicity over time
- CT:
    Initially high-attenuation mass that decreases in attenuation over time

- MRI:
    Generally increased signal on both T1- and T2-weighted images; is not suppressed with fat saturation techniques

ADRENAL MYELOLIPOMA

Clinical

- Rare, benign tumor that originates from myeloproliferative cells and includes fat
- Usually small and discovered incidentally at autopsy

Imaging

- May contain hemorrhage and calcify
- Ultrasound:
    Hyperechoic
- CT:
    Fat attenuation
- MRI:
    Similar to retroperitoneal fat, bright on both T1- and T2-weighted images, suppresses with fat saturation techniques, may show chemical shift artifact

ADRENOCORTICAL ADENOMA

Clinical

- Cords of clear cells separated by fibrovascular trabeculae
- Typically contain fatty elements
- Incidental finding on 1% of CT examinations, 3% of autopsies
- Nonhyperfunctioning type most common
- Hyperfunctioning type can cause primary hyperaldosteronism, Cushing's syndrome, or virilization

Imaging

- CT:
    Usually small, homogeneous, low-attenuation masses (HU less than 0 is 100% specific for benignity); minimal enhancement
- MRI:
    Typically less bright than metastases on T2-weighted images, chemical shift imaging can be used to identify associated fat

ADRENOCORTICAL CARCINOMA

Clinical

- Uncommon (1:1,000,000 incidence); ratio of males to females is 1:1
- Usually large at presentation
- 50 to 80% functional (Cushing's syndrome more common than virilization, which is more common than feminization)
- Prognosis poor

Imaging

- Radiograph:
    Large abdominal mass displacing kidney inferiorly; calcification may be seen
- Ultrasound:
    Small lesions usually homogeneous, large lesions heterogeneous
- CT:
    Central areas of necrosis; calcification in 30%; heterogeneous enhancement; invasion into renal vein and IVC may be visible
- MRI:
    Signal intensity on T2-weighted images high but not as high as that of pheochromocytoma

ADRENOCORTICAL HYPERPLASIA

Clinical

- Diffuse adrenocortical overgrowth (no focal mass)
- Causes include idiopathic, inborn error of metabolism, pituitary tumor, ectopic hormone production, and exogenous hormone source
- Cushing's syndrome/disease, Conn's syndrome, virilization

Imaging

- Bilateral adrenal enlargement without focal mass (adreniform shape maintained)

AIDS NEPHROPATHY (HUMAN IMMUNODEFICIENCY VIRUS [HIV] NEPHROPATHY)

Clinical

- Combination of renal insufficiency, nephrotic syndrome, and glomerular changes secondary to HIV infection
- Interstitial infiltrates and fibrosis, focal/segmental glomerulosclerosis, microcystic dilatation of tubules, and intratubular casts
- Proteinuria and progressive renal failure

Imaging

- Kidneys normal in size or enlarged
- Ultrasound:
    Increased cortical and medullary echogenicity (focal or global)
- CT:
    May see medullary hyperattenuation
- MRI:
    Loss of corticomedullary differentiation on T1-weighted images

AMYLOIDOSIS

Clinical

- Extracellular deposition of proteinaceous material
- Multiple organs involved in 85%
- Primary: renal involvement in 35%, idiopathic
- Secondary: renal involvement in more than 80%, causes include rheumatoid arthritis, TB, leprosy, chronic osteomyelitis, and malignancy

Imaging

- Early: kidneys normal in size to enlarged
- Late: small kidneys
- IVU/CT:
    Diminished nephrogram; attenuation of collecting system may be seen
- Ultrasound:
    Echogenic cortex
- Angiography:
    Tortuosity and irregularity of interlobar arteries

ANGIOMYOLIPOMA (RENAL HAMARTOMA)

Clinical

- Benign mesenchymal tumor composed of fat, smooth muscle, and blood vessels
- Females affected more often than males; 0.07 to 0.3% overall incidence
- 80% of patients with tuberous sclerosis (TS) have angiomyolipomas (AMLs); fewer than 40% of patients with AML have TS
- Usually asymptomatic; painful if hemorrhage occurs
- Usually only large or complicated lesions are resected

6

Imaging

- Radiograph:
    Fat lucency in less than 10%
- Ultrasound:
    Hyperechoic mass
- CT:
    Demonstration of fat virtually diagnostic (rare case reports of fat within renal adenocarcinoma and Wilms' tumor)
- MRI:
    Bright on T1-weighted images, suppression with fat saturation techniques
- Angiography:
    Vascular mass

ASHERMAN'S SYNDROME (UTERINE SYNECHIAE)

Clinical

- Intrauterine adhesions that partially or completely obliterate endometrial cavity
- Causes include surgery or instrumentation, infection, pregnancy, amenorrhea, and oligomenorrhea
- Complications include infertility and spontaneous abortion

Imaging

- HSG:
    Irregular filling defects in endometrial cavity
- Ultrasound:
    Nonspecific; thin endometrial stripe, echogenic endometrial focus may be seen

AUTOSOMAL DOMINANT POLYCYSTIC KIDNEY DISEASE

Clinical

- High penetrance, 1 in 1000 symptomatic (higher autopsy prevalence)
- Ratio of males to females is 1:1; usually manifests by middle age; may occur in neonates
- Responsible for 10 to 12% of dialysis patients
- Cysts also seen in liver (30 to 70%), pancreas (less than 10%) and, less commonly, thyroid, testes, seminal vesicles, and ovaries
- 60% hypertension, 30 to 50% cerebral aneurysms (cause of death in 10%), possible increased incidence of renal cell carcinoma

Imaging

- Bilaterally enlarged kidneys
- Multiple bilateral cortical cysts of varying sizes
- Cyst walls may be calcified and urolithiasis may occur
- Cysts may contain protein and debris from prior hemorrhage
- Ultrasound:
    Debris in cysts may appear as dependent sludge
- CT:
    Cysts of variable attenuation
- MRI:
    Cysts bright on T2-weighted images, variable signal intensity on T1-weighted images

AUTOSOMAL RECESSIVE POLYCYSTIC KIDNEY DISEASE

Clinical

- 1:6000 to 1:14,000 live births; ratio of males to females affected is 1:2
- Small saccular enlargement of medullary collecting ducts
- Associated hepatic disease: fibrosis and cyst formation
- In infantile form, renal disease more common than hepatic disease, causes renal failure at birth
- In childhood form, hepatic disease more common than renal disease, causes portal hypertension and varices

Imaging

- Bilaterally enlarged kidneys, calcifications common
- Ultrasound:
    Diffusely increased echogenicity, cysts too small to be individually visualized without high-resolution equipment
- IVU/CT:
    Streaky nephrogram

BENIGN PROSTATIC HYPERTROPHY

Clinical

- Hyperplasia of transition and periurethral zones (central gland)
- Rare before age 50 years; more than 50% of men aged more than 60 years, nearly 100% aged more than 80 years affected
- Symptoms present in 20%, secondary to bladder outlet obstruction

Imaging

- IVU:
    Elevation of bladder base and distal ureters ("J" hooking), round filling defect at bladder base
- TRUS:
    Prostate weight (g) = volume (cc) = length (cm) $\times$ width (cm) $\times$ height (cm) $\times$ 0.52 (normal = 20 g in a young man, up to 40 g in an older man); heterogeneous echotexture, echogenic calcifications frequently seen at surgical capsule (corpora amylacea)
- CT:
    Enlarged gland, calcifications common
- MRI:
    Enlarged, heterogeneous central gland

BLADDER RUPTURE

Clinical

- Extraperitoneal: more common (80%); typically occurs at base secondary to pelvic fracture; can usually be treated with indwelling catheterization
- Intraperitoneal: less common (20%); typically occurs at dome secondary to iatrogenic injury or blunt trauma; usually requires surgical treatment

Imaging

- IVU/cystogram/CT:
    Extraperitoneal: streaky, stationary contrast outside bladder; "pear-shaped" bladder
    Intraperitoneal: free peritoneal contrast surrounding bowel loops, liver, and spleen

CALYCEAL DIVERTICULUM

Clinical

- Outpouching of calyx into corticomedullary region
- Congenital or acquired (reflux, obstruction, infection)
- Usually asymptomatic, may predispose patient to infection or calculi

Imaging

- IVU/retrograde:
    Collection of contrast extending eccentrically from fornix of affected calyx; communicating channel usually not directly visualized

- Ultrasound:
    Indistinguishable from cyst
- CT:
    Indistinguishable from cyst on unenhanced images; accumulates contrast

CERVICAL CARCINOMA

Clinical

- Third most common primary gynecologic malignancy
- 95% squamous cell carcinoma, 5% adenocarcinoma
- Associations: multiple sexual partners, increased parity, human papillomavirus, smoking
- FIGO staging:
    IA   Microinvasion of stroma
    IB   Stromal invasion
    IIA   Extension into upper two thirds of vagina
    IIB   Parametrial invasion
    IIIA Extension into lower third of vagina
    IIIB Hydronephrosis or pelvic sidewall invasion
    IVA   Invasion of bladder/rectal mucosa, extension out of true pelvis
    IVB   Distant metastases

Imaging

- Cervical enlargement or mass
- Fluid-filled uterus if obstructed
- MRI:
    High-signal intensity focus within normally low-signal cervical stroma on T2-weighted images

CONN'S SYNDROME

Clinical

- Hyperaldosteronism; ratio of males to females is 1:2
- Hypertension, hypokalemia, hyperkaluria
- Adenoma 75%, hyperplasia 20 to 25%, carcinoma less than 1%

Imaging

- Bilateral enlargement in hyperplasia, small mass in adenoma, large mass in carcinoma
- Nuclear medicine: adrenal uptake by NP-59
- Venography or venous sampling often required to establish diagnosis

CORPUS LUTEUM CYST

Clinical

- Failure of resorption or bleeding into corpus luteum (residual follicle after ovulation)
- Most resolve spontaneously; may or may not be associated with pregnancy
- Most common adnexal mass in pregnancy, usually involutes by 14th week
- May cause pain or be asymptomatic

Imaging

- Ultrasound:
    Three- to 15-cm hypoechoic adnexal cyst; may have low-level echoes secondary to hemorrhage

CUSHING'S SYNDROME

Clinical

- Hypercorticolism; ratio of males to females affected is 1:4
- Central fat deposition (truncal obesity, moon facies, buffalo hump)
- Hypertension, hirsutism, diabetes, acne, abdominal striae
- Diagnosis made by dexamethasone suppression test
- Hyperplasia 70% (Cushing's disease is hyperplasia secondary to adrenocortico-tropic hormone-producing pituitary adenoma), adenoma 20%, carcinoma 10%

Imaging

- Bilateral enlargement in hyperplasia, small mass in adenoma, large mass in carcinoma
- Nuclear medicine:
    Adrenal uptake by NP-59

END-STAGE RENAL DISEASE

Clinical

- Uremic renal failure requiring dialysis
- Several causes, including diabetes, hypertension, glomerulonephritis, hereditary chronic nephritis (Alport's syndrome), acute cortical necrosis, connective tissue/autoimmune diseases, drugs (analgesics, aminoglycosides), infection, reflux, amyloidosis, storage diseases, and others
- Complications: acquired cystic disease of uremia and renal adenocarcinoma

Imaging

- Bilaterally small kidneys often with cortical thinning
- May see acquired cysts or tumor

ENDOMETRIAL CARCINOMA

Clinical

- Most common gynecologic malignancy, fourth most common malignancy overall in women
- 85% adenocarcinoma; uncommon histologies: clear cell carcinoma, papillary serous carcinoma, and adenocarcinoma with squamous differentiation
- Associated with nulliparity, early menarche or late menopause, breast cancer, hypertension, diabetes, and obesity
- Usually diagnosed clinically by dilatation and curettage (one third of patients with postmenopausal bleeding will be diagnosed with endometrial carcinoma)
- FIGO staging:
    IA   Limited to endometrium
    IB   Invasion into less than half of myometrium
    IC   Invasion into more than half of myometrium
    IIA Endocervical glandular invasion
    IIB Cervical stromal invasion
    IIIA Serosal or adnexal involvement; positive peritoneal cytologic studies
    IIIB Vaginal involvement
    IIIC Pelvic or periaortic lymph node involvement
    IVA Invasion of bladder or bowel mucosa
    IVB Distant metastases

Imaging

- Uterus normal in size or enlarged
- Ultrasound:
    Focal endometrial mass in larger lesions; widening of endometrial stripe (nor-

mally less than 14 mm during menstrual years, less than 8 mm in postmenopausal years) is the only finding in some cases
- MRI:
    Darker than endometrium and brighter than junctional zone/myometrium on
    T2-weighted images; differential enhancement with gadolinium (useful for
    assessing depth of myometrial invasion)

ENDOMETRIAL POLYP

Clinical

- Pedunculated or sessile excrescences of endometrial tissue
- May be single or multiple, small or large (may protrude through cervix)
- Common, found in 10% of women
- Bleeding is typical symptom, but many are asymptomatic
- Rarely undergo malignant transformation

Imaging

- Cannot be reliably differentiated from endometrial carcinoma
- HSG:
    Intrauterine filling defect(s)
- Ultrasound:
    Widening of endometrial stripe, focal echogenic endometrial mass (may be
    surrounded by fluid); mass often contains cysts

ENDOMETRIOSIS

Clinical

- Presence of functional endometrial tissue outside of endometrial cavity
- Affects 25% of women in third and fourth decades
- Causes pelvic pain, dysmenorrhea
- Forms include small implants, endometriomas (complex cystic mass, "chocolate
  cyst"), or adhesions
- Common locations: pouch of Douglas, surface of ovary, fallopian tubes, uterus,
  and broad ligament
- Unusual locations: urinary tract (1%, bladder more common site than ureter),
  bowel and pleura (may result in catamenial pneumothorax)

Imaging

- Ultrasound:
    About 50% of endometriomas are unilocular cysts with diffuse low-level inter-
    nal echoes; the other 50% are more heterogeneous in appearance
- IVU/barium enema:
    May see implants on ureters, bladder, bowel
- MRI:
    Endometriomas and implants bright on T2-weighted images; also bright on T1-
    weighted images if hemorrhage is present (not suppressed with fat satura-
    tion techniques)

EPIDIDYMAL CYST

Clinical

- Dilatation of tubules in epididymis
- Up to 2 cm in size, often multiple; may occur throughout epididymis
- Contain serous fluid

Imaging

- Ultrasound:
    Anechoic mass or masses in epididymis

EPIDIDYMOORCHITIS

Clinical

- Occurs in postpubertal men via retrograde spread of infection
- Organisms include *Neisseria gonorrhoeae*, *Chlamydia* spp, *Escherichia coli*, *Proteus* spp, and mumps virus
- Symptoms include pain, swelling (differential diagnosis to torsion)

Imaging

- Ultrasound:
    Head and body of epididymis enlarged, heterogeneous, and predominantly hypoechoic; focal or diffuse hypoechoic areas in testis if orchitis; increased vascular flow by Doppler ultrasound
- Nuclear medicine:
    Increased perfusion on dynamic and static images

FOLLICULAR CYST

Clinical

- Results when mature follicle fails to ovulate or involute
- Usually does not cause symptoms; patient may have pain, hemorrhage, rupture, or torsion
- Cyclic changes, usually regress spontaneously

Imaging

- Ultrasound:
    Smooth, round, anechoic ovarian cyst measuring more than 2.5 cm (range: 1 to 10 cm; 2.5-cm cut-off chosen because normal follicles may attain this size); may have internal echoes if hemorrhage present

FRALEY SYNDROME

Clinical

- Obstruction of an upper pole infundibulum by a crossing vessel
- Symptoms include pain, which may be severe enough to require surgery

Imaging

- Dilated upper pole collecting system; extrinsic compression by crossing vessel; upper pole parenchyma may atrophy

GLOMERULONEPHRITIS

Clinical

- Usually autoimmune as a result of streptococcal infection, IgA nephropathy, Goodpasture's syndrome
- Hematuria, proteinuria, urinary casts
- Most patients recover from acute poststreptococcal glomerulonephritis (5 to 20% show progressive renal damage); prognosis poorer for IgA nephropathy and Goodpasture's syndrome

Imaging

- Acute: kidneys normal in size or slightly enlarged
- Chronic: small, smooth kidneys; cortical calcification may occur but is uncommon

HEREDITARY CHRONIC NEPHRITIS (ALPORT'S SYNDROME)

Clinical

- Fat-filled macrophages ("foam cells") in corticomedullary junction and medulla
- Probably autosomal dominant
- In males: progressive renal insufficiency occurs, death usually before age 50 years
- In females: not progressive
- Classic clinical triad: hematuria, nerve deafness, and ocular abnormalities

Imaging

- Small, smooth kidneys; cortical calcifications
- IVU/CT:
    Diminished contrast concentration

HYDROCELE

Clinical

- Simple: fluid collection in tunica vaginalis; can be idiopathic or secondary to inflammation, tumor, trauma, or torsion; small idiopathic hydrocele present in 60% of normal men
- Congenital: ascites that enters scrotum through open processus vaginalis (associated with hernia)
- Infantile: extends to funicular process but no peritoneal communication

Imaging

- Ultrasound:
    Anechoic extratesticular scrotal fluid; internal echoes can be seen with infection or hemorrhage
- MRI:
    Low signal on T1-weighted images, high signal on T2-weighted images; increased signal on T1-weighted images with infection or hemorrhage

JUXTAGLOMERULAR TUMOR (RENINOMA)

Clinical

- Rare benign tumor arising from renin-producing cells of juxtaglomerular apparatus
- Hypertension, hypokalemia, headaches, polyuria, and polydipsia
- Measures 2 to 7 cm, located just beneath renal capsule

Imaging

- Ultrasound:
    Echogenic mass
- CT:
    Mass enhances less than normal parenchyma
- Angiography:
    Hypovascular mass, high ipsilateral renal venous renin

LEUKOPLAKIA

Clinical

- Keratinizing squamous metaplasia of transitional epithelium
- Premalignant, may develop into squamous cell carcinoma

- Bladder affected most often, followed by renal pelvis, then ureter
- Males affected more often than females; associated with frequent urinary tract infections and long-standing calculi

Imaging

- Poorly defined filling defects in bladder, ureter, and collecting system/pelvis
- May become large in bladder and pelvis

MALACOPLAKIA

Clinical

- Chronic inflammatory response to *E. coli* infection
- Periodic acid–Schiff (PAS)-positive histiocytes containing Michaelis-Gutmann inclusion bodies
- Females affected more often than males; associated with diabetes
- Bladder most common site, followed by ureter, then renal pelvis
- Renal parenchymal involvement in 16%
- Not premalignant

Imaging

- Multiple smooth, scalloped filling defects in urothelium

MEDULLARY CYSTIC DISEASE

Clinical

- Autosomal recessive (nephronopthesis): most common, onset between ages 3 and 5 years
- Autosomal dominant: less common, adult onset
- Renal failure with salt wasting and polyuria
- Multiple small (less than 2 mm) cysts in collecting tubules at corticomedullary junction and medulla

Imaging

- Kidney size normal or small, no calcifications
- IVU:
    Streaky parenchyma
- Ultrasound:
    Hyperechoic parenchyma with thin cortex; cysts seen if sufficiently large
- CT:
    Streaky parenchyma; cysts seen if sufficiently large

MEDULLARY SPONGE KIDNEY

Clinical

- No definite hereditary pattern; men affected slightly more often than women
- Occurs in young to middle-aged adults
- May be bilateral, unilateral, or unifocal
- Cystic or fusiform dilatation of collecting tubules with calculi in more than 50%
- Often asymptomatic; mild form seen incidentally on 0.5% of IVUs

Imaging

- Radiograph:
    Medullary intratubular calcifications in 40 to 80%
- IVU:
    Streaky "paint-brush" appearance of contrast-filled, dilated tubules

MEGAURETER (PRIMARY MEGAURETER)

Clinical

- Deficient longitudinal muscle in distal ureter leading to nonobstructive dilatation
- Occurs at all ages; ratio of males to females affected is 2:1
- Mostly asymptomatic; associated with other genitourinary anomalies in 40%

Imaging

- IVU:
  - Grade 1 Distal ureter dilated
  - Grade 2 Entire ureter dilated, with or without mild caliectasis
  - Grade 3 Entire ureter dilated and moderate to severe caliectasis; characteristic "beak-like" configuration at ureterovesical junction; ureter usually not tortuous (differential diagnosis to obstruction/reflux)
- VCUG: no vesicoureteral reflux

MULTICYSTIC DYSPLASTIC KIDNEY

Clinical

- Second most common abdominal mass in neonate after hydronephrosis
- Males affected slightly more often than females
- Ureteric bud division is arrested, causing pelvoinfundibular atresia
- Collection of irregularly sized cysts and fibrous tissue
- Contralateral anomalies in 30%, most commonly ureteropelvic junction obstruction

Imaging

- Radiograph:
  - Curvilinear calcifications in 30% of adults, rarely in children
- IVU:
  - Typically no function; "puddling" may be seen on 24-hour delayed film if some normal parenchyma is present
- Retrograde atretic ureter
- Angiography:
  - Absent or severely hypoplastic renal artery
- Ultrasound/CT:
  - Renal parenchyma replaced by multiple cysts with distinct septa

MULTILOCULAR CYSTIC NEPHROMA

Clinical

- Well-circumscribed septated cystic mass; individual cysts do not communicate
- Males: peak incidence between ages of 3 months and 4 years
- Females: bimodal distribution with peak incidences between ages of 4 and 20 years and above age 40 years
- Cause unclear; may be congenital or related to Wilms' tumor or multicystic dysplastic kidney
- Treated with partial nephrectomy (cannot entirely exclude cystic renal adenocarcinoma or Wilms' tumor in children)

Imaging

- Ultrasound:
  - Mass of multiple anechoic cysts separated by septa
- CT:
  - Mass of multiple water attenuation cysts separated by septa, which may contain calcifications and enhance with contrast
- MRI:
  - Mass of multiple cysts separated by septa; cyst fluid follows urine dark on

T1-weighted images, bright on T2-weighted images; septa may enhance with contrast
- Angiography:
    Hypovascular mass

MULTIPLE MYELOMA

Clinical

- Precipitation of Bence Jones protein leads to renal failure in 30 to 50% of patients with myeloma
- Secondary amyloidosis develops in 10%
- Urographic contrast media controversial (may increase Bence Jones protein deposition)

Imaging

- Smooth, enlarged kidneys; may become small with progression of renal failure
- Radiograph:
    May develop medullary nephrocalcinosis secondary to hypercalcemia associated with bone lesions
- IVU:
    Diminished nephrogram; collecting system may be attenuated
- Ultrasound:
    Normal to increased echogenicity

MYCETOMA (RENAL FUNGAL INFECTIONS)

Clinical

- Relatively common: candidiasis; rare: actinomycosis, aspergillosis, blastomycosis, coccidioidomycosis, cryptococcosis, and histoplasmosis
- Usually opportunistic infections in patients with altered immunity, diabetes, or indwelling catheters
- Symptoms include flank pain, passage of debris with urination (hematuria rare)

Imaging

- IVU:
    Nonvisualization (focal, multifocal, entire kidney); papillary necrosis; irregular mucosa; filling defects in collecting system, ureter, and bladder
- Ultrasound/CT:
    Masses in parenchyma, collecting system, ureter, and bladder

NEPHROGENIC ADENOMA

Clinical

- Rare metaplastic response to urothelial injury, calculi, or infection
- Males affected more often than females; usually involves bladder

Imaging

- Filling defect in bladder

NEUROGENIC BLADDER

Clinical

- Hyperactive detrusor: more common; upper motor neuron lesion; involuntary bladder contractions, usually associated with sphincteric dysfunction
- Hyporeflexic detrusor: less common; lower motor neuron lesion; absence of bladder contractions with associated sphincteric dysfunction

Imaging

- Hyperactive detrusor: small capacity, trabeculated, "Christmas tree" appearance
- Hyporeflexic detrusor: large volume bladder with large postvoid residual

OBSTRUCTIVE NEPHROPATHY

Clinical

- Renal parenchymal loss secondary to chronic obstruction
- Causes include congenital anomaly, calculi, intrinsic or extrinsic mass, retroperitoneal fibrosis, and radiation

Imaging

- Dilated collecting system, pelvis, or ureter with parenchymal loss

ONCOCYTOMA

Clinical

- Benign renal adenoma of proximal tubular cell origin
- 4 to 7% of all renal tumors
- Usually does not cause symptoms; patient may have hematuria
- Surgery required for diagnosis (cannot exclude renal adenocarcinoma by fine-needle aspiration or biopsy)
- Pathologic diagnosis requires several sections showing no clear cell carcinoma

Imaging

- Cannot be differentiated from renal adenocarcinoma reliably
- CT:
    Central scar classic but seen in only 30%
- Angiography:
    "Spoke wheel" pattern of vessels seen in 80%

OVARIAN EPITHELIAL ADENOMA

Clinical

- Benign ovarian tumors
- Serous cystadenoma more common than mucinous cystadenoma, which is more common than Brenner tumor
- Serous cystadenoma is less common than serous cystadenocarcinoma; mucinous cystadenoma is more common than mucinous cystadenocarcinoma
- Bilateral lesions: 20% of serous cystadenomas, 5% of mucinous cystadenomas

Imaging

- Cystic/complex mass: serous cystadenoma, mucinous cystadenoma
- Solid mass: Brenner tumor

OVARIAN EPITHELIAL CARCINOMA

Clinical

- Second most common primary gynecologic malignancy; incidence increases with age
- Highest mortality rate of gynecologic malignancies (two thirds of patients present with advanced disease)
- Associations: nulliparity, breast cancer, family history
- Serous cystadenocarcinoma most common type followed by endometrioid carcinoma, mucinous cystadenocarinoma, undifferentiated carcinoma, and clear cell carcinoma

- FIGO staging:
    - IA   One ovary
    - IB   Both ovaries
    - IC   IA or IB with positive peritoneal cytologic studies
    - IIA   Implants on fallopian tubes/uterus
    - IIB   Extension to other pelvic tissues
    - IIC   IIA or IIB with positive peritoneal cytologic studies
    - IIIA Microscopic peritoneal implants beyond pelvis
    - IIIB Peritoneal implants less than 2 cm in size beyond pelvis
    - IIIC Peritoneal implants more than 2 cm in size beyond pelvis
    - IV   Distant metastases
- CA-125: positive in 80% of patients with advanced disease, in 35% with stage I disease, and in many patients with benign disease (e.g., pelvic inflammatory disease, endometriosis) or pregnancy; useful as a marker for assessing recurrent or metastatic disease

Imaging

- Ultrasound:
    Cystic mass with thick septations, wall irregularity, septal nodules, or mural nodules
- CT:
    Complex cystic mass; can assess peritoneal disease; calcifications associated with serous cystadenocarcinoma
- MRI:
    Complex cystic mass; can assess peritoneal disease

OVARIAN GERM CELL TUMORS (OTHER THAN MATURE TERATOMA)

Clinical

- Most common primary malignant ovarian tumors in adolescent and young women
- Dysgerminoma (5% of all ovarian neoplasms, counterpart to seminoma in males) most common histologic type, followed by immature teratoma, endodermal sinus tumor, yolk sac tumor, primary ovarian choriocarcinoma, enbryonal carcinoma, and mixed tumors

Imaging

- Predominantly solid but may be complex

OVARIAN HYPERSTIMULATION SYNDROME

Clinical

- Exogenous hCG given for infertility
- Symptoms include abdominal pain, nausea, vomiting, ascites, and anasarca

Imaging

- Enlarged ovaries with multiple cysts; ascites may be seen

OVARIAN MATURE TERATOMA (DERMOID CYST)

Clinical

- Generally benign tumor (malignant transformation in 2 to 3%) containing at least ectodermal elements
- Usually presents in adolescents and young women
- Most common ovarian neoplasm (20% of all)
- May present with pain secondary to torsion and hemorrhage

Imaging

- Radiograph:
    Fat density; bone, tooth may be seen
- Ultrasound:
    Complex cystic mass; highly echogenic focus ("dermoid plug"); shadowing distal to hair, bone, tooth; may mimic bowel
- CT:
    Complex cystic mass; fat attenuation material; bone, tooth, other calcifications
- MRI:
    Complex cystic mass (fluid-fluid layers often seen secondary to floating proteinaceous debris); high-signal intensity fat on T1-weighted images (suppresses with fat saturation techniques; chemical shift artifact may be seen)

OVARIAN METASTASES

Clinical

- Ovary most common site of intraperitoneal pelvic metastases
- Primary tumors: stomach, pancreas, breast, liver, biliary tract, or uterus
- Krukenberg's tumor: metastasis to ovary from mucin-producing signet ring cells, usually gastric primary

Imaging

- Usually solid adnexal mass(es); ascites frequent

OVARIAN STROMAL TUMORS

Clinical

- Rare, generally benign tumors of stromal origin
- Histologic types include fibroma, thecoma, fibrothecoma, granulosa cell, and Sertoli-Leydig cell
- Meigs' syndrome: ascites and pleural effusion associated with benign fibroma or fibrothecoma (50% incidence with lesions more than 5 cm)

Imaging

- Nonspecific ovarian masses, generally solid

OVARIAN TORSION

Clinical

- May be idiopathic or caused by hypermobility (usual cause in children) or ovarian mass or cyst
- The right side is more frequently involved than the left
- Symptoms include pain, nausea, vomiting

Imaging

- Ultrasound:
    Enlarged ovary, engorged vessels at periphery, decreased or absent flow with Doppler ultrasound

OXALOSIS

Clinical

- Hyperoxalemia causing precipitation of oxalate crystals in several tissues (e.g., kidneys, myocardium, lung, spleen, arterial walls) and formation of calcium oxalate renal calculi

- Primary: rare autosomal recessive enzymatic defect; patients present with renal calculi early in life
- Secondary: usually results from increased colonic absorption of oxalate secondary to small bowel disease (e.g., resection, celiac disease, Crohn's disease)

Imaging

- Renal cortical or medullary (or both) calcification
- Urolithiasis

PAGE KIDNEY

Clinical

- Renin-angiotensin mediated hypertension from perinephric or subcapsular renal compression
- Usually caused by subcapsular hematoma; can also occur secondary to cyst or tumor

Imaging

- Renal compression secondary to hematoma, cyst, or tumor

PAPILLARY NECROSIS

Clinical

- Papillary ischemia resulting in necrosis and sloughing, unifocal or multifocal
- Causes include analgesic abuse, sickle cell disease, infection (bacterial, TB, fungi), diabetes, renal vein thrombosis, obstruction, cirrhosis, dehydration, and alcoholism
- Symptoms include pain, fever, dysuria, hematuria

Imaging

- IVU:
    Widened/club-shaped calyx (contrast collection usually extends centrally from calyx); intraluminal filling defect
- Ultrasound/CT:
    Medullary cystic spaces

PARAOVARIAN CYST

Clinical

- Arises from wolffian duct remnants (Gartner's duct) within broad ligament
- Common, up to 10% of all adnexal masses
- May cause no symptoms or cause pain, hemorrhage, rupture, or torsion
- No cyclic changes

Imaging

- Ultrasound:
    Smooth, round, anechoic adnexal cyst; may have internal echoes if hemorrhage present; can be diagnosed reliably only if cyst is seen separate from ipsilateral ovary

PELVIC INFLAMMATORY DISEASE

Clinical

- Spectrum includes endometritis, salpingitis, oophoritis, pelvic peritonitis, pyosalpinx, and tuboovarian abscess
- Affects 10% of menstruating women

- *Chlamydia* spp and *N. gonorrhoeae* most common organisms; *E. coli* and *Enterococcus*, *Bacteroides*, and *Streptococcus* spp also seen
- Complications: hydrosalpinx, ectopic pregnancy, infertility

Imaging

- Pelvic fluid, endometrial fluid, fibrosis, adhesions
- Tuboovarian abscess: complex pelvic/adnexal mass
- Pyosalpinx or hydrosalpinx: dilated, fluid-filled tubular structure in adnexa

PELVIC LIPOMATOSIS

Clinical

- Abundant fat in pelvis; may contain inflammatory and fibrotic tissue
- Rare; males and females affected equally; debatable increased incidence in blacks
- Often does not cause symptoms; patient may have pain, frequency, outlet obstruction
- Rarely results in ureteral or IVC obstruction

Imaging

- Radiograph:
    Increased lucency may be seen in pelvis
- IVU/cystogram:
    Narrowing or cephalad displacement of bladder ("inverted pear" sign); medial displacement of distal ureters; ureteral obstruction may be seen
- Barium enema:
    May see elevation of sigmoid colon
- CT/MRI:
    Abundant fat in pelvis; ureteral or IVC obstruction may be seen

PHEOCHROMOCYTOMA

Clinical

- Functional tumor of chromaffin tissue (paraganglioma)
- 0.001 to 0.01% incidence in general population; 0.6% in hypertensive patients
- Hypertension (50% episodic, 50% sustained); palpitations, sweating, headache, pallor
- Elevated 24-hour urine vanillylmandelic acid in 50%
- Associations: multiple endocrine neoplasia (MEN) IIA, MEN IIB, neurofibromatosis, von Hippel-Lindau disease
- 10% malignant, 10% extraadrenal (30% in children), 10% bilateral, 10% familial

Imaging

- Hypertensive reaction a risk with iodinated contrast media
- CT:
    Solid mass; sensitivity 95% for adrenal mass, 90% overall
- MRI:
    Hyperintense mass on T2-weighted images; sensitivity near 100% for adrenal mass, 91% overall
- Nuclear medicine:
    Uptake of MIBG; sensitivity 75% for adrenal mass, 80% overall; specificity more than 90% (better than that of CT or MRI)
- Angiography:
    Hypervascular

POLYCYSTIC OVARIAN DISEASE (STEIN-LEVENTHAL SYNDROME)

Clinical

- Enzyme deficiency leading to androgen excess, luteinizing hormone excess, follicle-stimulating hormone deficiency

- Affects 5% of menstrual age women
- Infertility, oligomenorrhea, obesity, hirsutism

Imaging

- Enlarged ovaries with numerous small (5 to 8 mm), peripheral cysts

PROSTATE ADENOCARCINOMA

Clinical

- Most common malignancy in men (microscopic foci in 30% over age 50 years, 50% over age 75 years; 1 in 5 lifetime risk of being diagnosed with prostate cancer)
- Second most common cause of cancer death in men (cause of death in 3%) after lung cancer
- Associated with advanced age, elevated prostate-specific antigen (normal is less than 4 on the Hybritech scale or less than 2.5 on the Yang scale)
- Screening, imaging, and treatment controversial
- Origin: 70% peripheral zone, 20% central zone, 10% transition zone
- Jewett-Whitmore staging:
    A1 Nonpalpable, less than 5% of glandular tissue
    A2 Nonpalpable, more than 5% of glandular tissue
    B1 Palpable, less than 1.5 cm
    B2 Palpable, more than 1.5 cm
    C Extracapsular extension, seminal vesicle invasion, or both
    D1 Regional lymph node metastases
    D2 Bone or visceral metastases, or both
- Likelihood of metastases related to tumor volume and histologic grade (Gleason score)

Imaging

- Central/transition zone (central gland) lesions cannot be detected reliably
- TRUS:
    60% hypoechoic, 35% isoechoic, 5% hyperechoic
- CT:
    Isodense to normal prostate
- MRI:
    Low-signal intensity lesion within bright signal peripheral zone on T2-weighted images

PUERPERAL OVARIAN VEIN THROMBOPHLEBITIS

Clinical

- Bacterial seeding of ovarian vein from puerperal endometritis with secondary thrombosis
- Abdominal/flank pain, fever, palpable thrombosed ovarian vein
- 80 to 90% right sided

Imaging

- Ultrasound:
    Difficult to perform; dilated ovarian vein may be seen with thrombus
- CT/MRI:
    Dilated ovarian vein with thrombus, peripheral enhancement

PROSTATITIS

Clinical

- Organisms: *E. coli; Proteus, Klebsiella, Enterobacter, Enterococci* spp; *N. gonorrhoeae;* fungi; TB

- Symptoms are fever, pain, urinary frequency and urgency, dysuria, outlet obstruction
- Acute: suppurative infection, may cause focal abscesses
- Chronic: associated with benign prostatic hypertrophy

Imaging

- Enlarged prostate
- TRUS:
    Heterogeneous gland; focal hypoechoic areas if abscesses; echogenic focal calcifications associated with chronic prostatitis
- CT:
    Heterogeneous gland with heterogenous enhancement; focal low-attenuation areas if abscesses; calcifications associated with chronic prostatitis
- MRI:
    Heterogeneous gland with heterogenous enhancement; abscesses result in focal areas of low signal on T1-weighted images and high signal on T2-weighted images

PYELONEPHRITIS

Clinical

- Upper urinary tract/renal parenchymal infection
- Encompasses emphysematous pyelonephritis, focal bacterial nephritis, lobar nephronia, and renal abscess
- Acquired via ascending pathway more commonly than hematogenously
- Females affected more often than males; reflux causes predisposition to pyelonephritis in general, diabetes to emphysematous pyelonephritis
- Common organisms: *E. coli; Proteus, Klebsiella,* and *Pseudomonas* spp

Imaging

- Kidneys normal in size or enlarged; foci of gas in emphysematous pyelonephritis; focal fluid or gas collections, or both, if abscess
- IVU:
    Delayed, persistent, striated nephrogram
- Ultrasound:
    Decreased/heterogeneous echogenicity of cortex, loss of corticomedullary differentiation
- CT:
    Decreased, heterogeneous, striated enhancement
- MRI:
    Loss of corticomedullary differentiation on T1-weighted images; increased signal intensity on T2-weighted images
- Nuclear medicine:
    Severely decreased DMSA uptake

RADIATION NEPHRITIS

Clinical

- Early: degenerative process affecting glomeruli/tubules
- Late: fibrinoid necrosis of arcuate/interlobar arteries
- Typical threshold dose: 2000 to 2500 rads over 5 weeks, may occur after only 1000 rads
- Proteinuria, hypertension
- Complications: uremia, malignant hypertension, mortality (50%)

Imaging

- Early: kidneys normal in size or enlarged
- Late: small kidneys

REFLUX NEPHROPATHY (CHRONIC ATROPHIC PYELONEPHRITIS)

Clinical

- Vesicoureteral reflux of infected urine leads to intratubular reflux
- Most common cause of parenchymal scarring
- Occurs before age of 4 years; girls are affected more often than boys

Imaging

- Small, scarred kidney; upper pole most commonly affected
- Parenchymal thinning adjacent to clubbed calyx

RENAL ADENOCARCINOMA (RENAL CELL CARCINOMA)

Clinical

- Arises from proximal convoluted tubular epithelial cells: 95% clear cell, 5% papillary
- Males are affected more often than females; can occur at any age, but peak incidence between ages of 45 and 60 years
- Associations include family history, acquired cystic disease of uremia, phenacetin or tobacco use, and von Hippel-Lindau disease (usually multiple tumors)
- 50% of patients have hematuria, 40% anemia, 33% flank pain, 25% weight loss; paraneoplastic syndromes may be seen
- 30% discovered incidentally at imaging (small lesions formerly called *benign adenomas* now considered malignant)
- Robson staging:
  - I   Confined to renal capsule
  - II   Confined to Gerota's fascia
  - IIIA Renal vein/IVC invasion
  - IIIB Local lymph node invasion
  - IIIC Both IIIA and IIIB
  - IVA Extension through Gerota's fascia
  - IVB Distant metastases
- 5-year survival: 50% stages I and II, 35% stage III, 15% stage IV
- Stauffer syndrome: elevated liver function test results without liver metastases

Imaging

- 8 to 18% have calcifications (87% of nonperipherally calcified renal masses are malignant); frequently necrotic; unusually truly cystic
- IVU:
  Decreased function, mass
- Ultrasound:
  Heterogeneous, predominantly isoechoic mass; can assess vascular invasion
- CT (examination of choice if performed with contrast):
  Heterogeneous mass, enhances less than normal parenchyma; can assess vascular invasion
- MRI:
  Heterogeneous mass, gadolinium assists detection (mass enhances less than normal parenchyma); useful for assessing vascular invasion (direct coronal/sagittal images)
- Angiography:
  95% Hypervascular; neovascularity and enlarged feeding vessels usually seen; venous shunting and "puddling" common

RENAL ANOMALIES

Clinical

- Formation: complete or partial nondevelopment of kidney
  Hypoplasia: kidney small, has less than normal number of calyces

Unilateral agenesis: 0.07 to 0.2% incidence, associated with ipsilateral adrenal agenesis (8 to 10%), contralateral renal anomalies (twofold increased incidence), and ipsilateral genital anomalies
Bilateral agenesis: rare and incompatible with life
- Malrotation: failure of rotation on vertical axis, pelvis more often anteriorly directed than laterally directed
- Ectopy: failure of ascent
   Pelvic kidney: 0.08 to 0.2% incidence
   Thoracic kidney: 0.007% incidence
- Fusion: postulated to result from abnormally situated umbilical artery
   Horseshoe: 0.25% incidence; ratio of males to females affected 2 to 1; associated with obstruction, infection, and calculi
   Crossed fused: 0.1% incidence
   Crossed nonfused: 0.01% incidence
   Disc/pancake/lump/cake: rare

Imaging

- IVU:
   Assesses renal presence and position well
- Ultrasound/CT/MRI:
   Better assesses orientation and degree of fusion

RENAL CORTICAL CYST (SIMPLE)

Clinical

- Acquired lesion: rare in children, 50% incidence over age 50 years
- Contains clear serous fluid, does not communicate with collecting system
- Majority asymptomatic; can have associated hemorrhage or infection

Imaging

- IVU:
   Lucent mass in renal parenchyma, smooth margin of displaced parenchyma ("claw" or "beak" sign)
- Ultrasound:
   Anechoic; uniformly thin, smooth wall (can have thin internal septation); posterior acoustic enhancement
- CT:
   Water attenuation (0 to 20 HU); uniformly thin, smooth wall (can have thin internal septation); no enhancement after contrast
- MRI:
   Homogeneous signal intensity (isointense to urine, dark on T1-weighted images, bright on T2-weighted images); uniformly thin, smooth wall (can have thin internal septation); no enhancement after contrast

RENAL INFARCTION/ISCHEMIA

Clinical

- Can be focal or diffuse, acute or chronic
- Causes include trauma, thrombosis, embolism, atherosclerosis, vasculitis, infection, and neoplasia

Imaging

- Early:
   Kidney normal in size or enlarged
- Late:
   Focal or diffuse parenchymal loss (relative sparing adjacent to collecting system)

- IVU/CT/angiography:
    Decreased or absent perfusion to affected areas, subcapsular rim sign acutely
        (1- to 2-mm thin enhancing rim of parenchyma, supplied by capsular arteries)

RENAL LEUKEMIA

Clinical

- Renal involvement usually asymptomatic
- Kidneys involved in 50% of patients at autopsy
- Interstitial foci or infiltrates, occasional masses

Imaging

- Bilateral renal enlargement, occasional masses
- Ultrasound:
    Hypoechoic areas may be seen

RENAL LYMPHOMA

Clinical

- Non-Hodgkin's lymphoma more common than Hodgkin's disease
- Renal involvement in 5% at diagnosis, 33% at autopsy
- Primary renal lymphoma rare (kidneys do not normally contain lymphoid tissue)
- Patients usually asymptomatic, can have renal failure and obstruction

Imaging

- Renal enlargement typical
- Multiple masses most common (45%), followed by invasion from adjacent nodal mass (25%), solitary mass (15%), diffuse infiltration (10%), and perinephric involvement (5%)
- Ultrasound:
    Hypoechoic mass(es)
- CT:
    Hypodense mass(es) that enhance slightly
- MRI:
    Nonspecific; high-signal intensity on T2-weighted images, generally isointense to renal parenchyma on T1-weighted images

RENAL METASTASES

Clinical

- Autopsy incidence: 12 to 20% of cancer patients (metastasis: primary tumor ratio, 4:1)
- Incidence at imaging much lower
- Most common tumors to metastasize to kidney: lung, breast, gastrointestinal tract, lymphoma, and melanoma
- Patients usually asymptomatic; occasional pain, hematuria

Imaging

- Typically multiple small renal masses
- CT/angiography:
    Mostly hypovascular except carcinoid, choriocarcinoma, and melanoma

RENAL SINUS CYST
Clinical

- Parapelvic: originates from renal parenchyma and expands into renal sinus
- Peripelvic: originates within sinus, probably lymphatic in origin or secondary to extravasated urine
- Does not communicate with collecting system

Imaging

- Seldom perfectly round because of displacement by other sinus structures
- IVU:
    Displaced/attenuated collecting system and pelvis, occasional obstruction
- Ultrasound:
    Hypoechoic mass in renal sinus, can be confused with hydronephrosis
- CT:
    Low-attenuation mass in renal sinus, does not enhance or opacify with contrast
- MRI:
    Renal sinus mass with urine signal characteristics (dark on T1-weighted images, bright on T2-weighted images); no enhancement with contrast

RENAL SINUS LIPOMATOSIS
Clinical

- Increase in peripelvic adipose tissue associated with obesity and aging
- No clinical consequence

Imaging

- Increased amount of fat in renal sinus
- IVU:
    Attenuated "spidery" appearance to collecting system

RENAL TRANSPLANT: FLUID COLLECTIONS
Clinical

- Hematoma/urinoma: can occur acutely
- Abscess: clinical signs of infection, develops within weeks
- Lymphocele: most common (10 to 20% of transplant patients), typically develops after 4 to 6 weeks; treated with long-term catheter or surgical drainage

Imaging

- Ultrasound:
    Urinoma/lymphocele: anechoic (lymphocele may have fine septa); hematoma/abscess: complex
- CT:
    Lymphocele is low density, nonenhancing: urinoma is low density, enhances if leaking; hematoma is 40 to 60 HU; abscess is complex, may contain gas
- MRI:
    Urinoma, lymphocele, and abscess all have dark signal on T1-weighted images, are bright on T2-weighted images (abscess may contain signal voids secondary to gas); hematoma has bright signal on T1-weighted images and T2-weighted images

RENAL TRANSPLANT: FUNCTIONAL COMPLICATIONS
Clinical

- Acute tubular necrosis: develops over first 1 to 2 days, then shows gradual improvement; incidence greater with cadaver allografts than with living-related allografts

- Rejection: *hyperacute* (preformed antibodies, occurs within minutes), *accelerated acute* (mechanism debated, occurs during first 2 to 3 days), *acute* (cellular-mediated, occurs after first week), *chronic* (fibrosis and scarring, occurs after months to years)
- Cyclosporine toxicity: can be acute or chronic, related to serum cyclosporine level

Imaging

- Difficult to reliably differentiate without biopsy; allograft enlargement in acute tubular necrosis and rejection; normal allograft size in cyclosporine toxicity
- Ultrasound:
  Loss of corticomedullary distinction in rejection, normal morphology in acute tubular necrosis or cyclosporine toxicity; elevated RI in acute tubular necrosis, elevated or decreased RI in rejection, normal RI in cyclosporine toxicity
- MRI:
  Loss of corticomedullary distinction on T1-weighted images in acute tubular necrosis or rejection, normal corticomedullary distinction in cyclosporine toxicity
- Nuclear medicine:
  Perfusion (DTPA) relatively well preserved in acute tubular necrosis and cyclosporine toxicity, impaired in rejection; function (hippuran/MAG3) decreased in acute tubular necrosis, rejection, and cyclosporine toxicity

RENAL TRAUMA

Clinical

- Can be caused by blunt or penetrating trauma
- Category I injuries: 75 to 85%; mild injuries, treated conservatively; no communication with collecting system; contusion, cortical lacerations, segmental infarction, small subcapsular or intrarenal hematoma
- Category II injuries: 10 to 20%; intermediate injuries, often do not require surgery; communicate with collecting system; large subcapsular hematoma, corticomedullary laceration or fracture
- Category III injuries: 5%; major injuries requiring surgery; shattered kidney, vascular pedicle injuries, avulsion or laceration of renal pelvis/ureteropelvic junction

Imaging

- Depends on type of injury, findings include global/segmental delayed or absent function, laceration or fracture, blood or urine extravasation
- IVU:
  Understages severe injuries, normal in 40% of patients with moderate injuries
- CT:
  Most sensitive and specific modality for evaluating renal trauma when performed with contrast
- Angiography:
  Useful for evaluating vascular injury and for embolization

RENAL TUBULAR ACIDOSIS

Clinical

- Metabolic acidosis, secondary inability of kidneys to excrete acidic urine
- Type I (distal): impaired ability of distal tubule to secrete hydrogen ion; autosomal dominant, sporadic and acquired causes; 70% of patients female; likely to cause symptoms or findings and require treatment (70% develop urolithiasis promoted by hypercalciuria and lack of urinary citrate)
- Type II (proximal): impaired ability of proximal tubule to absorb bicarbonate ion; often transient in infants, usually acquired in adults; hereditary in a few families; unlikely to cause symptoms or findings, treatment often not necessary

Imaging

- Medullary nephrocalcinosis, urolithiasis

RENAL VEIN THROMBOSIS

Clinical

- Causes include dehydration; hypercoagulable states; renal disease, infection, or tumor; and extrinsic mass
- Acute symptoms: hematuria, proteinuria, flank pain, palpable mass
- Chronic disease usually asymptomatic

Imaging

Acute
- Enlarged kidney
- IVU:
    Delayed pyelogram, stretched "spidery" infundibula
- Ultrasound/CT/MRI:
    Thrombus may be seen

Chronic
- Kidney small or normal in size
- IVU:
    Notching secondary to collaterals may be seen
- Ultrasound/CT/MRI:
    Collateral veins may be seen

RENOVASCULAR HYPERTENSION

Clinical

- Decreased renal blood flow leads to renin-mediated hypertension
- Responsible for less than 5% of hypertension cases
- More likely to be the cause of hypertension in patients who become hypertensive before age of 20 years or after age of 50 years
- Causes include atherosclerosis, fibromuscular dysplasia, connective tissue disease, and compression (mass, Page's kidney)

Imaging

- Affected kidney may be small
- IVU:
    Delayed or prolonged nephrogram; vascular notching in ureter from collaterals
- Ultrasound:
    Elevated peak velocity, decreased diastolic flow, prolonged acceleration time distal to stenosis
- CT:
    May directly evaluate renal arteries with spiral/helical CT
- Nuclear medicine:
    Delayed perfusion with captopril
- Angiography/MR angiography:
    Focal, multifocal, or diffuse arterial narrowing

RETROCAVAL URETER

Clinical

- Abnormal persistence of right subcardinal vein in formation of IVC forces right ureter to pass medial and dorsal to IVC
- Incidence is 0.07%; ratio of males to females affected is 3:1
- May cause obstruction of right ureter, otherwise asymptomatic

Imaging

- Right ureter lies medial to vertebral pedicle at L2–L3 level

RETROPERITONEAL FIBROSIS

Clinical

- Retroperitoneum enveloped between kidneys and pelvic brim by fibrous tissue, which can obstruct ureters and blood vessels
- Primary: most cases, idiopathic or possibly autoimmune
- Secondary: aortoiliac aneurysm (desmoplastic reaction, not leakage), drugs (classically methylsergide), radiation, trauma, tumor, infection or connective tissue disease

Imaging

- IVU/retrograde:
    Medial ureteral deviation, hydroureteronephrosis with gradual tapering or "rat-tail" appearance at site of obstruction
- Ultrasound:
    Homogeneous hypoechoic periaortic mass
- CT/MRI:
    Homogeneous periaortic mass that may be enhanced

SALPINGITIS ISTHMICA NODOSA (SIN)

Clinical

- Overgrowth of epithelium surrounded by hypertrophied muscle
- Seen in 4% of HSGs
- Cause unknown, may be related to previous infection
- Increased risk of infertility and ectopic pregnancy

Imaging

- HSG:
    Multiple 1- to 2-mm pseudodiverticula; honeycomb appearance of contrast in wall of fallopian tube

SCHISTOSOMIASIS (BILHARZIOSIS)

Clinical

- Infection by fluke *Schistosoma haematobium*; eggs excreted into urinary tract cause granulomatous reaction
- Endemic in Middle East, India, central and south Africa; rare in United States
- Typically infects bladder, but ureter involvement seen in 30%
- Males affected more often than females; age usually less than 30 years
- Predisposes to squamous cell carcinoma of urothelium

Imaging

- Radiograph:
    Calcifications in wall of bladder and distal ureters
- IVU/retorograde/cystogram:
    Mucosal irregularity, inflammatory pseudopolyps, ureteritis cystica, ureteral dilatation and stricture, reduced bladder capacity, fistulas
- CT:
    More sensitive for calcifications than radiograph

SEMINAL VESICLE CYST

Clinical

- Congenital: associated with ipsilateral renal/ureteral agenesis and ectopic insertion of ipsilateral ureter
- Acquired: much less common, possibly delayed presentation of congenital lesion
- Patients often asymptomatic; may have pain, dysuria, frequency

Imaging

- Cystic mass posterior or posterolateral to bladder

SPERMATOCELE

Clinical

- Retention cysts of small tubules in epididymal head
- Contains sperm-filled fluid

Imaging

- Ultrasound: cystic mass in epididymal head, may be loculated and have internal echoes

TESTICULAR GERM CELL TUMORS

Clinical

- Most common malignancy in adolescent and young men
- Seminoma most common histology (40 to 50%); sensitive to radiation therapy and chemotherapy; good prognosis
- Nonseminomatous: embryonal cell carcinoma (10 to 20%), teratoma (5 to 10%), choriocarcinoma (1%); rare tumors: yolk sac tumor, epidermoid cyst; prognosis not as good as for seminoma
- Mixed histology: common pattern, probably occurs in at least 40% of cases
- Burned-out (Azzopardi) tumors: "healed" primary lesion, may still metastasize
- Elevated AFP level: all yolk sac tumors, some embryonal cell carcinomas and teratomas
- Elevated hCG level: all choriocarcinomas, some seminomas
- Staging:
  - I   Limited to testis and spermatic cord
  - IIA Less than 5 cm retroperitoneal lymph node metastases
  - IIB More than 5 cm retroperitoneal lymph node metastases
  - IIIA Lymph node metastases above diaphragm
  - IIIB Extranodal metastases

Imaging

- Ultrasound:
  - Seminomas homogeneously hypoechoic; embryonal cell cystic/heterogeneous; others mixed echogenicity; "burned-out" (Azzopardi) tumors highly echogenic, often with posterior acoustic shadowing
- MRI:
  - Hypointense lesions on T2-weighted images, enhancement with gadolinium

TESTICULAR MICROLITHIASIS

Clinical

- 1- to 2-mm calcifications within seminiferous tubules
- Rare, cause unknown
- Patients usually asymptomatic

- Associations: germ cell tumors, infertility, undescended testes, Kleinfelter's syndrome, male pseudohermaphroditism

Imaging

- Ultrasound:
    Multiple small echogenic foci in testes, usually too small to cause shadowing; testes otherwise have normal echotexture

TESTICULAR STROMAL CELL TUMORS

Clinical

- Much less common than germ cell tumors, usually benign
- Leydig's cell tumor, Sertoli's cell tumor, gonadoblastoma (mixed stromal and germ cell elements)

Imaging

- Ultrasound:
    Usually hypoechoic, may have associated cysts

TESTICULAR TORSION

Clinical

- Complete encirclement of the epididymis and testis by tunica vaginalis ("bell-and-clapper" deformity) causes predisposition to torsion
- Most common between ages of 12 and 18 years
- Sudden, severe pain (often occurs at night); testis tender and swollen
- Ideally treated surgically in first 4 hours; fewer than 20% salvageable after 12 hours, 0% salvageable after 24 hours

Imaging

- Ultrasound:
    Absent or decreased testicular and epididymal flow at color Doppler ultrasound; enlarged testis and epididymis and spermatic cord; decreased echogenicity may be seen in testis, with increased echogenicity of swollen epididymis
- Nuclear medicine:
    Diminished ipsilateral perfusion (rim of increased activity on blood pool images indicates late torsion)

THECA LUTEIN CYST

Clinical

- Develops secondary to elevated hCG levels
- Associated with exogenous hCG administration, gestational trophoblastic disease, choriocarcinoma, multiple pregnancies, Rh incompatibility, and diabetes

Imaging

- Ultrasound:
    Multiple large (up to 20 cm) bilateral ovarian cysts, may have septations

TUBERCULOSIS

Clinical

- Kidney initially infected hematogenously (25% of cases are bilateral); ureter and bladder secondarily involved by passage of infected urine

- Renal TB affects 10% of patients with pulmonary TB
- Symptoms include hematuria, sterile pyuria, dysuria, and urinary frequency
- 30% of patients have abnormal chest radiograph, fewer than 5% have active pulmonary disease

Imaging

- IVU:

    Parenchymal calcification and scarring, papillary necrosis, irregularity and stenoses in collecting system/pelvis (Kerr's sign) and ureter, small volume bladder, bladder calcifications
- CT:

    Low attenuation renal masses, autonephrectomy, extrarenal spread to spine and psoas

TUBEROUS SCLEROSIS

Clinical

- Autosomal dominant phakomatosis, 50 to 80% sporadic
- Kidneys involved by angiomyolipomas in 80%, by cortical cysts less commonly
- Several organs involved (e.g., cysts, tumors); characteristic involvement of central nervous system (seizures, ocular phakomas, cortical hamartomas, giant cell astrocytomas) and skin (adenoma sebaceum)

Imaging

- Renal angiomyolipomas and cortical cysts
- Multiorgan masses and cysts

UNDESCENDED TESTIS (CRYPTORCHIDISM)

Clinical

- Affects 33% of premature males, 3% of normal term males, less than 1% of boys and young men
- Testis may be in inguinal canal (80 to 90%), abdomen, or pelvis
- Complications: sterility, torsion, malignancy (incidence of seminoma increased tenfold in both undescended and normally descended contralateral testes)

Imaging

- Undescended testis smaller than normal
- Ultrasound:

    Round or oval homogeneous medium echogenicity soft tissue mass; sensitive only for inguinal testis
- CT:

    Round or oval homogeneous soft tissue mass; sensitive for all locations
- MRI:

    Round or oval homogeneous mass; medium intensity on T1-weighted images, bright on T2-weighted images

URACHAL CARCINOMA

Clinical

- 0.4% of bladder carcinomas, 40% of bladder adenocarcinomas
- Arises in urachus (musculofibrous band extending from umbilicus to anterior superior bladder surface)
- Prognosis is worse than that for other bladder carcinomas
- 70% mucin-producing adenocarcinomas, 15% nonmucin-producing adenocarcinomas; remainder transitional cell carcinomas, squamous cell carcinomas, and sarcomas

Imaging

• Midline mass anterosuperior to bladder dome; cystic or solid; calcification common

URETERAL DUPLICATION

Clinical

• Incomplete: includes bifid pelvis and ureters that join proximal to ureterovesical junction
• Complete: two separate ipsilateral ureters with separate ureterovesical junctions
• Weigert-Meyer rule: upper pole moiety inserts medial and caudal to normal ureterovesical junction and is prone to obstruction; lower pole moiety inserts normally but is prone to reflux

Imaging

• Ipsilateral renal enlargement
• IVU:
  Best modality to assess level of duplication if both moieties function; with upper pole obstruction, displacement of lower pole by poorly functioning hydronephrotic upper pole gives "drooping lily" appearance
• Ultrasound:
  Two separate renal sinuses separated by junctional parenchyma; with upper pole obstruction, fluid-filled upper pole "mass" with parenchymal loss
• CT:
  Two separate opacified ureters can be seen on delayed images if both moieties function; with upper pole obstruction, fluid-filled upper pole "mass" with parenchymal loss

URETERITIS CYSTICA (PYELITIS CYSTICA, CYSTITIS CYSTICA)

Clinical

• Multiple subepithelial cysts in urothelium
• Causes include chronic infection, calculi, and stents
• Patients asymptomatic; females affected more often than males
• Bladder (cystitis cystica) most common site, followed by ureter (ureteritis cystica), then collecting system/pelvis (pyelitis cystica)

Imaging

• IVU/retrograde:
  Multiple smooth, round filling defects 2 to 4 mm in size; may be larger in collecting system/pelvis and bladder

URETEROCELE

Clinical

• Prolapse of dilated distal ureter into bladder
• Simple: normally located ureterovesical junction, usually discovered incidentally in an adult
• Ectopic: most commonly involves abnormal insertion of upper pole moiety of duplicated system; usually presents clinically during childhood; in males inserts proximal to external sphincter, continence preserved; in females may insert distal to external sphincter, incontinence possible

Imaging

• IVU:
  Opacified dilated distal ureter appears as "cobra head"; unopacified dilated distal ureter appears as round filling defect

- Cystogram:
    Round filling defect at site of insertion
- Ultrasound:
    Round cystic mass in bladder

URETHRAL CARCINOMA

Clinical

- Squamous cell carcinoma (SCC) most common type, followed by transitional cell carcinoma (TCC), then adenocarcinoma (ADC)
- SCC usually involves bulbus portion; TCC usually involves posterior portion
- Bleeding common, associated with stricture

Imaging

- VCUG/RUG:
    Often indistinguishable from focal stricture
- MRI:
    Periurethral mass may be seen with carcinoma and can be used to differentiate it from stricture

URETHRAL STRICTURE

Clinical

- Acquired more common than congenital
- Acquired secondary to infection (usually *N. gonorrhoeae),* trauma, instrumentation, or indwelling catheter

Imaging

- VCUG/RUG:
    Diffuse or localized area of narrowing in urethra; congenital, usually short and weblike

URETHRAL TRAUMA

Clinical

- Associated with pelvic fracture and other organ system injury
- Blood at external meatus should raise suspicion; blind catheterization contraindicated (perform RUG before catheterization)
- Type 1: urethra stretched but intact
- Type 2: urethral rupture above urogenital diaphragm at prostatomembranous junction
- Type 3: urethral rupture below urogenital diaphragm, disruption of urogenital diaphragm

Imaging

- RUG:
    Type 1 Narrowed urethra, no extravasation
    Type 2 Contrast extravasation into retroperitoneum
    Type 3 Contrast extravasation into perineum/scrotum and retroperitoneum

UROLITHIASIS

Clinical

- Causes include hypercalcemic states, hypercalciuria, renal tubular acidosis, stasis, infection, foreign bodies, indwelling stents or catheters, hyperoxaluria, cystinuria, medullary sponge kidney, and others

- 5% of women and 12% of men have an episode of renal colic by age 70 years
- Calcium oxalate and calcium phosphate: 75% of all calculi; 50% hypercalcemic, 50% normocalcemic
- Struvite (magnesium ammonium phosphate): 15% of all calculi; associated with alkaline urine caused by proteus infection; forms staghorn calculi
- Uric acid: 5 to 10% of all calculi; associated with acidic urine, hyperuricosemia
- Cystine: 3% of all calculi, associated with congenital cystinuria
- Matrix: rare calculi, associated with infection

Imaging

- Radiograph:
    Calcium oxalate, calcium phosphate, and struvite are *radiopaque,* account for 92% of stones; cystine is *minimally radiopaque*; matrix and uric acid are *radiolucent*
- IVU:
    Delayed or persistent nephrogram if obstructing; radiolucent calculi seen as filling defects, tend to lodge at ureteropelvic junction, iliac vessel crossing, and ureterovesical junction
- Ultrasound:
    Echogenic focus with posterior shadowing; 96% sensitive overall, can detect calculi as small as 0.5 mm; less sensitive for proximal and mid-ureteral stones
- CT:
    Most sensitive modality, nearly all appear denser than water or urine

UROTHELIAL CARCINOMA

Clinical

- Transitional cell carcinoma (TCC) most common type, followed by squamous cell carcinoma (SCC), then adenocarcinoma (ADC)
- Associations: *TCC:* aniline dye, cyclophosphamide, tobacco, analgesic abuse, previous or synchronous TCC; *SCC:* calculi, chronic infection, leukoplakia, schistosomiasis; *ADC:* bladder exstrophy, cystitis glandularis, urachal remnant
- Symptoms are hematuria and pain
- Bladder is the most common site of TCC (92%), followed by collecting system/pelvis (6%), then ureter (2%)
- 40 to 80% of patients with upper urinary tract TCC develop bladder TCC, 3 to 5% with bladder TCC develop upper urinary tract TCC
- 30% of collecting system/pelvic TCCs are multifocal; more than 30% of bladder TCCs are multifocal
- Bladder carcinoma staging:
    A   Mucosal/submucosal lesion
    B1 Superficial (less than 50%) muscle invasion
    B2 Deep (more than 50%) muscle invasion
    C   Perivesical fat invasion
    D1 Extension to perivesical organs
    D2 Lymph node/distant metastases

Imaging

- IVU/retrograde/cystogram:
    Filling defect(s), dilatation distal to ureteral lesion (Bergman or "goblet" sign); proximal obstruction may be seen
- Ultrasound/CT/MRI:
    Solid mass, proximal obstruction may be seen

UTERINE ANOMALIES

Clinical

- Congenital malformations range from agenesis to aplasia (including T-shaped) to unicornous, didelphic, bicornuate, septate, or arcuate uterus

- Associations: ipsilateral renal anomalies (agenesis, ectopia), infertility, spontaneous abortion, maternal diethylstilbestrol (DES) exposure (T-shaped uterus, also associated with clear cell vaginal carcinoma)

Imaging

- HSG:

    Aplasia; rudimentary cavity; *unicornous*: single horn and fallopian tube; *didelphysis*: two vaginas, two cervices, two separate horns; *bicornuate* and *septate*: two separate horns; *arcuate*: smooth indentation at fundus (horns not divided)
- MRI:

    Best modality to differentiate bicornuate (horns separated by myometrium) from septate (horns separated by fibrous band)

UTERINE LEIOMYOMA (FIBROID)

Clinical

- Benign smooth muscle neoplasm, estrogen dependent
- Affects 20 to 50% of all women, including 40% of women over age 35 years; usually multiple
- Most common location is intramural (more than 95%), followed by subserosal (may be pedunculated), then submucosal (most likely to cause symptoms and complications)
- Patients usually asymptomatic: may have pelvic pain, pelvic mass, or bleeding
- Complications: infertility (35%), spontaneous abortion

Imaging

- Radiograph:

    Soft tissue pelvic mass, calcifications frequent
- HSG:

    Filling defect for submucosal; endometrial cavity distortion for intramural or subserosal if large enough
- Ultrasound:

    Heterogeneous uterine mass, classically hypoechoic but often isoechoic or echogenic; contour abnormality
- CT:

    Uterine enlargement, calcifications, enhances to same degree as myometrium
- MRI:

    Best modality to assess presence and position; well-defined, low-signal intensity mass on T2-weighted images; isointense or hypointense to myometrium on T1-weighted images

VARICOCELE

Clinical

- Dilated veins in pampiniform plexus
- Idiopathic: related to incompetent valves and drainage of left testicular vein into left renal vein; 98% left-sided, occasionally bilateral; affects 15% of normal men, 40% of infertile men
- Secondary: extrinsic compression, no definite side predominates (right-sided varicocele should raise suspicion of intraabdominal tumor causing extrinsic venous compression)

Imaging

- Ultrasound:

    Pampiniform plexus measures more than 3 mm in diameter with increase in size or transient increase in flow with Valsalva maneuver

VON HIPPEL-LINDAU DISEASE

Clinical

- Autosomal dominant (chromosome 3p) with incomplete penetrance
- Renal: cysts, renal adenocarcinomas (occur in 40%, usually multiple, less aggressive than in other patients)
- Adrenal: pheochromocytomas (occur in 10%)
- Central nervous system: hemangioblastomas (cerebellar and spinal), retinal angiomatosis
- Pancreas: cysts, islet cell tumors
- Epididymis: cystadenoma

Imaging

- Multiple renal cysts and solid masses
- Cysts in other organs

XANTHOGRANULOMATOUS PYELONEPHRITIS (XGP)

Clinical

- Rare chronic suppurative renal infection
- 85% diffuse, 15% focal
- Organisms: *Proteus* spp, *E. coli, Staphylococcus* spp
- Characterized by presence of lipid-laden macrophages (xanthoma cells)
- Nearly all cases associated with calculi
- Classic triad: staghorn calculus (75%), absent or diminished contrast excretion, poorly functioning mass
- 10% of patients are diabetic

Imaging

- Enlarged kidney and staghorn calculus typically seen
- IVU:
    Absent or reduced contrast excretion
- Ultrasound:
    Hypoechoic inflammatory masses often with "ground-glass" appearance
- CT:
    Low-attenuation inflammatory masses

6

Breast Imaging

■ **Steven D. Frankel,** M.D.

OVERVIEW

Breast cancer is the second most frequently diagnosed malignancy in the United States (skin cancer is first). The American Cancer Society (ACS) estimates that 186,000 women were diagnosed with and approximately 46,000 women died from breast cancer in 1996. Since 1985, breast cancer has rated second (after lung cancer) as the leading cause of cancer deaths in women. Statistics for the incidence of breast cancer are based on the National Cancer Institute's (NCI) Surveillance, Epidemiology, and End Results (SEER) program, which obtained information from nine cancer registries. The annual incidence of age-adjusted invasive breast cancer increased less than 1% per year from 1973 to 1980, according to NCI data. The age-adjusted incidence of breast cancer showed a relative increase of 32% from 1980 to 1987, or approximately 3% per year. Since 1987, NCI data suggest that breast cancer in the United States may be stabilizing or perhaps even declining.

The incidence of breast cancer increases with age. It is rare before the age of 25 years and seems to peak between the ages of 75 and 79 years, after which the age-specific incidence declines. Nevertheless, there is the impression that the incidence of breast cancer continues to increase among women younger than 50 years of age, which may correspond to the expansion in the number of women in this age group.

The increase in incidence and diagnosis of breast cancer may also be the result of increased screening and availability of mammography. Between 1978 and 1983, only 15 to 20% of American women had ever had a mammographic examination. By 1992, approximately 75% of women older than 40 years had had at least one mammographic examination. Most important, there are now more women who regularly use screening.

According to some, the apparent growing prevalence of breast cancer may be attributed to the improved ability to detect it. The benefit of early detection cannot be underestimated, because it can decrease breast cancer mortality. Despite this ability to decrease mortality, paradoxically, the age-adjusted mortality rate from breast cancer has not changed significantly over the last 30 years.

Since 1980, cancer of the breast has been diagnosed at a more localized stage, an advance that parallels the improved performance of x-ray mammography. The proportion of cancers detected when in situ (DCIS) has also increased, but controversies about the true significance of DCIS abound. Only within the last few years has there been a decline in the rate of breast cancer detected at regional and distant stages. Five-year survival rates have also improved during this period. (Longer-term, disease-free survival rates remain to be established.) Clinical trials have unequivocally demonstrated that earlier detection of breast cancer (often smaller, lower-stage tumors) improves the rate of survival.

The ACS currently estimates that one in nine women will be diagnosed with breast cancer within her lifetime. This statistic should be viewed with caution, however, because it reflects lifetime risk, calculated to at least age 85 years. This lifetime risk is cumulative, and demographics may contribute to this statistic. More correctly, a woman aged 50 years has a 1 in 500 likelihood of developing breast cancer in the next year, whereas by the age of 75 years, the likelihood increases to 1 in 30.

Risk factors for breast cancer include a history of certain benign breast diseases and a family history of breast cancer. Other factors include early age at menarche, late age of menopause, late age of first live birth, and high-dose radiation exposure. The most important risk factor is a family history of breast cancer, especially in a mother or sister. Excluding family history and age, none of the other risk factors is particularly strong. Because less than 20% of women with breast cancer give a positive family history, all women in appropriate age categories should be screened. The greatest potential for reducing the mortality rate lies with early detection, via appropriate screening. This requires a high rate of participation in conjunction with competence and expertise in interpretation. For instance, a prior history of breast cancer (in situ or invasive) increases a woman's risk for a second breast cancer by approximately 1% per year.

MAMMOGRAPHY

Mammography is the most effective noninvasive means of examining the breast. It has two basic applications, screening and diagnosis. The purpose of screening is to search for cancer in asymptomatic women. A high number of "normal" screening studies is expected. Screening should be used only to detect abnormalities requiring further study or work-up, which may include diagnostic mammography (using other views or techniques), as well as breast sonography or needle biopsy. Diagnostic mammography is used to better characterize the nature of the abnormality in previously detected disease.

Mammography is the most sensitive and accurate method for detecting early occult breast cancer. Unfortunately, mammography may have less success with the radiographically dense breast. Additionally, it is not always diagnostically specific. Distinguishing benign from malignant processes is not always possible, and biopsy is then necessary to confirm the diagnosis. Most biopsies reveal various benign entities that have caused changes on the mammographic images that arouse suspicion. Occasionally, mammography fails to detect some tumors. As a diagnostic technique, it complements but cannot replace appropriate, regular physical examination (along with self-examination of the breast). The most convincing demonstration of screening benefits comes from eight randomized, controlled trials that have shown that screening reduces mortality from breast cancer. These studies include the Health Insurance Plan (HIP) of New York study and the Swedish study.

The risk of radiation from screening is quite negligible. Current estimates show an absolute risk in women over the age of 35 years of 0.4 to 0.7 excess cancers per million women per year per screening examination. With these data, the benefit:risk ratio is highly favorable. In women aged 40 to 49 years, the benefit is anywhere from 40 to 80 times greater than the risk. In women aged 50 years and over, the benefit:risk ratio is more than 100:1. The current ACS screening recommendations are for all women age 40 and older to have a screening mammogram every year. Controversy, however, persists about the under 50 years age group as to the usefulness of mammographic screening. A Canadian trial (NBSS) argues against screening in this age range, but these results remain controversial.

Diagnostic breast imaging is used as a problem-solving modality in situations that include evaluation of screening abnormalities, imaging of symptomatic patients, analysis of abnormal physical findings, or short-term follow-up of "probably benign" lesions. Patients with palpable breast neoplasms should be imaged to search for occult (nonpalpable) lesions in both breasts. In general, mammography's ability to characterize the palpable breast abnormality is not as accurate or as important as the search for nonpalpable early cancer. Palpable masses are sometimes benign and occult breast cancers could exist in the same or the opposite breast.

When diagnostic mammography is used to characterize lesions detected by either screening mammograms or physical examination, the evaluation should be tailored to the individual findings. Abnormalities that can be seen on mammograms include masses (calcified or noncalcified), focal asymmetric densities, architectural distortion, calcification, densities (seen on one view only), prominent ducts, skin thickening, or nipple retraction. The majority of abnormal mammographic findings are classified as either masses or calcifications.

Thus, mammography serves two purposes: it detects previously unsuspected disease, usually by screening mammography, and diagnoses previously detected disease. Screening mammography can demonstrate the presence of many nonpalpable breast lesions months or years before they would have been found by other means. In addition to detecting disease early, it is cost effective, available, and accepted; moreover, screening mammography decreases mortality. Screening mammograms are interpreted as normal (requiring no additional evaluation) or abnormal (requiring additional evaluation, usually more imaging or an invasive procedure).

Diagnostic mammography is individualized for each woman. The basic approach is to distinguish between benign and malignant lesions. The findings relate to either masses or calcifications, which are interpreted as benign, malignant, or indeterminate.

OTHER TECHNIQUES

Ultrasound has a limited role in the diagnosis of breast disease. It can be used to distinguish cystic from solid lesions, if rigid interpretive criteria are used, but cannot reliably distinguish benign from malignant lesions. It does not detect small calcifications. When a mass is sonographically detected, ultrasound can be used for needle aspiration, core biopsy, or wire localization procedures. Ultrasound is not adequate as a screening procedure.

Galactography, or *ductography,* is used to search for lesions in patients who have bloody nipple discharge from a single duct. This technique can determine if lesions are single or multiple and assist in their localization; however, the procedure usually does not change the management of the patient with nipple discharge. Some surgeons prefer to cannulate the involved duct and remove it en mass, thereby removing the offending lesion.

Breast *magnetic resonance imaging* (MRI) is usually performed with a dedicated, double-well phased array coil while the patient is in the prone position. Other protocols involve supine imaging and use of a body coil or surface coil. Artifacts typical of MRI include cardiac motion ("phase" direction of the image recommended to avoid the breast); respiratory motion (considered worse in supine imaging); and aliasing (signal averaging may have to be increased and "no-wrap" choices used). Currently, breast MRI is used routinely for implant evaluation. For this application, it is important to know before the study is done whether the implant is silicone or saline and whether it has a double lumen. Many sequence protocols are possible. The most specific finding for intracapsular rupture is the appearance of the low-signal, curvilinear implant shell floating within the sea of silicone ("linguini" sign). Fat and silicone peaks are very close, generally requiring manual prescanning before imaging.

Imaging of parenchymal lesions currently is experimental. Dynamic MRI may improve the specificity of mammographically detected lesions, but several benign entities (including fibroadenomas) are enhanced with intravenous contrast. The use of three-dimensional volume sequences before and after intravenous contrast yield sensitive, high-resolution, thin-section images. Some lesions may not have been noted during physical examination or mammography but are detected with MRI. In such cases, MRI-guided interventional procedures may become important for further analysis.

Fine-needle aspiration or *core biopsy* (providing cytologic and histologic information, respectively) can reduce the need for surgery in benign diseases and assist in treatment planning when results show that malignant disease is present. These biopsy techniques use sonographic or stereotactic localization. Stereotactic localization can be performed with the use of detachable units, in which case the patient sits, or with dedicated units, in which case the patient is prone. The prone units are expensive and cannot be used for diagnostic imaging or screening. The units with the patient upright are less expensive and can be detached so that the machine can be used for a routine screening or diagnostic examinations.

MAMMOGRAPHIC ANALYSIS

Masses. Mammographic analysis of masses includes differentiation of a true mass from a benign, asymmetric increased density or summation of shadows; description of size, location, density, shape, and margins of a mass; and assessment of interval change. Features such as calcifications and architectural distortion are important. The features that distinguish benign masses from malignant ones are summarized in Table 7–1. Table 7–2 outlines a systematic approach to a mammogram.

The first step in mammographic analysis is the distinction between true masses and asymmetric density and superimposition of normal fibroglandular tissue. True masses have convex borders and generally are denser toward the center. They tend to displace the breast's architecture. They are seen in multiple projections and are unchanged in appearance when spot compression views are obtained. Asymmetric breast parenchyma or superimposition has an amorphous quality. The tissue spreads apart on compression views. Additionally, summation shadows can resemble masses but generally are visible in one view only and disappear with additional views, especially on coned compression mammograms.

Next, size is evaluated. The size of the mass does not predict whether it is benign or malignant, but it can play a role in determining the next step in the evaluation. Larger masses are more likely to be palpable and therefore are more likely to permit tissue diagnosis from fine-needle aspiration (as opposed to excisional biopsy). In breast cancer, the size of the tumor helps determine staging and therefore is an important prognostic factor.

A third feature is the location of the lesion and the presence of other lesions, because some cancers present as multifocal or multicentric disease.

Skin lesions can project over the parenchyma and appear to lie within the breast. A skin lesion may have air around it, which produces a dark halo. If uncertainty exists, a radiopaque marker may be placed on the skin lesion and another image obtained.

The fourth step is evaluation of the density of the mass, which is classified as fatty, water density, or mixed. Masses that are fatty or mixed fat and soft tissue density are invariably benign, requiring no further evaluation. These include lipomas, galactoceles, posttraumatic oil cysts, hamartomas, and intramammary lymph nodes. Significant breast mass lesions are isodense with the parenchyma or of higher density than the parenchyma. These may be benign or malignant and the differential diagnosis includes cysts, fibroadenomas, and carcinomas. With vigorous compression

Table 7–1. Typical Findings for Benign and Malignant Breast Masses

Feature	Benign	Malignant
Radiographic density	Fatty or mixed; water	Water
Shape	Round, oval, gently lobulated	Irregular
Margins	Well circumscribed	Ill defined (indistinct), microlobulated, spiculated
Change	Stable	Any change in appearance
Number	Solitary or multiple	Usually solitary
Associated calcifications	Benign types	Malignant types

Table 7–2. How to Approach a Mammogram

Tissue Characteristics

BIRADS terminology
Mostly fatty, scattered fibroglandular densities, heterogeneously dense, dense

Describe Abnormality or Abnormalities

Type of abnormality, location, which breast, associated findings, change (if prior films)
Masses
Shape: round, oval, lobulated, irregular, tubular
Margins: well circumscribed, microlobulated, indistinct, spiculated
Size

Calcifications
Distribution: clustered, linear, segmental, regional, scattered
Shape: punctate, amorphous, pleomorphic, linear, branching
Size of area containing calcifications

Other main types of abnormality
Architectural distortion, focal asymmetric density (abnormality seen in two
   projections), not definitely a mass, density (seen in one projection only), neodensity,
   single dilated duct (especially if associated with blood nipple discharge), skin
   thickening

Assessment

Benign, probably benign (if worked up), needs further work-up (i.e., magnification
   images, ultrasound), somewhat suspicious (consider biopsy, but still may get additional
   views first to see better detail and full extent of abnormality), very suggestive of
   malignancy (can go straight to biopsy)

Management

Routine follow-up, short-term follow-up (i.e., 6 months), further imaging including
   ultrasound in appropriate cases, obtain tissue (fine-needle aspiration, core biopsy
   stereotactic or ultrasound guided, needle localization/excisional biopsy). Know how
   and why these procedures are done.

and high-resolution techniques, some carcinomas appear higher in density than water.

One of the most important aspects in evaluating a mass is to look at its shape and margins. In general, benign masses are round or oval in shape, well circumscribed, and have smooth or slightly lobulated margins. Malignant masses classically have irregular shapes and ill-defined margins, sometimes with a spiculated appearance. Some malignancies have multiple lobulations (microlobulations are more common than macrolobulations). Most small cancers are simply poorly defined or somewhat irregular in shape. Multiple mammographic projections and use of spot compression magnification mammography may help in elucidation of the margins of a mass lesion.

Finally, interval change should be assessed by the use of prior studies for comparison. Stability is an indicator of benignity, especially when the time between mammograms is long. Most stable masses are followed with periodic mammograms. Any change suggests malignancy and indicates the need for prompt evaluation.

Mammographic interpretation also includes a consideration of the physical examination, risk profile, and history.

Calcifications. Many mammograms show calcifications, which are the smallest structures demonstrated. Many of these are clearly benign, requiring no further evaluation. Analysis includes morphologic features, size, distribution, location, and interval changes or stability. The typical distribution of calcifications seen in breast cancer includes clusters of microcalcifications, which are characterized as morphologically linear, branching, or pleomorphic. Many other small microcalcifications may not be characteristically malignant in shape and therefore offer difficulties in interpretation and evaluation.

The first step is to identify those calcifications that are obviously benign. In general, benign calcifications are typically scattered, round, and uniform in size and shape (monomorphic). The various types of benign calcification are summarized in Table 7–3. Typical benign calcifications include those caused by a secretory disease known as *ductal ectasia*. These calcifications are benign secretions within a duct and generally are tubular, thick, and solid. They are likely to be present bilaterally. Fibroadenomas showing degeneration often have coarse "popcorn" calcifications that often are quite dense. They may be seen at the center or the periphery of the mass; however, when calcifications occur within clefts of the fibroadenoma or when the calcifications are early in the course of degeneration, they may be difficult to distinguish from malignant calcifications. Vascular calcifications are characterized by a linear parallel "railroad track" configuration when well developed; however, they, too, can be indeterminate in the early stages of formation. Dermal calcifications are usually low in density and can have central lucency. Radiopaque markers and tangential views can be obtained in questionable cases. Calcified cysts develop an eggshell appearance, whereas milk of calcium has free-floating calcifications within small cysts on the lateral view (i.e., the "tea-cup" appearance) but a more smudgy appearance on the craniocaudal view. The crescentic appearance of classic milk of calcium is best seen on a 90-degree lateral view. Other calcifications that are clearly benign are foreign body granulomas from injection of silicone or paraffin and dystrophic calcifications, which generally are large and amorphous clumps or streaks at sites of previous surgery. Fat necrosis and oil cysts also may occur in areas of previous trauma or surgery. The irregularly shaped calcifications sometimes seen in fat necrosis may simulate malignant calcifications.

Care should be taken to recognize artifactual "calcifications," such as those from deodorant, sprays, talc, electrocardiogram paste, and tattoos. Artifacts on the film (including fingerprints) and the screen or from quantum mottle noise may also resemble calcifications.

Suspicious microcalcifications can occur with or without an associated tumor mass. Virtually all breast carcinomas that contain calcifications have some features that suggest malignancy. Malignant calcifications are typically numerous, grouped or clustered, and pleomorphic, linear, or branching. In general, a cluster is defined as more than five microcalcifications within an area of 1 cm^2 or three or more within an area of 0.5 cm^2. The greater the number, the greater the likelihood of malignancy. Once a typical cluster has been identified, the initial interpretation is "suspicious for malignancy."

More than 70% of DCIS is manifested by mammographically detected microcalcifications, which are generally the result of two mechanisms. First, the cancer fills the lumens of the ducts, then it undergoes necrosis and calcification. Comedocarcinoma is often characterized by microcalcifications that form casts of the ducts and reveal elongated rod-shaped and branching patterns. Cribriform or micropapillary in situ

Table 7–3. Benign Calcifications

Ductal ectasias: large linear or ovoid, round, or ring-like calcifications in or adjacent to dilated ducts; caused by secretory disease or plasma cell mastitis; calcifications often oriented toward the nipple, are in the subareolar area, and are bilateral

Benign tumoral calcifications: "rocks," popcorn, amorphous clumps; seen mainly with fibroadenomas; typically located at the periphery of the mass

Arterial calcifications: parallel lines ("tram tracks")

Eggshell calcifications: radiolucent centers; may be scattered in the breast parenchyma or on the skin

Sedimented calcifications: semilunar or curvilinear on lateral projection and "smudgy" or poorly seen on craniocaudal projection; consists of milk-of-calcium in tiny cysts

Granulomatous calcifications: partial or complete rim calcification; similar to eggshell calcification; occurs at the borders of some granulomas; seen as a foreign body phenomenon after direct injection of silicone or paraffin or implant rupture

Dystrophic calcifications: large, amorphous streaks or clumps; occur at sites of prior biopsies or trauma

Fat necrosis: ring-like around a radiolucent oil cyst or can be malignant looking

Artifactual "calcifications": various shapes and sizes; scratches, talc, deodorant, paste from electrocardiogram, and tattoos all can simulate calcifications

carcinoma, which is thought to be the result of stagnated secretions within the interstices of these tumors, may be manifested by numerous smaller calcifications that are variable in shape and size.

Other distributions of calcifications describing their arrangement within the breast are found. Calcifications arranged in a line that may have branch points (i.e., linear distribution) are suggestive of malignancy. A segmental distribution is a wedge-shaped area pointing toward the nipple; it can be worrisome for malignancy when the morphology of the calcifications is not specifically benign.

Bilateral, scattered calcifications (which may be randomly clustered) that tend to appear similar to each other are generally benign. This "rule of multiplicity" can be applied with great confidence, but the calcifications should be followed for any interval changes. Regional calcifications are scattered in a large volume of breast tissue but not everywhere in the breast and not conforming to ductal distribution. This type of distribution probably is benign.

Fine-detail magnification mammography is recommended as the best means of evaluating the shape and number of calcific particles. Adequate breast compression decreases the thickness of breast tissue and reduces scatter radiation. Appropriate kVp as well as use of grids and optimal processing (including extended processing) can also improve visualization. Optimal viewing conditions in a dark reading room with elimination of extraneous light and the use of a magnifying lens and high-intensity view box help in image evaluation. The best way to increase resolution and analyze microcalcifications is through spot compression magnification mammography.

Indeterminate calcifications have a 20 to 30% incidence of malignancy and must be investigated by biopsy or spot compression magnification images so that the shape of the individual calcifications can be evaluated. Those that can be determined to be benign (round or oval, grouped tightly) can be followed with serial mammography. Biopsy samples must be taken from the others.

Other Signs of Carcinoma. *Focally asymmetric tissue* is commonly seen and usually benign. However, if this asymmetry has a similar shape on two projections, is quite dense, is associated with secondary findings (such as architectural distortion), or is palpable, further work-up and possible tissue diagnosis is recommended. *Architectural distortion*, usually seen as a disturbance of the normal orientation of the tissue toward the nipple, can be manifested as a spiculation without a mass or some puckering of the parenchyma. Additional imaging should be obtained for further analysis.

Sometimes two-view screening mammography produces inconclusive results. One finding that requires further work-up is a lesion demonstrated on only one standard projection. It must be determined whether this is a true lesion, superimposition, or focus of normal fibroglandular tissue. A lesion seen on only one projection is generally referred to as a *density*. Spot compression and magnification techniques can be combined with any of the standard or nonstandard views to produce finer, detailed images and to eliminate some overlap of adjacent dense tissue.

Secondary signs of breast cancer include focal skin thickening or retraction, as well as nipple or areolar thickening and retraction. A single dilated duct, especially associated with (bloody) nipple discharge, may be a sign of malignancy. Several dilated ducts, especially when noted bilaterally, usually are not indicative of malignancy.

False-Negative Mammography. Ten to 15% of breast carcinomas are not seen on mammography. There are several factors that can result in a higher false-negative rate. One such factor is dense parenchymal tissue. Technical factors, including positioning, penetration, developing, and so forth, also may be responsible for a higher false-negative rate. Finally, any of the following can cause an error in interpretation:

Inadequate searching
Inadequate clinical information
Misinterpretation of detected masses
Failure to detect subtle indirect features of malignancy
Failure to detect change from prior mammogram

TECHNICAL FACTORS IN MAMMOGRAPHY

Detailed discussion of the physics of breast imaging, the techniques for obtaining adequate film screen mammography, appropriate positioning, as well as quality control, data collection, and outcome assessment are beyond the scope of this text, but some of the main technical points of mammography are reviewed here.

Virtually all current mammographic imaging is performed with film screen technique. Xeromammography rarely is performed. The technical requirements of appropriate film screen mammography include molybdenum anode and filter using low kVp techniques (26 to 32 kVp). The kVp controls the x-ray beam spectrum and thus can alter image (subject) contrast via the penetrating power of the beam. Too high a kVp results in a loss of contrast, so that the image is too dark. Too low a kVp results in high contrast for the medium densities, but the overall image loses detail. The appropriate mA for the breast tissue yields proper density. If the mA is too high, the image is overexposed (too dark); if the mA is too low, the image is underexposed (too light).

Dedicated mammography equipment uses a C-arm tube stand with an x-ray tube designed specifically for mammography. Most have rotating anodes. There are specialized tungsten targets with the appropriate K-edge filtration with molybdenum, radium, or yttrium. Small focal spots are necessary: approximately 0.4 mm for routine work and 0.15 mm or smaller for magnification mammography. (The actual focal spot is that region on the anode bombarded by electrons, whereas the effective focal spot is the x-ray beam projected toward the patient and the film.) Grids are used to improve radiographic image contrast by decreasing scatter radiation, but at the cost of increased dose. Grid imaging in mammography generally requires an increase in exposure of 2.5 compared with nongrid mammography. This is dependent on the grid ratio. The grid is especially helpful in dense breast tissue or in thick breast tissue. Adequate tissue compression is necessary to help decrease superimposition of breast tissue, to ensure imaging position conformity as much as possible, and to decrease motion artifacts. The compression surface should be parallel to the film receptor.

Magnification views are obtained by increasing the distance of the x-ray source (anode) from the patient's breast and also of the breast from the x-ray film. The magnification factor is usually 1.5, but certain units have the ability to perform other degrees of magnification. The greater the magnification, the greater the skin dose to the patient. For higher resolution, the smallest focal spot must be used for magnification mammography; otherwise, the image will be blurred. Because of lower effective mA, the exposure time increases, which increases the chance of patient motion. Scatter is reduced as the distance between the breast and the film increases during magnification; therefore, a grid generally is not used.

The film is placed on top of a single screen (rare-earth phosphors) to take advantage of low scatter from the screen. Higher speed screens may decrease exposure by 40% versus standard screens; however, quantum mottle increases. The emulsion side of the film must be in contact with the screen. Single-emulsion, high-contrast film is recommended. The dark side of the film is the nonemulsion side.

Proper film processing is essential in producing quality images. Because processing conditions affect speed and contrast, a dedicated processor is recommended. Processing occurs as film goes through developer solution, then fixer, then is washed and finally dried. Temperature, time in developer, and chemical milieu are all very important. The recommended temperature is 35°C; a lower temperature may result in decreased contrast that requires increased exposure and dose. If the temperature is too high, speed increases, as does quantum mottle. Standard developing time is 90 seconds, but extended processing can be done. Advantages of extended processing may include increased speed, lower patient dose, reduced patient motion, and increased contrast. A problem with extended processing is increased film fog. Also, care must be taken to recognize artifacts; screen artifacts include dust and abrasions; film artifacts include static electricity, fingerprints, and improper processing; and system artifacts include compression device and grid in suboptimal condition.

In summary, virtually all mammograms are now obtained with a film/screen technique, which uses low kVp (molybdenum anode and filter; 26 to 32 kVp), single-emulsion film, rare-earth screens, small focal spot (0.4 mm for routine views; 0.1

mm for magnification views), marked compression, grids (often, especially for dense or thick breasts), optimal processing, adequate penetration, and optimal viewing (high-intensity light, dark room, magnifying lens, etc.). The advantages of this technique are its low dose of radiation and better contrast; its disadvantages are lower latitude.

Positioning. Because the chest wall has a curved contour and the film or image receptor has a straight edge, portions of the posterior breast will not be well imaged. Multiple projections minimize this limitation. The greatest amount of tissue is visualized with the oblique projection (usually the mediolateral oblique [MLO]). A properly positioned MLO view displays the pectoralis major muscle to the level of the nipple (mid-breast) and the inframammary skin fold. The central ray is aimed in a superior-medial to an inferior-lateral direction. The MLO view tends to miss the posterior medial portion of the breast.

The other standard projection is the craniocaudal (CC) view. By obtaining a CC view with slight medial orientation, the technologist can try to compensate for the deficiency of the MLO view. For the CC view, the central ray is directed from superior (cranial) to inferior (caudal). An optimal CC view shows some skin thickening toward the cleavage and visualizes the pectoralis muscle.

Some mammographers prefer a straight lateral projection (usually, lateral-medial is used because more of the breast is included compared with the medial-lateral view) instead of the MLO (note that the MLO and CC are the two standard views usually recommended). For the lateral-medial (LM) projection, the central ray is directed from lateral to medial at 90 degrees (perpendicular to the CC). With the LM projection, the posterolateral portion of the breast tends to be missed; to compensate for this deficiency, the CC should be obtained with a slightly exaggerated lateral orientation.

Body habitus may vary considerably among patients. The technologist must assess how to best image as much breast tissue as possible. Often, mammographic positioning must be tailored to the individual patient.

Additional views may be necessary to better evaluate an abnormality or to exclude a significant lesion. Additional views are many and varied and often depend on the artistry and creativity of the technologist. The special views that can be helpful include exaggerated CC, caudal-cranial, rolled lateral or rolled medial CC, tangential, lateromedial oblique, 90-degree medial-lateral, Cleopatra, cleavage, Eklund or implant displacement, spot compression, and spot compression magnification. Discussion of each of these is beyond the scope of this text. Suffice it to say that well-trained technologists are key to excellent mammography. Radiologists need to understand positioning so they can better evaluate images and make intelligent requests of the technologists.

TRIANGULATION

Apparent movement of the lesion achieved by rolling the breast about the nipple axis while the patient is in a craniocaudal position or by slightly angling the x-ray tube can reveal the location of a lesion within the upper, middle, or lower breast. It also assists in determining the lesion location in the lateral projection. Keeping the following in mind also helps in localization: a lesion in the lateral portion of the breast appears to move inferiorly when viewed first from an oblique projection, then from a true lateral projection; however, it appears to move inferiorly if it is medial within the breast.

Lesions can be fairly accurately triangulated by alignment of the straight lateral, oblique, and craniocaudal views with the nipple on a horizontal line. The lesion should be located along a straight-line path through all three projections.

NEEDLE LOCALIZATIONS

Needle localizations are performed to accurately localize a nonpalpable mammographic lesion before excisional biopsy. The breast surgeon can then remove the appropriate lesion and the appropriate amount of surrounding breast tissue. There are essentially two techniques for needle localization procedures: the procedure can be done free hand or with an alphanumeric grid device. For all techniques, local anesthesic can be applied to the skin.

The free-hand procedure is generally more difficult and requires better three-dimensional understanding of the breast. A needle is passed into the breast perpendicular to the chest wall using scout CC and true lateral projections as a map. After the needle is placed, films are obtained to ensure proper position of the needle tip (approximately 1 cm beyond the lesion). If necessary, the needle may be adjusted, or a second needle may be placed using the first as a guide. A hooked wire is then advanced through the needle or a preloaded wire is inserted and the needle is removed. Some physicians administer 0.1 mL methylene blue dye into the lesion before the wire is deployed. Radiographs should always be acquired of the excised specimen.

With the alphanumeric compression device, the procedure is faster. The breast is placed in the compression device with the shortest distance to the lesion nearest the opening of the compression grid. A needle is passed into the breast parallel to the chest wall after an image has been obtained. The needle advances in the direction of the x-ray beam. Another film is taken to confirm that the position is appropriate, then a film is taken in the orthogonal plane (i.e., 90 degrees to the first film). Wire is placed and dye may be used as in the free-hand technique. Again, a radiograph is obtained of the specimen to ensure that the lesion has been removed.

In summary, masses or suspicious calcifications detected only by mammography must be localized mammographically so that a sample can be removed for biopsy. The technique involves (1) insertion of a needle under mammographic control into or through the suspected site, (2) exchange of the needle for a marker (hooked or curved wire or vital dye), (3) surgical excision of the lesion, and (4) radiograph of the specimen. For this technique to be successful, it must be established that the lesion is in the parenchyma of the breast (tangential views if uncertain) and is not superimposition of normal structures (spot compression magnification). Localization should not be accepted unless the marker is less than 1 cm from the lesion. The distance is closer for small breasts, small lesions, and lesions not clearly seen at 90 degrees. Excision of the mass must be confirmed by histologic tumor, specimen radiographs, or mammography of the biopsied breast.

Stereotactic localization and fine-needle aspiration or core biopsy of nonpalpable breast lesions is now widely available. This procedure can replace excisional biopsy in many cases and radiologists should be familiar with this alternative.

PATHOLOGY

Approximately 99% of breast cancers are adenocarcinomas, 90% of which are ductal in origin and 10% of which are lobular in origin. Ductal carcinomas may be further classified as in situ or invasive. In situ tumors are subclassified as comedocarcinoma or noncomedocarcinoma. Comedocarcinoma is generally more aggressive. Invasive ductal carcinomas may be subclassified as colloid, papillary, tubular, medullary, adenoid cystic, or "not otherwise specified" (the majority). Tumors of lobular origin are infiltrating lobular carcinoma and lobular carcinoma in situ (LCIS), which is thought to be premalignant without specific mammographic findings. The diagnosis of LCIS confers a 30% risk of cancer (ductal or lobular) within 15 to 20 years (i.e., 15% per breast). Rarer breast malignancies include lymphoma, sarcoma, and metastatic disease (most commonly from contralateral breast, melanoma, lymphoma, lung cancer, and renal cancer).

Many special studies can supplement routine histologic tumor evaluation. These include flow cytometry and other methods to assess DNA content and proliferative rates, electron microscopy, immunohistochemical studies, and hormonal receptor analysis. Measuring estrogen and progesterone receptors yields information about prognosis and the potential for response to endocrine therapy. Tumors that histologically have lymphatic or vascular invasion as well as necrosis have a more unfavorable prognosis.

BREAST CANCER STAGING

Generally, breast cancer can be categorized as local (growth within the breast), regional (tumor in the axillary nodes), and distant (metastatic disease). The American

Table 7–4. Breast Cancer Staging

Stage 0	In situ
Stage I	Cancer less than 2 cm; no axillary node disease or metastasis
Stage II	Cancer 2–5 cm or positive axillary lymph nodes present, ipsilateral, mobile
Stage III	Cancer more than 5 cm, fixed to the pectoralis fascia, or has positive nodes matted together in the axilla
Stage IV	Any cancer with distant metastasis

Joint Committee on Cancer (AJCC) has staged breast cancer using the TNM (tumor, nodes, metastases) classification. Breast cancer stages are described in Table 7–4.

Axillary lymph nodes are grouped into "levels." Level I nodes lie within the axilla itself and are inferior and lateral to the relatively vertically oriented pectoralis minor muscle. Level II nodes are high within the apex of the axilla, deep to the pectoralis minor muscle. Level III nodes are infraclavicular, medial to the pectoralis minor muscle. Surgical node sampling generally involves level I and II only to minimize the chances for upper extremity lymphedema. Other nodes, such as supraclavicular or internal mammary, are considered as distant metastases. Lymph node involvement increases with tumor size and survival rates (Table 7–5) decrease with positive nodes.

TREATMENT OF BREAST CANCER

Mastectomy. The indications for mastectomy include patient preference, pregnancy, expected poor cosmetic result from lumpectomy, diffuse or multicentric disease, or contraindications to or inavailability of radiation therapy. These are all relative contraindications for breast-sparing surgery. Patients undergoing mastectomy may have immediate reconstruction through the use of breast implants or expanders, as well as musculocutaneous flaps of the patient's own tissue (e.g., latissimus dorsi or transverse rectus abdominis muscle myocutaneous flap).

Breast-Conserving Therapy. Breast-conserving therapy (i.e., lumpectomy, quadrantectomy) requires careful evaluation of the presurgical mammogram, status of the margins of the excision, and the presence or absence of an extensive intraductal component (EIC). The risk of recurrence of EIC tumors after 5 years is approximately 25%; however, a subsequent wider reexcision seems to decrease this recurrence rate. The risk of recurrence of EIC-negative tumors is approximately 6% after 5 years.

In early cancer, breast conservation requires resection of the tumor with a surrounding region of normal tissue, with or without axillary node dissection, and radiation therapy (XRT). The survival rate of well-selected patients who have had breast-conserving surgery and XRT is equal to that of patients who have had mastectomies. Postoperative mammography is useful for assessing completeness of

Table 7–5. Survival Rate for Different Stages of Breast Cancer

	5 Year (%)	10 Year (%)
DCIS or invasive cancer less than 5 mm	98	95
Axillary nodes negative	85	75
Axillary nodes positive	55	40
Metastases	10	2

DCIS, ductal carcinoma in situ.

Table 7–6. Recommendations for Adjuvant Therapy

Axillary Node	Age < 50 Years		Age > 50 Years	
	ER Negative	ER Positive	ER Negative	ER Positive
Negative	Uncertain	Uncertain	Uncertain	Tamoxifen (5 y)
Positive	Chemotherapy (6 m)	Chemotherapy (6 m)	Chemotherapy (6 m)	Tamoxifen (5 y)

ER, estrogen receptor; m, months; y, years.

excision, especially in tumors defined primarily by microcalcifications. Shorter interval follow-up of the involved breast (i.e., every 6 months) for 3 to 5 years is recommended after breast-conserving surgery. Mammograms must be carefully evaluated because postsurgical and postradiation changes can obscure or mimic cancer. Early stage cancer treated with breast-sparing surgery and XRT has a 5 to 10% recurrence rate at 5 years and a 7 to 20% recurrence rate at 10 years.

Most therapeutic radiologists treat the entire breast (less than 50 Gy over 5 to 6 weeks). The need for a boosting dose (10 to 20 Gy) to the primary site is controversial. A boost is probably less important in tumors treated with a wide excision or quadrantectomy.

It is controversial whether axillary nodal dissection is necessary in all patients treated with conservative surgery and XRT. If the axillary nodes are not palpable, dissection is still preferred by many because of the information it provides; if nodes are not dissected, XRT to the axillary nodes is suggested.

Adjuvant Systemic Therapy. Adjuvant systemic therapy includes chemotherapy and hormonal therapy in patients without grossly detectable recurrence but with evidence of micrometastasis. Unfortunately, none of the agents used is specific to cancer cells. Most agents work on cells in an active stage of the cell cycle. The most commonly used chemotherapeutic agents for breast cancer are alkylating agents (e.g., cyclophosphamide), antimetabolites (e.g., 5-fluorouracil), anthracyclines (e.g., doxorubicin), and vinca alkaloids (e.g., vinblastine). The most common combination regimens are cyclophosphamide, methotrexate, and 5-fluorouracil (CMF) or cyclophosphamide, Adriamycin (doxorubicin), and 5-fluorouracil (CAF).

Tumors positive for expression of estrogen (ER) and progesterone (PR) receptor proteins generally have a better prognosis than tumors without expression of these proteins. ER or PR positivity also indicates the potential for a good response to hormone therapy. As a patient's age increases (especially over 50 years), the chances of being ER positive increase. Hormonal therapy techniques act by eliminating estrogen production (oophorectomy, luteinizing hormone-releasing hormone analogue, progestin therapy) or blocking the estrogen effect at the cellular level (tamoxifen). Tamoxifen has weak estrogen-like effects and may be protective against osteoporosis and coronary artery disease while increasing uterine cancers.

Randomized trials have shown delay in time to relapse and a decreased likelihood of dying from breast cancer in those treated with adjuvant therapy. Adjuvant therapy appears more effective than therapy given when a relapse occurs. Recommendations for adjuvant therapy are given in Table 7–6.

Additional Reading Section

American College of Radiology Committee on Quality Assurance on Mammography: Mammography Quality Control, 1992.

The ACR and Society of Breast Imaging Syllabus: The First Meeting and Postgraduate Course, April 1993. Amelia Island, FL: Society of Breast Imaging.

American Society of Radiologic Technologists: Fundamentals of Mammography: The Quest for Quality: Positioning Guidebook.

Andolina VF, Lille SL, Willison KM: Mammographic Imaging: A Practical Guide. Philadelphia: JB Lippincott, 1992.

Bassett LW, Jahanshahi R, Gold RH, et al: Film-Screen Mammography: An Atlas of Instructional Cases, 1991.

Beahrs OH: CA—A Cancer Journal for Clinicians. American Cancer Society, 41: 1991.

Breast Imaging, Current Status and Future Directions. Radiologic Clinics of North America, January 1992. Philadelphia: WB Saunders.

Eastman Kodak Company: Medical Radiography and Photography: Mammography in Clinical Practice, volume 62, number 2. Rochester, NY: Eastman Kodak Company, 1986.

Harris JR, Hellman S, Henderson IC, et al: Breast Diseases, 2nd ed. Philadelphia: JB Lippincott, 1991.

Haus AG, Yaffe MJ (eds): Syllabus: A Categorical Course in Physics, Technical Aspects of Breast Imaging. RSNA, 1993.

Kopans DB: Breast Imaging. Philadelphia: JB Lippincott, 1989.

Wentz G: Mammography for Radiologic Technologists. New York: McGraw-Hill, 1992.

BREAST IMAGING DIFFERENTIAL DIAGNOSES

Calcifications, malignant appearance
Calcifications, benign appearance
Mass, well-circumscribed margins
Mass, ill-defined (indistinct) margins
Mass, spiculated margins
Mass, obscured margins
Masses, multiple
Masses, fat-containing
Architectural distortion
Asymmetry
Diffusely increased breast density, trabecular thickening, and skin thickening
Axillary lymph nodes
Single dilated duct bloody nipple discharge
Gynecomastia

7

CALCIFICATIONS, MALIGNANT APPEARANCE

List five causes of malignant-appearing calcifications.

Invasive ductal carcinoma
Ductal carcinoma in situ (DCIS)
Fat necrosis
Early vascular disease
Early fibroadenoma degeneration
Fibrous capsule adjacent to implant
Other benign conditions

Invasive ductal carcinoma (not otherwise specified [NOS])

· Most common form of breast cancer (approximately 80%)
· Usually a mass on mammograms
· Calcifications are common

FIGURE Radiol Clin North Am: 98

Ductal carcinoma in situ (DCIS)

What type of DCIS generally has the worst prognosis? Describe the classic shape of calcifications in comedocarcinoma and noncomedocarcinoma.

· Confined to ductal structures
· Typically, large number of calcifications (pleomorphic, fine, and branching forms are more likely to be malignant than punctate or amorphous/indistinct forms)
· Distribution: clustered, linear, or segmental
· Comedocarcinoma often undergoes necrosis with calcifications

forming casts of ducts, often rod-like or branching; generally has poor prognosis
- Cribriform and micropapillary calcify from stagnations of secretions; are usually punctate

FIGURES   Radiol Clin North Am: 96–97; Bassett et al.: 29–31

Fat necrosis

What are the mammographic findings of fat necrosis?

- Often secondary to trauma or surgery
- Findings include ill-defined mass, radiolucent oil cyst, branching irregular or rim calcifications
- Can mimic cancer
- May decrease in size with time (cancer tends to grow)

FIGURES   Radiol Clin North Am: 102, 131, 135; Bassett et al.: 48–51, 109–113

Early vascular disease

- Classic description: parallel "railroad" tracks or linear tubular calcifications associated with blood vessel
- Early fine, irregular calcifications can mimic malignant calcifications

Early fibroadenoma degeneration

Are fibroadenomas ever biopsied because of their associated calcifications?

- Classic description: coarse or "popcorn-like"
- Early in degenerative course, calcifications in clefts of fibroadenomas can mimic malignant calcifications
- Calcifications can wax and wane
- Associated mass usually seen

FIGURES   Radiol Clin North Am: 100; Bassett et al.: 106–108

Fibrous capsule adjacent to implant

Do all breast implants form fibrous capsules?

- Breast implants all tend to form fibrous capsules, especially those that are prepectoral (subglandular) in position
- If associated calcifications occur, usually they are of a long, curvilinear or "sheet-like" configuration; thin, linear, slightly suspicious calcifications also can be seen
- Implant displacement (Eklund) views can help in visualization of more of the native parenchyma, but imaging becomes more difficult when significant encapsulation occurs

Other benign conditions

Are biopsies often done for benign entities?

Name five artifacts that can simulate calcifications.

- Calcifications of various forms of fibrocystic change often cannot be distinguished mammographically from those of a malignancy
- Positive biopsy rate for calcifications ranges from 15 to 30%; procedures such as core biopsy are being used to decrease the number of benign excisional biopsies
- Artifacts (e.g., scratches, dust, fingerprints, static, deodorant, talc, electrocardiogram paste, tattoos, gold treatment for rheumatoid arthritis, crystallization of processing chemicals, others) can simulate benign or malignant calcifications

FIGURES   Radiol Clin North Am: 103; Bassett et al.: 227–232, 260–264, 281–286

CALCIFICATIONS, BENIGN APPEARANCE

List five causes of benign-appearing calcifications.

Skin (dermal)
Vascular
Degenerating fibroadenoma
Secretory calcification
Oil cyst
Milk of calcium
Adenosis
Foreign body

Skin

- Typically have lucent centers; are low density and spherical
- If atypical, tangential projections can be obtained for confirmation

Vascular

- Usually have linear, tubular, parallel, railroad track appearance
- Associated with blood vessels
- Related to other vascular disease, including coronary artery disease

FIGURES Bassett et al.: 276–280

Degenerating fibroadenoma

What distinguishes pericanalicular fibroadenoma from intracanalicular fibroadenoma?

- Coarse, popcorn-like, often associated with mass
- *Coarse* means larger than 1 mm; often measures several mm or cm
- Most common benign solid breast lesion prompting biopsy
- Produced by overgrowth of stromal connective tissue of lobule
- *Pericanalicular*: collagen proliferates around tubular structures; *intracanalicular*: growth into lumen
- Usually involute after menopause; also may atrophy, hyalinize, and infarct
- Calcifications usually begin centrally and increase outwardly but can calcify at periphery first

FIGURES Kopans: 147–149, 262–266

Secretory calcification

- Coarse linear calcifications, solid or ring-like, often bilateral
- Also known as *mammary duct ectasia, plasma cell mastitis*
- Inspissated intraluminal contents calcify and can be surrounded by periductal fibrosis
- Most often occurs in perimenopausal or postmenopausal women

FIGURES Kopans: 91, 150; Bassett et al.: 276–280, 292–294; Kodak: 35

Oil cyst

- Postsurgical fat necrosis
- Lucent lesion
- May have ring-like curvilinear calcifications peripherally (eggshell calcification)

FIGURES Kopans: 71, 222

Milk of calcium

- Sedimented calcium with "tea-cup" crescentic appearance on true lateral view and round or amorphous on CC view
- Usually bilateral; can be clustered or scattered

FIGURES   Radiol Clin North Am: 101; Kopans: 269; Kodak: 36

Adenosis

- Comprises a range of lobular lesions
- Proliferates within terminal lobular unit
- Can be confusing to pathologist and appear similar to cancer
- Rarely a visible mass; occasionally an indeterminant cluster of microcalcifications, thus requiring biopsy, but usually indistinguishable from normal breast tissue
- Sometimes present as diffuse bilateral calcifications, relatively round and regular

FIGURE   Kopans: 273

Foreign body

- Usually in vicinity of prior surgery; most common after radiation
- Usually tubular calcifications
- Some types of suture material can develop calcifications

FIGURE   Kopans: 96

MASS, WELL-CIRCUMSCRIBED MARGINS (sharp demarcation with abrupt transition between the mass and the adjacent tissue)

What is the definition of well circumscribed?

Cyst
Fibroadenoma
Cystosarcoma phyllodes
Other benign conditions
    Intramammary lymph node
    Papilloma
Carcinoma
    Medullary carcinoma
    Colloid carcinoma (mucinous carcinoma)
    Papillary carcinoma
    Invasive ductal carcinoma (NOS)
Metastasis

Cyst

True or false: A cyst can be differentiated from a solid lesion by mammography. What are the sonographic criteria of a cyst?

- Probably results from dilation of terminal ducts
- When mammographically apparent, often multiple and bilateral
- Usual mammographic appearance: well defined (round, oval, lobulated), partially obscured, or focal increased density
- Cannot be distinguished mammographically from solid mass; sonography or needle aspiration needed
- Although intracystic cancer is rare, pneumocystogram is recommended after aspiration to rule out nodular component
- Natural history: waxes and wanes with menstrual cycle and over time
- Most common in premenopausal women (age 30 to 50)
- Use strict sonographic criteria: anechoic, sharp margins, posterior acoustical enhancement

- Occasional thin, peripheral, egg-shell calcifications occur
- Usually asymptomatic but can be painful and tender

FIGURES   Bassett et al.: 22–26; Radiol Clin North Am: 76, 172–174;
           Kopans: 74, 163, 165, 171, 216, 270, 271; Kodak: 25–26

Fibroadenoma

Do fibroadenomas generally arise in postmenopausal women?

- Well-circumscribed masses with round, oval, or lobular borders
- Frequently multiple and bilateral, usually 3 cm or less
- Most common in women aged 35 years or less; rarely appears or grows after menopause
- Degenerative calcification described under Calcifications, Benign Appearance (512)

Degenerating fibroadenoma

- Mammographically not distinguishable from cysts or other solid tumors unless associated classic calcifications are present

FIGURES   Radiol Clin North Am: 76; Kodak: 33; Kopans: 73,
           161–163, 191–192, 217–218, 263–265

Cystosarcoma phyllodes (phyllodes tumor)

Is cystosarcoma phyllodes a malignant diagnosis?

- Composed of stromal and epithelial elements, similar to fibroadenomas
- Stromal elements more cellular and cells more pleomorphic than those of fibroadenomas
- Most nonmetastastic (90%); limited local invasion
- Approximately 15% are malignant
- Hematogenous metastases to lung, pleura, and bones
- Can grow to large sizes; can recur (approximately 25%) if incompletely excised
- Rarely calcify
- Often present as (soft) palpable lump; often grow rapidly
- Mammogram cannot distinguish from "giant fibroadenoma," which is usually seen in teenagers or women in their 20s
- Smooth, round, oval, lobulated

FIGURES   Bassett et al.: 131–134; Kopans: 79, 302; Kodak: 24

Intramammary lymph node

True or false: Mammography can always distinguish intramammary lymph nodes from other lesions.

- Round, ovoid, or reniform
- Fatty hilus confirms diagnosis
- Seen mammographically in upper outer quadrant, but can be found anywhere in the breast
- Enlargement beyond about 1 cm and loss of fatty hilus may raise suspicion, but infection and inflammatory processes can cause enlargement, as can primary breast cancer, lymphoma or metastasis

FIGURES   Bassett et al.: 253–257; Kopans: 108

Papilloma

True or false: Papilloma and papillomatosis are synonymous. Is papillomatosis a form of hyperplasia? Is it true that it may be premalignant?

- (Solitary) papillomas of large ducts are not the same as (multiple) papillomatosis of distal ducts
- Solitary papillomas are always benign and are a common cause of serous or bloody nipple discharge

- Solitary papillomas occasionally grow large enough to be visible mammographically (usually well circumscribed and lobulated within the anterior retroareolar region of the breast)

FIGURE Kopans: 274

Medullary carcinoma

True or false: Medullary carcinomas often present when small (i.e., less than 2 cm). Do they have a better or worse prognosis than typical invasive ductal carcinomas?

- Uncommon (10%) among the invasive carcinomas
- Well differentiated; can get very large (up to 10 cm) before being found
- Cellular; minimal stroma; prominent infiltration of lymphocytes and other inflammatory cells; large cells with large, atypical nuclei; syncytial growth pattern
- Calcifications typically do not occur
- Has varying degrees of lobulation or is round
- Relatively soft by palpation
- Carries a better prognosis than typical invasive ductal carcinomas (NOS)

FIGURES Bassett et al.: 223–226; Kopans: 299

Colloid carcinoma (mucinous carcinoma)

True or false: Colloid carcinomas are relatively common.

- Uncommon (2%) among invasive carcinomas
- Large amount of mucin within cystic spaces of the tumor is characteristic
- Generally firm but not hard mass by palpation
- Pure colloid carcinoma has a better prognosis than typical invasive cancers
- Tends to present mammographically as a well-circumscribed mass, but can have microlobulations, sometimes ill defined or spiculated
- Tumors that contain a large quantity of mucin may be radiographically hypodense

FIGURE Kopans: 299

Papillary carcinoma

- Uncommon (less than 1%) among invasive carcinomas
- Tend to occur in perimenopausal women
- Papillary or cribriform growth pattern, epithelium with villous-like proliferation
- Tends to present with serosanguineous discharge; usually well-circumscribed mammographic masses or multiple small masses
- Rare intracystic papillary carcinoma; can be confused with atypical papillomatosis
- Slow growing with good prognosis

FIGURE Kopans: 298

Invasive ductal carcinoma (NOS)

- Can present as well-circumscribed mass, but microlobulated, indistinct, or spiculated margins are more suggestive from an imaging standpoint
- A well-circumscribed, noncalcified, solid mass should be considered for biopsy if it is new, growing, or palpable

FIGURES Bassett et al.: 115–119

Metastasis

Excluding lymphoma, what are the most common hematogenous cancers to metastasize to the breast? Are metastases usually solitary?

- Lymphoma, melanoma, and lung are most common hematogenous cancers metastatic to the breast
- Ovarian cancer, sarcomas, gastrointestinal (GI) malignancies (e.g., gastric) and genitourinary (GU) malignancies (e.g., renal cell) also metastasize to the breast
- Metastases may be solitary (85%) or multiple (15%); unilateral (75%) or bilateral (25%); most occur in the upper outer quadrant
- Usually round and well circumscribed

FIGURE Kopans: 308

MASS, ILL-DEFINED (INDISTINCT) MARGINS (obscuring by adjacent tissue does not explain the poorly defined margins of the mass)

Define indistinct margins.

Carcinoma
Biopsy scar
Fat necrosis
Abscess
Hematoma
Sclerosing adenosis and fibrosis

Carcinoma

- Ill-defined margins should raise more suspicion than well-defined ones
- Invasive NOS, medullary, mucinous, papillary, and invasive lobular may present with ill-defined margins
- Spot compression magnification may better characterize margins and clarify cases in which superimposition of tissue simulates a mass
- Postoperative scarring can simulate carcinoma (history is important!)

FIGURES Kopans: 188, 194, 198, 199

Biopsy scar

Are scars usually similar in appearance on different mammographic projections? What problems can occur when a scar is first imaged a year or more after the surgery?

- Can vary in appearance on different projections and have a planar (not three-dimensional) configuration
- Usually diminishes with time
- New baseline mammography several months after surgery can help avoid another biopsy for possible residual or recurrent carcinoma
- If central lucency is present to suggest fat necrosis, more likely that lesion is the result of prior surgery

FIGURES Radiol Clin North Am: 73

Fat necrosis

- Wide spectrum of mammographic appearances (mass-like, cyst-like with fat density, architectural distortion, and calcifications)
- Helpful to find central fatty lucency
- Clinical history of surgery or trauma helpful but not always present
- Clinically can have palpable mass, skin thickening, and skin retraction

FIGURES Kodak: 20, 21

Abscess

In what group of patients do abscesses typically occur?

- Clinical history is helpful but inflammatory signs are often absent (pain, swelling, erythema)
- Most located in retroareolar area; may or may not have associated skin thickening
- Usually occur in young women during lactation
- Mastitis from infection of sebaceous glands may proceed to abscess formation
- Abscess usually staphylococcal or streptococcal
- Abscess appears mass-like or as focal increased density
- Needle aspiration can be performed
- Follow-up mammography recommended to ensure that lesion is diminishing or gone and that no underlying cancer is present

Hematoma

- May appear as subtle tissue infiltration; can produce increased trabeculation and architectural distortion
- True hematoma usually presents as an ill-defined or fairly well-circumscribed, mass-like lesion; may be found after surgery or blunt trauma or in those with bleeding disorders
- Resolution usually within weeks or months, but can persist
- May be sonolucent, but usually has some low-level internal echoes
- Follow-up recommended to ensure lesion diminishes or is gone
- Can calcify at later stages

FIGURES Kopans: 79, 190, 191; Kodak: 21

Sclerosing adenosis and fibrosis

- Sclerosing adenosis is a late stage of proliferation of acinar elements characterized by extensive fibrosis
- A local region of sclerosing adenosis uncommonly presents as a mass or density
- Focal fibrous breast disease or fibrous mastopathy, characterized by fibrosis with minimal glandular components, may represent further progression of sclerosing adenosis

FIGURE Radiol Clin North Am: 80

MASS, SPICULATED MARGINS (lines radiating from the margins of the mass; irregular border)

Define spiculated margins.

Invasive carcinoma (including tubular carcinoma)
Radial scar
      Sclerosing duct hyperplasia
      Elastosis
      Indurative mastopathy
Biopsy scar (*See Mass, Ill-defined margins*)
Fat necrosis (*See Mass, Ill-defined margins*)
Breast abscess (*See Mass, Ill-defined margins*)
Sclerosing adenosis (*See Mass, Ill-defined margins*)

Invasive carcinoma

Are tubular carcinomas relatively rapid growing tumors?

- Spiculated margins are more worrisome than well-circumscribed or ill-defined ones

True or false: Invasive lobular carcinoma is generally distinguishable from invasive ductal carcinoma mammographically.

- Usually implies invasion of adjacent tissue (invasive lobular or invasive ductal) but occasionally is seen in DCIS
- The irregular border is consistent with a desmoplastic reaction
- Approximately 90% of invasive cancers are ductal in origin
- A small number of invasive ductal cancers contain enough well-differentiated ductal elements to be subclassified as tubular carcinoma, the most benign and slow-growing of all invasive breast carcinomas
- Invasive lobular often indistinguishable from invasive ductal carcinoma, but compared with invasive ductal carcinoma presents more often as asymmetric densities or architectural distortion and less often as spiculated masses

FIGURES Radiol Clin North Am: 71, 72, 73; Kodak: 19; Kopans: 117; Bassett et al.: 12–14

Radial scar

True or false: It is inappropriate to take a biopsy sample from a radial scar.

- Not from surgery or trauma, but a condition in which ductal elements are surrounded by radiating bands of fibrous connective tissue
- Most consider it benign; some think it is a precursor of tubular carcinoma
- Usually without central definable mass or has a lucent central area; radiating lines seen in one or both projections but tend to be planar at histology
- Lucent streaks between the spicules suggestive of this diagnosis; often appears similar to focal architectural distortion with no mass
- Despite findings suggesting the diagnosis, biopsy is required because it mimics carcinoma
- Lesions usually are small but can be relatively large
- Can contain calcifications

FIGURES Radiol Clin North Am: 75; Kodak: 22; Kopans: 289

7

MASS, OBSCURED MARGINS

What do obscured margins mean?

- Can include any of the previously discussed entities that are partially or completely "silhouetted" by adjacent isodense fibroglandular tissue
- Mass is (partially) hidden by superimposed or adjacent breast tissue

MASSES, MULTIPLE

Are multiple masses usually benign or malignant?

Cysts
Fibroadenomas (*See Mass, well-circumscribed margins*)
Intramammary lymph nodes (*See Mass, well-circumscribed margins*)
Papillomas (*See Mass, well-circumscribed margins*)
Metastases (*See Mass, well-circumscribed margins*)
Multifocal or multicentric breast cancer
Skin lesions

Management of multiple well-circumscribed lesions

- Closely evaluate each lesion and its margins
- Correlate with physical examination
- If none is clearly dominant or palpable, follow-up in 6 months or 1 year at most

• Avoid ultrasound unless only a few lesions present

Cysts

• Often multiple and bilateral
• Wax and wane
• If palpable or symptomatic, aspiration often recommended
• Ultrasound not recommended for multiple masses: analysis of all easily missed, difficult to correlate with mammogram
• If one of the multiple masses grows out of proportion to the others, further analysis is warranted

FIGURES Kopans: 216, 217

Multifocal or multicentric breast cancer

Why is it important to make this diagnosis?

• Multifocal: same breast quadrant but more than 2 cm apart from each other
• Multicentric: different breast quadrants
• If several lesions are suspicious mammographically, tissue diagnosis of all is recommended because definitive treatment can be effected
• Either diagnosis usually precludes breast-sparing surgery

FIGURES Kopans: 218, 219, 220

Skin lesions

Are skin lesions ever distinguishable from parenchymal breast lesions?

• Includes moles, neurofibromatosis, keratosis, sebaceous cysts
• Lucent halo of air sometimes seen around skin lesion(s)
• Tangential projections, radiopaque markers, clinical history, and physical examination can be helpful

FIGURES Kodak: 30; Kopans: 216

MASSES, FAT-CONTAINING (radiolucent or mixed density)

Name five radiolucent or mixed density lesions.

Oil cyst (*See Calcifications, benign appearance*)
Fat necrosis (*See Mass, ill-defined margins*)
Lipoma
Galactocele
Hamartoma (fibroadenolipoma)
Intramammary lymph node (*See Mass, well-circumscribed margins*)

Lipoma

Are lipomas encapsulated?

• Completely fatty (lucent), well-circumscribed mass with a very thin capsule that infrequently calcifies
• Occurs mostly in fatty breasts
• May splay adjacent breast tissue and trabeculae but does not infiltrate
• Can be difficult to distinguish from normal fatty tissue of the breast
• Usually located superficially and at the periphery of the breast
• Lipomas are soft, but liposarcomas are typically firm and radiographically dense
• Lipomas occasionally have central calcifications, which indicates some infarction

FIGURES Radiol Clin North Am: 79; Kopans: 71, 222, 279, 281

Galactocele

Are galactoceles generally found in young women?

- Milk-containing cyst that develops in women during lactation; often presents 6 to 10 months after breast feeding has stopped
- Probably caused by duct obstruction
- Can have fat or fluid level on MLO or true lateral projection; in some patients the densities can be mixed and appear mottled
- If fat content is high, galactocele can be very lucent and look like a lipoma
- If palpable, is soft and mobile
- Resolves with aspiration

FIGURES   Bassett et al.: 39–42; Kopans: 71, 223

Hamartoma

Is it true that between 10 and 15% of breast harmartomas undergo malignant degeneration?

- Contain varying combinations of fatty and soft tissue densities, usually with a thin surrounding capsule
- Benign; malignant degeneration not reported
- Approximately 50% have the typical appearance at mammography; 35% present as nonspecific masses; nearly 20% had some finding, such as ill-defined margins, to raise suspicion
- Caused by proliferation of fibrous and adenomatous nodular elements in fat
- Relatively uncommon
- Large (up to 5 cm) and usually palpable

FIGURES   Bassett et al.: 245–248; Radiol Clin North Am: 79; Kopans: 108, 285

7

ARCHITECTURAL DISTORTION

Give five reasons for architectural distortion.

Carcinoma
Radial scar
Posttraumatic fat necrosis
Prior surgery
Prior radiation
Fibrocystic change

Definition

- Normal breast pattern is distorted
- Includes spiculations radiating from a point and focal retraction of superficial structures or distortion of the parenchyma
- Tissue appears pulled toward a point eccentric from the nipple; normal breast structures are arranged along duct lines flowing toward the nipple
- Abnormal arrangement of Cooper's ligaments can be seen

Carcinoma

- Architectural distortion can be primary finding or associated finding
- Comparison with previous mammographic examinations may reveal subtle distortion and subtle changes

FIGURES   Kopans: 67, 125, 212–215; Bassett et al.: 125–130

Radial scar

- Dense radiating lines can be interspersed with trapped fat
- Cannot be differentiated from cancer: biopsy necessary

FIGURES   Kopans: 126, 210, 211

Posttraumatic fat necrosis

- Usually asymptomatic; found mammographically as an oil cyst, density or mass, area of architectural distortion, or calcification
- Can present as a painful or palpable mass
- Histologic examination: damaged adipocytes without nuclei and phagocytized fat in cytoplasm of histiocytes; fibrotic response and calcifications also seen
- Tends to regress with time

Prior surgery

How can postsurgical changes be distinguished from carcinoma?

- Scar production after surgical procedure can yield architectural distortion, trabecular thickening, and skin thickening
- Distortion in a region of previous surgery should be carefully assessed at subsequent mammographic examinations
- May mimic or obscure cancer scarring; suggested when central region of distortion contains fat
- Distortion common in immediate postoperative period; fades, usually in 6 to 12 months, occasionally longer, especially if patient also had radiation therapy
- Occult cancer developing in region of a completely benign biopsy is rare

FIGURES   Kopans: 126, 281

Prior radiation

- Response of breast to radiation therapy varies
- Skin and trabecular thickening can be seen acutely; generally resolves but can progress to fibrosis
- Mammography can be difficult to perform because edematous radiated breast cannot be compressed
- Architectural distortion can be significant, especially with coexistent extensive surgery
- Distortion usually diminishes after 12 to 18 months; if persistent, biopsy may be needed
- Changes from surgery plus radiation can last longer than changes from either surgery or radiation alone
- Dystrophic calcifications can develop, usually after several years

FIGURES   Kopans: 109, 225

Fibrocystic change

- Comprises a group of proliferative disorders, usually in women aged 35 to 50 years
- Includes cysts, fibrosis, apocrine metaplasia, epithelial hyperplasia, and papillomatosis
- *Fibrocystic change* is a histologic term, not a mammographic one
- If there is a significant fibrotic component, architectural distortion can occur

FIGURES   Bassett et al.: 191–195

ASYMMETRY

Asymmetric dense glandular tissue
Carcinoma (especially invasive lobular)

Asymmetric dense glandular tissue

- Breasts normally can show some degree of asymmetry
- Previous surgical removal of tissue can lead to an asymmetric appearance of the tissue
- Reduction mammoplasty often results in asymmetry, as can breast reconstructions using patient's own tissue or muscle flaps
- Asymmetry alone is not cause for suspicion unless associated with microcalcifications, architectural distortion, or a palpable mass
- Asymmetric breast tissue is not equal to (focal) asymmetric density

FIGURES   Kopans: 128, 129, 206–209

Carcinoma

- Invasive ductal and invasive lobular carcinoma can look alike mammographically
- Invasive lobular carcinoma presenting as focal asymmetric density (with architectural distortion) more common than invasive ductal carcinoma presenting as focal asymmetric density; invasive ductal carcinoma usually presents as a mass
- Invasive lobular carcinoma is bilateral in up to 20% of cases; invasive ductal carcinoma less frequently bilateral
- 80% of invasive lobular carcinomas have associated foci of LCIS; the relationship of these entities is not clear
- Invasive lobular carcinomas may be missed more often on mammograms
- Lobular carcinoma can present with single rows of cells diffusely infiltrating the breast tissue, little or no distortion of the normal breast anatomy, and no central tumor nidus

FIGURES   Bassett et al.: 63–68, 215, 218

DIFFUSELY INCREASED BREAST DENSITY, TRABECULAR THICKENING, AND SKIN THICKENING

Diffuse carcinoma and inflammatory carcinoma
Surgical biopsies or axillary dissection
Radiation therapy
Mastitis or inflammation
Dermatologic disorders
Generalized edema

Diffuse carcinoma and inflammatory carcinoma

- Some patients with angiolymphatic cancer spread present clinically with inflammatory carcinoma, not a discrete mass or microcalcifications
- Easy to misinterpret clinical presentation as mastitis
- Diffuse changes suggest advanced disease
- Inflammatory carcinoma is aggressive with early tumor invasion of the lymphatics of the skin; clinical evidence of erythema, heat,

What are some of the clinical manifestations of inflammatory carcinoma?

and peau d'orange should be sought; axillary adenopathy is often present
- Inflammatory carcinoma can be difficult to diagnose; biopsy often required
- Pure inflammatory carcinoma has a poorer prognosis than an infiltrating ductal carcinoma that has secondarily invaded the skin

FIGURES   Kopans: 130, 224, 300; Kodak: 39

Surgical biopsies or axillary dissection

- Breast biopsies can cause breast edema for a few months, even when disease is benign
- Axillary node dissection almost always causes breast edema from disruption of lymphatic drainage
- Lumpectomy for cancer causes changes (including increasing density and skin thickening) that are more pronounced and last longer if patient also has radiation therapy

Radiation therapy

What is the typical time course for radiation changes of the breast?

- Typical dose: 50 Gy to the breast; up to 20 Gy boost to the lumpectomy site
- Overall increase in breast density peaks at about 6 months and is nearly gone by 2 years
- Skin thickening and trabecular prominence (from engorged dermal and parenchymal lymphatics) diminish within a few months unless fibrosis and architectural distortion ensue; these changes mimic carcinoma
- It can be difficult to adequately compress a radiated breast
- Recurrence of breast edema after it has subsided is reason to evaluate for cancer recurrence, although other causes, including infection, are possible
- Possible increased incidence of leukemia or other tumors such as sarcomas

FIGURES   Kopans: 109, 225; Radiol Clin North Am: 119

Mastitis or inflammation

- Can produce generalized breast edema, but process typically is localized
- Acute mastitis usually is related to lactation
- Plasma cell mastitis is an aseptic process occurring in the subareolar region; may result from extravasated ductal secretions causing a reactive inflammatory process; usually occurs in older women
- Rare to have mastitis from tuberculosis

FIGURE   Kopans: 224

Dermatologic disorders

- Includes conditions such as psoriasis
- Skin thickening seen; may have a reticular pattern subcutaneously
- Underlying breast parenchyma usually not affected

FIGURE   Kopans: 224

Generalized edema

- Causes: cardiac failure, hypoalbuminemia (e.g., cirrhosis of the liver, nephrotic syndrome), other causes of anasarca

FIGURES   Kodak: 39; Kopans: 225

AXILLARY LYMPH NODES

Breast cancer metastatic to lymph node
Lymphoma
Other malignant neoplasms
Hyperplasia
Inflammation or infection
Drugs or systemic diseases

Definition

Is mammography an appropriate method for evaluation of axillary adenopathy?

- Axillary lymph nodes abnormal if larger than 2 cm or abnormally dense, or if size increases on serial studies
- If fatty hilus present, even large nodes can be benign
- Mammographic analysis of axillary lymph nodes often is not optimal; physical examination and other imaging techniques (e.g., CT or MRI) are more reliable

Breast cancer metastatic to lymph node

True or false: When breast cancer spreads to lymph nodes, the most common chain is internal mammary.

- Uncommon for lymph node metastases to present as spiculated mass or to contain microcalcifications despite the appearance of the primary
- Axillary lymph nodes may appear normal mammographically, yet contain tumor foci; surgical sampling required
- Prognosis worse and survival decreased if tumor spreads to axillary nodes
- Breast cancer can spread to contralateral as well as ipsilateral axillary nodes
- Breast cancer spread to internal mammary or supraclavicular chains is less common

FIGURES   Kodak: 29; Kopans: 104, 105, 131

Lymphoma

- Bilateral axillary adenopathy raises the possibility of lymphoma
- Primary lymphoma of the breast itself is unusual
- Secondary lymphoma of the breast is more frequent; can present as a mass or a diffuse increase in breast density

FIGURES   Kopans: 106, 133; Kodak: 29

Other malignant neoplasms

- Metastasis to axillary nodes less common than breast cancer (or lymphoma)

Hyperplasia

- Nonspecific enlargement of axillary nodes
- Not mammographically distinct from malignant causes of nodal enlargement

FIGURES   Kopans: 105, 132

Inflammation or infection

- Cannot be differentiated from other causes
- Clinical examination and history important

FIGURE Kodak: 28

Drugs or systemic diseases

- Gold therapy for rheumatoid arthritis can cause calcifications within axillary lymph nodes
- Other systemic causes of enlarged axillary lymph nodes include psoriatic arthritis and systemic lupus erythematosus
- History is important

SINGLE DILATED DUCT/BLOODY NIPPLE DISCHARGE

Duct ectasia
Papilloma
Malignancy

Comment

- Single dilated duct not a significant mammographic finding unless other signs that raise suspicion are present, including bloody nipple discharge; multiple dilated ducts are not worrisome
- Bloody nipple discharge is nonspecific; patient often has normal mammogram; diagnosis usually is benign intraductal papilloma, but malignancy cannot be ruled out by mammography or galactography

Duct ectasia

- Primarily involves major ducts in subareolar region
- Filled with secretions and cellular debris
- Cause of dilation unknown but may be related to periductal inflammation, which causes weakening of duct wall and subsequent dilation
- Characteristic calcifications can be seen

FIGURE Kopans: 278

Papilloma

- Common cause of bloody discharge
- Usually in subareolar region
- Can grow large enough to be seen mammographically
- No increased risk of cancer with solitary intraductal papillomas

FIGURE Kopans: 275

Malignancy

- 5% of single duct discharge is caused by breast cancer
- Usually a clinical finding (discharge), not mammographic
- Mammography and galactography usually not helpful; lesion usually occult mammographically

GYNECOMASTIA

Drugs
Tumors
Cirrhosis

Definition

- Nonneoplastic enlargement of the male breast
- Male breast normally fatty, but in gynecomastia some increased density may be seen, often fan-shaped in the retroareolar region, and may extend toward the upper outer quadrant
- Male breast cancer usually is eccentric in location, not subareolar

Drugs

- Include marijuana, cimetidine, reserpine, cardiac glycosides, and exogenous estrogens
- Nipple secretions can be associated with exogenous estrogens (given for prostate cancer)

Tumors

- Testicular tumors including seminoma, embryonal cell carcinoma, and choriocarcinoma can cause gynecomastia
- Testicular examination is mandatory when male breast enlargement is present
- Gynecomastia results from increased estrogen produced by testicular tumors

Cirrhosis

- Chronic liver disease may result in gynecomastia caused by poor hepatic degradation and elimination of estrogens

FIGURES   Kopans: 344, 345

7

Figure References

Bassett LW, Jahanshahi R, Gold RH, et al: Film-Screen Mammography: An Atlas of Instructional Cases, 1991.
Breast Imaging: Current Status and Future Directions. Radiologic Clinics of North America January 1992.
Eastman Kodak Company: Medical Radiography and Photography: Mammography in Clinical Practice 62, (2): 1986.
Kopans DB: Breast Imaging. Philadelphia: JB Lippincott, 1989.

BREAST IMAGING: DISEASE ENTITIES

ABSCESS

Clinical

- Two subtypes: nonlactational and lactational
- Nonlactational (nonpuerperal) abscesses more commonly seen in clinical practice than lactational (puerperal) abscesses

Nonlactational abscess
- Mostly subareolar; indolent and relapsing course; may have tenderness, induration, and erythema
- Usually contains multiple organisms when cultured; requires broad-spectrum antibiotic treatment, including coverage for anaerobic organisms
- Has a high recurrence rate despite incision and drainage, possibly because underlying causative factor of obstructed ducts persists after incision and drainage

Lactational abscess
- Accounts for less than 10% of the breast abscesses seen in clinical practice; more often peripheral (not subareolar); predisposing conditions include steroid use or diabetes
- *Staphylococcus aureus* most common organism, often the only organism present
- Can usually be treated appropriately with incision and drainage and correct antibiotics
- After treatment, usually heals promptly; only rarely develops fistulas (in contrast to subareolar nonlactational abscesses)

Imaging

- Appears as focal mass
- Margins can be indistinct mammographically
- Sonogram shows complex fluid

ADENOSIS

Clinical

- Benign proliferation of stromal and epithelial elements of the breast lobule
- Can occasionally be confused with malignant changes, especially at frozen section
- Hypertrophic changes of epithelium can occur, as can overgrowth of myoepithelial cells
- Secretory activity can increase
- Locally infiltrative appearance, but is benign with no malignant predisposition
- Can be palpable if large volume of tissue is involved

Imaging

- Usually not distinguishable from normal glandular breast tissue
- Rarely forms a visible mass
- Round and uniform or malignant-appearing calcifications can be present
- Calcifications can be diffuse, segmental, or clustered when they occur

ADENOID CYSTIC CARCINOMA

Clinical

- Generally associated with salivary glands
- Rarely occurs in the breast (less than 0.1% of all breast carcinomas)
- Indolent; death from this entity is rare
- Special stains at histology to reveal mucin
- Prone to microscopic invasion of perineural spaces
- Occurs in central or subareolar region of breast

Imaging

- Lobulated mass, indistinct margins
- Not distinguishable from other breast masses

APOCRINE METAPLASIA

Clinical

- Apocrine glands are normal cutaneous appendages
- Ductal or lobular epithelial cells undergo structural alteration and resemble cells found in apocrine glands
- Occurs mostly in cyst lining but also associated with fibroadenomas and sclerosing adenosis
- Precancerous?

AXILLARY ADENOPATHY

Clinical

- Major regional drainage for the breast
- Likelihood of nodal tumor involvement related to size of primary breast tumor
- Axillary adenopathy occurs more often in lateral breast cancers than in medial breast cancers; some medial tumors have preferential drainage to the internal mammary nodal chain
- Clinical assessment of axillary adenopathy has high false-positive and false-negative rates
- Malignant adenopathy correlates with prognosis: patients with negative nodes do better than those with one to three positive nodes, who do better than those with four or more positive axillary nodes
- 20 to 30% of patients with negative nodes develop distant metastases within 10 years, which suggests hematogenous spread bypassing the regional nodes

Imaging

- Mammography generally provides a limited view of the axilla
- Level I nodes can be seen with the MLO projection or special axillary projections, but status of the nodes is not accurate
- Nodes more than 2 cm, dense, without fatty hilus, or enlarging are considered abnormal
- CT better images the axilla and the internal mammary chain
- Enlarged nodes can be secondary to reactive hyperplasia; small, normal-appearing nodes can contain tumor
- Nodal dissection (level I and II) is more accurate than mammography or physical examination
- Calcifications within the nodes rarely seen but can occur in gold therapy for rheumatoid arthritis, primary breast cancer, lymphoma, or metastases from other primary cancers

BLOODY NIPPLE DISCHARGE

Clinical

- Pathologic discharge usually unilateral, spontaneous, and often from a single duct
- Pathologic discharge may be bloody, serous, serosanguineous, or greenish
- Most common cause: benign diseases, including intraductal papilloma and papillomatosis; carcinoma much less common
- Role of cytologic evaluation of discharge controversial; probably has little value

Imaging

- Mammography may reveal single dilated duct or multiple ducts; occasionally an occult lesion may be found (such as a mass)
- Galactography (injecting offending duct with contrast): may reveal an intraductal lesion but does not differentiate benign from malignant; probably does not affect surgical approach (some believe it allows excision of a smaller amount of tissue); can identify a mass that would be missed at a standard duct excision (e.g., an unusual peripheral lesion causing bloody discharge)

COLLOID CARCINOMA

Clinical

- 1 to 2% of breast carcinomas
- Pure colloid carcinoma has a better prognosis than other ductal carcinomas
- Initial symptom usually a mass, but some smaller lesions initially detected by mammography
- Abundant extracellular mucin is characteristic
- Better differentiated than other ductal carcinomas; relatively slow growth rate

- Approximately 60% of pure colloid carcinomas are estrogen-receptor positive; nearly all are diploid by flow cytometry
- Histologically, gland formation is uncommon
- Intraductal component exists in many cases

Imaging

- Mammography: no particular features distinguish colloid carcinoma from other breast carcinomas
- Colloid carcinoma usually better circumscribed than other breast carcinoma but can present with ill-defined or spiculated margins
- When copious amount of mucin present, these tumors can be radiographically hypodense

COMEDOCARCINOMA

Clinical

- Term for an indraductal carcinoma with a large amount of necrosis filling the ducts and often calcifying
- Can be confined to ducts (characteristic) or exhibit some invasion

Imaging

- Characteristically produces numerous calcifications that tend to be pleomorphic and branching ("dot-dash" pattern)
- Calcifications occur in the areas of necrosis
- Calcifications typically distributed along duct lines, which can produce segmental appearance; alternatively, may be clustered

CYSTS

Clinical

- Arise from terminal acinar structures; enlarge because of obstruction or excessive secretion
- Cuboidal epithelial lining found at histology
- May be asymptomatic, palpable, painful, or tender
- May wax and wane, especially with menstrual cycle and hormonal status
- Peak age of occurence: women aged 30 to 50 years; may regress after menopause
- May be solitary but usually multiple (and often bilateral)
- Intracystic carcinoma extremely rare
- No increased risk of carcinoma with simple cysts
- Needle drainage may help painful or tender cysts, but fluid often reaccumulates

Imaging

- Multiple, rounded masses; can be lobulated and can overlap
- Portions of margins can be obscured by adjacent glandular tissue
- If some cyst fluid leaks into surrounding tissue and causes reactive fibrosis, the margins of the mass can appear ill defined (more typical to be well circumscribed)
- Cannot be distinguished from solid masses by mammography; aspiration or sonography needed
- Occasionally, the wall may calcify producing rim calcification
- Strict sonographic criteria must be adhered to for appropriate diagnosis: anechoic, sharply marginated, posterior acoustical enhancement

CYSTOSARCOMA PHYLLODES (PHYLLODES TUMOR)

Clinical

- Probably related to fibroadenoma
- Most benign; 25% recur locally if not completely treated; about 10% metastasize

- Peak ages: 30 to 50 years
- Can grow rapidly
- Hypercellular overgrowth produces cystic spaces
- Histologic differentiation of benign from malignant based upon mitotic activity, atypia, infiltrative margins, and characteristics of stroma
- Most are well circumscribed at gross pathology but without true capsules
- Histologically, epithelial elements and connective tissue stroma are present
- Most discovered as painless breast masses

Imaging

- Mammography: not distinguishable from other well-circumscribed breast masses; appearance may resemble that of fibroadenoma with smooth or lobulated margins
- Microcalcification not a feature of these lesions
- Sonography: appearance of fluid-filled clefts may suggest the diagnosis

DERMAL CALCIFICATIONS

Clinical

- Cause not known in most cases
- Folliculitis or inspissated material in sebaceous glands can produce these calcifications

Imaging

- Round or polygonal shaped; lucent centers; near breast periphery
- If classic lucent center not present, can mimic parenchymal calcifications
- Tangential projections of the skin can confirm dermal location

DESMOID

Clinical

- Extraabdominal desmoids do not metastasize but are locally invasive; tend to recur
- Rare in the breast
- Usually arise in the fascia and muscle of the abdominal wall
- Consists of hypocellular dense, fibrous tissue that invades local muscle
- In the breast, tends to occur adjacent to the pectoralis major
- Wide excision is the appropriate treatment

Imaging

- Can have spiculated margins and therefore not distinguishable from breast cancer
- Calcifications are not seen

DUCT ECTASIA

Clinical

- Also known as *plasma cell mastitis, secretory disease*
- Mononuclear cell infiltrate seen, often with plasma cells
- Generally affects major ducts in the subareolar region but can involve smaller segmental ducts
- Duct(s) distended by secretions and cellular debris
- Periductal fibrosis (periductal mastitis) is associated with an inflammatory infiltrative process that may cause the ductal dilation; alternatively, dilation may cause the inflammation
- Palpable mass may occur; also may have subareolar tenderness, nipple retraction, or discharge
- No predisposition to malignancy
- Patients presenting with mass may require biopsy to rule out malignancy

- If frozen section suggests periductal mastitis, broad-spectrum antibiotics are often prescribed

Imaging

- Dilated, thick ducts are common; if symmetric in distribution, are of no concern
- Accompanying mastitis may result in distinctive spherical and tubular (rod-shaped) calcifications (often called *secretory*) in the lumen and walls of the duct(s)
- Calcifications can be confined to a single ductal network but are usually diffuse and bilateral in distribution
- Sonography of dilated duct shows tubular structures: if fluid filled, may appear relatively sonolucent; if debris filled, may have a homogenous echotexture

DUCTAL CARCINOMA IN SITU (DCIS)

Clinical

- Heterogeneous group of lesions
- Cells of ductal carcinoma distend the duct
- Noncomedocarcinoma (micropapillary, cribriform, solid, large cell type) probably has better prognosis than comedocarcinoma
- Comedocarcinoma more frequently expresses the Her2/neu oncogene
- Continuum model: intraductal carcinoma grows for a varying length of time until it ultimately penetrates the basement membrane and invades
- Dual theory: invasive cancer and intraductal disease may be separate entities
- Approximately 30 to 50% of women who undergo biopsy for intraductal cancer (DCIS) but not definitive treatment progress to invasive cancer; both continuum model and dual theory can be used to support these data
- Mammography detects many preinvasive cancers and screening trials have shown decreased deaths from breast cancer; this seems to support the continuum model
- Mastectomy is standard treatment; cure rate is close to 100%
- Breast-conserving surgery must be carefully evaluated mammographically and pathologically so that adequacy of resection can be judged
- Breast-conserving therapy usually also consists of radiation therapy

Imaging

- Since advent of screening mammography, incidence of DCIS has markedly increased
- Breast Cancer Detection Demonstration Project (BCDDP) data showed that 31% of the cancers detected by mammography alone were noninvasive
- *Comedocarcinoma*: extent of lesion well correlated with extent of calcifications noted mammographically; calcifications often casting, linear, branching, or coarse and granular with quite irregular shapes
- *Noncomedocarcinoma*: extent of disease often greater than predicted by calcifications seen at mammography; calcifications often fine and granular with relatively regular oval and circular forms
- Less frequently, DCIS presents as a mass on mammograms, with or without associated calcifications

DYSTROPHIC CALCIFICATIONS

Clinical

- Benign calcifications can occur up to 4 years after surgery or radiation

Imaging

- Usually measure 1 mm or less
- Usually easy to distinguish from smaller calcifications that may suggest a new cancer or a recurrence
- Can have lucent centers

FAT NECROSIS

Clinical

- Results from blunt trauma, biopsy, surgery, or infection; however, such a history not always present
- Nonsuppurative inflammatory response to lipocyte damage
- Can produce palpable, painful mass indistinguishable from carcinoma (or other entities)
- May have skin thickening or retraction, or both
- Most often clinically occult
- Damaged fat cells without nuclei; histiocytes phagocytize fat; inflammation can cause a fibrotic reaction
- If history of trauma is present, observation may be appropriate; size may initially increase, but gradual regression or no change can be expected

Imaging

- Spectrum of findings: architectural distortion, lobulated mass, spiculated mass, oil cyst, calcified walls of small cysts, malignant-appearing microcalcifications, or any combination
- Can mimic cancer
- Easiest form of fat necrosis to diagnose is the oil cyst: usually round, lucent lesion defined by its capsule
- Without absolute evidence of trauma (history, ecchymosis, palpable lump), biopsy often is required because fat necrosis is not always reliably distinguished from carcinoma clinically or mammographically

FIBROADENOMA

Clinical

- Produced by stromal connective tissue overgrowth of the lobule with variable epithelial overgrowth
- Collagen proliferation is *pericanalicular* if growth is around the lumen; is *intracanalicular* if growth is into the lumen
- May produce a palpable mass
- Usually freely mobile at palpation
- Most are hormone dependent; therefore, tend to occur postmenarche and premenopause, often enlarging during pregnancy and lactation
- By itself, fibroadenoma benign, with no malignant potential; rare reports exist of malignancy within a fibroadenoma (0.1 to 0.3%)
- Relationship to phyllodes tumor unclear
- Atrophy, hyalinization, or infarction can occur, usually after menopause when hormonal support ceases
- Most common benign solid lesion prompting a biopsy
- Most common breast mass in adolescents
- Juvenile fibroadenomas (giant or cellular fibroadenomas) enlarge rapidly; are differentiated from adult fibroadenomas by size and histology

Imaging

- Mammography: usually round or oval, sharply circumscribed mass; may have lobulations, occasionally microlobulated margins
- If fibroadenoma involutes and hyalinizes, calcification may occur
- Calcifications usually begin centrally and increase outward (centripetal); may start from the periphery (centrifugal)
- Pathognomonic classic calcification is popcorn-like and coarse
- Early fine calcifications occasionally resemble malignancy
- Sonography: appearance variable, but typically well-circumscribed, hypoechoic lesions often with posterior acoustical enhancement; however, shadowing can occur

FIBROCYSTIC CHANGE

Clinical

- Pathologically heterogeneous population, therefore not a useful term
- Risk of breast cancer significantly elevated (fivefold) only in patients with atypical hyperplasia (if family history of breast cancer, risk increases to elevenfold)
- Most patients whose biopsies show fibrocystic change have nonproliferative lesions and are not at increased risk of developing cancer
- Terms such as *fibrocystic disease* and *mammary dysplasia* are nonspecific

Imaging

- Atypical hyperplasia (the only clinically meaningful subcategory) diagnosed only by breast biopsy; cannot be predicted by mammography
- *Fibrocystic change* should be eliminated from imaging lexicon and replaced with specific histologic categories:
    Nonproliferative lesions (cysts, apocrine change, epithelial-related calcifications, mild hyperplasia)
    Proliferative lesions without atypia (moderate or florid hyperplasia, intraductal papillomas, sclerosing adenosis)
    Atypical hyperplasia (ductal or lobular)

FIBROSIS

Clinical

- Cause of focal or diffuse fibrosis unknown
- Focal forms may mimic cancer; diagnosis by biopsy
- Often palpable; freely mobile, rubbery consistency
- Isolated regions of abundant fibrous stroma
- No association with cancer

Imaging

- May present as a clinically occult, ill-defined mass that cannot be distinguished from cancer
- Can appear well circumscribed

FIBROUS CAPSULE (ENCAPSULATION)

Clinical

- The body reacts to silicone with a minor inflammatory response; implant becomes encapsulated with fibrous tissue
- Natural, polyurethane-covered implants less likely to become encapsulated than other implants
- Prepectoral (subglandular) implants more likely to become encapsulated than retropectoral implants
- Baker classification of capsular contracture semiquantitative but useful:
    Grade I   No palpable capsule, breasts are soft
    Grade II   Minimal firmness, breast less soft than normal
    Grade III   Moderate firmness, breast feels harder, implant easily palpated
    Grade IV   Severe, breast is very hard, may be painful and tender
- As the capsule contracts, implant beneath becomes more spherical
- Capsulotomy procedures (closed and open) may be performed

Imaging

- Implant may appear more round
- Breast difficult to compress, thus mammography difficult
- Implant-displacement (Eklund) views difficult to obtain
- Crenulated margins suggest contracture

FOREIGN BODY CALCIFICATION

Clinical

- Foreign bodies can cause calcification
- Granulomatous inflammatory reaction has been described after injection of silicone or paraffin
- Silicone or paraffin nodules are firm and tender

Imaging

- Some suture material can cause tubular-appearing calcifications
- Paraffin nodules often smaller than silicone nodules and usually less dense
- Both may have thin-rim or thick-rim calcifications

GALACTOCELE

Clinical

- Milk-containing mass
- Occurs during or after lactation
- May be caused by obstruction of a duct
- Inspissated milk composition varies depending on fat and protein content
- Clinically indistinguishable from any other palpable mass
- Always benign
- Can resolve if aspirated

Imaging

- When fat content is high, radiolucent, well-circumscribed mass may be seen
- Fat-fluid levels can sometimes be seen on lateral projections
- Sonography: well circumscribed with low-level internal echoes

GRANULAR CELL TUMOR

Clinical

- Uncommon in breast; usually occurs in tongue
- Simulates carcinoma clinically
- Firm or fibrous by palpation; skin retraction occasionally seen
- More common in blacks than whites
- More often in the upper inner quadrant
- Gritty when cut with a knife
- Invariably benign; may be locally infiltrative, thus requires wide excision
- Initially thought to be myogenic in origin, hence the name *granular cell myoblastoma*
- Recent studies support neurogenic origin

Imaging

- Mammography: may appear spiculated
- Margins irregular, appear infiltrative
- Indistinguishable from carcinoma

GYNECOMASTIA

Clinical

- Nonneoplastic enlargement of the male breast, usually reversible
- Most common in adolescents and men over 50 years of age
- Usually asymmetric; unilateral (left more often affected than right) or bilateral
- Breasts can be soft or firm; can be sore
- Usually presents as palpable mass or enlarged breast
- Proliferation of stromal, epithelial, myoepithelial, vascular elements

- Secretions can be produced, especially when gynecomastia caused by exogenous hormone administration
- Rare cases have foci of intraductal epithelial hyperplasia
- Number of ducts decreases with time, as does epithelial component; stromal hyalinization and fibrosis then dominate
- Causes: drugs including marijuana; testicular tumors; chronic hepatic disease; lung diseases including lung cancer; Kleinfelter's syndrome; exogenous estrogens; also may be idiopathic
- When persistent, underlying disease process needs to be identified
- Medical treatment usually effective for idiopathic gynecomastia; i.e., dihydrotestosterone
- Surgery indicated, especially in elderly men when differential diagnosis includes carcinoma
- Other treatment: suction lipectomy

Imaging

- Standard mammographic projections (MLO and CC) are obtained
- Spectrum of mammographic appearance: diffuse fat deposition; small density in subareolar region; fan- or flame-shaped density extending from nipple eccentrically toward upper outer quadrant (most common appearance); spherical increased density; female-like appearance of breast (e.g., from exogenous hormones)

HAMARTOMA

Clinical

- Proliferation of fibrous and adenomatous nodular elements in fat with a connective tissue capsule
- Also called *fibroadenolipoma*
- Relatively uncommon benign lesion
- May present as a palpable mass or may be clinically occult

Imaging

- May be indistinguishable from surrounding breast tissue unless capsule is appreciated
- Lesion "lucent" or mixed fatty–soft tissue density
- Characteristic appearance: lobulated nodular densities within encapsulated fat

HEMATOMA

Clinical

- Breast trauma; usually self-limited and manifested by pain, breast edema, and ecchymosis
- Sequelae of trauma are hematoma and fat necrosis
- Management varies with clinical picture: support of breast (e.g., brassiere) and analgesics in smaller lesions, drainage sometimes required in larger lesions

Imaging

- Mammographic appearance can be ominous, i.e., mass with poorly defined margins simulating carcinoma
- Opacity of the hematoma can obscure adequate visualization of other parts (or all) of the breast
- Tenderness after acute event (blunt trauma or biopsy) can make breast compression difficult, which also limits usefulness of mammography
- Mammography repeated within approximately 1 to 2 months to make sure lesion regressing or totally resolved
- May be sonolucent, but usually shows low-level echoes at ultrasound

• Small (few mm) subcutaneous microhematomas with peripheral eggshell calcifications are liponecrosis microcystica calcificans

HEMANGIOMAS

Clinical

• Benign vascular breast lesions are relatively uncommon
• Lesions must be distinguished from angiosarcomas
• Benign angiomatous lesions lack atypia and endothelial proliferation
• Excision recommended

Imaging

• Calcifications small and varied in shape and size or large and bizarrely shaped
• Lobulated mass can also be seen with or without calcifications

HYPERPLASIA

Clinical

• Benign epithelial proliferation of distal (prelobular) terminal ducts, but may develop in lobular epithelium
• Overgrowth of epithelial cells may fill duct
• Common entity: probably affects 20% of population
• Uncommon before age 40 years
• Usually discovered by histologic study in association with other lesions
• No apparent increase in risk of subsequent cancer development unless atypia present (*see Fibrocystic change*)

Imaging

• No mammographic findings
• Hyperplasia is found associated with other lesions detected by mammography or by clinical examination

IMPLANTS

Clinical

• Many types: single-lumen silicone gel, saline; double-lumen with silicone in the inner compartment and saline in the outer compartment or silicone in the outer compartment and saline in the inner compartment (expander type of prosthesis, valuable in reconstruction after mastectomy)
• Location: prepectoral (subglandular) or retropectoral
• Possible complications: capsular contracture, infection, hematoma or seroma, and human adjuvant disease (possible relationship to autoimmune diseases including scleroderma? This remains very controversial)
• Estimated 1.5 to 2 million women in the United States have breast implants
• No clear evidence of increased breast cancer, but imaging and interpretation may be more difficult than in nonaugmented breasts
• Implants may rupture from trauma (including closed capsulotomy for encapsulation) or from aging
• Bag (or shell) porous to some degree: microscopic egress of silicone from the bag (silicone gel bleed) occurs and fluids and fat (from the body) sometimes are found within the bag

Imaging

• Standard mammographic projections plus implant-displacement (Eklund) views recommended
• Film-screen mammography visualizes only anterior portion (perhaps half) of implant

- Xeromammography may image deeper but currently is not used
- Rupture suggested by shape change (clinical and mammographic), contour bulge, silicone in breast parenchyma
- Sonographic suggestion of silicone leak: echogenic noise
- MRI findings in rupture: *intracapsular rupture* suggested by "linguini sign" (bag floating within sea of silicone but contained within fibrous capsule); *extracapsular rupture* suggested by presence of silicone outside of the capsule
- MR spectroscopy may have a future role in finding silicone and byproducts within capsule, breast parenchyma, lymph nodes, and distant organs

INFLAMMATORY CARCINOMA

Clinical

- Rare entity
- Clinical evidence: increased warmth from inflammation, erythema, induration, and thickened skin with peau d'orange appearance
- Median duration of symptoms before diagnosis is less than 3 months
- Benign inflammatory process can present similarly; therefore, biopsy is needed
- Nipple retraction with crusting may also be seen; axillary lymph nodes may be palpable (are involved with cancer in more than 85% of cases)
- Antibiotics may improve clinical course
- Histologic findings: early diffuse invasion of dermal lymphatics; diffuse involvement of the breast without defined tumor margins
- Most lethal of the variants of locally advanced breast cancer
- American Cancer Society (Beahrs, 1991) classifies this as T4d
- Chemotherapy has been used before, with, and after radiation therapy
- Chemotherapy may be appropriate initial treatment because inflammatory carcinoma is considered a systematic process
- Surgical treatment is not curative; mastectomy is used as adjunctive treatment for local control
- Radiation therapy important for local control

Imaging

- Skin thickening from carcinomatosis of skin lymphatics
- Trabecular thickening
- Diffuse increased breast attenuation density may be present
- Mammographic findings should be correlated with symptoms and clinical evaluation

INTRAMAMMARY LYMPH NODES

Clinical

- Extremely common
- Found in all regions of breast at histologic examination
- Usually at the edge of the parenchyma, not deep in the breast
- Usually have reniform shape with hilar indentation

Imaging

- Seen only in upper outer quadrant mammographically
- Lucent fatty hilar notch may be seen; can be almost entirely replaced by fat
- Should be viewed cautiously if hilar notch is lost or node grows beyond 1 cm
- Enlargement from breast cancer, lymphoma, infection, hyperplasia (e.g., dermatologic conditions such as psoriasis)

INVASIVE DUCTAL CARCINOMA (NOS)

Clinical

- Several other subtypes discussed elsewhere
- Most common form of breast cancer, accounting for approximately 80%

- Desmoplastic reaction with cicatrization and fibrosis causes a hard mass on palpation
- Nuclear grading (structural features of tumor cell nuclei) and histologic grading (growth pattern) correlate: higher grade (more poorly differentiated) lesions have higher frequency of positive axillary lymph nodes, are more likely to recur, and have higher mortality rate
- Tumor also assessed for lymphatic, vascular, and perineural invasion
- Immunohistochemical markers (i.e., carcinoembryonic antigen [CEA], S-100, vimentin, etc.): potential indicators of prognosis?

Imaging

- Main finding usually a mass (circumscribed, lobulated, microlobulated, ill defined, or spiculated)
- Desmoplastic response can cause spiculations, which may be visible mammographically
- Desmoplastic reaction can also cause architectural distortion and, later, nipple or skin retraction
- Calcifications are a relatively common associated finding

INVASIVE LOBULAR CARCINOMA
Clinical

- 10 to 15% of invasive breast carcinomas are invasive lobular carcinoma
- Clinical and gross pathology: not distinguishable from infiltrating (invasive) ductal carcinoma
- Prognostically similar to invasive ductal carcinoma
- Relationship with LCIS is unclear, although about 80% of infiltrating lobular carcinomas have associated foci of LCIS
- Cells resemble those of the breast lobule
- Tumor cells arranged linearly ("Indian file")
- Tumor tends to grow circumferentially around ducts and lobules
- Higher frequency of bilaterality and multicentricity than found in invasive ductal carcinomas

Imaging

- No features to distinguish infiltrating lobular from infiltrating ductal
- Presents more often as asymmetric density or architectural distortion (or both) than does infiltrating ductal carcinoma
- Associated calcifications not as common as in infiltrating ductal carcinoma

LIPOMA
Clinical

- Common tumor; slow growing; found in older patients
- Location usually superficial
- Soft and easily movable
- Always benign
- Mature adipose tissue

Imaging

- Lucent lesion with thin capsule (which can calcify)

LOBULAR NEOPLASIA OR LOBULAR CARCINOMA IN SITU (LCIS)
Clinical

- Incidence not known
- No gross morphologic changes clinically or mammographically

- Diagnosis based on histologic findings
- Indicator of increased cancer risk (premalignant or marker?): 30% risk of developing infiltrating ductal or infiltrating lobular carcinoma within 15 to 20 years; equal risk for each breast (15% per breast)
- Because both breasts are at risk, therapy is controversial: use "careful" clinical and mammographic follow-up, mirror-image biopsy, or prophylactic mastecomies?
- Solid; many small cells with uniform nuclei; more of the terminal duct or lobule (or both) involved than in atypical hyperplasia (cells similar)
- More common in dense breast?

Imaging

- No findings; diagnosis based on incidental finding in breast tissue removed for another reason

LYMPHOMA

Clinical

- Primary breast lymphoma uncommon (less than 0.1% of breast malignancies)
- When lymphoma is found in the breast, usually it is present elsewhere in the body
- Other tests (e.g., CT, lymphangiography, isotope scans) should be performed to search for lymphoma elsewhere
- Can grow rapidly
- Involvement of lymphatic structures, including axillary adenopathy, suggests the diagnosis (differential diagnosis includes inflammatory carcinoma, "benign" inflammation)
- For stages I and II, 5-year survival approximately is 75%
- Treatment: adequate surgical biopsy followed by radiation or chemotherapy, or both
- Radical surgery not recommended

Imaging

- Characteristics vary: diffuse increase in radiographic density, mass (circumscribed or ill defined), or multiple masses
- Not associated with microcalcifications
- Well-circumscribed mass(es) can mimic benign tumors such as fibroadenomas

MALE BREAST CANCER

Clinical

- 1% of all breast cancer, but less than 1% of cancers in men
- Predisposing factors include prior breast irradiation and Kleinfelter's syndrome
- Poorer prognosis than female breast cancer?
- Normal male breast contains ducts similar to those found in prepubescent girls
- Palpable mass most common presentation
- Most are infiltrating ductal carcinomas
- Lobule formation rare in men; therefore, infiltrating lobular carcinomas rare
- Lymphoma can occur in male breast
- Primary local management: modified radical mastectomy

Imaging

- Findings resemble those in female breast cancers
- Most occur away from subareolar region (as opposed to gynecomastia)

MASTITIS

Clinical

- Puerperal or lactational mastitis is an acute cellulitis that can progress to abscess formation

- Irritated nipple may be entry site for bacteria
- Affected wedge of breast tissue is warm, tender, and red
- Infection is around the ducts
- Resolves completely with appropriate antibiotics
- Patient should continue breast-feeding or pumping

Imaging

- Diagnosed on clinical findings

MEDULLARY CARCINOMA

Clinical

- Can grow large (5 to 10 cm) before discovery
- Relatively uncommon (less than 5% of breast carcinomas)
- Fairly soft to palpation
- Relatively favorable prognosis
- Patients often younger (majority aged less than 50 years)
- Histologic findings: cellular with minimal stroma
- Prominent lymphocytic infiltration and other inflammatory cells
- Syncytial growth pattern (cells grow in broad sheets)
- Regions of necrosis seen

Imaging

- Mass (often well circumscribed), round or lobulated
- Usually no calcifications present

METAPLASTIC BONE FORMATION

Clinical

- Unusual
- Occurs in benign processes such as hematoma and fat necrosis
- Occurs in malignant processes such as sarcoma and adenocarcinoma
- Mechanism probably cellular metaplasia

Imaging

- Matrix of calcifications quite coarse
- Biopsy necessary to confirm diagnosis
- May have positive uptake on bone scans

METASTASES TO BREAST

Clinical

- Most common tumors metastatic to breast: melanoma, followed by sarcoma, lymphoma, lung, and gastric carcinoma
- Less common metastases: ovarian, renal, and prostatic cancer
- History of primary extramammary malignancy helpful
- Metastatic tumor suggested when neoplastic cells are fairly homogenous, there is no desmoplastic reaction, no in situ carcinoma is seen, and transition from tumor to normal breast tissue is sharp

Imaging

- Often round or oval
- Usually well circumscribed
- Can be multiple and bilateral
- Calcifications not typical

MILK OF CALCIUM

Clinical

- Tiny cysts containing fluid-like calcium
- Small calcific particles gravitate to dependent portion of the cyst

Imaging

- Concave, crescentic appearance of calcium on true lateral projection
- Round, amorphous, "smudged" appearance on CC projection (viewed en face)
- Appearance is pathognomonic
- Can be scattered or clustered (or both)
- Usually bilateral
- Routine screening adequate; 6-month follow-up not necessary; biopsy not indicated when appearance is classic

MULTIFOCAL OR MULTICENTRIC BREAST CANCER

Clinical

- These terms often used synonymously; however, some define *multifocal* as cancers 2 cm apart and *multicentric* as cancers more than 5 cm apart or in different quadrants
- Incidence of multifocal/multicentric breast cancer in sites distinct from the biopsy site in mastectomies range from 10 to 75%
- Wide range because of imprecise definition of multicentricity, technique used to examine mastectomy specimens, and extent of tissue evaluated
- Recent data suggest quadrantectomy leaves less multicentric disease in the breast than a wide excision (i.e., 2-cm margins)
- Some multifocal and most multicentric cancers are not appropriate for breast-conserving surgery

Imaging

- Recent data: approximately 45% incidence of multicentricity in mammographically detected, clinically occult breast cancers
- Sloan-Kettering reported that, in patients receiving mastectomies for in situ cancer, 60% had multicentric disease
- 1993 RSNA abstract reported that mammography detected multifocal/multicentric lesions in 20%, whereas breast MRI did so in 80% of serially sectioned mastectomies

PAGET'S DISEASE OF THE NIPPLE

Clinical

- Relatively uncommon (5% of breast carcinomas)
- Tends to occur in older women
- Clinically, eczematoid changes with occasional serous or bloody nipple discharge; can have palpable mass
- Early detection because of early clinical presentation; thus, good prognosis
- Ductal carcinoma (in situ or infiltrating)
- Tumor cells involve the nipple (epidermal infiltration)
- Punch biopsy or incisional biopsy should be obtained for clinically suspicious nipple changes

Imaging

- May have no mammographic findings
- Occasionally tumor may be seen deeper within the breast (which has spread via ducts to the nipple)
- Microcalcifications can be seen within subareolar ducts

• In patients with biopsy-proven Paget's disease, bilateral mammography, including subareolar magnification views, is recommended

PAPILLARY CARCINOMA

Clinical

• World Health Organization (WHO) definition: rare, invasive pattern predominantly in form of papillary structures
• Papillary carcinoma arising within a cyst: separate WHO classification referred to as *noninvasive intracystic carcinoma*
• Approximately 1 to 2% of all breast carcinomas
• Microscopically, frond-like growth pattern seen
• Distinction from papilloma depends on cytologic features of the cells and their growth pattern
• Considered a form of ductal carcinoma with slower growth and better prognosis than NOS

Imaging

• Although intraductal, probably not evident by mammography
• As neoplasm enlarges, well-circumscribed mass can be seen
• Fibrotic desmosplastic reaction not produced; ill-defined or spiculated margins therefore are not characteristic

PAPILLOMA

Clinical

• Usually in women aged 30 to 50 years
• Benign lesions usually are found within dilated subareolar duct
• Most common cause of bloody or serous nipple discharge
• Occasionally palpable
• No increased risk of cancer
• Microscopically, hyperplastic epithelium on a fibrovascular stalk or sessile

Imaging

• Small subareolar mass (lobulated and usually fairly well circumscribed) occasionally seen
• Dilated duct may be evident
• Associated calcifications rare
• Galactography may help localize lesion but cannot reliably distinguish it from cancer

PAPILLOMATOSIS (EPITHELIOSIS)

Clinical

• Thought to represent a different process than solitary papillomas of large (more central) ducts
• Multiple, peripheral papillomas found within the duct just proximal to lobule
• Suggested increased risk of malignancy (could be related to finding atypia)
• Do not have a fibrovascular core
• Diagnosis usually based on histology only

Imaging

• Can produce mammographic clustered microcalcifications
• Some can be linear and raise suspicion for malignancy

POSTSURGICAL CHANGES

Clinical

- Skin changes including scar
- Distortion of breast appearance may be extreme or nonexistent, depending on type of surgery or biopsy, surgical technique, time since procedure, and associated procedures such as radiation treatment
- Reduction mammoplasty yields a typical skin scar pattern: tilting and elevation of the nipple; skin changes more prominent inferiorly

Imaging

- Most postsurgical changes involute with time
- Without clinical history, postsurgical changes (especially early ones) cannot be distinguished reliably from carcinoma
- Types of findings: skin changes, architectural distortion, loss of parenchymal and fatty tissue, parenchymal scarring, calcifications (of any shape or size), fat necrosis (including oil cyst), and foreign body
- Features that can distinguish scar from cancer: planar rather than three-dimensional, fat interspersed, often superficial in location, spicules may extend to the skin
- Some features of reduction mammoplasty: much of the residual dense tissue is seen inferiorly, areolar skin thickening and calcifications, fat in retroareolar region

RADIAL SCAR

Clinical

- Benign
- On rare occasions when palpable, usually freely mobile
- Histologic study: may be difficult to distinguish from cancer
- Predominantly elastic tissue surrounded by terminal lobular proliferation (elastosis)
- Occasionally contains calcifications
- Sclerosing adenosis and apocrine metaplasia frequently seen with this lesion

Imaging

- Appears similar to carcinoma (cannot be reliably distinguished); requires biopsy
- Area of architectural distortion with radiating spiculations
- May appear different on different projections (e.g., planar)
- No central mass
- Spicules can be long and thin
- Sometimes see radiolucent linear structures between spicules
- No skin thickening

RADIATION THERAPY

Clinical

- Overall survival and recurrence rates similar in patients treated with mastectomy and those treated with breast-conserving surgery and subsequent radiation therapy
- "Appropriate" patient: has early stage lesion
- National Surgical Adjuvant Breast Project (NSABP) B-06 trial showed that disease recurred in 40% of women treated with lumpectomy alone (tumor-free margins)
- Additional cancer foci found mainly in the area of the primary tumor
- Purpose of radiation therapy after breast-conserving surgery: control of primary tumor, and eradication of microscopic foci of (multicentric) cancer
- Recurrence rates increase in tumors with extensive intraductal component
- Complications from radiation: brachial plexopathy, arm edema, decreased arm mobility, radiation pneumonitis, rib fractures, soft tissue necrosis, and carcinogenesis
- Typical dose to breast: 45 to 50 Gy (4500 to 5000 rads) given over 5 weeks

- Radiation boost may be given at lumpectomy site (i.e., electrons or iridium implants, which can increase the breast dose to 60 to 65 Gy); more important after excisional biopsy than after wide excision
- Controversy exists over management of axilla
- Postradiation palpation may be soft or firm

Imaging

- Careful mammographic analysis to assess extent of any calcifications and to define other cancer foci helpful before decision made about breast conservation plus radiation versus mastectomy
- Postradiation mammography every 6 months for 3 to 5 years, then yearly
- Postradiation changes: edema results in diffuse increased breast density (maximum at about 6 months; gone by 24 months), skin and trabecular thickening, scarring of parenchyma
- Postradiation calcifications from residual tumor calcifications, necrosis of original tumor, benign dystrophic calcifications

RECONSTRUCTION

Clinical

- Types of reconstruction after mastectomy: *local tissue* plus implant (submuscular implant, tissue expansion, or permanent expander); *distant tissue* with or without implants (latissimus dorsi, transverse rectus abdominis myocutaneous flap, or microvascular free flaps)
- Preservation of nipple not recommended
- Several flap techniques for nipple reconstruction
- Areola refashioned from donor skin (hidden site) then tattooed to match normal coloration
- Uninvolved breast may require augmentation, mastopexy, or reduction to become relatively symmetric
- Optimal timing of reconstruction controversial: some prefer immediate reconstruction, others prefer delayed reconstruction

Imaging

- No value in imaging mastectomy site
- Recurrences found by palpation
- Implant, expander, muscle, and subcutaneous tissue may be seen on the site of prior mastectomy

SARCOMA

Clinical

- Uncommon (less than 1% of all malignant breast tumors)
- Includes angiosarcoma, malignant fibrous histiocytoma, malignant phyllodes tumors, liposarcoma, fibrosarcoma, and others
- Rare malignancies arising from hormonally sensitive breast stroma sometimes called *stromal sarcoma*
- Angiosarcoma probably most common sarcoma of the breast

Imaging

- Masses may be lobulated
- Often well-circumscribed margins
- Microcalcifications generally not a component of these lesions

SCLEROSING ADENOSIS

Clinical

- Adenosis comprises a range of lobular lesions (*see Adenosis*)
- *Sclerosing* refers to occurence of dense hyalinization

- Hyalinization may compress and distort epithelium and be mistaken for malignancy
- If large volume is involved, may be palpable (usually firm and less than 1 cm)
- Most often an incidental microscopic finding
- Microscopically, must be distinguished from tubular carcinoma

Imaging

- Sometimes associated with calcifications that can be detected mammographically
- Core biopsy and needle aspiration biopsy may yield false-positive results for carcinoma

SECRETORY CARCINOMA

Clinical

- Rare form of ductal carcinoma
- May occur in adults, but has been described in preadolescents
- Usually presents as hard, painless mass
- Low-grade clinical behavior
- Histologic findings: eosinophilic-staining material from secretions that resemble lactation
- Has solid and papillary regions
- Prognosis favorable

Imaging

- Often not imaged because of occurrence in children
- If imaged in adult, no distinctive characteristics

SKIN LESIONS

Clinical

- Many skin processes can project over the breast, including neurofibromatosis, seborrheic keratoses, sebaceous cysts, pimples, warts, and moles
- Clinical evaluation and observant mammography technologist are important

Imaging

- Radiopaque marker can be placed on skin lesion before imaging to clarify whether dermal or parenchymal
- Tangential projections also may be performed
- Lucent halo of air sometimes can be seen around skin lesion, which can trap powder and mimic calcification
- Seborrheic keratosis has typical verrucoid appearance with air trapped in the interstices
- Calcifications in sebaceous glands are same size as skin pores and have central lucencies
- Warts rarely calcify, usually have lobulated contour

TUBULAR CARCINOMA

Clinical

- Trend toward younger women
- Elements of tubular carcinoma may be found in other invasive ductal carcinomas
- Pure tubular carcinoma: at least 75% of the tumor must be tubular
- Not common (less than 2% of all breast carcinomas)
- Some believe these evolve from radial scars
- Microscopically, proliferation of small ducts and tubules seen in haphazard arrangement yielding irregular tumors with poorly defined boundaries
- Calcifications in about 50% (usually within an intraductal component)

- Microscopically, must be distinguished from benign entities such as sclerosing adenosis
- Favorable prognosis in pure tubular carcinomas
- May be the slowest growing breast carcinoma

Imaging

- Indistinguishable from other malignant tumors (margins ill defined or spiculated)
- Tends to be small because of slow growth rate (majority less than 1 cm at time of diagnosis)
- Some contain visible microcalcifications, although not a characteristic feature

VASCULAR CALCIFICATIONS

Clinical

- Deposits in the intima
- Generally a consequence of patient age
- In younger women, may be associated with diabetes or dialysis

Imaging

- Characteristic parallel appearance, as in arterial deposits seen elsewhere in the body
- Tubular serpiginous vascular structure is usually visible
- Early calcification may be more difficult to diagnose; magnification views are helpful

7

8

Heart and Great Vessel Imaging

■ **Gordon Gamsu,** M.D.

OVERVIEW

INTERPRETATION

The chest radiograph is often the first examination obtained in suspected cardiac disease. It can provide the first indication of disease or determine the severity of known disease.

Significant cardiac disease is sometimes accurately reflected on the chest radiograph and sometimes present without causing alterations in the size and shape of the heart or of the pulmonary vessels.

A systematic approach allows the radiologist to narrow the diagnostic possibilities. The six entities that must be evaluated are

> Pulmonary vasculature
> Cardiac size and configuration
> Great arteries (aorta and main pulmonary artery)
> Musculoskeletal structures
> Abdominal situs
> Pericardium

The six-step evaluation presented below covers the salient features.

Pulmonary Vasculature. With heart disease, the pulmonary vasculature can show six patterns, as follows:

> Normal
> Increased flow
> With cyanosis
> Without cyanosis
> Increased arterial pressure
> Increased venous pressure
> Decreased flow
> Systemic collaterals

Each pattern must be evaluated for type, severity, and distribution of the abnormality.

> *Normal Pulmonary Vasculature.* The normal pulmonary vessels on a chest radiograph show the following:

Progressive tapering from central to peripheral (arteries branch like an oak tree and veins branch like a pine tree)
Symmetric vascular caliber in the two lungs
Larger vessels in the dependent portions of the lung (bases in the upright patient)
Absence of vessels in the outer 1 to 2 cm of the lung

Normal pulmonary artery (PA) pressure is less than 30/14 mm Hg; normal venous pressure is less than 12 mm Hg.

Differential diagnosis of normal pulmonary vessels includes the following:

Normal
Coronary artery disease without heart failure
Mild left heart obstruction (i.e., mitral/aortic stenosis)
Mild left heart regurgitation (i.e., mitral/aortic regurgitation)
Mild left-to-right shunt (e.g., atrial septal defect, ventricular septal defect, tetralogy of Fallot)

Enlarged heart chambers can be a clue to the correct diagnosis of the cause of a shunt or valvular lesion.

Increased Flow. Increased flow is characterized by the following:

Increased size of pulmonary vessels (arteries and veins) with preservation of the upper lobe: lower lobe differences in caliber
Some increase in the number of visible vessels (recruitment)
Vessels visible to the periphery of the lung

Caveats include the following:

> *It is essential to know whether cyanosis is present.*
> Increased caliber is a slow adaptive change to at least a doubling of pulmonary blood flow (2-to-1 shunt)
> With increased cardiac output (high-output state) such as that seen in anemia or renal failure, the pulmonary vessels can be prominent but do not show features of shunt vessels

The differential diagnosis of *acyanotic increased flow* includes the following:

Atrial septal defect (ASD): right heart and main PA are enlarged; left atrium (LA) is not enlarged unless one of the following is present: a septum primum defect, a cushion defect, or associated mitral disease, e.g., cleft valve or stenosis. The aorta is normal or small. In adults, an ASD is by far the most common cause of a left-to-right shunt.
Ventricular septal defect (VSD): the LA, right ventricle (RV), and main pulmonary artery are enlarged, the right atrium (RA) is normal, and the aorta is normal or small. By adulthood, almost all VSDs have closed or become symptomatic; thus, they are uncommon.
Patent ductus arteriosus (PDA): the LA, left ventricle (LV), and aorta are enlarged.
Arteriovenous malformation (AVM): is a low-pressure system that can handle a large flow. Pulmonary artery hypertension and flow vessels are very rare.
High-output states: with increased cardiac output (e.g., anemia, renal failure), the pulmonary vessels can be prominent but do not show features of shunt vessels.

The differential diagnosis of *cyanotic increased flow* (e.g., admixture lesions, bidirectional/reversed shunts, right-to-left shunts) includes the following:

Transposition of the great vessels (TGV): absence of the main pulmonary artery segment and a narrow vascular pedicle giving an "egg-on-string" appearance to the heart

Truncus arteriosus: prominent vascular pedicle at the base of the heart and often a right aortic arch

Total anomalous pulmonary venous return (TAPVR): shows different features depending on the type (e.g., with the supracardiac type the "snowman" appearance is seen); if venous obstruction is present the appearances can be those of heart failure.

Increased Arterial Pressure. The cardinal feature of increased arterial pressure (i.e., pulmonary hypertension) is an increase in the size of the central fibrous pulmonary arteries. With primary increased pressure, the peripheral arteries taper rapidly and are small. With increased pressure secondary to increased flow (shunt), the peripheral arteries may remain increased in caliber for a long time or permanently.

Increased Venous Pressure. Increased venous pressure is characterized by an increase in the caliber of the pulmonary veins in the upper (nondependent) lungs. The other findings depend on the acuteness of the pressure change and may include:

Acute raised venous pressure (left heart failure): lower lobe vessels are obscured by perivascular edema; the hila show lack of definition from perihilar edema; other findings include loss of the right hilar angle, interstitial edema (septal lines, bronchial cuffs), followed by alveolar edema (flooding).

Chronic raised venous pressure (e.g., mitral stenosis): vascular caliber changes are present, but the lower lobe vessels and hila remain better defined. (Fibrosis can cause thin, sharply defined septal lines.)

Long-standing raised venous pressure: perivascular fibrosis causes the vessels to lose their compliance and they become reduced in caliber. The radiograph then looks more normal and vascular caliber does not reflect intravascular pressures.

Pulmonary hemosiderosis with long-standing left heart failure/venous hypertension: hemosiderin deposition, fibrosis, and even ossification in the lungs occurs (small dense nodules, predominantly at the lung bases).

Caveat: never diagnose left heart failure on the basis of vessel caliber changes alone; other features must also be present.

Decreased Arterial Flow: Decreased arterial flow is characterized by small central and peripheral vessels. Regional decrease in vessel size is seen in emphysema or Swyer-James syndrome. It is more difficult to recognize a global than regional decrease in pulmonary vessel caliber.

Caveat: you are more likely to be wrong than right in detecting global decreased pulmonary vessel size, so do it with great reservation.

Systemic Collaterals to the Lungs. Systemic collaterals to the lungs are characterized by a lacy, almost interstitial appearance to the lungs. Central pulmonary artery or arteries are small. Collaterals can be unilateral or bilateral.

Cardiac Evaluation. In evaluation of the heart, the size of the whole organ and enlargement of specific chambers are assessed.

Heart Size. Both posteroanterior and lateral chest radiographs should be used. On the posteroanterior view, the cardiothoracic ratio is moderately sensitive but reasonably specific (i.e., some large hearts are missed, but few normal-sized hearts are called large). It is the best tool available, so use a cardiothoracic ratio (C/T) of 0.50 or 0.55 (C is the total transverse diameter of the heart, i.e., the horizontal distance between the most right and left cardiac margins; T is the transverse diameter of the thorax from inner rib margins measured at the level of the apex of the right hemidiaphragm).

Always factor in the size of the heart from the lateral radiograph (even though specific measurements or ratios are not available for this projection). If a discrepancy appears between the posteroanterior and lateral views, the lateral should be used, because it is less likely to be misleading.

More sophisticated measurements of heart size can be obtained from the frontal radiograph, but these are not often used.

Specific Chamber Enlargement. The different chambers are best evaluated with specific views.

The LV is evaluated with lateral and left anterior oblique (LAO) views. On the lateral view, find where the inferior vena cava (IVC) intersects the left hemidiaphragm, go up 2 cm, then measure back to the posterior border of the heart (LV); this should not be more than 1.7 cm (Rigler's sign). If the RV is enlarged, it is impossible to assess the LV. Also, the projection must be a true lateral; there cannot be a pectus. On the 60-degree LAO view, the enlarged LV forms a hemispheric projection over the spine, instead of pointing downward.

The RV is evaluated with lateral and right anterior oblique (RAO) views. Lateral is the best. The enlarged RV forms a convex bulge, filling the retrosternal space and contacting the sternum for more than one third of the distance from the diaphragm to the sternomanubrial junction. In most circumstances, a large RV is accompanied by large main or central pulmonary arteries, caused by pulmonary valvular stenosis or pulmonary hypertension (i.e., if no large pulmonary arteries are present, skepticism should exist about the presence of a large RV).

The LA is evaluated by posteroanterior and lateral views. On the posteroanterior view, an enlarged LA shows the following:

Convex bulge to the upper left heart border
"Double density" to the right of the spine, caused by the LA projecting behind the RA
Elevation of the left main bronchus
Calcification of the wall of the LA (this and left atrial appendage enlargement both suggest a rheumatic origin for the LA enlargement)

On the *lateral* view, findings include the following:

Posterior bulge above the position of the LV. A useful measurement is the left atrial-anteroposterior diameter (LA-APD). Find the posterior border of the ascending aorta and drop a perpendicular downward to the middle of the heart. The right-angle distance from this line to the posterior border of the LA, excluding the pulmonary veins, should not exceed 4.5 to 5 cm.
Posterior displacement of the left main bronchus (the dark circle)
Posterior (and usually to the right) displacement of the barium-containing esophagus

Be careful about diagnosing LA enlargement in the absence of pulmonary venous hypertension.

The RA is evaluated by posteroanterior and LAO views. There is no good view to assess the RA. A focal lateral bulge of the right heart border on the posteroanterior view suggests isolated RA enlargement from Ebstein's anomaly. If any other chambers are enlarged, it is *not* possible to detect RA enlargement from plain radiographs.

Great Arteries. The aorta is assessed for the following:

Side (left, right, or both)
Size (normal, small, or large)

In the adult, the ascending aorta should be less than 5 cm in diameter and the descending aorta less than 4.5 cm (more liberality is called for with these measurements in anyone over the age of 50 years).

The central pulmonary arteries are assessed for the following:

Size (normal, unilateral enlargement, bilateral enlargement)
Presence (present, absent)

Musculoskeletal Structures. The bony thorax can show features that are associated with specific entities, as follows:

Sternum/pectus	Mitral valve prolapse
	Marfan's syndrome
	Cardiac compression
Bifid manubrium	Endocardial cushion defects (Down syndrome)
Median sternotomy	Prior surgery, often cardiac

Narrow anteroposterior (AP) diameter of the thorax (less than 8 cm sternum to anterior vertebral bodies) can indicate "straightback" syndrome, with associated murmurs.

Rib notching indicates

> Coarctations of several types (you need to know the differential for bilateral, unilateral left, and unilateral right rib notching)
> Neurofibromatosis
> Idiopathic
> After surgical shunts, e.g., Blalock-Taussig
> Surgical defects: most thoracotomies are through the fifth rib, unless the surgeon can't count; sometimes coarct repairs are higher
> Expansion: anemia, rarely cyanotic congenital heart disease (CHD)
> Infarcts: sickle cell anemia with cardiomyopathy or crisis and cardiomegaly

Cardiac and Abdominal Position (Situs). The atria determine cardiac situs. The IVC usually enters the morphologic right atrium. The liver, spleen, and stomach determine abdominal situs. Cardiac and abdominal situs can be concordant (the same) or discordant (opposite). Organ situs can be

> Situs solitus ("usual position")
>> Cardiac and abdominal organs in normal left-right position
> Situs inversus (with dextrocardia)
>> All cardiac chambers have a left-right inverted position
>> Cardiac anomalies in 5 to 10%
> Situs ambiguous
>> Abdominal organ position is neither right sided nor left sided
>> Lungs are either bilaterally right-sided or left sided
>> Tendency to bronchiectasis and sinusitis (Kartagener syndrome)
>> Splenic abnormalities (asplenia or polysplenia) always present
>> Atria often a common chamber
>> Tendency for bilateral left-sidedness with polysplenia (mnemonic: **left-p**oly); IVC interruption with a big azygous vein
>> Bilateral right-sidedness with asplenia (mnemonic: **right-a**splenia); very severe cardiac defects (e.g., cushion defects, transpositions, pulmonary atresia)

Cardiac (atrial) solitus can be distinguished from inversus in the following way. Look for the position of the stomach bubble. (The IVC invariably is on the opposite side, even though you can't see it.) The IVC is always on the side of the right atrium, and the atria (*not* the aorta) determine cardiac situs. This method does not work in situs ambiguous. Thus, whenever the position of the heart or abdominal organs (or both) looks unusual, first look for the length of the main bronchi and for the minor fissure(s) to be certain that situs ambiguous (two left or two right lungs) is not present. Then look for the stomach bubble.

Dextro refers to the position of the cardiac apex, not to the atria and thus not to situs. The three dextros (not a left-handed jazz band) to be aware of are

> Dextroversion
> Abnormal rotation of the cardiac loop during development, i.e., situs solitus with a right-sided cardiac apex
> High incidence of CHD, especially cyanotic
> Dextroposition
> Rightward displacement of the cardiac apex from a congenital or acquired small right lung such as seen in scimitar (venolobar/hypoplastic right lung) syndrome
> Dextrocardia: the position of the heart is inverted left to right; this can occur as:
>> An isolated anomaly
>> Part of situs inversus totalis
>> Dextrocardia with the asplenia syndrome (bilateral right-sidedness)
>> Dextrocardia with the polysplenia syndrome (bilateral left-sidedness)
>> Dextrocardia with one of the immotile cilia syndromes (exactly 50% have dextrocardia)

An isolated right arch is not a significant anomaly by itself.

8

Pericardium. Evaluation of the pericardium by chest radiographs is limited. Any suspicion of abnormality indicates the need for an echocardiogram. Radiographic features suggesting pericardial disease are calcifications and effusions.

Calcification within the cardiac silhouette occurs at the following six sites:

Pericardium: should extend over more than one chamber; linear/plate-like; often multifocal

Myocardium: linear; conforms to one chamber, most commonly the LA (rheumatic) or LV (ischemic)

Thrombus with the heart chambers: most commonly the LV (especially within an aneurysm) or in an enlarged LA

Coronary arteries: much better seen on computed tomography (CT) or fluoroscopy; linear/tubular; proximal around the aortic root and in the left anterior descending (LAD)

Valves: the most common is the mitral (rheumatic heart disease with mitral stenosis); next is the aortic (congenital bicuspid valve, suggests stenosis); others are rare

Valve annulus: most common is the mitral (1% of elderly women, slightly increased incidence of valvular disease); second is the aortic (degenerative)

There are no reliable findings of a pericardial effusion. Signs that have been described are

"Pericardial stripe:" this is a water-density stripe about 5 mm in thickness and several centimeters long (at least), paralleling the heart border and outlined by two fat-density lines formed by epicardial fat and mediastinal fat. It is much better seen on the lateral radiograph, although even then only in about 20% of large effusions.

Cardiomegaly: cardiac silhouette frequently is enlarged with a pericardial effusion; supposed to have a water-bottle shape (rarely seen).

Dominant or isolated left pleural effusion: is as common as a pericardial stripe and equally predicative.

Therefore, think of a pericardial effusion in any patient with a large heart, a pericardial stripe, or a dominant left effusion.

CONGENITAL HEART DISEASE

In most instances, it is not possible to diagnose a specific congenital heart anomaly or anomalies from chest radiographs. However, one can list probable lesions from the radiographic findings interpreted in conjunction with knowledge of the clinical history, especially whether or not cyanosis (oxygen saturation less than 90%) is present.

Most important in CHD is the assessment of the pulmonary circulation and an understanding of the meaning of any alterations. The three factors that control the caliber of the pulmonary veins and arteries are

Transmural pressure difference, i.e., the difference between the pressure inside the vessel (PA or PV pressure) and that outside the vessel (alveolar pressure)

Compliance of the vessel wall (muscle, elastic tissues, etc.)

Adaptive changes to long-standing alterations in flow (acute changes in flow [within physiologic range] through a vessel have minimal effect on its caliber)

ACQUIRED HEART DISEASE

Acquired heart disease is divided into two groups, depending on whether substantial cardiomegaly is present.

In small heart disease the heart size is normal, or mild cardiomegaly (i.e., cardiothoracic ratio of 0.55 or less) is present. Pathophysiologic mechanism is pressure overload or diminished ventricular compliance.

The differential diagnosis includes the following:

Aortic stenosis

Arterial hypertension
Mitral stenosis
Acute myocardial infarction (MI)
Hypertrophic cardiomyopathy
Restrictive cardiomyopathy
Constrictive pericarditis

In large heart disease, cardiomegaly is substantial (i.e., cardiothoracic ratio more than 0.55). Pathophysiologic mechanism is volume overload and myocardial failure. The differential diagnosis is

Aortic regurgitation
Mitral regurgitation
Tricuspid regurgitation
High-output states
Congestive cardiomyopathy
Ischemic cardiomyopathy
Pericardial effusion

CORONARY ARTERIOGRAPHY

Coronary arteriography is the only method presently available for defining precisely the pathomorphology of the coronary arteries.
The indications for coronary arteriography are

Before surgery for ischemic heart disease
Before angioplasty for ischemic heart disease
Before open heart surgery in patients older than 40 years
Intractable ventricular arrhythmias/"sudden death syndrome"
Congestive cardiomyopathy

Technique.   There are three approaches, as follows:

Percutaneous transfemoral (Judkins): used in almost all cases
Brachial arteriotomy (Sones): used only if severe ileofemoral obstruction prevents use of the femoral route
Axillary: rarely used

The catheters used are either Judkins or Amplatz. Different catheters are used for the left and right coronary arteries. A special catheter is used for coronary bypass grafts.
Four to 8 mL of high-iodine content, nonionic contrast is injected by hand. Recording is on cine at 30 to 60 frames per second.
Positioning requires various degrees of obliquity (LAO or RAO) and angulation (cranial or caudal) of the tube, depending on the portion of the circulation being evaluated:

Cranial LAO for ostial lesions of the left coronary artery (LCA); proximal LAD; and circumflex
Caudal LAO for the origin of the circumflex and proximal ramus intermedius
Caudal RAO for the proximal circumflex
Cranial RAO for the origin of the acute diagonals
Cranial LAO for the proximal posterior descending (PD) and posterolaterals

Coronary Artery Anatomy.   The coronary arteries are on the epicardial surface of the heart within the atrioventricular (AV) or interventricular grooves.

Left Coronary Artery (LCA).   The LCA originates from the left sinus of Valsalva and is 1 to 2 cm long. It gives rise to two or three branches, as follows:

LAD: courses in the interventricular groove, terminates just past the apex; visible face-on in LAO view and in profile in RAO view; its branches are
Septal arteries: run at a right angle to the LAD and supply the upper two thirds of the ventricular septum
Diagonal arteries: run from the LAD to supply the anterolateral wall of the LV

Circumflex: courses in the left half of the AV groove and usually terminates at the junction of the AV and interventricular grooves (the groovy crux [cross]); visible face-on in the RAO view and in profile in the LAO view; branches are the obtuse marginal arteries supplying the LV wall not supplied by diagonal arteries

Ramus intermedius: about 15 to 30% of the time the LCA trifurcates; the third branch is the ramus intermedius (medianus), whose branches supply that portion of the lateral wall of the LV not supplied by the diagonals or obtuse marginals

Right coronary artery (RCA).   The RCA originates from the right sinus of Valsalva and courses in the right half of the AV groove. It gives rise to five or six branches, as follows:

Conus (50% of patients): runs anteriorly over the RV outflow tract
Sinoatrial (SA) node: runs posteriorly to supply the SA node
Acute marginals: supply the lateral wall of the RV
AV node: a branch arising at the crux supplies the atrioventricular node
Posterior descending: at the crux, the PD artery lies in the posterior interventricular groove and terminates near the apex of the heart; it has small septal branches supplying the lower third of the septum

The RCA is seen face-on in the RAO and in profile in the LAO; the PDA is seen face-on in the LAO and in profile in the RAO. Table 8–1 summarizes the vessels seen in the RAO and LAO views.

In dealing with coronary arteriograms, dominance (a question often asked) refers to which coronary artery supplies the diaphragmatic surface of the LV and the interventricular septum. In *right dominance* (which occurs in 85% of people), the RCA supplies the diaphragmatic surface of the LV and interventricular septum via the PDA and posterior LV branches. In *left dominance* (8%), the LCA via the circumflex supplies most of the heart. In *codominance* (7%), the RCA supplies the PDA and the LCA supplies the LV branches via the circumflex.

Interpretation.   Coronary angiograms are reviewed for the following findings:

Anatomic variants: for example, the most common is anomalous origin of the circumflex from the RCA
Stenoses: usually described as a percent reduction from normal luminal diameter: a reduction of more than 50% is considered hemodynamically significant; a 50% decrease in diameter is a 75% decrease in cross-sectional area; a 75% decrease in diameter is a 95% decrease in cross-sectional area
Morphology of the stenosis: especially ulceration of plaques, which are considered ominous for occlusion
Collateral vessels: the common collaterals are from:
LAD occlusion/stenosis
RCA to distal LAD via marginal branches
Proximal LAD to distal LAD via septal branches
RCA to LAD via conus branch
RCA occlusion/stenosis:
LAD to PDA via septal branches
Circumflex to distal RCA at the crux

Table 8–1. Vessels Seen in Left and Right Anterior Oblique Views

View	Seen Face-on	Seen in Profile
Left anterior oblique (LAO)	LAD*	Circumflex
	PDA	Right coronary artery
Right anterior oblique (RAO)	Circumflex	LAD
	Right coronary artery	PDA

* Mnemonic: the LA-PD go together and are in your face in (the) LA(O).
LAD, left anterior descending artery; PDA, posterior descending artery.

Marginal branches of the circumflex to posterior LV branches
Circumflex occlusion/stenosis:
Proximal circumflex to distal circumflex
High marginals to low marginals

LV VENTRICULOGRAM

The following features must be described:

LV size and the ejection fraction
Competence and status of the mitral/aortic valves
Regional LV function, divided into:
Akinesis: no systolic wall motion
Hypokinesis: reduced systolic wall motion
Dyskinesis: paradoxical outward systolic wall motion
Asynchrony: wall motion normal in direction but out of phase with the rest of the LV
Complications of prior MIs, e.g., LV aneurysm, mural thrombus, papillary muscle dysfunction (usually mitral regurgitation), VSD from septal infarction

CARDIAC NUCLEAR MEDICINE

Clinical applications are continuing to expand as a result of newer, function-specific radiopharmaceuticals; the evolution of single photon emission tomography (SPECT), with its improved spatial resolution giving better sensitivity and specificity; and the evolution of positron emission tomography (PET), with its metabolic tracers.

Myocardial Perfusion. The information obtained allows for inferential conclusions on the territorial supply of the coronary arteries and regional viability of the myocardium. The technique is performed under stress (induced by exercise or pharmacologic agent) and, if results are abnormal, under rest conditions.

Stress Protocol. The stress protocol is

Standardized exercise treadmill or intravenous (IV) infusion of pharmacologic stress agent
One minute before completion of exercise or plateau of stress agent effect, 3.0 to 3.5 mCi of thallium-201 injected via an indwelling catheter
After a 15- to 20-minute delay, SPECT imaging started
Thallium SPECT acquisition performed over a 180-degree arc from RAO to LPO; anterior only approach because of attenuation of low energy from thallium (mercury: 68–83 KeV)
Patient is supine, decubitus, or prone
Usual method uses a single-detector, rotating-head SPECT system
Matrix usually 64 × 64, and 60 to 64 images are collected using filtered, backprojection algorithms
Tomographic slices are in long and short cardiac axes, through the LV myocardium

Rest Protocol. The rest protocol is

Three- to 4-hour delayed images ("redistribution images")/second injection/ separate rest studies are all employed
Imaging parameters are otherwise the same as for poststress images

Interpretation. The radiologist looks for defects. Emphasis is placed on the contiguous oblique short-axis slices, and results are categorized as follows:

Normal (no defects)
Reversible ischemia (stress-induced defects)
Prior infarction/severe stenosis (persistent defects)
Ischemia (reverse redistribution—rapid wash-out from normal myocardium)
LV failure (increased lung activity with exercise)

Causes of Misinformation. False-positive results may be caused by:

> Coronary spasm
> Other heart disease (e.g., bundle branch block)
> Systolic bridging
> Patient motion
> High diaphragm
> Pacemaker
> Ascites
> Large breasts

False-negative results may be caused by

> Peripheral arterial disease
> Inadequate stress
> Excessive delay to imaging
> Developed collaterals
> Diffuse uniform ischemia ("triple-vessel disease")

Agents to Induce Stress. Stress-inducing agents are

> Dipyridamole (IV, 0.14 mg/kg/min)
> Thallium given with increased heart rate, symptoms, or decreased blood pressure
> Adenosine (IV, 0.14 mg/kg/min); higher incidence of side effects

Agents for Myocardial SPECT Imaging. The agents used for myocardial SPECT imaging are

> Thallium-201 (3.0 mCi)
> Technetium-99m Sestamibi (7–30 mCi)

Myocardial Infarct Imaging. The agent used is technetium-99m pyrophosphate (20 mCi); pyrophosphate is a calcium analogue that enters the damaged myocardial cell. Maximal abnormality is seen at 2 to 3 days. The study can be abnormal with increased deposition for 7 to 10 days after an infarct.

Blood Pool Imaging. Red blood cells are labeled with technetium-99m pertechnetate or stannous pyrophosphate. The technique is

> Electrocardiogram (ECG)-gated
> R wave triggered
> R-R interval divided into 20 frames, 150,000 to 200,000 counts per frame
> Supine rest study in different projections
> Sitting rest-exercise study in LAO view

The following information is provided:

> Ventricular volumes
> Ejection fraction (normal: more than 0.50)
> Wall motion, which is classified as
> > Normal
> > Hypokinesis: reduced motion
> > Akinesis: no motion
> > Dyskinesis: paradoxical systolic motion
> Aneurysm: focal diastolic bulge with akinesis or dyskinesis and a "gooseneck" effect (not to be confused with the "gooseneck" deformity found with an AV canal)

HEART AND GREAT VESSELS DIFFERENTIAL DIAGNOSES

Shunt lesions
> Acyanotic, increased pulmonary blood flow, with or without increased heart size

Left-to-right shunts
Cyanotic, decreased pulmonary blood flow, "normal" heart size
Right-to-left shunts
Cyanotic, increased pulmonary blood flow, big heart
Admixture (bidirectional) shunts
Cyanotic, decreased pulmonary blood flow, big heart
Pulmonary hypertension
Acquired large heart disease
Acquired small heart disease

SHUNT LESIONS

ACYANOTIC, INCREASED PULMONARY BLOOD FLOW, WITH OR WITHOUT INCREASED HEART SIZE

LEFT-TO-RIGHT SHUNTS

Name five causes of a left-to-right shunt.

Atrial septal defect (ASD)
Ventricular septal defect (VSD)
Patent ductus arteriosus (PDA)
Partial anomalous pulmonary venous return
AP window
Coronary artery-to-pulmonary artery shunt
Systemic AV fistula
SV aneurysm
Cushion defect

Radiographic features

• Increased pulmonary vasculature with or without cardiomegaly

Atrial septal defect (ASD)

• Right heart and main PA enlarged
• LA not enlarged unless there is septum primum defect, cushion defect, or associated mitral disease (e.g., cleft valve or stenosis)
• Aorta normal or small
• Most common cause of left-to-right shunt in adults

Ventricular septal defect (VSD)

• LA, RV, and main pulmonary artery enlarged
• RA normal
• Aorta normal or small
• By adulthood, almost all closed or corrected because symptomatic; thus, uncommon

Patent ductus arteriosus (PDA)

• LA, LV, and aorta enlarged

Partial anomalous pulmonary venous return

• Low-pressure system that can handle large flow
• Pulmonary artery hypertension does not occur
• Shunt vasculature not evident

CYANOTIC, DECREASED PULMONARY BLOOD FLOW, "NORMAL" HEART SIZE

RIGHT-TO-LEFT SHUNT

Name four causes of CHD with cyanosis and a normal-sized heart.

Tetralogy of Fallot
Pulmonary atresia type I
Double-outlet right ventricle (DORV) with pulmonary stenosis (PS)
Transposition of great vessels (TGV) with PS
Corrected transposition of great vessels (CTGV) with PS
Single ventricle (SV) with PS
PS with ASD (or PVC)
Hypoplastic RV
Tricuspid atresia (some types)

Radiographic features

• Normal or "decreased" pulmonary vasculature
• Heart size normal or slightly enlarged

CYANOTIC, INCREASED PULMONARY BLOOD FLOW, BIG HEART

ADMIXTURE (BIDIRECTIONAL) SHUNT

List five causes of CHD with cyanosis and a large heart.

TGV
Truncus arteriosus
Total anomalous pulmonary venous return (TAPVR)
DORV
SV
SA
Hypoplastic left heart
Tricuspid atresia without PS
AV canal
Large/multiple pulmonary AVMs

Clinical features

• Cyanosis (often mild)
• CHF

Radiographic features

• Increased pulmonary vasculature
• Increased heart size

Transposition of great vessels

• Absence of main pulmonary artery segment and narrow vascular pedicle give "egg-on-string" appearance to heart

Truncus arteriosus

• Prominent vascular pedicle at base of heart, and often a right aortic arch

Total anomalous pulmonary venous return

- Shows different features depending on type
- "Snowman" appearance in supracardiac type
- If venous obstruction is present, appearance can be that of heart failure

CYANOTIC, DECREASED PULMONARY BLOOD FLOW, BIG HEART

Ebstein anomaly
Tricuspid atresia (some types)
Pulmonary atresia type II
Severe PS with ASD

Radiographic features

- Normal or "decreased" pulmonary vasculature
- Heart size increased (often markedly)

PULMONARY HYPERTENSION

Causes

- Secondary to increased flow (reversal of VSD or ASD to produce Eisenmenger's syndrome physiology)
- Secondary to increased pressure caused by abnormalities:
    - ¶ In vessel lumen, e.g., embolic blood clots, parasites (schistosomiasis most common cause of pulmonary hypertension in the world), or foreign substances (e.g., talc)
    - ¶ In vessel wall, e.g., vasculitis, some poisons
    - ¶ In lung parenchyma; caused by obstructive or restrictive lung disease, e.g., emphysema, chronic bronchitis, sarcoid, interstitial fibrosis
    - ¶ In inhaled air, e.g., hypoxia, sleep apnea syndromes
    - ¶ In chest wall, e.g., scoliosis
    - ¶ Idiopathic, i.e., essential (primary) pulmonary hypertension

NONCARDIOGENIC PULMONARY EDEMA

Causes

List six causes of noncardiogenic pulmonary edema.

- Via blood stream
    - ¶ Septicemia (toxins)
    - ¶ Drugs (cocaine, heroin, aspirin overdose, valium, methadone)
    - ¶ Anaphylactic reaction (blood, contrast, antibiotics, etc.)
    - ¶ Poisons (parathion)
    - ¶ Reexpansion (lung must be atelectatic for at least 72 hours)
- Via airway
    - ¶ Near drowning
    - ¶ Asphyxia
    - ¶ Inhalation of noxious gases (nitrous oxide, sulfur dioxide [N_2O, SO_2, smoke, etc.])
    - ¶ Upper airway obstruction
- Via nerves
    - ¶ High altitude

¶ Increased intracranial pressure

"LARGE HEART" HEART DISEASE

Aortic regurgitation
Mitral regurgitation
Tricuspid regurgitation
High-output states
Congestive cardiomyopathy
Ischemic cardiomyopathy
Pericardial effusion

Clinical

- Substantial cardiomegaly, i.e., cardiothoracic ratio more than 0.55
- Pathophysiology: volume overload and myocardial failure

"SMALL HEART" HEART DISEASE

Aortic stenosis
Arterial hypertension
Mitral stenosis
Acute myocardial infarction
Hypertrophic cardiomyopathy
Restrictive cardiomyopathy
Constrictive pericarditis

Clinical

- Normal to mild cardiomegaly, i.e., cardiothoracic ratio 0.55 or less
- Pathophysiology: pressure overload or diminished ventricular compliance

HEART AND GREAT VESSEL DISEASE ENTITIES

CONGENITAL HEART DISEASE

AP Window

Clinical
- Shunt is ascending aorta to main PA

Imaging
- Findings same as in PDA

Atrial Septal Defect

Clinical
- Several types exist

Septum Secundum
- Most common form of CHD
- Most frequent CHD to present in adulthood
- Defect in middle of septum
- Not uncommonly asymptomatic
- Sometimes mistaken for long-standing mitral stenosis with pulmonary hypertension

Septum Primum
- Much less common; part of partial cushion defect and thus often has associated mitral defects, e.g., cleft mitral valve with regurgitation
- Defect is low and anterior in septum

Sinus Venosus
- Defect is high, near SVC
- Usually partial anomalous pulmonary venous connection (PAPVC) (findings depend on the degree of pulmonary venous obstruction)

Lutembacher Syndrome
- ASD with acquired mitral stenosis; now rare, so it is not necessary to know details

Imaging
- Enlarged RA, RV, central pulmonary arteries
- Shunt vessels
- Normal to small LA, aortic arch

Coarctation of the Aorta

Clinical
- Usually presents in childhood
- Upper limb hypertension
- Obstruction at the aortic isthmus
- Associated bicuspid aortic valve
- Systolic murmur

Imaging
- Enlarged ascending aorta, great arteries, internal mammary arteries (retrosternal opacities on lateral view), intercostal arteries (rib notching), superior intercostal arteries (masses over the apices)
- "Three" sign (formed by dilated left subclavian and aortic nob)
- "Reverse three" sign (impression on the barium-filled esophagus from the prestenotic and poststenotic dilatation of aorta)
- Bicuspid aortic valve (stenosis, calcification later in life) (85%)

Ebstein Anomaly

Clinical
- Should not be confused with Eisenmenger syndrome, which is pulmonary hypertension and reversal of a left-to-right shunt that causes cyanosis

Imaging
- Enlarged (massively) RV and RA (from the ventricular insertion of the septal and posterior leaflets of the tricuspid valve); tricuspid insufficiency; and tremendous overload of RV and RA
- Pulmonary vasculature normal to decreased

Endocardial Cushion Defect

Clinical
Complete (AV Canal)
- ASD, VSD, cleft mitral valve, cleft tricuspid valve

Partial
- Primum ASD, cleft mitral valve

Imaging
Complete
- Enlarged RA, RV, LA, and LV
- CHF
- Eisenmenger syndrome
- Mitral regurgitation
- Tricuspid regurgitation

Partial
- ASD with or without mitral regurgitation
- Enlarged LV

PAPVC

Clinical
- Three types:
  - Right upper pulmonary vein to SVC
  - Left upper pulmonary veins to persistent left SVC (straight vein) to left brachio-cephalic veins to SVC
  - All or most of right lung pulmonary veins to IVC or hepatic veins (scimitar syndrome)
- Components of scimitar syndrome: hypoplastic right lung (decreased number of segments), PAPVC, and systemic arterial supply to right lower lung, with or without the following: proximal interruption of the right PA, large left PA, bronchiectasis in the right lung, bilateral left sidedness
- Scimitar syndrome is an important entity; its components must be known

Imaging
- Enlarged RV and RA
- Shunt vessels
- ASD

Patent Ductus Arteriosus (PDA)

Clinical
- Continuous "machinery" murmur
- Usually diagnosed shortly after birth or childhood
- Shunt is descending aorta to main pulmonary artery
- Physiology is left heart overload

Imaging
- Enlarged LA, LV, aorta, central pulmonary arteries
- Shunt vessels
- RA, RV normal

Tetralogy of Fallot

Clinical
- Consists of VSD, RV hypertrophy, infundibular PS, and aorta overriding the VSD (increasing right-to-left shunt)

Imaging
- Chest radiograph:
  - "Boot-shaped" heart; lower left heart border on PA sticks out and has rounded contour from the big RV, displacing and distorting the LV
  - Concave main PA segment (enhancing toe of boot)
  - Dilated aorta
  - Decreased to normal pulmonary vasculature
  - Right aortic arch with mirror-image great vessels (25%)

Ventricular Septal Defect

Clinical
- 10% of congenital heart disease
- Left-to-right shunt at level of ventricles
- Large shunts result in dyspnea and pansystolic murmur

Imaging
- Enlarged LA, LV, RV, central pulmonary arteries
- Shunt vessels
- Normal RA, aortic arch

- CHF in infancy
- Spontaneous closure in 50% by age of 5 years and in 75% by age of 10 years
- Adults have asymptomatic small defects or were symptomatic in infancy/childhood and had surgery

ACQUIRED HEART DISEASE

HEART DISEASE WITHOUT CARDIOMEGALY ("SMALL HEART" HEART DISEASE)

Acute Myocardial Infarction

Clinical
Papillary muscle rupture
- Dramatic in onset with acute intractable pulmonary edema
- Caused by infarction of one of the papillary muscles of mitral valve, resulting in acute mitral regurgitation
- Partial rupture with less severe mitral regurgitation and no pulmonary edema can also occur

Rupture of interventricular septum
- Uncommon and frequently fatal

Imaging
First 24 hours
- 50% normal
- 50% show some features of acute pulmonary venous hypertension or pulmonary edema (from decreased LV compliance); at early stage, degree of pulmonary venous hypertension (judged from chest radiographs) correlates with subsequent patient survival
- Cardiomegaly uncommon with first heart attack

After 24 hours
- Cardiac rupture; contained rupture may not be fatal; may present with pericardial effusion
- LV aneurysm, both true and false (pseudoaneurysm)
  True LV Aneurysm
     Most patients have normal chest radiograph; entity suspected from ECG changes or persistent LV failure (or both) and confirmed with echocardiography, CT, or magnetic resonance imaging (MRI)
     If present, radiographic abnormality is a bulge along lower-mid left heart border or in region of cardiac apex (usual sites for true LV aneurysms)
     Myocardial calcification as manifestation of LV aneurysm rare from radiographs but not infrequent on CT or fluoroscopy
     Occlusion usually affects LAD
  False LV Aneurysm
     If bulge is posterior, more likely to be a false aneurysm
     Other features suggesting false aneurysm: large size and projection on posterior and/or diaphragmatic surfaces of heart
     Occlusion usually affects circumflex or right coronary artery

Papillary muscle rupture
- Pulmonary edema
- Little or no cardiomegaly or left atrial enlargement in patient with mitral regurgitation murmur

Rupture of interventricular septum
- Findings varied
- Mild cardiac enlargement
- Shunt vessels (after time)
- Left heart failure
- Cardiomegaly increases if patient survives weeks or months

8

Aortic Stenosis

Clinical
- Mechanism: pressure overload; initially compensated for by concentric hypertrophy of LV, which reduces size of LV chamber but does not cause cardiomegaly
- Causes: congenital; degeneration of a bicuspid (rarely unicuspid or tricuspid) valve; rheumatic heart disease, hypertension in older patients

Imaging
- Pulmonary vasculature normal until LV decompensation occurs; this is the turning point in aortic stenosis
- LV failure results in cardiac enlargement, pulmonary venous hypertension, and pulmonary edema
- Pulmonary venous hypertension occasionally seen with normal-sized heart compromised by reduced LV compliance
- Key finding: enlargement of ascending aorta; present in almost all cases but without enlargement of aortic arch or descending aorta
- With aortic regurgitation, the entire aorta frequently is enlarged; in older patients, the aorta may be enlarged from atherosclerosis and useless for cardiac evaluation
- Calcification of aortic valve seen on chest radiographs in minority of patients
- On fluoroscopy, extent of calcification of aortic valve relates to severity of pressure gradient across valve
- Chest radiograph poor for detecting LV hypertrophy
- Echocardiography and MRI: can measure ventricular wall thickness and better detect LV hypertrophy; can measure LV mass and gradient across valve
- Caliber of aorta has no relationship to severity of stenosis; probably consequence of eccentric jet across stenotic valve

Constrictive Pericarditis

Clinical
- Increasing in frequency
- Causes:
    Iatrogenic from postoperative bleeding, especially with cardiac revascularization procedures
    Mediastinal radiation
    Repeated episodes of viral pericarditis
    Uremic pericarditis (less common) and is more likely to be effusive
    Tuberculosis used to be common cause; now rare, but increasing because of acquired immunodeficiency syndrome (AIDS)
- Mechanism of left heart failure is restriction to LA emptying during diastole; important fact, frequently asked
- Most patients do not have pericardial effusion
- In *effusive constrictive pericarditis*, both clinical and functional constriction and pericardial effusion are present; after drainage of effusion, constriction persists, indicating that fluid was not the cause (? visceral pericardial constriction)

Imaging
- If hemodynamically significant, chest radiograph likely to be abnormal
- Pulmonary venous hypertension
- Various degrees of pulmonary edema
- Normal or near-normal heart size
- LA can enlarge out of proportion to ventricular enlargement
- In small number of patients, right and less commonly left heart borders show "flattening," reputed to be pathognomonic of constrictive pericarditis and supposedly from scarring with flattening of atrial contours
- Pericardial calcification: generally spans more than one chamber; more dense in interatrial and interventricular grooves; best method of detection is rapid CT
- Pleural effusion: classically, isolated left or dominant left effusion, especially without left heart failure, suggestive of pericardial constriction
- SVC distention: difficult to detect and to determine its significance

Dressler Syndrome

Clinical
- Caused by disruption of heart muscle after infarction; release of antigens and autoimmune response
- Occurs in days to months after MI

Imaging
- Pleural and pericardial effusions (unilateral or bilateral) in patient with fever, pain, and malaise

Hypertensive Heart Disease

Clinical
- Pressure overload; heart size is normal as long as it is compensated
- Presence and severity of LV hypertrophy cannot be determined from chest radiograph

Imaging
- Normal heart size
- Normal pulmonary vessels
- No specific cardiac chamber enlargement
- Prominent thoracic aorta, especially arch and descending aorta

Hypertrophic Cardiomyopathy

Clinical
- Approximately 30% of symptomatic patients have mitral regurgitation with LA enlargement
- Cardiomegaly with hypertrophic cardiomyopathy caused by mitral regurgitation or end-stage failing heart (enlarged LA should be evident)
- Can occur as isolated entity or with neurofibromatosis, Noonan syndrome, or lentiginosis syndrome

Imaging
- In 50%, chest radiograph is normal
- In 50%, chest radiograph is not specific for the disease; in those with reduced ventricular compliance, lungs may show features of pulmonary venous hypertension (usually mild)
- In a small minority, left heart border is squared-off because of extreme enlargement of outflow portion of interventricular septum
- Echocardiography or MRI used to judge severity and distribution of hypertrophied myocardium
- With obstructive form of cardiomyopathy, AS-type ejection murmur usually is present, without prominence of the ascending aorta (a pretty flimsy piece of evidence to establish a diagnosis, but it at least can explain the findings and get one off the hook)

Mitral Stenosis

Clinical
- Pressure overload lesion that does not cause generalized cardiomegaly, but enlargement of LA
- Normal 4 to 6 cm² surface area of mitral valve reduced to 1.5 to 2 cm²
- About 50% of patients develop venous hypertension and have hemoptysis; 50% develop arterial hypertension and RV enlargement
- Pulmonary venous hypertension (sequential): increase in upper lobe vein caliber, reduction in lower lobe vein caliber, septal lines and bronchial cuffs, pulmonary hemosiderosis, pulmonary calcification, interstitial fibrosis
- Pulmonary arterial hypertension: RV enlargement and right heart failure; occasionally RV enlargement from concomitant tricuspid regurgitation, usually from rheumatic heart disease
- Radiographic findings diagnostic and correlate with severity of stenosis

8

Imaging
- Heart size normal
- LA enlarged (big LA appendage indicative of rheumatic cause for mitral stenosis)
- Minor or no obscuration of vessels; no alveolar edema
- When right heart enlarged and main PA normal in size, think of tricuspid regurgitation or, rarely, pulmonic stenosis
- When LV is enlarged with mitral stenosis, think of mitral regurgitation with mitral stenosis (mixed mitral valve disease); rarely, LV enlargement is caused by active rheumatic myocarditis (unusual in the United States today)
- When LV and thoracic aorta are enlarged with mitral stenosis, think of aortic regurgitation
- When LV and only ascending aorta are enlarged with mitral stenosis, think of the less common rheumatic aortic stenosis

Restrictive Cardiomyopathy

Clinical
- Rarer than hypertrophic cardiomyopathy
- Causes: idiopathic or infiltrative diseases, e.g., sarcoidosis, hemochromatosis, amyloidosis

Imaging
- Early: heart size normal; pulmonary venous hypertension (from decreased LV compliance); and, uncommonly, LA enlarged; radiographic findings can thus closely mimic those of mitral stenosis
- Late: LA and LV enlargement causes moderate cardiomegaly; pulmonary venous hypertension; pleural effusions
- If restrictive cardiomyopathy progresses to congestive cardiomyopathy, considerable generalized heart enlargement occurs

HEART DISEASE WITH CARDIOMEGALY ("BIG HEART" HEART DISEASE)

Aortic Regurgitation

Clinical
- Causes: bacterial endocarditis, rheumatic heart disease, myxomatous degeneration of valve; also secondary to aortic root dilatation in Marfan syndrome, syphilitic aortitis, and aortic dissection
- Severity of disease as manifest by heart size on chest radiographs correlates with prognosis:

Cardiothoracic Ratio	Survival
Less than 0.55	85% 5-year survival after surgery
More than 0.60	45% survival

Imaging
- Enlarged left ventricle
- Enlarged ascending, arch, and descending aorta
- Pulmonary vasculature normal until LV fails
- When LV fails, pulmonary venous hypertension and pulmonary edema occur (both poor prognostic findings)

Congestive (Dilated) Cardiomyopathy

Clinical
- Causes: ischemic heart disease (in fact, to be pedantic, congestive cardiomyopathy is really classified as "dilated cardiomyopathy of unknown etiology")
- Usually diagnosis of exclusion; radiologist must be sure no systemic disease is present that could be the cause (e.g., sarcoid, hemochromatosis, connective tissue disease, diabetes mellitus, thyroid dysfunction, acromegaly, peripheral myopathy)

Imaging
- Findings relatively nonspecific
- Substantially enlarged heart

- Pulmonary venous hypertension/edema (most patients)
- No features to indicate mitral, tricuspid, or aortic valvular disease
- Differential diagnosis: pericardial effusion

Mitral Regurgitation

Clinical
- Causes:
    Rheumatic heart disease
    Mitral valve prolapse
    Postinfarction papillary muscle dysfunction
    Infectious endocarditis
    Degenerative disease causing rupture of chordae tendineae
    Systematic diseases such as Marfan syndrome
    Associated with annular calcification
    Secondary to LV dilatation in CHF, cardiomyopathy

Imaging
- Enlarged LV, LA, and sometimes RV and RA; LA appendage is enlarged when the cause is rheumatic heart disease (90%); giant LA can be found with mitral stenosis or, more commonly, with regurgitation
- Pulmonary venous hypertension (mild when compensated, unlike that in mitral stenosis)
- Aorta normal in size

Pericardial Effusion

Clinical
- Causes: infection (viral, bacterial), malignancy, autoimmune disease, uremia, CHF, trauma, and postsurgical

Imaging
- Findings relatively nonspecific
- Cardiomegaly (about 40% of cases)
- "Water-bottle"–shaped heart difficult to recognize
- Pericardial stripe (approximately 15% of cases; literature incorrectly states 50%)
- Dominant or unilateral left effusion (approximately 20% of cases)
- "Varying density" sign seen on frontal radiograph as lesser density to heart silhouette laterally than centrally; I think this is an impossible sign to appreciate with high kVp chest radiographs
- Echocardiography, CT, and MRI: only reasonable way to diagnose a pericardial effusion

Tricuspid Regurgitation

Clinical
- Incidence increasing because of bacterial endocarditis associated with IV drug abuse; other causes: rheumatic heart disease and various RV dysplasias

Imaging
- Can be difficult to detect, especially enlargement of RA, until substantial
- Best signs:
    RA enlargement (elongation and rightward bulge to right heart border)
    Normal or reduced pulmonary vascularity
    Generalized cardiomegaly
    Occasionally SVC or IVC enlargement (the latter readily detected with ultrasound)
- Most likely diagnosis for cardiomegaly with RA enlargement is tricuspid regurgitation; differential diagnosis: congestive cardiomyopathy and pericardial effusion

ACQUIRED AORTIC DISEASE

Aortic Dissection

Clinical
- Caused by spontaneous bleeding/rupture into media of aorta, with dissection of hematoma in proximal or distal direction
- Communication with lumen of aorta at one or more sites
- Most common origin just distal to left subclavian artery; also found in aortic root, ascending aorta, descending aorta
- 2 to 5% focal (only a few centimeters long)
- Classification:
  - Type A: involves ascending aorta with or without descending aorta (usually requires surgical repair)
  - Type B: involves only descending aorta (usually treated medically, unless features of impending aortic rupture are present)

Imaging
- Chest radiographs
  - Frequently show surprising paucity of abnormalities
  - Never exclude clinically suspected diagnosis because the chest radiograph is negative!
  - Aortic widening; usually only mild (5 to 10 cm) and unimpressive
  - Discrepancy can be present in size of ascending and descending aorta but is difficult to detect
  - Displaced intimal calcification more than 4 to 5 mm from outer wall of aorta useful but not common; beware of this sign on frontal view in aortic arch: frequently it is falsely positive because of curvature of aorta
  - Most other findings seen only when dissection leaks into mediastinum or starts to rupture; then mediastinal widening, displaced trachea or esophagus, left effusion, obscured arch, widened paraspinous line can be seen, as in other causes of rupture
- MRI/MRA: best modality (in experienced hands) for stable patient; false lumen and flap can be imaged as well as extension of dissection to abdomen or great arteries off aorta
- CT, especially spiral CT: probably as good as MRI; findings:
  - Two lumens; with chronic (? 20%) or even acute dissection, second lumen (false) may be thrombosed
  - Displaced calcium in flap between the lumens; beware of calcium within aortic mural thrombus
  - Enlarged aortic contour (nonspecific)
  - Other findings relate to leaking and mediastinal hematoma
- Angiography: reserved for type A dissections and only when thoracic surgeon wants to know status of coronary arteries, great arteries, and abdominal aortic branches

Aortic Rupture

Clinical
- Important to know all about this entity
- Causes:
  - Trauma, most commonly deceleration in motor vehicle accident or fall from a height
  - After surgical repair of aneurysm or dissection
  - As complication of aortic dissection or aneurysm
- If cause is unspecified, then one is referring to the traumatic variety
- More than 85% of patients are dead on arrival; mortality increases with continued delay before treatment
- 2% are missed and present later with focal false aneurysm at the aortic isthmus (region between left subclavian artery and ligamentum arteriosum)

Imaging
- Obscuration of aortic arch (most common finding)
- Upper mediastinum generally widened

- Widened left paraspinous line
- Left apical cap (extrapleural dissection of blood)
- Rightward displacement of the trachea or esophagus or their contained tubes
- Left pleural effusion
- Widened right paraspinous line
- Thickened right paratracheal stripe
- Depressed left main bronchus
- All radiographic findings can be simulated by venous bleeding; diagnosis must be confirmed by aortography unless spiral CT is diagnostic
- Spiral CT: used in patients in whom there is low clinical suspicion of rupture, few or no clinical findings, and raised suspicion of widened mediastinum; under these circumstances CT can exclude hematoma as cause of radiographic appearance (usually fat in mediastinum), and in stable patients raising a high clinical suspicion
- In these patients, spiral CT can demonstrate aortic tears, flaps, and ruptures in a reasonably high percentage of patients

8

Interventional Radiology

■ Scott Schultz, M.D.

OVERVIEW

Angiography is used to answer specific clinical questions that cannot be answered by noninvasive methods (such as spiral computed tomography [CT], ultrasound, and magnetic resonance [MR] angiography). The first goal of any angiographic procedure is to ascertain the anatomy of the area of interest. Once the anatomy is portrayed clearly, the next step can be undertaken. A diagnostic arteriogram is the cornerstone of all vascular interventions. The patient may need only a diagnostic arteriogram from an interventional radiologist before an operative procedure. When the diagnostic arteriogram reveals a problem that can be treated with interventional therapy, that procedure can be performed. The basic vascular interventions performed include thrombolysis, angioplasty, atherectomy, vascular stents, inferior vena cava (IVC) filters, and transjugular intrahepatic portosystemic shunts (TIPS).

The vast array of interventional procedures performed today can be overwhelming to the radiology resident. All angiographic procedures involve the same principle, which requires three basic tools: a needle, a guidewire, and a catheter. All arterial and venous catheterizations employ standard Seldinger technique. Although there are several types of needles, numerous types of guidewires, and innumerable types of catheters, the basic procedure is always the same. The specific combination used in each case depends on the patient and the specific clinical situation.

The standard approach to arterial catheterization involves a double-wall puncture using a double-wall needle and Seldinger technique. Double-wall puncture is used for femoral and transaxillary approaches. The axillary approach is used when there is no femoral pulse. The axillary approach is also used in the setting of severe pelvic trauma, groin infections, or recent groin surgery.

EQUIPMENT

Catheters. Important variables involved in the selection of a catheter include material, size, shape, length, and presence of side holes. Catheter size is measured by outside diameter (OD): 1 French is one third of a millimeter (6 Fr = 2 mm). Catheter material is typically polyethylene or braided nylon. Catheter shapes and their uses are as follows:

Pigtail	Aortography
Cobra	Visceral angiography
Simmons	Visceral angiography and cerebral angiography
Chuang	Contralateral iliac angiography

A microcatheter is a special catheter, measuring 3 Fr, that is used coaxially through a larger catheter for subselective angiography and embolization.

Wires. Guidewires have two functions: they support the passage of the catheter through the soft tissues into the lumen of the vessel and they guide the catheter safely through tortuous vessels to a desired location. Most guidewires are constructed in the same way: the outer portion is a coil of wire, inside which are two additional wires, a safety wire to hold the wire together and a core or mandril wire that provides stiffness or support. Specific wires vary in size, length, stiffness, torque, material, and distal end. The most frequently used wires are as follows:

15J	Standard angiography wire
Rosen	Stiffer wire with a tight J tip
Glide	Hydrophilic-coated wire for tough angles
Amplatz Super Stiff	Stiffest wire available
Lunderquist	High-torque wire used in the biliary tree

Contraindications. If noninvasive imaging has been performed and does not answer the clinical question or the referring physicians have determined that angiography is necessary regardless of the noninvasive images, angiography is performed. Thus, there are no absolute contraindications to angiography if it is clinically indicated. Relative contraindications include the following:

1. Poor renal function. The higher the serum creatinine level, the higher the risk of contrast-induced renal failure. The risk of contrast-induced renal failure can be minimized by use of a carbon dioxide angiogram, hydrating the patient before and after the procedure, and use of a diuretic such as mannitol immediately before the procedure.
2. Coagulopathy. Coagulopathies should be corrected with fresh frozen plasma (FFP) or platelets. Heparin should be stopped 1 hour before the procedure. Aspirin and coumadin should be stopped 7 to 10 days before an angiogram, if the patient is able to discontinue therapy for a short period.
3. Active bleeding from an aneurysm. For a patient with a known aortic aneurysm who is bleeding, surgical exploration and treatment are the standards of care.
4. Severe hypertension. Patients with severe hypertension (systolic blood pressure more than 185, diastolic blood pressure more than 100) require pharmacologic manipulation (e.g. nifedipine, nitroprusside) to lower the blood pressure before angiography.
5. History of severe allergic reaction. Patients with a history of severe allergic reaction to radiographic contrast material should undergo angiographic procedures only if there is no other alternative. If the patient needs an angiographic procedure and has had a history of a severe allergy, he or she needs to be premedicated for the allergy and may need an anesthesiologist to stand by during the procedure.

Complications. The Society for Cardiovascular and Interventional Radiography standards for complications of diagnostic arteriography are shown in Table 9–1. The rate of complications for angioplasty and other vascular interventions is only slightly higher.

Normal Anatomy and Common Anomalies. In the *thoracic aorta,* a normal arch is seen in 70% of individuals. Common anomalies include a common origin of the

Table 9–1. Society for Cardiovascular and Interventional Radiology (SCVIR) Standards for Complications of Diagnostic Arteriography

Puncture site hematoma	<3%
Puncture site pseudoaneurysm	<0.5%
Vessel occlusion or arteriovenous fistula	<0.5%
Distal emboli (CVA, gastrointestinal, extremities)	<0.5%
Arterial dissection	<2.0%
Subintimal injection	<1.0%

CVA, cardiovascular accident.

brachiocephalic artery and left common carotid artery (seen in 22% of individuals), left vertebral origin from arch (1%), left arch with aberrant right subclavian artery (1%), mirror-image branching in the right arch (high association with congenital heart disease), and aberrant left subclavian artery in the right arch (low association with congenital heart disease).

There are no common anomalies of the *abdominal aorta;* anomalies seen in this area involve the visceral and renal arteries and include left hepatic branches from left gastric artery (23%), replaced right hepatic artery from superior mesenteric artery (SMA) (10%), completely replaced hepatic artery from SMA (1%), and more than one renal artery per kidney (10%).

Mesenteric collaterals are important in maintaining circulation to the entire gastro-intestinal tract. The most important collaterals run between the superior mesenteric artery and the inferior mesenteric artery (IMA). The marginal artery of Drummond runs in the antimesenteric border of the left colon between the IMA and the middle colic artery, which is a branch of the SMA. The arch of Riolan is a meandering artery that runs just lateral to the spine between the IMA and the middle colic artery. The collateral circulation between the celiac artery and the SMA is primarily through the pancreaticoduodenal arcade. The inferior pancreaticoduodenal artery is a branch of the SMA and communicates with the superior pancreatic artery, which is a branch of the gastroduodenal artery. Rarely, a persistent embryonic communication is present between the celiac artery and the superior mesenteric artery. This communication is known as the arc of Buehler.

ANGIOGRAPHIC FILMING AND INJECTIONS

The basic principle of angiography is to clearly determine the clinically relevant vascular anatomy. Usually, for accurate definition the anatomy must be seen in two different projections (e.g., anteroposterior [AP] and lateral); oblique and magnification views also can be helpful. The technique of catheterization was described earlier. Board examiners also like to ask about injection rates and volumes as well as film rates. Table 9–2 shows common injection rates and volumes and filming rates, describing the techniques for cut film. For digital filming, a good rule of thumb is to cut the injection rates and volumes in half.

As an example, for a study of the portal venous system, the superior mesenteric artery should be injected with a large volume over 10 to 11 seconds (e.g., 6 mL/sec for a total of 60 mL). Filming is typically one every other second for 20 films. Initially, portal flow is hepatopetal (toward the liver); as it slows (e.g., in cirrhosis), flow is to and fro; finally flow is hepatofugal (away from the liver), and sometimes even portal vein thrombosis occurs.

ANGIOPLASTY

The basic principle of angioplasty is to enlarge, with a balloon, the lumen of a vessel narrowed by plaque. The mechanisms by which angioplasty enlarges the vessel include compression, remodeling, and redistribution of the plaque; fracture of the plaque with or without intraplaque hemorrhage; and stretching of the tunica media. Basically, angioplasty involves a controlled traumatic event to the vessel wall that generally results in an increase in luminal diameter.

Table 9–2. Common Injection Rates and Volumes and Filming Rates for Cut Film

Vessel	Injection Rate/Volume (mL/sec)	Filming Sequence (1 Frame/ sec)
Aortic arch	30/60	3/4 then 1/5
Common carotid	7/14	3/3 then 1/5
Subclavian	7/14	2/3 then 1/5
Abdominal aorta	20/40	2/3 then 1/5
Aortic bifurcation for pelvis	15/30	1/10
Aortic bifurcation for runoff	7/77	Delay and filming depend on flow
Renal	5/10	2/3 then 1/4
Splenic	5/50	1/4 then 0.5/16
Hepatic	5/40	2/5 then 1/10
Superior mesenteric artery	6/60	0.5/30
Pulmonary artery	20/40	3/3 then 1/4
Inferior vena cava	20/40	2/3 then 1/4

Indications.   The common indications for angioplasty include:

Symptomatic stenosis or occlusion of a vessel. Symptoms may range from mild claudication to rest pain to a nonhealing ulcer in the lower extremities. A significant stenosis is generally believed to be one that narrows luminal diameter more than 50% or has a peak systolic pressure drop of at least 10 mm Hg.

Fibromuscular dysplasia (FMD) involving the renal arteries is one of the most classic indications for angioplasty because of its excellent response to angioplasty. FMD involving the carotid arteries is also now being treated with angioplasty at some institutions with encouraging results.

Stenoses at graft anastamoses often undergo angioplasty. This is particularly true for dialysis grafts. Vascular grafts to the lower extremities must be evaluated on an individual basis with consultation from the vascular surgeon. Grafts less than 4 to 6 weeks old should not be treated with angioplasty. Table 9–3 shows criteria that indicate which lesions have a better or worse response to angioplasty.

Contraindications.   There are several contraindications to angioplasty. A stenosis adjacent to an aneurysm should not be dilated because of the increased risk of rupture. Occlusions caused by an embolus generally require either surgical thrombectomy or thrombolysis. Ostial renal artery stenoses actually are caused by disease in the aorta and typically do not respond well to angioplasty. A stenosis in a fresh graft (less than 4 to 6 weeks old) should not be dilated. Finally, if adequate surgical back-up is not available, angioplasty should not be undertaken.

Technique.   Once it has been determined that a patient is a candidate for angioplasty, the approach must be considered. Generally, an ipsilateral approach is recommended. The most difficult part of an angioplasty is crossing the stenosis or occlu-

Table 9–3. Criteria for Predicting Response of Lesion to Angioplasty

Better Prognosis	Worse Prognosis
Short lesions	Long lesions (more than 4 cm)
Concentric	Eccentric
Noncalcified	Calcified
Large vessel	Small vessel
Proximal lesion	Distal lesion
Stenosis	Occlusion
Single lesion	Multiple lesions

sion with a guidewire. A torqueable guidewire and roadmapping can be used to help cross lesions. The balloons used in angioplasty vary in diameter and length, and some balloons are stronger than others. The balloons all cross the lesion over a guidewire. Before inflation, the proper balloon size is determined from the diagnostic arteriogram; determination should take into account the 20% magnification factor on cut film arteriograms. After the arterial system has been entered but before angioplasty is done, the patient should receive 5,000 units of heparin. We also give 100 µg of nitroglycerin intraarterially before and after angioplasty is performed. Some interventionalists give 10 mg of nifedipine before renal and below-the-knee angioplasties. Once the balloon is at the lesion, three serial dilatations are performed. The balloon is inflated by hand, using a syringe containing half saline and half contrast. If full-strength contrast is used, the balloon may not deflate all the way because of the high viscosity of the contrast. After the angioplasty is performed, a completion angiogram is performed through the vascular sheath, with the wire still across the lesion, to check the result. The overall luminal diameter should be enlarged as a result of the procedure. Initially, the area that undergoes angioplasty usually has an irregular appearance, which improves with time. The presence of an intimal flap is not unusual and is generally of no concern. If the flap significantly narrows the lumen, additional steps must be taken. First, the angioplasty can be repeated. If the flap still narrows the lumen, a stent may be placed across the lesion. Rarely, an atherectomy may need to be performed.

Because an atherectomy catheter rarely is used today in the peripheral circulation, it is discussed briefly here. For board examination purposes, an atherectomy catheter is used for eccentric calcified lesions or an eccentric intimal flap. We use the atherectomy catheter only for eccentric lesions and use stents for flaps. The atherectomy device is on a 7- to 9-Fr system and has an electric motor that actually chips away plaque. The device looks like a large angioplasty catheter with a motor attachment.

Postangioplasty care usually involves an overnight stay in the hospital with a noninvasive ultrasound the next day. Most interventionalists start their patients on aspirin (325 mg daily), and obtain another noninvasive test at 6 months.

Complications. The overall complication rate after angioplasty is approximately 5%. Complications are listed in Table 9–4. A typical board examination question is "What do you do if a vessel ruptures during angioplasty?" The answer is that the balloon is placed back across the lesion and reinflated while the nurse calls the vascular surgeon. If the rupture occurs in an extremity, direct pressure should be applied over the injury.

Patency rates reported in most large series 3 to 5 years after angioplasty are shown in Table 9–5.

STENTS

Vascular stents are becoming more and more popular as their success is published in the literature. Vascular stents are short metallic tubes that are deployed across vascular lesions (e.g., stenoses refractory to angioplasty).

Table 9–4. Complications of Angioplasty

Complication	Incidence
Distal emboli	Less than 4%
Dissection with intimal flap narrowing lumen	Less than 4%
Spasm refractory to nitroglycerin	Less than 1%
Arterial rupture	Less than 1%
Acute occlusion caused by thrombus, spasm, or dissection	Less than 1%
Groin hematoma	5–10%
Retroperitoneal hematoma	Less than 2%

Table 9–5. Patency Rates Reported 3 to 5 Years After Angioplasty

Vessel	Percent Patent
Common iliac artery	85–95
External iliac artery	75–90
Superficial femoral artery	60–75
Renal artery	70–80
Renal artery for fibromuscular dysplasia	85–95
Below the knee	40–60

Indications for stent placement are changing rapidly, and new applications are found regularly. The following are the most common indications:

Stenoses refractory to angioplasty, particularly iliac lesions
Vascular dissections or flaps after percutaneous transluminal angioplasty (PTA) are often stented
Venous stenoses caused by tumor, particularly in the superior vena cava (SVC)
Central venous stenoses refractory to angioplasty in dialysis patients
TIPS require the placement of vascular stents

As far as contraindications are concerned, septic patients should not receive stents because of the risk of infection. An adjacent aneurysm is a relative contraindication.

Stents placed in the femoral arteries and in vessels smaller than the iliacs have *not* shown adequate long-term patency. Iliac stenoses have demonstrated excellent long-term patency rates (up to 94% at 4 years) after stent placement. These results are comparable to those of primary angioplasty alone.

Many types of stents exist; however, only two are used frequently enough to be important for boards, the Palmaz stent (Johnson and Johnson, Warren, NJ) and the Wallstent (Schneider USA, Minneapolis, MN). The only vascular stents approved for use in the United States are the Palmaz stent and the Wallstent. The Palmaz stent is deployed on a balloon; it is placed across the lesion and the balloon is inflated. The Wallstent is a self-expanding stent that is more flexible than the Palmaz. A new type of stent that is beginning to attract attention is the "stent-graft," which is a large stent covered with a synthetic fiber such as Dacron. It is used to treat thoracic and abdominal aortic aneurysms, primarily in lieu of surgery, and also to treat aortic dissections.

Technique. The technique for placement of both the Palmaz stent and the Wallstent is similar to that for performing an angioplasty. First, the patient is heparinized. Next, a wire is used to cross the lesion. Immediately before the procedure an angiogram is performed, and nitroglycerin is administered with every manipulation. The stent is manipulated across the lesion over the wire within a sheath, then deployed by withdrawal of the sheath and inflation of the balloon (Palmaz) or by deployment of the stent device (Wallstent). A completion angiogram is then performed, and both stents can be dilated further if necessary.

Complications. Complications of stent placement are almost identical to those of angioplasty. The overall complication rate is less than 5%, and less than 1% of these require surgical intervention. The only additional complication with stents is the risk of stent migration; this occurs in less than 1% of cases.

TRANSJUGULAR INTRAHEPATIC PORTOSYSTEMIC SHUNTS

TIPS are a relatively new way to treat portal hypertension using interventional radiology and vascular stents. TIPS are shunts created through the liver between the portal vein and the hepatic vein. The shunt functions like a surgical shunt in that it decompresses variceal flow and thus stops variceal bleeding. The technique is complex but basically involves an internal jugular vein approach to catheterize a hepatic vein, use of a special needle to create a tract to the portal vein, and dilatation and stenting of this tract. The patients are followed in the intensive care unit (ICU) overnight, then the shunt is studied the next day with ultrasound. The success of TIPS versus surgical shunts is shown in Table 9–6.

Table 9–6. Success of TIPS versus Surgical Shunts

	% Rebleeding at 1 year	% Encephalopathy
TIPS	10–20	18
Surgical shunt	25–30	25–40

TIPS, transjugular intrahepatic portosystemic shunts.

The indications for TIPS are acute or recurrent variceal bleeding refractory to sclerotherapy. The contraindications for TIPS are acute systemic infection, severe hepatic failure, and severe pulmonary hypertension. Complications of TIPS include death (less than 0.5%) from bleeding or pulmonary hypertension—bleeding can be from a capsular puncture, an IVC injury, or a mesenteric venous injury; stent malposition, for example, in the IVC or renal artery (less than 5%); and neck hematoma (less than 5%).

IVC FILTERS

IVC filters are used by radiologists to prevent pulmonary emboli in selected patients. Various types of filters are available for placement, all of which are permanent. Several retrievable IVC filters are currently undergoing clinical trials.
The indications for IVC filter placement are

Development of pulmonary embolism or deep venous thrombosis despite adequate anticoagulation
Pulmonary embolism or deep venous thrombosis in a patient with a contraindication to anticoagulation. Contraindications to anticoagulation include recent stroke or gastrointestinal bleeding; recent surgery or upcoming surgery; metastatic lesions, particularly of the brain; bleeding diathesis; a patient prone to falling.
Free-floating iliofemoral thrombus
Massive pulmonary embolism
Diminished respiratory reserve

There are no contraindications to IVC filter placement as long as the placement is indicated as determined by the referring physician in consultation with the interventional radiologist.
The complications of IVC filter placement are

Recurrent pulmonary embolism (approximately 3% for all filters)
Caval thrombosis is seen with all filters with varying percentages (5 to 20%); most are asymptomatic, but about 5% are symptomatic with all filters
Filter migration (less than 5%), which is generally asymptomatic; rarely, a filter migrates to the right atrium and requires surgical removal
Caval perforation by the filter (less than 1%)

No large randomized studies have been performed on the complications or indications for filters.
The technique for filter placement at our institution involves the following. A right common femoral vein (CFV) approach is used if ultrasound shows that it is patent. Initially, a vena cavogram is performed to locate the renal veins and evaluate caval size. If the cava is greater than 28 mm, a bird's nest filter must be placed. The filter is then deployed in an infrarenal location. Alternative approaches for placement include the right internal jugular vein (IJV), left CFV, and antecubital veins (Simon Nitinol filter only). The left IJV generally is not used because of the difficult angles through the heart that are required.
The types of filters commonly used are listed on the following page.

Vena Tech (Braun, Inc., Evanston, IL): 12 Fr; can be deployed from the femoral or jugular approach; occasionally incomplete opening occurs, which can be adjusted by using a Rosen wire

Titanium Greenfield (Boston Scientific, Watertown, MA): 14 Fr; tends to tilt, significance unknown; also tends to incompletely open and cross legs; best suprarenal filter

Bird's nest filter (Cook, Bloomington, IL): only filter good in large venae cavae (more than 28 mm); involves more complex deployment

Simon Nitinol filter (Bard Radiology, Covington, GA): 8 Fr; can be deployed from an arm vein; works using thermal memory technology.

Greenfield filter: 24 Fr; thus, is generally used in the operating room; not used at our center for the last 10 years

EMBOLOTHERAPY

Embolization of a vessel is one of the most important procedures performed by an interventionalist. It is most often performed to arrest active bleeding and is thus life saving. The procedure is performed through an angiographic catheter after an angiogram has revealed the bleeding site.

The following factors must be considered before embolization:

What are the other clinical options available?

What is the anatomy of the vessel? Are there collateral vessels? Should the collaterals be embolized?

Is the embolization to be permanent or should it be able to recanalize? What type and size of material should be used to perform the embolization? Gelfoam allows for recanalization; other materials are permanent.

Should the embolization be more proximal or more distal in the vessel? The more proximal the embolization, the more likely that collaterals will reconstitute the lesion and allow rebleeding. The more distal the embolization, the more likely there will be tissue necrosis. Pseudoaneurysms require embolization proximal and distal to the lesion. Arteriovenous fistulas often require embolization proximal and distal to the lesion.

Will a microcatheter (3-Fr coaxial) be required? Polyurethane catheters cannot be used to place coils.

Materials. The commonly used embolization materials include:

Coils: permanent; metallic with thrombogenic material embedded in them. Gianturco coils go through 0.035-inch lumens. Hilal and Tracker coils go through 0.018-inch lumens. All coils are available in different lengths and diameters. Coils are either pushed out through catheters with wires or, less commonly, injected using saline.

Balloons: detachable balloons are available in different diameters; they are primarily used in neurointerventional procedures. They are a permanent embolization material. None are approved by the Food and Drug Administration (FDA) for use in the United States.

Gelfoam pledgets: wafers of Gelfoam that are cut to the desired size, then injected through the catheter into the desired vessel. Vessels embolized exclusively with Gelfoam can recanalize within 2 weeks.

Ivalon: permanent small particles (250 to 1,000 μ) that are injected through the catheter after they are suspended in contrast. The smaller the particle, the more distal the embolization and the higher the risk of tissue necrosis.

Ethanol: liquid ethanol acts as a permanent sclerosant. It can be quite painful when injected. Typically, it is injected into varices and venous malformations.

Glue (cyanoacrylate): injected as a permanent embolic material, particularly into arteriovenous malformations of the central nervous system and other central nervous system lesions. The glue can polymerize slowly and travel to the lung or polymerize rapidly and occlude the catheter.

Other rarely used embolic materials include: dura mater, autologous clot, bucry-late, Oxycel, and Avitene.

Indications and Contraindications. Indications for embolization include the following:

Bleeding secondary to trauma, tumor, and inflammatory processes. Examples include pelvic fractures requiring internal iliac embolization, hemoptysis in cystic fibrosis patients requiring bronchial artery embolization, and tumors that have become hemorrhagic or that require debulking before surgery.

Symptomatic arteriovenous malformations can be embolized, although they can be difficult and the central nidus must be embolized; a typical example is a pulmonary arteriovenous malformation.

Arteriovenous fistulas (AVFs) that are iatrogenic or traumatic are often treated with embolization.

Chemoembolization of tumors is a burgeoning interventional procedure in which a chemotherapeutic agent is mixed with Gelfoam and the embolization is performed. It typically is used for hepatic lesions (e.g., hepatoma) that require hepatic artery embolization.

If embolization is indicated clinically, there are no specific contraindications.

Complications. Complications from embolization include:

Accidental embolization of nontargeted tissues. Preventive measures include a familiarity with the anatomy before the procedure is done; for example, the interventionalist should make sure that no spinal artery arises from the bronchial artery to be embolized. The interventionalist also should always watch the catheter tip during embolization, to be certain that it does not fall out. A further measure is frequent puffing with contrast to determine when flow has slowed considerably, which decreases the likelihood of reflux of embolic material distally.

Postembolization infection of tissues distal to the embolized vessel. Prophylactic antibiotics are often given to reduce the risk of this complication.

Postembolization syndrome is a common complication. It is seen within days after the procedure; lasts for less than 5 days; and involves pain, fever, and leukocytosis. Treatment is symptomatic relief with nonsteroidal antiinflammatory drugs.

Although pain is not a complication after embolization, it is not unusual for patients to complain of pain after tissue has been embolized. Treatment is, again, symptomatic.

VASOPRESSIN

At some institutions vasopressin is not used for gastrointestinal (GI) bleeding and subselective embolization is the treatment of choice.

Vasopressin is still used at many hospitals, however, for the management of GI bleeding. The technique involves placing the catheter in the appropriate vessel (e.g., SMA), performing a diagnostic angiogram, then initiating the vasopressin infusion. Initially, the rate is 0.2 unit per minute. The patient needs to be studied again in 20 minutes so that vasospasm or continued bleeding can be sought. If vasospasm is seen, the dose must be decreased by 0.1 unit per minute, and the patient must be studied again in 20 minutes to determine whether the spasm has gone or further reductions need to be made. If the patient is still bleeding, the vasopressin rate may be increased up to 0.4 unit per minute at increments of 0.1 to 0.2 unit per minute. The infusion is continued for 12 to 24 hours after the patient has stopped bleeding. At the end of this period, the vasopressin dose must be tapered over a 12- to 24-hour period, during which the rate is decreased at increments of 0.2 unit per minute every 8 hours.

Patients with significant coronary artery disease or hypertension generally should not undergo vasopressin infusion.

The complications of vasopressin are significant and include the following:

Coronary artery spasm resulting in myocardial infarction

Exacerbating hypertension

Bowel infarction (occurs in less than 10%)

Hyponatremia severe enough to result in seizures (vasopressin is an antidiuretic hormone analog)

Diarrhea from promotion of peristalsis

Complications from prolonged catheter placement (e.g., groin hematoma)

Obviously, patients receiving vasopressin need to be closely monitored in the ICU. Particular attention should be paid to hematocrit, sodium level, and urine output.

THROMBOLYSIS

Lysis of arterial and venous thrombi is becoming more and more prevalent as the initial therapy for acute and subacute thrombi. The most commonly used thrombolytic agent is urokinase (UK), which is administered directly into the thrombus via an intravascular infusion catheter or wire. Streptokinase and tissue plasminogen activator (TPA) are the other two thrombolytics used in the United States.

Thrombolysis is the result of plasmin digesting fibrin into its degradation products. A commonly asked question on the board examination is "How does UK work?" UK directly activates circulating plasminogen, resulting in plasmin formation. Streptokinase indirectly activates plasminogen. Plasmin is a nonspecific proteolytic enzyme whose primary purpose is to digest fibrin contained in thrombus (thus *fibrinolysis* is another commonly used term for UK infusion). The half-life of UK is 16 minutes.

Technique. The technique for thrombolysis involves performance of a diagnostic angiogram to define the anatomy. Once the anatomy has been defined and thrombolysis is clinically indicated, the following basic technique is used. First, the thrombosed segment of the vessel is entered from the contralateral or ipsilateral side using a wire (we always use a guide wire). Next, a catheter with several sideholes is buried in the thrombus and the therapeutic agent is introduced. Numerous infusion catheters are available (Mewissen; Boston Scientific, Watertown, MA); alternatively, infusion wires (Katzen; Boston Scientific, Watertown MA) may be used. The clot is laced with about 200,000 units of UK initially, then the infusion is started. Infusion rates vary from institution to institution. We infuse at 200,000 units per hour for 2 hours, then switch to 100,000 units per hour for the duration of the infusion. The patient must be in the ICU during the infusion in order to be monitored for bleeding and other complications. The patient is routinely heparinized while the infusion catheter is in place. Because the patient must remain flat, a Foley catheter is routinely placed. The patient must be watched closely for bleeding from the GI or genitourinary (GU) tract. Every 4 to 6 hours prothrombin time, partial thromboplastin time, hematocrit, and fibrinogen level are assessed. The level of fibrinogen is kept above 100 mg/dL by titrating the UK dose.

The patient must have a follow-up angiogram in less than 24 hours to ensure that the catheter is in the proper location and to determine what progress has been made. If no progress has been made at 24 hours, we terminate the infusion. Often the follow-up angiogram reveals the reason for the thrombosis, such as stenosis. If a stenosis is found, we perform angioplasty. Follow-up angiograms are also undertaken if the patient develops bleeding, hematoma, or any other complication. A decision must then be made about continuation of the infusion, based on the clinical situation and the angiographic appearance. UK infusions are almost never carried out for more than 48 hours at our institution.

Factors that predict a successful outcome include

A treatable underlying lesion (e.g., stenosis responds better than occlusion)

Relatively recent thrombosis (less than 4 months)

Successful placement of the catheter *within* the thrombus

Significant progress within the first 12 to 24 hours

Indications. Indications for thrombolysis are based on the clinical presentation and angiographic appearance of the lesion. The single indication is vascular thrombosis. Both acute and chronic thromboses can be thrombolysed; the more recent the occlusion, the better the result with UK. Often the thrombosed vessel is a surgical graft, and after a course of UK an underlying distal stenosis that requires angioplasty is revealed. Embolic occlusions originating from the heart or aorta are candidates for thrombolysis at some institutions; however, this is controversial.

Contraindications. Contraindications for thrombolysis include the following:

Recent surgery (less than 4 weeks)
Active bleeding from another site (e.g., gastrointestinal bleeding or hematuria)
Pregnancy
History of allergy to UK
Clinical status of patient; that is, can patient survive ongoing ischemia to the affected extremity? If the patient loses sensation or motor function (or both) in the affected extremity, prompt surgical intervention is indicated.
Recent stroke
Metastatic disease, particularly intracranial metasases

Complications. Complications of thrombolysis include

Distal embolization as the thrombus breaks up. This is seen in approximately 15% of cases and is managed by continuing the UK infusion and treating the symptoms (analgesia). Rarely do distal emboli require surgery (less than 1%).
Bleeding around the catheter is seen in about 20% of cases, often requiring placement of a larger sheath or even termination of the infusion.
Pericatheter thrombus is seen in about 15% of cases. It can be prevented by heparinization of the patient.
Severe bleeding from a distant site (e.g., GI tract) is seen in up to 15% of cases and almost always requires termination of the infusion.

INTERVENTIONAL RADIOLOGY DIFFERENTIAL DIAGNOSES

Aortic aneurysms
Aortic dissection
Budd-Chiari syndrome
Gastrointestinal bleeding
Mesenteric ischemia
Middle aortic syndrome
Popliteal artery disease
Portal vein thrombosis
Portal hypertension
Renal artery disease
Visceral/renal microaneurysms

AORTIC ANEURYSMS

List the causes of abnormal enlargement of the thoracic or abdominal aorta.

Atherosclerotic
Infectious/syphilitic
Traumatic
Congenital
Cystic medial necrosis

Which is the most common?

Atherosclerotic aneurysms

Where are atherosclerotic aneurysms typically found?

When is surgery indicated?

- Most common cause of aortic aneurysms
- Typically fusiform in appearance
- Location typically infrarenal; suprarenal aneurysms seen occasionally; thoracic aneurysms less common

- Surgery performed on aneurysms that are more than 5 cm, symptomatic, and rapidly expanding (growing more than 0.5 cm in 12 months)
- Angiography should show the relationships of the visceral and renal arteries to the aneurysms

Infectious aneurysms

What are the common organisms involved in mycotic aneurysms?

- Mycotic aneurysms can involve the aorta or smaller vessels (e.g., renal)
- Causative agents include *Staphylococcus aureus*; *Escherichia coli*; and *Salmonella, Candida,* and *Aspergillus* spp
- Syphilitic aneurysms are rare today; seen with tertiary syphilis
- Syphilitic aneurysms affect the ascending aorta
- Syphilitic aneurysms have tree-bark appearance on angiography

Traumatic aneurysms

What is the most common cause of a traumatic pseudoaneurysm?

Where do traumatic aneurysms occur?

- Aortic pseudoaneurysms usually the result of a motor vehicle accident with sudden deceleration
- Most traumatic aneurysms occur at aortic isthmus; rarely found at aortic root or diaphragm level
- These contained ruptures are surgical emergencies
- These pseudoaneurysms result from aortic transections
- Chest radiograph signs associated with aortic laceration include mediastinal widening, obscured aortic arch, displaced nasogastric tube or trachea, left apical cap, upper rib fractures

Congenital aneurysms

Where do congenital aortic aneurysms occur?

- Congenital aneurysms occur at aortic sinuses; all are asymptomatic until they rupture

Cystic medial necrosis

What types of patients have cystic medial necrosis?

Where does cystic medial necrosis affect the aorta most commonly?

What conditions, other than aortoannular ectasia, are patients with cystic medial necrosis at risk for developing?

- Seen in patients with Marfan syndrome, Ehlers-Danlos syndrome, and homocystinuria
- Typically affects ascending aorta; classically results in aortoannular ectasia
- Patients with cystic medial necrosis also at high risk for aortic dissection

AORTIC DISSECTION

What are the findings in aortic dissection?

- Intimal tear, compression of lumen, thick wall, abnormal catheter position, inability to advance catheter
- Most often occurs in aorta of normal size
- DeBakey classification:
1 Involvement of ascending and descending aorta (30%)
2 Involvement of ascending aorta only (20%)
3 Involvement of descending aorta beyond left subclavian (50%)

What are the different classification systems for dissections?

- Stanford classification:

A Involves ascending aorta
B Involves descending aorta only
- If ascending aorta is involved, treatment is surgery
- If descending aorta only is involved, treatment is medical therapy (e.g., antihypertensives)

How are dissections treated?

Which renal artery is most commonly involved in aortic dissections?

- Left renal artery often is occluded by the false lumen as it dissects down the aorta

9

BUDD-CHIARI SYNDROME

What are the causes of Budd-Chiari syndrome?

- Hepatic vein thrombus from hypercoagulable states: polycythemia vera, pregnancy, sickle cell anemia, oral contraceptives
- IVC membranes/webs
- Tumor growth into IVC or hepatic vein: hepatoma, renal cell

GASTROINTESTINAL BLEEDING

What are the common causes of gastrointestinal bleeding?

Upper GI tract
    Mallory-Weiss tear
    Gastritis
    Ulcers
    Tumors
    Pancreatitis or other inflammatory processes causing
        pseudoaneurysms
    Varices
Lower GI tract
    Tumors
    Arteriovenous malformations
    Varices
    Pseudoaneurysms

Treatment

How are the various causes of gastrointestinal bleeding typically treated?

- GI bleeding is treated as follows:
  - ¶ Mallory-Weiss tear: embolotheraphy or vasopressin
  - ¶ Gastritis: medical therapy
  - ¶ Ulcers: embolotherapy, surgery, medical therapy, or vasopressin
  - ¶ Upper GI tract tumors: surgery, embolotherapy
  - ¶ Pancreatitis, other inflammatory processes: embolotheraphy
  - ¶ Varices: sclerotherapy, embolotherapy, TIPS
  - ¶ Lower GI tract tumors: surgery, embolotherapy, vasopressin
  - ¶ Arteriovenous malformations: sclerotherapy, embolotherapy, surgery
  - ¶ Varices: sclerotherapy, embolotherapy, TIPS
  - ¶ Pseudoaneurysms: embolotherapy

9

MESENTERIC ISCHEMIA

What are the causes of mesenteric ischemia?

- Embolic occlusion; typically emboli from the left atrium
- Arterial occlusion in patients with underlying atherosclerotic stenoses that suddenly become occluded; similar to coronary arteries that are occluded
- Low-flow states: hypotension, dehydration, poor cardiac output, mesenteric vasculitis from radiation therapy or polyarteritis nodosa (PAN)
- Less than 10% caused by venous thrombosis, seen with volvulus or intussusceptions

What are the symptoms of mesenteric ischemia?

- Symptoms: severe postprandial abdominal pain, weight loss, and changing bowel habits

MIDDLE AORTIC SYNDROME

- Narrowing of abdominal aorta; often also involves narrowing of renal arteries

What are the causes of narrowing of the mid-abdominal aorta?

- Causes include radiation vasculitis, rubella-associated vasculitis, Takayasu syndrome, neurofibromatosis, and Williams syndrome

POPLITEAL ARTERY DISEASE

What are the diseases that involve the popliteal artery and have similar appearances?

Entrapment
Atherosclerotic disease
Embolic occlusion
Aneurysmal disease
Adventitial cystic disease
Buerger disease

Appearance

- Many of these entities look the same when they involve the popliteal artery

Entrapment

- Caused by anomalous insertion of medial head of gastrocnemius
- Severely narrows the popliteal artery with plantar flexion

Atherosclerotic disease

- Often involves the popliteal artery, typically resulting in narrowing at its origin, distal occlusion, or both

Embolic occlusion

- Emboli from heart or aorta

Aneurysmal disease

How often are popliteal aneurysms bilateral?

- Can result in occlusion of vessel or rupture of aneurysm
- 50% of popliteal aneurysms bilateral
- 30% of patients with popliteal aneurysms also have abdominal aortic aneurysms

Adventitial cystic disease

- Adventitial cystic disease of popliteal artery results in stenoses and occlusions of the vessel
- Rare idiopathic disease
- Mucinous cysts form in media of vessel wall
- Diagnose with ultrasound or CT showing cyst

Buerger disease

Who gets Buerger disease?

- Also known as *thrombangiitis obliterans*
- Idiopathic vasculitis of small arteries below knee or elbow
- Classically seen in young male and female smokers aged 30 to 40 years
- Results in tortuous small collaterals below knee or elbow

PORTAL VEIN THROMBOSIS

What are the causes of portal vein thrombosis?

Bland thrombus
    Portal hypertension (most common)
    Pancreatitis
    Septicemia

Trauma
Hypercoagulable states
Budd-Chiari syndrome
Tumor thrombus in portal vein
Hepatoma (most common)
Pancreatic cancer
Renal cell cancer
Gallbladder cancer

Ultrasound

How is tumor thrombus distinguished from bland thrombus?

- Tumor thrombus can show color flow on Doppler ultrasound, whereas bland thrombus cannot

Budd-Chiari syndrome

- 20% of patients with hepatic vein thrombus eventually develop portal vein thrombus

PORTAL HYPERTENSION

What are the common causes of portal hypertension?

Presinusoidal
Portal vein thrombosis
Splenic/mesenteric venous occlusion
Sinusoidal
Cirrhosis
Sclerosing cholangitis
Postsinusoidal
Budd-Chiari syndrome

RENAL ARTERY DISEASE

What are the common causes of renovascular hypertension?

Atherosclerosis
Fibromuscular dysplasia
Arteritides
Takayasu
PAN
Neurofibromatosis

Renal artery disease

- Typically found on routine abdominal aortic angiography or in work-up of renovascular hypertension
- All causes symptomatic as result of stenoses in main or segmental renal arteries

Atherosclerosis

- Causes 70% of cases of renal artery disease
How is renal artery atherosclerosis treated?
- Can be treated with angioplasty or endarterectomy

Fibromuscular dysplasia

- Classically affects women aged 30 to 40 years
- Second most common cause of renal artery stenoses
- Excellent results with angioplasty (85% patent at 5 years)

VISCERAL/RENAL MICROANEURYSMS

What are the causes of visceral and renal arterial microaneurysms

PAN
Intravenous drug abuse–associated vasculitis
Systemic lupus erythematosus–associated vasculitis
Radiation vasculitis
Septic emboli

Figure References

1. Darcy MD, LaBerge JM, eds: Peripheral Vascular Interventions. Society of Cardiovascular and Interventional Radiology syllabus, 1994.
2. Kadir S, ed: Current Practice of Interventional Radiology. Philadelphia: B. C. Decker, 1991.
3. Standards of Practice Committee of the Society of Cardiovascular and Interventional Radiology: Guidelines for Percutaneous Transluminal Angioplasty. Radiology 1990;177:619–626.
4. Van Breda A, Strandness DE Jr, eds: *Vascular Diseases: Surgical and Interventional Therapy.* New York: Churchill Livingstone, 1994.

INTERVENTIONAL RADIOLOGY DISEASE ENTITIES

AORTIC ANEURYSM

Clinical

- Atherosclerosis most common cause of aneurysm
- Other causes include infection, syphilis, cystic medial degeneration, and trauma
- Abdominal aortic aneurysms (AAA) are the most common; typically infrarenal in location
- Pulsatile abdominal mass in asymptomatic patient
- When patient presents with abdominal pain that radiates to the back and hypotension, ruptured AAA should be in the differential diagnosis

Imaging

- Ultrasound:
  Used to follow AAA; surgery indicated if aneurysm measures 5 cm or increases 0.5 cm in 12 months because risk of rupture increased
- CT:
  Used to identify AAA in patient with back pain and suspected AAA; spiral CT increasingly being used to diagnose AAAs, and often can visualize visceral vessels well enough to allow the surgeon to operate without an angiogram
- Angiography:
  The gold standard; critical to image origins of visceral and renal arteries as they relate to the aneurysm; the surgeon also needs to see proximal and distal extent of aneurysm and infrarenal neck of aneurysm; typically, aneurysms are fusiform in appearance: few are saccular, and saccular appearance suggests mycotic aneurysm

AORTIC DISSECTION

Clinical

- Intimal tear leads to dissection of blood into media; dissection may or may not exit distally, resulting in a false channel
- Classifications:

Stanford A	Involves ascending aorta
Stanford B	Involves descending aorta only (70%)
DeBakey 1	Involves ascending and descending aorta (30%)
DeBakey 2	Involves ascending aorta only
DeBakey 3	Involves descending aorta only

- Cystic medial necrosis often cited as cause of dissection; patients also tend to be hypertensive
- Can also be iatrogenic; e.g., subintimal dissection caused by wire during angiography or occurring after aortic valvular surgery
- Symptoms: severe back pain (same as rupturing aneurysm) and hypotension; symptoms related to dissection occluding great vessels or left renal artery
- Therapy: if dissection involves ascending aorta, patient requires surgery because of risk of dissection involving coronary arteries and great vessels

Imaging

- CT:
    Modality of choice in patient with suspected dissection; should be dynamic and contrast enhanced at the levels of the aortic root, aortic arch, mid-thoracic aorta, and the level of the diaphragm.
    Findings same as in angiography: identification of an intimal flap and two separate lumens; false lumen may or may not have flow and thus be enhanced with contrast
- Spiral CT angiography can be performed to diagnose dissection; is becoming the screening examination of choice
- MRI:
    Also used in some centers, findings the same as in CT
- Transesophageal echocardiography:
    Can be done portably in emergency room or ICU; is accurate for detecting dissections
- Angiography:
    Now rarely done to diagnose dissections; may be difficult to perform because of catheterization of false lumen; may require transaxillary catheterization; key to help surgeon determine extent of involvement of great and visceral vessels
- Chest radiography:
    Most dissections have normal aorta on chest radiograph; if calcified intima is displaced inward when compared with prior chest radiograph, dissection can be suspected; rarely, widened mediastinum is associated with dissection

AORTIC TRANSECTION/PSEUDOANEURYSM

Clinical

- Contained tear of aortic wall; generally contained by adventitia
- Typically results from high-speed motor vehicle accident or fall
- Rarely progresses to pseudoaneurysm if patient survives initial injury
- More than 80% occur at the aortic isthmus, fewer than 20% occur at the aortic root; because these are the relatively fixed portions of the aorta, tears occur in these locations with sudden deceleration
- New osseous pinch theory: aorta injured when pinched between ribs and clavicle anteriorly and spine posteriorly
- Surgical emergency: most patients die at the accident scene; if patient survives accident and tear is not discovered, most patients die in the next 24 hours

Imaging

- Chest radiography:
    Signs of aortic transection include widened mediastinum on upright chest radiograph (more than 8 cm), obscured arch, displaced nasogastric tube or trachea, displaced left mainstem bronchus, left apical cap, hemothorax, and fracture of rib 1 or 2 (or both)
- CT/MRI:
    Hematoma around the aorta and same signs as for chest radiograph; it is rare to actually visualize the tear or pseudoaneurysm, but with contrast, active extravasation occasionally is seen
- Angiography:
    Always done at our institution if transection suspected clinically

Tear, intimal flap, luminal irregularity sought

Pseudoaneurysm may actually be seen

Ductus bump should not be confused with tear; both occur in region of ductus arteriosus; *ductus bump:* smooth and round, contrast washes out on venous-phase films; *tear:* sharp, irregular margins, contrast does not wash out on venous-phase films

ANGIODYSPLASIA

Clinical

- Acquired vascular dysplasia, probably postinflammatory; classically involves cecum or right colon
- Common cause of painless, chronic, intermittent GI bleeding; unclear association with aortic stenosis

Imaging

- Angiography:
    Shows vascular tuft and early persistent draining vein; active bleeding may or may not occur; seen in 15% of "normal" SMA angiograms
- Nuclear medicine:
    TcRBC study may show bleeding from right colon

Intervention

- Endoscopic sclerosis, transcatheter embolization, or surgical excision are all options; selection based on individual patient; surgical excision the definitive therapy; percutaneous interventions only temporizing measures

AORTITIS

Clinical

Giant cell arteritis
- Inflammatory changes in wall of vessel; diagnosed by temporal artery biopsy; typically seen in patients older than 55 years

Takayasu arteritis
- Intimal fibroproliferation of aorta, great vessels, pulmonary arteries, and renal arteries
- Occurs in young women (aged less than 30 years); all other types of aortitis occur in older patients

Syphilis
- Tertiary syphilis causes perivascular inflammation in vasa vasorum, which results in occlusion of vasa; consequently, arterial wall weakened and affected vessel (classically the ascending aorta) dilatated
- Ruptured ascending aortic aneurysms used to be cause of death in more than 30% of patients with untreated syphilis; with the advent of Venereal Disease Research Laboratory (VDRL) and fluorescent treponemal antibody absorption (FTA-ABS) tests, *Treponema pallidum* now is diagnosed much earlier

Imaging

Giant cell arteritis
- Angiography:
    Segmental occlusion and narrowing of small and medium-sized arteries; classically involves branches of external carotid artery; less than 10% involve aorta

Takayasu arteritis
- Angiography: aorta, great vessels, and renal arteries have segments of narrowing or, less commonly, occlusion

Syphilis
- Angiography: saccular (75%) or fusiform (25%) aneurysm of the ascending aorta (35%), arch (25%), or descending aorta (15%)

ARTERIOVENOUS FISTULA

Clinical

- AVFs typically are the result of penetrating trauma or secondary to an iatrogenic cause (e.g., renal needle biopsy, transhepatic abscess drainage, transfemoral arterial catheterization); all have a single feeding artery and one or more draining veins
- Presentation of AVF depends on its location, e.g.:

Liver AVF	Hemobilia
Renal AVF	Hematuria, hypertension, elevation of creatinine level
Groin AVF	Pulsatile mass

Imaging

- Angiography:
  Key is identification of a single feeding artery and a single draining vein

Intervention
- AVFs with large arteriovenous communication require surgery
- AVFs in liver or kidney that result from biopsies or other interventions can be embolized by placement of coils

ARTERIOVENOUS MALFORMATION (AVM), CONGENITAL

Clinical

- Result from persistence of arterial and venous communications of primitive vascular system
- Can be classified as follows:
  Cavernous/simple hemangiomas
  Microfistulous communications
  Macrofistulous communications
  Developmental anomalies
- AVMs in face, arms, and legs are clinically obvious when they become symptomatic as large pulsatile, blue-purple cutaneous structures
- Pulmonary AVMs often present in teenagers who develop dyspnea on exertion

Imaging

- Angiography:
  Varied appearance; some have clearly visible large tangle of arteries and veins; classically, single feeding artery supplies a tangle of vessels that then drain into single draining vein; some clinically large AVMs are angiographically occult (typically, these are the microfistulous malformations)

Intervention

- Key to embolization of AVMs is eradication of the central nidus; if eradication not possible, the feeding artery should be embolized
- In the central nervous system, neurointerventionalists embolize draining veins; however, in the body, venous embolizations of AVMs are not typically done
- To eradicate the nidus, we typically use Ivalon particles (Contour; Interventional Therapeutics, San Francisco, CA) or small coils; to embolize the feeding artery, we use large coils until complete stasis is achieved

9

ATHEROSCLEROSIS

Clinical

- Degenerative atherosclerotic plaques (cholesterol/lipid laden) build up on intima of vessels, typically resulting in vascular narrowing and degeneration and weakening of vessel wall
- Most common cause of aortic aneurysms in United States
- Unusual type of atherosclerotic disease results in vascular ectasia (arteriomegaly or arteria magna); almost exclusively seen in males
- Plaques can also rupture and result in acute occlusions, ulcerate, or break off and result in distal embolic occlusion
- Has several clinical presentations, ranging from claudication and diminished pulses to cutaneous ulcers and arterial occlusion

Imaging

- Noninvasive ultrasound:
    Often the screening test that diagnoses atherosclerosis: ankle-brachial index (ABI) most commonly used and suggests vascular disease of lower extremities if less than 0.9; the lower the ABI, the more severe the vascular disease
- Color Doppler:
    Used to directly image areas of narrowing, particularly in lower extremities and carotid arteries
- MR angiography:
    Used to study carotids at many institutions; used to screen for renal artery disease
- Angiography for atherosclerotic disease one of the most common procedures performed by interventionalists
- Angiography:
    Directly visualizes affected lumens; findings include aneurysms, stenoses, ulceration, embolic occlusions at bifurcations; atherosclerotic narrowing typically has irregular eccentric pattern; occasionally, webs and smooth concentric narrowings seen; atherosclerosis generally has one of the following distributions: aortoiliac, femoral-popliteal, or tibio-peroneal (trifurcation vessels); atherosclerotic aneurysms occur in aorta or iliac, common femoral, or popliteal arteries

Intervention

- Angioplasty of pelvis and lower extremities is a commonly performed procedure; stenting of atherosclerotic lesions also is becoming more common (particularly in the iliac arteries)

BUDD-CHIARI SYNDROME

Clinical

- Obstruction of hepatic venous flow results in hepatocellular congestion and progressive liver failure
- Causes: venous webs (hepatic veins are affected more often than the IVC), hypercoagulable states (polycythemia vera, oral contraceptive use, pregnancy, lupus anticoagulant, protein C deficiency), veno-occlusive disease, idiopathic
- Symptoms: right upper quadrant pain, ascites, hepatomegaly, and eventually cirrhosis

Imaging

- CT:
    Heterogeneous enhancement of liver with exception of caudate, which has separate venous drainage into IVC and usually is spared in Budd-Chiari syndrome, thus appearing normal; hepatic veins often are low in attenuation because of intraluminal thrombus

- Nuclear medicine:
    Sulfur colloid studies show normal activity in caudate and diminished activity in the rest of the liver, giving "hot caudate" appearance on liver-spleen scans
- Ultrasound:
    Visualization of venous thrombus, heterogeneous liver
- Angiography:
    Hepatic venous webs, varices and other signs of portal hypertension, and portovenous thrombus seen in 20% of patients with Budd-Chiari syndrome

Intervention

- Depending on underlying cause, treatments include liver transplantation, thrombolysis, thrombectomy, TIPS

BUERGER DISEASE (THROMBOANGIITIS OBLITERANS)

Clinical

- Idiopathic inflammatory vasculitis of medium and small arteries of extremities; classically, below the knee, but also seen beyond the elbow
- Typically seen in young male smokers (aged 30 to 40 years), who present with claudication or other signs of ischemia; becoming more common in young female smokers

Imaging

- Angiography:
    Shows multiple corkscrew collaterals below knee or elbow; areas of occlusion and spasm intermix with relatively normal arterial segments

EMBOLIC DISEASE

Clinical

- Atherosclerotic emboli arise from right atrium, aorta, iliac arteries, and superficial femoral arteries; patients with aneurysms that contain thrombus also can send emboli distally
- Emboli lodge at arterial bifurcations and result in acute arterial occlusions
- Symptoms ("five Ps") of acute arterial occlusion include pallor, pain, paralysis, paresthesia, and pulselessness
- "Blue toe syndrome" describes symptom that occurs when emboli arise from subfemoral or iliac arteries and occlude small vessels of the feet; patient has palpable pulses in affected extremity

Imaging

- Angiography: signs of emboli include
        Abrupt termination of a vessel, usually at bifurcations
        Occlusion with smooth, meniscus-like appearance at its termination
        Minimal collaterals around occlusion
        Embolic occlusions often multiple
        Asymmetrical occlusion
    Important to image regions proximal and distal to area of interest and contralateral extremity

Intervention

- Acute occlusion is an emergency, and time is of the essence; irreversible ischemia of tissue invariably is seen within 12 hours of occlusion
- Thrombolysis and surgical thrombectomy are the mainstays of therapy
- If embolic source is cardiac, some interventionalists do not even attempt thrombolysis; patient undergoes thrombectomy

9

- If embolic source unknown and interventionalists and clinicians desire it, thrombolysis can be instituted; underlying stenosis may be uncovered during thrombolysis, then subjected to angioplasty

FIBROMUSCULAR DYSPLASIA (FMD)

Clinical

- Idiopathic progressive fibromuscular proliferation of the arterial wall; can involve intima, media, and adventitia, resulting in strictures and aneurysms
- Medial FMD accounts for more than 90% of the FMD seen angiographically, with the classic string-of-beads appearance
- Intimal and adventitial FMD are less common types; result in webs and smooth, tapered stenoses
- Vessels involved include

Renal arteries	60%
Common and internal carotid arteries	35%
External iliac arteries	4%
Visceral arteries (SMA)	1%

- Typically presents in children or young women with renal failure or hypertension (or both)

Imaging

- Angiography:
  Medial FMD: classic string-of-beads appearance in involved vessels; this appearance is caused by web-like stenoses alternating with aneurysmal segments; *intimal and adventitial FMD:* webs and long, tapered stenoses, respectively; spontaneous dissection can occur in involved vessel and is particularly devastating when involved vessel is carotid artery; disease bilateral in more than 50% of renal FMD cases; multiple vessels often involved simultaneously (e.g., renal, SMA, and carotids)

Intervention

- FMD responds to angioplasty better than any other vascular lesion does: initial success seen in nearly 100% of cases; 5-year patency rates greater than 85%
- Angioplasty has been used in renal lesions with clinical success for years
- More recently, angioplasty has had excellent results in carotid FMD

GASTROINTESTINAL HEMORRHAGE

Clinical

- Cause of GI bleeding essentially determines treatment
- Causes of GI bleeding and therapeutic options typically employed are as follows:

UPPER GI TRACT	
Gastritis	Medical therapy; vasopressin in left gastric artery
Mallory-Weiss tear	Embolization of left gastric artery
Peptic ulcers	Embolization of feeders from celiac axis and SMA
Upper GI neoplasms	Surgery or embolization
Pseudoaneurysms of celiac branches resulting from pancreatitis, cholecystitis, etc.	Embolization
Varices	Sclerotherapy, embolization, TIPS
LOWER GI TRACT	
Neoplasms	Surgery or embolization as temporizing measure

Unknown cause   Surgery (catheter can be left in SMA and in operating room methylene blue injected to localize pathology with an angiographic abnormality), or vasopressin

Angiodysplasia   Surgical resection

Diverticuli   Surgery or embolization

Iatrogenic, status post biopsy   Embolization

- Divided into upper and lower GI bleeding angiographically and clinically by ligament of Treitz
- Upper GI hemorrhage presents with hematemesis and anemia; nasogastric tube lavage reveals coffee grounds or bright red blood; upper GI bleeding eventually results in melena, unless brisk and causes hematochezia; diagnosis and treatment of upper GI bleeding often accomplished with endoscopy
- Lower GI bleeding presents with melena or hematochezia, depending on rate and location of bleeding; rectal bleeding always presents with bright red blood per rectum, as does brisk cecal bleeding; oozing from cecum presents with melena; diagnosis and treatment of lower GI bleeding often accomplished with colonoscopy

Imaging

- Endoscopy:
    Required by some interventionalists before angiography for both upper and lower GI bleeding; often detects site and cause of bleeding; endoscopist can then either treat underlying cause or direct the surgeon or interventionalist to bleeding site
- Nuclear medicine:
    Tc-99m red blood cell studies or Tc-99m sulfur colloid studies can localize region of bleeding; can detect rates as low as 0.05 mL per second; study results usually direct angiographer to approximate location of bleeding, thus it can be determined which vessel to inject first
- Angiography:
    Gold standard for pinpointing bleeding source; however, patient must be actively bleeding at a rate of 1.0 mL per second for it to be seen angiographically

Intervention

- Two methods of treatment: embolization or vasopressin infusion; at the University of California, San Francisco, subselective embolization is the treatment of choice
- In addition to risks of embolization described earlier in this chapter, in GI tract embolization carries a 10 to 20% risk of bowel infarction that will require surgery
- Both coils and Gelfoam used, depending on patient and clinical situation; we use Gelfoam in gastric arteries, coils in gastroduodenal artery and SMA; we subselectively catheterize at least a third-order branch before we embolize in the SMA
- Vasopressin still used at many hospitals

LERICHE SYNDROME

Clinical

- Distal aortic occlusion, typically caused by atherosclerotic disease
- Entails three classic symptoms: thigh claudication, buttock claudication, and impotence, along with absence of femoral pulses

Imaging

- Angiography:
    Typically reveals occlusion of distal aorta and no filling of iliac arteries; often extensive pelvic and lumbar collaterals present that reconstitute femoral vessels

POLYARTERITIS NODOSA (PAN)

Clinical

- Idiopathic vasculitis involving small and medium-sized vessels, resulting in microaneurysms, occlusions, and strictures
- Involves renal arteries (85%), SMA (50%), and hepatic artery (50%)
- Symptoms related to kidney (hematuria, renal failure) or GI tract (GI bleeding); sedimentation rate elevated

Imaging

- Ultrasound:
    Microaneurysms appear as small hypoechoic structures; aneurysms typically so small that color flow is not seen on Doppler
- CT:
    Hepatic and renal aneurysms appear as multiple, small (less than 1 cm), low-attenuation structures; wedge-shaped infarcts may be seen in kidney, less often in liver
- Angiography:
    Typically appears as multiple microaneurysms located in affected organ; areas of vascular narrowing and occlusion also are revealed

PORTAL HYPERTENSION

Clinical

- Defined as portal venous pressure greater than 10 mm Hg
- Causes classified as follows:

Presinusoidal	Extrahepatic	
		Portal vein obstruction
		Lymphadenopathy
		Pyelophlebitis
		Pancreatic cancer
		Pancreatitis
		Thrombus in portal vein
	Intrahepatic	
		Primary biliary cirrhosis
		Congenital hepatic fibrosis
		Sarcoid
		Wilson disease
		Schistosomiasis
Sinusoidal	Cirrhosis (alcoholic, hepatitis)	
	Sclerosing cholangitis	
Postsinusoidal	Hepatic venous occlusion (Budd-Chiari)	
	IVC occlusion	
Arterioportal	Fistulas (posttraumatic or congenital)	

- Most common cause of portal hypertension in United States is cirrhosis from alcohol abuse or hepatitis
- As portal blood flow slows and varices develop, patients present with GI bleeding, ascites, jaundice, and other symptoms of liver failure

Imaging

- Ultrasound:
    Signs that suggest portal hypertension include small nodular echogenic liver, ascites, splenomegaly, slow flow or hepatofugal flow in portal vein, and periportal collaterals
- CT:
    Signs consistent with portal hypertension include small, heterogeneous, irregular liver; ascites; splenomegaly; and varices (esophageal, mesenteric, retroperitoneal, paraumbilical, etc.)

- Angiography:
     Findings vary, depending on severity and duration of portal hypertension
- Varices develop in early stages of portal hypertension but do not become symptomatic until after their appearance (time varies); varices develop in the following locations:
     Splenic vein to short gastric veins
     Coronary vein to paraesophageal veins
     Omental veins
     Umbilical vein
     Unnamed retroperitoneal varices
     Caput medusa (paraumbilical veins)
     Inferior mesenteric vein varices involving the hemorrhoidal plexus
- Other angiographic signs of portal hypertension include
     Corkscrew-like hepatic arteries
     Numerous periportal collateral veins in hilum of liver around portal vein, known as *cavernous transformation* of portal vein (seen in portal vein thrombosis)
     During hepatofugal flow, portal vein can be seen with hepatic arterial injections
     Development of spontaneous splenorenal shunt
- Other interventional techniques used to diagnose portal hypertension include
     Hepatic wedge pressure measured during hepatic vein catheterization (normal is 10 mm Hg or less)
     Direct splenic puncture and pressure measurement, rarely done today (normal is less than 9 mm Hg)
- Endoscopy often is the initial way portal hypertension is diagnosed because patients frequently are referred to a gastroenterologist; endoscopy reveals varices, which then confirm the diagnosis

Intervention

- Variceal bleeding is first controlled with endoscopic sclerotherapy
- Portal decompression is indicated when sclerotherapy fails to stop variceal bleeding after several tries; portal decompression can be accomplished via surgical shunts or TIPS (described earlier in this chapter); surgical shunts that decompress portal venous system include splenorenal shunts (Warren shunt is a distal splenorenal shunt), portocaval shunts, mesocaval shunts
- Varices can be embolized using interventional techniques either via a transhepatic approach to the portal vein or after placement of a TIPS

RENAL ARTERY HYPERTENSION (RAH)

Clinical

- Only 1% of adults with hypertension have an identifiable cause; majority of those with identifiable cause have renal artery hypertension (RAH)
- RAH caused by renal arterial stenosis or occlusion; stenosis most commonly result of atherosclerosis (70%), less commonly result of FMD (10%), Takayasu arteritis, or polyarteritis nodosa
- Hypertension obviously present in all patients; renal arterial compromise leads to elevated renin levels, believed to be underlying cause of hypertension in these patients
- Patients tend to be aged less than 30 years or more than 60 years and to have other symptoms suggestive of atherosclerotic disease; they tend to be smokers and have a family history of hypertension
- Sudden onset of hypertension also may suggest renal arterial cause of hypertension
- Laboratory abnormalities suggestive of renal arterial disease causing hypertension: elevated creatinine and renin levels, hypokalemia, and proteinuria
- On physical examination, bruit may be heard over midabdomen
- Angiotensin converting enzyme (ACE) inhibitors contraindicated in patients with RAH; can cause patients to go into renal failure and exacerbate the hypertension

9

Imaging

- Ultrasound:
    Can suggest renal arterial stenosis by identifying significant velocity shifts with Doppler studies; affected kidney often small
- CT:
    Helical CT angiograms undergoing promising evaluation for identification of renal arterial stenosis
- MRI:
    MR angiography now commonly used as a screening study
- Nuclear medicine:
    Captopril studies used as screening study for RAH in many hospitals
- Angiography:
    Renal arterial stenosis commonly identified on midstream aortograms in asymptomatic individuals; the following supportive findings can determine if a renal arterial stenosis is significant:
    Tight stenoses usually have some poststenotic dilatation
    Peak systolic gradient across the lesion of 10 mm Hg is significant; the higher the gradient, the more severe the lesion
    Renal vein renin levels can be obtained, although generally not necessary; levels elevated 50% more than those of opposite kidney are considered significant
- Exact number and location of stenoses important: ostial main renal artery lesions are less successfully treated by angioplasty than other lesions; if several intersegmental arterial stenoses are identified, all need to be treated

Intervention

- Surgical treatments include renal endarterectomy or bypass grafts
- Interventional treatment: angioplasty with or without stent placement
- Success rates of angioplasty vary depending on cause of stenosis; following data are based on several large studies that used guidelines suggested by the Society of Cardiovascular and Interventional Radiology:

Cause	Cured (%)	Improved (%)	Failed (%)
Atherosclerosis	20	50	30
FMD	40	40	<20

Cured = diastolic blood pressure <90 mm Hg; improved = diastolic blood pressure reduced but antihypertensive medication still required, although at reduced dose

TRAUMATIC INJURIES TO VESSELS OF EXTREMITIES

Clinical

- Blunt and penetrating trauma can result in vascular injuries ranging from vasospasm to transection; lesion depends on amount of force applied and the penetrating instrument
- There are hard and soft signs of vascular injury in an extremity; typically, angiogram not indicated unless one or more hard signs are present

Hard	Soft
Absent distal pulse	"Diminished" distal pulse
Posterior knee dislocation	Proximity of injury to vessel
Obvious arterial bleeding	History of arterial bleeding
Expanding hematoma	Stable hematoma
Bruit over injured site	
Neurologic deficit	"Possible" neurologic deficit

Imaging

- When vascular injury is suspected, angiogram typically is performed; sometimes ultrasound or CT performed initially reveals unsuspected injury

- Ultrasound:
    Can uncover AV fistulas or pseudoaneurysms, particularly with color Doppler
- CT:
    Can reveal hematomas as high-attenuation collections adjacent to site of injury
- Angiography: angiographic appearance of traumatic vascular injuries is the gold standard in reflecting true nature of injury; both blunt and penetrating injuries can result in an overlapping spectrum of findings; however, some injuries occur more often with blunt and others more commonly with penetrating trauma as follows:
    More common with *blunt* trauma from stretching and shear injuries:
        Spasm
        Displacement from mass effect from adjacent hematoma
        Intimal flap formation
    More common with *penetrating* injuries from direct vascular injury with an instrument (knife, bullet):
        Arterial transection
        AV fistula formation
        Arterial disruption
        Pseudoaneurysm formation
        Vascular occlusion

INTERVENTIONAL RADIOLOGY QUESTIONS AND DISCUSSIONS

For the various entities found in this section, a **film** is described, followed either by a list of questions (**Q**) that could be asked about the film and the appropriate answers (**A**) or by a discussion (**D**) of the film.

FEMORAL GRAFT OCCLUSION

Film: Angiography showing no opacification of a femoral graft.

Q: *What are the causes of an occluded femoral graft?*

A: Anastomotic stricture
Intraoperative clamp injury
Poor outflow/run-off
Patient noncompliance with anticoagulation medicine
Hypotensive condition (e.g., dehydration)
Hypercoagulable states

Q: *Name five hypercoagulable states.*

A: Pregnancy
Oral contraceptive use
Polycythemia vera
Protein C deficiency
Lupus coagulopathy

Q: *What options are available for treating an occluded graft?*

A: Surgical thrombectomy with Fogarty balloon catheters
Urokinase (UK) infusion

Q: *What type of catheter or wire would you use to administer UK?*

A: A multi-sidehole catheter such as a Mewissen, or a multi-sidehole infusion wire such as the SOS wire

Q: *What is the infusion dose?*

A: 100,000 units per hour

Q: *When should the patient undergo another study?*

A: In 24 hours or earlier if his or her pulse returns
The patient should also be studied again earlier if he or she develops any of the complications of UK infusion

Q: *What are the common complications of UK infusion?*

A: Bleeding around the catheter or internally (e.g., GI, CNS)
Distal embolization of the thrombus as it breaks up

GI BLEEDING

Q: *A patient is passing bright red blood per rectum; what is the source of the bleeding?*

A: The source may be either an upper or lower GI bleed. An upper GI source that is bleeding briskly may present with bright red blood per rectum.

Q: *How is the source identified?*

A: The screening study I would use is a Tc-99m red blood cell study.

Q: *What if it showed that the likely source was an upper GI bleed?*

A: If the referring physician requested, I would perform an angiogram; otherwise, endoscopy could be considered. An upper GI bleed would also have a bloody aspirate from a nasogastric tube.

Q: *What vessel would you inject first, and what type of catheter would you use?*

A: I would use a Cobra-type catheter for visceral injections. My initial injection for an upper GI bleed would be a celiac artery injection.

Q: *What should the injection rate and volume be?*

A: 5 mL/second for a total of 40 mL

Q: *What if that was negative?*

A: I would then selectively inject the gastroduodenal artery (GDA), left and right gastric arteries, and the hepatic artery.

Film: Bleeding source from the left gastric artery.

Q: *What would you do now?*

A: This film shows a selective injection into the gastroduodenal artery and a persistent collection of contrast that does not conform to a vascular structure. These findings are consistent with active bleeding from the GDA. I would consult with the referring physician and embolize the GDA if he or she desired.

Q: *How would you do that?*

A: I would embolize the vessel using Gelfoam pledgets. I would intermittently puff with contrast until complete stasis of flow was achieved. Then I would perform a superior mesentery artery (SMA) angiogram to identify the retrograde filling of the GDA from inferior pancreaticoduodenal branches. If active bleeding were identified from the SMA injection, I would then embolize it with Gelfoam pledgets.

Q: *What are the common causes of upper GI bleeding?*

A: Bleeding peptic ulcer or gastritis
Gastric or duodenal neoplasm
Bleeding pseudoaneurysms from pancreatitis or cholecystitis
Mallory-Weiss tear
Iatrogenic injuries from endoscopy and other procedures

Q: *What are common causes of lower GI bleeding?*

A: Diverticulosis
Angiodysplasia
Colonic neoplasms
Iatrogenic injuries

FIBROMUSCULAR DYSPLASIA

Film: Renal artery injection showing beaded vessel.

D: This film is a selective renal artery injection with a Cobra catheter. The midrenal artery has web-like stenoses alternating with segmental areas of dilatation. This gives the artery a beaded appearance that is most consistent with fibromuscular dysplasia (FMD) involving the renal artery. Atherosclerotic disease tends to have a more focal appearance and typically involves the more proximal portion of the vessel.

Q: *What other vessels does FMD typically involve?*

A: FMD typically involves the renal arteries and is often bilateral. FMD also can involve the carotid arteries and visceral vessels. Rarely, it involves other vessels.

Q: *How is this lesion treated?*

A: Typically, angioplasty is used to treat FMD because FMD has an excellent response to angioplasty. The success and patency rates for renal FMD angioplasty at 1 year are about 90%.

Q: *What type of patient would you suspect of having FMD?*

A: FMD classically affects young women, who suddenly develop hypertension.

Q: *What is the most common type of FMD?*

A: Medial FMD is the most common type. It is the type of FMD that has the beaded appearance seen in this case. Intimal and adventitial FMD are rare and have either a web-like stenosis or a smooth, tapered narrowing.

IVC FILTERS

Film: Ultrasound showing thrombus in right common femoral vein (CFV).

Q: *What are the findings?*

A: The film is labeled right CFV, and the vessel is filled with echogenic material. There is no flow seen with Doppler interrogation of the vessel. This is consistent with thrombus in the CFV.

Q: *If the referring physician asks for an IVC filter, would you put one in?*

A: Yes, if it is indicated.

Q: *What are the indications?*

A: 1. Pulmonary embolism in a patient with deep venous thrombosis despite adequate anticoagulation
2. Pulmonary embolism (PE) or deep venous thrombosis (DVT) in a patient with contraindication to anticoagulation, such as recent surgery or recent GI bleed or stroke
3. DVT in a patient who is going to undergo orthopedic surgery of the lower extremities
4. Free-floating caval thrombus
5. A patient with a history of pulmonary embolus or DVT who develops a complication while on adequate anticoagulation.

Q: *What type of filter would you put in?*

A: First, I would determine the extent of the thrombus, because if the clot extends into the iliac vein and then the IVC, the approach would have to be via the jugular vein.

Q: *What types of filters can be placed via the jugular vein?*

A: Vena Techs, Titanium Greenfields, Simon Nitinols, and bird's nest filters

Q: *What is the main complication of filter placement after the first week?*

A: The complication most frequently remarked on by patients is caval thrombosis. The incidence of this complication is up to 20% in reported studies that have looked at all filters.

Q: *Do you perform a vena cavagram before filter placement?*

A: Yes, because the extent of thrombus, the location of the renal veins, and the size of the cava have to be known.

Q: *Why is the size of the cava important?*

A: Because if the cava is more than 28 mm in diameter, a bird's nest filter must be placed. The bird's nest filter is the only one large enough to use in a cava of that size.

Q: *What is the rate of recurrent PE after filter placement?*

A: The rate of recurrent PE is about 3% for all filters.

SUBCLAVIAN ARTERIAL THROMBOSIS/SUBCLAVIAN STEAL

Film: Arch and great vessels with proximal subclavian occlusion and filling of the more distal subclavian artery (SCA).

D: This is a single film from a thoracic aortogram via a pigtail catheter in the ascending aorta. The proximal left SCA is occluded and reconstituted via the left vertebral artery. This entity is known as the "subclavian steal" phenomenon.

Q: *What direction does the flow follow in this entity?*

A: The flow is generally from the right vertebral artery to the basilar artery, then reversed flow down the left vertebral artery and into the left subclavian artery. Other collaterals include the thyrocervical trunk, thyroidal arteries, and internal mammary arteries.

Q: *What symptoms may this patient have?*

A: The symptoms are classically those of vertebrobasilar ischemia with exertion of the arm as a result of the reduction in central nervous system flow. Symptoms may include vertigo, headache, syncope, paresis, paralysis, paresthesias, diplopia, dysarthria, and homonymous hemianopia. Symptoms also involve the affected arm and include intermittent claudication, rest pain, paresthesias, weakness, and decreased temperature of the arm.

Q: *What are the causes of subclavian stenosis or occlusion?*

A:
1. Atherosclerosis is the most common cause of SCA stenosis and occlusion (>90%). More than half the patients with subclavian steal have subclavian occlusion, and the vast majority of these are caused by atherosclerotic disease.
2. Posttraumatic injury to the proximal SCA may result in subclavian occlusion.
3. If the patient has had surgery for a coarctation of the aorta, the shunt may necessitate a subclavian steal.
4. Congenital lesions such as an aberrant left SCA arising from the aorta distal to an aortic coarctation may result in subclavian steal.
5. If the patient has an apical lung neoplasm compressing the SCA, the result may be subclavian steal.
6. If the patient has Takayasu arteritis that is selectively affecting one of the SCAs out of proportion to the other great vessels, the result may be subclavian steal.

Q: *What is the treatment for SCA stenosis or occlusion?*

A: The treatment for subclavian steal depends on the cause of the stenosis/occlusion. If the lesion is caused by atherosclerosis, the therapeutic options include surgical and interventional techniques. The surgical options include endarterectomy and bypass grafts. The interventional options include angioplasty or stent placement, or both, for subclavian stenoses and occlusions.

AV FISTULA

Film: Renal arteriogram with an AV fistula.

D: This is a left renal arteriogram showing the left renal artery being injected with a Cobra catheter. In the left upper pole, a segmental renal artery is communicating with a large early filling vein. This is the typical appearance of an arteriovenous fistula (AVF).

Q: *What are some causes of AVFs?*

A: Penetrating trauma, such as a bullet
Iatrogenic causes, such as a renal biopsy
Neoplasm can erode tissues and create an AVF

Q: *What might the patient's symptoms be?*

A: Hematuria or laboratory abnormalities, such as an elevated creatinine level, or both

Q: *What therapeutic options are available?*

A: An AVF such as this could be treated using percutaneous interventions. The artery could be subselectively catheterized using a microcatheter. Then the AVF could be traversed and microcoils could be deployed across the AVF from the venous to the arterial side. A completion arteriogram should then be performed to confirm the success of the procedure.

Film: Renal arteriogram with coils in place, next case!

9

RENAL ARTERY STENOSIS

Film: Midstream aortogram.

D: This is an early film from a midstream aortogram performed through a pigtail catheter. There is a focal short-segment narrowing of the right renal artery.

Q: *What is the typical injection rate for this study?*

A: 20 mL/second for 40 mL

Q: *What projection would you film next?*

A: The renal arteries are best seen in the right posterior oblique (RPO) projection.

Film: RPO confirming the lesion.

Q: *What is the differential diagnosis?*

A: Atherosclerotic disease is the most common cause of this type of lesion, particularly in older patients.
FMD can also cause renal stenoses, but it typically has multiple areas of narrowing alternating with dilated segments.
Takayasu arteritis can also result in renal arterial stenoses, but typically the abdominal aorta is also involved.

Q: *What types of patients have FMD and Takayasu arteritis?*

A: Both are most common in young women.

Q: *What might the symptoms of this patient be?*

A: Renal arterial stenoses can result in hypertension, probably because of elevated renin levels from the affected kidney.

Q: *How could you confirm that this lesion was contributing to the patient's hypertension?*

A: A nuclear medicine captopril renogram could help confirm that this lesion was contributing to the patient's hypertension. Renal vein renin sampling could also be used.

Q: *What is an abnormal renal vein renin level?*

A: One and one half times the level in the contralateral kidney

Q: *What are the therapeutic options available to this patient, assuming that it is a symptomatic lesion?*

A: Renal endarterectomy or angioplasty is the treatment commonly used at our hospital.

Film: Renal arteriogram showing a postangioplasty film with a large flap almost occluding the renal artery; the wire is still across the lesion.

Q: *Based on the postangioplasty film, what would you do now?*

A: This postangioplasty film demonstrates a flap nearly occluding the vessel. The options include stent placement or repeat angioplasty, or both. The severity of this flap probably indicates stent placement.

Q: *What type of stent would you use?*

A: A Palmaz balloon expandable stent

Q: *Why?*

A: Because of its radial strength and radiopacity

Q: *What other stents are available in the United States?*

A: Wallstent and Gianturco stents, both self-expanding, are available.

RENAL VEIN THROMBOSIS

Film: Ultrasound showing no flow in the right renal vein.

D: This is a transverse sonogram labeled *right renal vein* with Doppler cursors in the vein demonstrating no flow. This finding is consistent with renal vein thrombosis.

Q: *What other studies could be done to confirm this finding?*

A: Renal venography
MR venography
Helical CT venography

Q: *What types of patients have this problem?*

A: Renal vein thrombosis is classically seen in adults with the nephrotic syndrome and in dehydrated neonates. Acute renal vein thrombosis is rare; it presents with acute renal failure and flank pain. Typically, patients are dehydrated or septic.

Q: *What therapeutic options are available?*

A: Typically, patients are anticoagulated for life. A suprarenal IVC filter may also be placed to prevent a pulmonary embolus.

VARICOCELES

Film: Left renal venogram with incompetent venous valves in the gonadal vein resulting in marked reflux of contrast down the gonadal vein into the pelvis.

Q: *What is this entity and what are the patient's symptoms?*

A: The film demonstrates reflux of contrast down the gonadal vein during a renal venogram. This is consistent with incompetent valves in the vessel resulting in a varicocele. The symptoms of varicoceles range from an asymptomatic scrotal mass to male infertility.

Q: *What other imaging modality can be used to identify varicoceles?*

A: Scrotal ultrasound can be used to identify a varicocele; Doppler interrogation identifies flow within the tubular structures.

Q: *What treatments are available?*

A: Percutaneous embolization and surgical ligation of the spermatic veins are the commonly employed treatments. Percutaneous embolization is performed by selective catheterization of the spermatic vein as distal as possible into the pelvis. Then several coils are deployed (in a standard case, we use about seven coils). When flow in the vein has been arrested, the procedure is complete. Semen quality and quantity are improved in 50 to 90% of reported cases. In 3 to 30% of cases, selective catheterization is not possible and surgical ligation is required.

UROKINASE

Film: Occluded right common iliac artery.

Q: *What are the findings?*

A: This is a single film from a pelvic arteriogram performed with a pigtail catheter in the abdominal aorta via the left transfemoral approach. The right common iliac artery is occluded at its origin and the right CFA is reconstituted via collaterals. The occlusion is abrupt and extends right up to the aortic bifurcation. Extensive pelvic collaterals are present. In particular, there is a large lumbar collateral as well as several pelvic collaterals. Also, the circumflex femoral arteries serve as a collateral pathway. The left common iliac artery and abdominal aorta show moderate atherosclerotic changes.

Q: *Are there any other collaterals present in addition to those already mentioned?*

A: The inferior epigastric artery probably is serving as a collateral here; however, I would need to see a series of films to ascertain exactly how it is filling.

Q: *Is this an acute or chronic occlusion?*

A: Chronic, because of the abrupt occlusion of the vessel at its origin, the straight margins of the occlusion, and the large extensive collaterals around the lesion.

Q: *What are the signs that suggest a relatively acute occlusion?*

A: Acute occlusions are typically embolic in nature. The angiographic signs of acute occlusions include abrupt termination of a vessel, usually at bifurcations; a smooth meniscus at the termination of the occlusion; and minimal collaterals present around the occlusion. Multiple embolic occlusions are not uncommon; thus, areas proximal and distal to the occlusion should be imaged, as should the contralateral extremity.

Q: *What are the therapeutic options available to this patient?*

A: Thrombolysis with UK or surgical thrombectomy

Q: *What are the contraindications to thrombolysis with UK?*

A: Contraindications for thrombolysis include recent surgery (less than 4 weeks); active bleeding from another site (e.g., GI bleeding or hematuria); pregnancy; history of allergy to UK; clinical status of patient (i.e., can patient survive ongoing ischemia during the infusion?); recent stroke; and metastatic disease, particularly intracranial metastases.

Q: *What are the complications of UK infusion?*

A: Complications of thrombolysis include

1. Distal embolization as the thrombus breaks up (seen in about 15% of cases), which is managed by continuing the infusion, treating the symptoms (analgesia), or surgery
2. Bleeding around the catheter (seen in about 20% of cases), which often requires placement of a larger sheath or even termination of the infusion
3. Pericatheter thrombus, seen in about 15% of cases, can sometimes be prevented by concomitant heparinization of the patient
4. Bleeding from a distant site (e.g., GI tract) is seen in up to 15% of cases and almost always requires termination of the infusion

Q: *How would you approach this vessel?*

A: I would enter the contralateral femoral artery, go over the horn, and embed a multi-sidehole catheter in the thrombosed iliac. I would then lace the thrombus with 250,000 units of UK and begin the infusion at 100,000 units per hour.

Q: *When would you study the patient again?*

A: When the patient's pulse returns, if a complication develops, or in 12 to 24 hours, whichever comes first.

Film: Follow-up angiogram at 24 hours shows a patent iliac artery; however; a distal stenosis is present.

Q: *What would you do now?*

A: I would perform an angioplasty of this lesion, which was probably the underlying cause of the occlusion.

Film: Completion angiogram showing the excellent result after angioplasty.

EMBOLIC DISEASE

Film: Occluded left popliteal artery.

D: The left popliteal artery is occluded just above the trifurcation of the run-off vessels. The vessel termination has a smooth meniscus and there are a few tenuous collaterals seen going beyond the occlusion. These findings suggest an acute embolic occlusion of the popliteal artery.

Q: *What are the symptoms of an acute embolic occlusion?*

A: The symptoms, or "five Ps," of acute arterial occlusion include pallor, pain, paralysis, paresthesia, and pulselessness.

Q: *What are the likely sources of this embolus?*

A: The most likely sources are the heart followed by the aorta and the pelvic vessels.

Q: *What would you do next?*

A: Image proximal to the lesion.

Film: Shows the left groin with an embolic occlusion of one of the branches of the deep femoral artery.

D: This film shows a similar-appearing occlusion of a muscular branch of the deep femoral artery. This supports the diagnosis of embolic occlusion, which is often multiple.

POPLITEAL ARTERY DISEASE

Film: Narrowing of the right popliteal artery at the knee joint with slight medial deviation of the vessel.

Q: *What is the differential diagnosis for narrowing of the popliteal artery?*

A: Popliteal artery entrapment syndrome
Atherosclerotic disease
Adventitial cystic disease
Popliteal aneurysm that has partially thrombosed
Embolic occlusion of the vessel

Q: *Which of these do you think is most likely?*

A: Entrapment, because of the smooth, tapered narrowing along with medial displacement of the vessel.

Q: *What causes entrapment syndrome?*

A: Entrapment is caused by the medial head of the gastrocnemius muscle displacing the popliteal artery, resulting in severe narrowing of the popliteal, particularly with plantar flexion.

Q: *What percentage of popliteal artery aneurysms are bilateral?*

A: Fifty percent of popliteal aneurysms are bilateral.

UPPER GI BLEEDING

Film: Left gastric angiogram with extravasation of contrast from the distal aspect of the vessel.

Q: *What is the differential diagnosis?*

A: This is a selective angiogram of the left gastric via a Cobra catheter. There is contrast at the distal aspect of the vessel that does not conform to any vascular structure and therefore represents active bleeding. The causes of active bleeding from the left gastric artery include Mallory-Weiss tear; gastric neoplasm, such as lymphoma, that has eroded the vessel; an iatrogenic cause, such as postendoscopic biopsy; and, rarely, severe gastritis has focal bleeding rather than the more common diffuse oozing.

Q: *How do you distinguish upper GI bleeds from lower GI bleeds?*

A: GI bleeds are divided into upper and lower GI bleeds angiographically and clinically by the ligament of Treitz. Upper GI bleeds present with hematemesis and anemia. Nasogastric tube lavage reveals coffee grounds or bright red blood. Upper GI bleeds eventually result in melena, unless they are brisk and cause hematochezia. An upper GI bleed can often be diagnosed and treated with endoscopy. Lower GI bleeds present with melena or hematochezia, depending on the rate and location of the bleed. Rectal bleeds always present with bright red blood per rectum, as do brisk cecal bleeds. Oozing from the cecum presents with melena. Lower GI bleeds are often diagnosed and treated with colonoscopy.

Q: *What diagnosis do you favor here?*

A: Diagnosis depends on the patient's history and presentation. If the patient is an alcoholic with retching, I would favor a Mallory-Weiss tear. If the patient has AIDS, the bleed may represent a high-grade lymphoma that has eroded into the vessel.

Q: *If bleeding were caused by gastritis, what would you do?*

A: Vasopressin is commonly used for bleeding caused by gastritis.

Q: *What is your regimen for vasopressin infusion?*

A: The technique involves placing the catheter in the appropriate vessel (LGA), performing a diagnostic angiogram, then initiating the vasopressin infusion. Initially, the rate is 0.2 units per minute. The patient should undergo another study in 20 minutes so that vasospasm or continued bleeding can be identified. If vasospasm is seen, the dose must be decreased by 0.1 unit per minute. The patient must be studied again in 20 minutes to ascertain whether the spasm has gone or further reductions need to be made. If the patient is still bleeding, the vasopressin rate may be increased up to 0.4 units per minute at increments of 0.1 to 0.2 units per minute. When the patient has stopped bleeding, the infusion is continued for 12 to 24 hours. When completed, the vasopressin dose must be tapered over a 12- to 24-hour period, the rate decreasing at increments of 0.2 units per minute every 8 to 12 hours.

Q: *What are the complications of vasopressin infusion?*

A: The complications of vasopressin are significant and include coronary artery spasm resulting in a myocardial infarction; exacerbation of existing hypertension; bowel infarction (less than 10%); hyponatremia severe enough to result in seizures (vasopressin is an antidiuretic hormone [ADH] analog); diarrhea from promotion of peristalsis; and complications from prolonged catheter placement. Patients with significant coronary artery disease or hypertension generally should not undergo vasopressin infusion. Obviously, patients receiving vasopressin need to be closely monitored in the ICU. Particular attention should be paid to the hematocrit, sodium level, and urine output.

PORTAL HYPERTENSION

Film: Venous phase from SMA arteriogram.

D: This is a venous-phase film from an SMA angiogram showing filling of large gastric and esophageal varices. The portal vein is also seen and is patent. The finding of varices is consistent with the diagnosis of portal hypertension.

Q: *What are the causes of portal hypertension?*

A: The most common cause of portal hypertension in the United States is cirrhosis caused by alcohol abuse and hepatitis. The causes of portal hypertension are divided as follows:

> *Presinusoidal*
> > Extrahepatic
> > > Portal vein obstruction
> > > Lymphadenopathy
> > > Pyelophlebitis
> > > Pancreatic cancer
> > > Pancreatitis
> > > Thrombus in portal vein
> > Intrahepatic
> > > Primary biliary cirrhosis
> > > Congenital hepatic fibrosis
> > > Sarcoid
> > > Wilson disease
> > > Schistosomiasis
> *Sinusoidal*
> > Cirrhosis (alcoholic, hepatitis)
> > Sclerosing cholangitis
> *Postsinusoidal*
> > Hepatic venous occlusion (Budd-Chiari)
> > IVC occlusion

Q: *What are the other angiographic signs of portal hypertension besides varices?*

A: (1) Corkscrew-like hepatic arteries; (2) with portal vein thrombosis, occasionally many periportal collateral veins develop in the hilum of the liver around the portal vein—this is known as *cavernous transformation of the portal vein*; (3) when hepatofugal flow is present, the portal vein is seen with hepatic arterial injections; and (4) with development of a spontaneous splenorenal shunt, the IVC is seen on the venous phase of an SMA injection.

Q: *What is another way an interventional radiologist could diagnose portal hypertension?*

A: Hepatic wedge pressures measured during hepatic vein catheterization; normal is 10 mm Hg or less.

Q: *What therapeutic options are available for treating variceal bleeding caused by portal hypertension?*

A: Generally, variceal bleeding is first controlled with endoscopic sclerotherapy. When sclerotherapy fails to stop variceal bleeding after several tries, portal decompression is indicated. Portal decompression can be accomplished via surgical shunts or transjugular intrahepatic portosystemic shunts (TIPS), which are described in the **Overview** section of this chapter. The surgical shunts used to decompress the portal venous system include splenorenal shunts (Warren shunt is a distal splenorenal shunt), portocaval shunts, and mesocaval shunts. Varices can also be embolized using interventional techniques either via a transhepatic approach to the portal vein or after placement of a TIPS.

EMBOLIZATION OF AN ANTERIOR TIBIAL PSEUDOANEURYSM

Film: Single film from a right lower extremity angiogram showing a 1-cm pseudoaneurysm off the anterior tibial artery.

Q: *What is the most likely cause of this pseudoaneurysm?*

A: Trauma is the most common cause of pseudoaneurysms in the extremities.

Q: *How would you treat this patient?*

A: By placing a catheter down into the pseudoaneurysm and deploying coils.

Q: *What size coils would you use?*

A: Coil size is based on the overall size of the aneurysm. This aneurysm appears to measure about 1 cm in its largest dimension; thus, the coil diameter should be about 10 mm. The coil should be as short as possible to prevent the coil from protruding into the normal vessel.

Q: *What complications could occur in this case?*

A: The most worrisome complication is distal embolization of the coil, resulting in distal ischemia. The other complication could be deployment of the coil into the native vessel, resulting in a more proximal occlusion. In this case, it would probably be all right, because the posterior tibial and peroneal arteries are widely patent and would supply the foot. It is important to completely occlude flow in the pseudoaneurysm with as many coils as necessary.

Film: Angiogram showing three coils deployed in the pseudoaneurysm resulting in complete stasis of flow into it.

9

Pediatric Imaging

■ **Tracy Samples,** M.D.

OVERVIEW

Pediatric radiology is a unique subspecialty in radiology. Unlike other subspecialties, pediatric radiology encompasses the evaluation of the entire patient. In addition, it emphasizes congenital lesions, which present less commonly in the adult population. For the purposes of this review, the assessment is broken down into organ-specific discussions and differential diagnoses. This method of categorization is artificial and not ideal, because many of the diseases fall into several categories. In those cases, the entity is discussed in the most common location and references are made to other possible manifestations of the disease. In addition, the preferred work-up and evaluation of various diseases are described. The evaluation of a pediatric patient often requires the use of sedation. Familiarity with sedation protocols for children is mandatory.

CHEST

In the neonatal population, respiratory distress is the most common indication for a chest radiograph. Pertinent clinical information is essential to help with a differential diagnosis. The gestational age, presence of meconium-stained amniotic fluid, history of traumatic delivery, or maternal fever can limit the diagnostic possibilities. In older children, chest films often are obtained to exclude an infection or to evaluate wheezing, stridor, or chest pain. Pertinent clinical information and prior films are essential for appropriate interpretation. The chest film should be interpreted using a systematic approach. Many radiologists advocate the "ABC" approach (A for airway and abdomen, B for bones and soft tissues, and C for the rest of the chest).

Airway and Abdomen. Because respiratory distress is a common presentation, evaluation of the intrathoracic airway can indicate intraluminal masses, intrinsic narrowing, and deviation or extrinsic mass effect on the trachea. The trachea normally deviates away from the aortic arch, so the presence of a right or double arch can be ascertained. Although the abdomen may not be the primary area of interest, the appearance of the visualized bowel loops, the abdominal situs, or the presence of free intraperitoneal air can offer useful information.

Bones and Soft Tissues. Evaluation of the bones can offer many clues to help limit an extensive differential diagnosis. For instance, 11 ribs or extrasternal ossification centers can point toward the diagnosis of Down syndrome. Vertebral anomalies can suggest Langerhans cell histiocytosis or differentiate between the mucopolysaccharidoses. The characteristic appearance of the ribs can point to a systemic disorder such as Hurler disease or neurofibromatosis. The ribs may show expansion or destruction from chest wall tumors such as Ewing sarcoma or Askin tumor (primitive neuroectodermal tumor).

Chest. Finally, the appearance of the lung parenchyma, cardiomediastinal silhouette, and pleural space should be assessed. The lung parenchyma is evaluated for the presence of infiltrates. Infiltrates that are detected should be characterized as to extent and symmetry and, if possible, it should be determined whether the infiltrate is interstitial or alveolar. The latter distinction may be possible only in the older child. The presence of a pleural effusion should be noted.

Pulmonary nodules may be solitary or multiple. Multiplicity suggests metastatic disease, papillomatosis, or a fungal infection. Because primary carcinoma is very rare, a solitary lesion commonly represents a round pneumonia, hamartoma, or arteriovenous malformation. Lung masses are uncommon, but the presence of air within the mass suggests a connection with the tracheobronchial tree. This connection explains why a mass that appears solid in the immediate newborn period can later appear cystic as fetal lung fluid is expelled. Cystic changes in childhood may be seen with congenital lesions, Langerhans cell histiocytosis, bronchiectasis, or pneumatoceles.

The location of mediastinal masses can help limit the possible differential considerations because various lesions have a predilection for a specific mediastinal compartment. The mediastinum usually is subdivided into anterior, middle, and posterior compartments. Most mediastinal lesions in childhood are malignant. The thymus in the anterior mediastinum can compromise the assessment of the chest. It is normal to see a prominent thymus until approximately 4 years of age. The undulating margins (wave sign) and characteristic interface with the minor fissure (sail sign) can help distinguish the thymus from other anterior mediastinal masses. An ectopic thymus can even mimic a posterior mediastinal mass. Pneumomediastinum lifts up the limbs of the thymus, causing an angel-wing appearance.

In infants, the anterior mediastinum can be evaluated using ultrasound, which limits exposure to ionizing radiation. Ultrasound is also useful to evaluate diaphragmatic motion in infants as long as both diaphragms can be seen simultaneously with one transducer. Ultrasound can be useful to look for the aberrant vascular supply if the diagnosis of sequestration is being considered. It can demonstrate normal thymus and show the side of the aortic arch before surgical repair of esophageal atresia.

Computed tomography (CT) is used to initially evaluate most pediatric thoracic masses. However, if there is a question of invasion into a vascular structure or the spinal canal, magnetic resonance imaging (MRI) can be of particular value.

It is important to check the position of tubes and lines, particularly in neonates. It is not uncommon for the radiologist to first recognize an esophageal intubation in a premature infant. The tip of an umbilical venous catheter should be just within the right atrium, and the tip of an umbilical arterial catheter can be high (between T6 and T10) or, more commonly, at the L3 vertebral body or below.

UPPER AIRWAY

The child with stridor has a lengthy list of possible differential diagnoses. It is usually most convenient to try to localize the portion of the airway that is involved. In general, inspiratory stridor is caused by an extrathoracic lesion, whereas expiratory stridor points to an intrathoracic lesion. When a lesion is large enough to occlude the airway during both phases of respiration, the stridor is biphasic. In an acute presentation, the possible considerations usually include epiglottitis. In the classic case, further radiographic studies are not indicated. If doubt exists, a lateral neck film is obtained. It is important to know the normal anatomy of the lateral neck in order to avoid calling unnecessary attention to normal variants. For example, adenoidal tissue in children can be very prominent. In addition, the retropharyngeal soft tissues in a child are relatively thicker than those in an adult. The rule of thumb is that the soft tissues in front of the C4 vertebral body should be no wider than one and a half times the vertebral body in a child under 6 months. This gradually decreases in width until the soft tissues are approximately one third the width of the C4 vertebral body by age 6 years. The radiograph must be obtained with the neck in full extension and in full inspiration; otherwise, pseudothickening can be produced. If doubt still exists about the diagnosis, the child can be evaluated with fluoroscopy or a barium swallow. Ultrasound is an excellent way to evaluate neck masses in children. It can help distinguish solid from cystic masses and help localize the mass to a compartment of the neck. However, most lesions are further evaluated with CT or possibly MRI to determine total extent of the lesion or other foci of disease within the mediastinum.

GASTROINTESTINAL TRACT

In evaluation of the neonatal abdomen, it is important to appreciate when the normal bowel fills with air. Air should be seen in the stomach within minutes from birth. The bowel progressively fills over the next 12 to 24 hours. In the neonatal period, the distinction between small and large bowel cannot be made with any certainty. If an obstruction exists, usually it is classified as either proximal or distal, based on the number of loops visualized. The presence of intramural air, pneumoperitoneum, abnormal calcifications, ascites, or portal venous gas is important corollary information. A clinical history of passage of meconium or imperforate anus can help limit the differential diagnosis.

In most children, a diagnostic enema can be performed with barium. Barium is a common contrast agent with a long record of safety and is an appropriate agent in most situations because it usually gives better anatomic detail. Retention of barium for more than 24 hours after a diagnostic enema is suggestive of Hirschsprung disease. If an enema is required in a neonate, an ionic or nonionic water soluble contrast material may be used. This can help with diagnosis as well as treatment if meconium ileus or meconium plug is determined to be the cause of an obstruction. Water soluble contrast agents also are used if there is a suspicion of bowel perforation. In addition, air can be used as a contrast agent, particularly in cases of intussusception. A vigorous preparation usually is not required for a pediatric enema. In fact, a child with the possible diagnosis of Hirschsprung disease should undergo no preparation because the diagnostic transitional zone may be obscured. A more thorough cleansing may be needed if a search for a juvenile polyp is being conducted.

During an upper gastrointestinal (GI) tract barium examination, the location of the ligament of Treitz and the presence of gastroesophageal (GE) reflux should always be ascertained. In infants, the ligament of Treitz is most easily detected when barium first passes through the duodenum. As the small bowel fills with contrast, it may be difficult to visualize the duodenum. Barium usually is used in the evaluation of the upper GI tract unless perforation is a possibility, such as in ingestion of a caustic agent or a sharp foreign body. Hypertonic water soluble agents are not indicated if there is a risk of aspiration. In these cases, a nonionic agent diluted to isotonicity or barium is the agent of choice.

If there is a history of bilious emesis, the differential possibilities include malrotation with midgut volvulus. Evaluation of this entity is an emergency and requires further studies, even if the plain film is unremarkable in appearance. In these cases, an upper GI series is the study of choice. A barium enema is less specific for identifying a malrotation because the pediatric cecum may not be located in the right lower quadrant as the result of a lax mesenteric attachment.

Ultrasound is a useful first line of evaluation in any child with a palpable abdominal mass, a history of nonbilious projectile vomiting, or possible appendicitis. The pylorus can be imaged easily in children with pyloric stenosis. It is important to be familiar with the ultrasound criteria for the diagnosis of an abnormal pylorus. Intussusceptions have characteristic findings on ultrasound. Absence of blood flow in the intussusceptum with Doppler ultrasound has been described in nonreducible cases. It is also advisable to know the graded compression technique for the evaluation of appendicitis.

Nuclear medicine pertechnetate scans can identify the presence of a Meckel diverticulum or intestinal duplication by accumulating isotope in foci of ectopic gastric mucosa. Hepatobiliary imaging is crucial in the evaluation of jaundice. Characteristic imaging patterns can help distinguish between biliary atresia and neonatal hepatitis. The radiopharmaceutical also accumulates in a choledochal cyst.

GENITOURINARY TRACT

In the pediatric patient, genitourinary (GU) lesions often present as an abdominal mass. Clinical history and the age of the patient are important in the evaluation. In infants and young children, the most likely cause of an abdominal mass is hydronephrosis, followed by multicystic dysplastic kidney. In older children, neoplasms such as Wilms tumor and neuroblastoma are relatively more common. Syndromes such as Beckwith-Wiedemann and hemihypertrophy are associated with an increased risk of Wilms tumor. Nephroblastomatosis and mesoblastic nephroma are lesions found only in infancy.

After an initial plain film of the abdomen, ultrasound usually is the first modality used for evaluation of a suspected urinary tract mass. If hydronephrosis is present, the child should undergo a voiding cystourethrogram (VCUG) to exclude the possibility of vesicoureteral reflux or posterior urethral valves and a nuclear medicine renal scan to exclude obstruction. Posterior urethral valves are present in approximately 50% of male infants with bilaterally dilated collecting systems. If hydronephrosis is diagnosed prenatally, an ultrasound scan performed in the first few days of life may be falsely negative, because the newborn infant is relatively oliguric. Therefore, a follow-up ultrasound scan should be performed at 4 to 6 weeks of life to exclude a false-negative examination. Ultrasound can also identify a duplicated system with an obstructed upper pole moiety. These children also need a VCUG and renal scan during their work-up.

CT and MRI both are used in the evaluation of solid GU masses. CT can better delineate the presence of calcifications and the extent of metastases in the case of neoplasms. However, MRI is valued because of its multiplanar imaging capabilities and its ability to identify vascular invasion by a tumor.

In the evaluation of the young child with a first urinary tract infection (UTI) or pyelonephritis, a renal ultrasound scan is performed to exclude an underlying congenital abnormality and to evaluate possible renal scarring. A VCUG is performed to determine whether reflux is present, because a high percentage of children with UTIs are found to have reflux. If reflux is present, therapy is based on the age of the child and the degree of reflux. Radionuclide cystography is used for follow-up assessment of reflux because the radiation dose is considerably smaller. If there is a question of surgical intervention, a nuclear medicine dimercaptosuccinic acid (DMSA) scan can be performed, because ultrasound can underestimate the extent of scarring. Older children or adolescents with a first UTI usually require only ultrasound examination. If the findings are normal, no further studies are needed unless it is imperative to exclude reflux. In that case, radionuclide cystography usually is performed. In addition, the young siblings of children with documented reflux can be screened with radionuclide cystography.

Ultrasound is used to evaluate renal transplants, localize undescended testicles, and characterize children with ambiguous genitalia. Duplex Doppler can assess renal blood flow and determine the resistive index in the evaluation of renovascular hypertension and renal vein thrombosis and in the assessment of transplants for signs of rejection.

The type of contrast agent used in excretory urograms varies from institution to institution. Some use nonionic agents for all pediatric patients, whereas others use ionic agents except in children with specific risk factors. Be familiar with the protocols used in your institution. It is imperative for a radiologist administering contrast to be able to recognize and to treat adverse contrast reactions in children.

The adrenal gland is much more prominent in infants and young children than in adults. It usually is easily identified with ultrasound. Unfortunately, it may be difficult to distinguish between a benign hemorrhage and congenital neuroblastoma. In these instances, follow-up studies are invaluable.

Bladder masses in childhood can be evaluated by ultrasound or during the filling phase of a VCUG; however, CT or MRI is required to determine the extent of disease. The most common bladder mass is rhabdomyosarcoma. Ectopic ureteroceles associated with a duplex system also are clearly seen. A dilated posterior urethra suggests the presence of posterior urethral valves.

SKELETAL SYSTEM

Conventional radiographs usually depict bone adequately and are the initial imaging study in most children with skeletal disorders. In cases of trauma, at least two perpendicular views are required. Imaging of the opposite side for comparison is not routinely required and should be reserved for those cases in which an injury or abnormality cannot be easily distinguished from a normal variant.

Skeletal surveys commonly are obtained to evaluate for nonaccidental trauma, to examine metabolic or genetic abnormalities, or to look for metastatic disease in children with neuroblastoma, leukemia, or Langerhans cell histiocytosis. In a skeletal survey for child abuse, it is important to use meticulous bone technique and to visualize every bone in the body, including the hands and feet.

CT is useful in the evaluation of the spine and casted structures and to determine the extent of an osseous abnormality identified on plain films.

Because of its ability to image in multiple planes, MRI may be required to fully determine the extent of a lesion. It is the best method for determining vascular or marrow involvement. In early infection and infiltrative processes, the marrow signal often is abnormal even when plain films are normal. MRI also is the procedure of choice for evaluating pediatric joints.

Ultrasound is currently the examination of choice in the evaluation of the immature hip and also for the detection of hip and knee effusions. It also has been described for the detection of acute subperiosteal hemorrhage in child abuse. In addition, it can help in the evaluation of soft tissue lesions by determining vascularity using duplex and color Doppler. Ultrasound is also invaluable in the assessment of the newborn spine and spinal cord.

Radionuclide bone scans are used to help identify early osteomyelitis, characterize bone lesions, identify metastatic disease, and screen for nonaccidental trauma. Bone scans can be less sensitive than a skeletal survey for the detection of some lesions such as neuroblastoma and Langerhans cell histiocytosis. In the evaluation of nonaccidental trauma, skull films should always be obtained because the bone scan is not considered as sensitive for the detection of fractures in the skull.

10

PEDIATRIC IMAGING DIFFERENTIAL DIAGNOSES

Chest
   Unilateral opacified hemithorax in neonate
   Cystic lung lesions
   Miliary interstitial disease
   Anterior mediastinal masses
   Posterior mediastinal masses
Upper airway
   Retropharyngeal mass
   Enlarged epiglottis
Gastrointestinal tract
   Gasless abdomen
   Double bubble
   Dilated bowel in newborn
   Esophageal strictures
   Right upper quadrant cystic mass
   Focal hepatic masses

Genitourinary tract
  Adrenal masses
  Renal masses
  Hydronephrosis
  Bilateral enlarged kidneys
Musculoskeletal system
  Periosteal reaction
  Vertebra plana
  Tibial bowing

CHEST

UNILATERAL OPACIFIED HEMITHORAX IN NEONATE

List causes of a unilateral opacified hemithorax in the neonate.

Chylothorax
Congenital cystic adenomatoid malformation
Congenital lobar emphysema
Pulmonary agenesis
Congenital diaphragmatic hernia
Neoplasm

Chylothorax

What is the most common cause of a large pleural effusion in the neonate?

Is one side more commonly affected?

Is chylothorax more frequent in males or females?

- Most common cause of large pleural effusion in neonate
- Cause unknown but thought to be secondary to birth trauma causing damage of the thoracic duct
- Right side more commonly affected (>50%)
- Males affected twice as often as females

FIGURE Caffey: 1998

Congenital cystic adenomatoid malformation

When can a cystic adenomatoid malformation appear solid?

Which is the most common type?

Which type has a higher incidence of associated anomalies?

- Congenital cystic adenomatoid malformations have a connection to the bronchial tree (unlike sequestrations)
- Delay often occurs in clearance of fetal lung fluid from the affected lung, giving an opaque appearance
- Type III has microscopic cysts and appears solid
- Type I the most common form, but type II has 30 to 50% incidence of associated anomalies, which can lead to early demise

FIGURE Kirks: 580

Congenital lobar emphysema

What lobe is most frequently affected in lobar emphysema?

What is the usual treatment?

What percent have associated heart disease?

- As in adenomatoid malformations, clearance of fluid from involved lobe can be delayed, leading to an opaque appearance
- Left upper lobe is most frequently affected; treatment is usually surgical excision
- Congenital heart lesions (patent ductus arteriosus or ventricular septal defect) seen in 15%

FIGURE Caffey: 2009

10

Pulmonary agenesis

What can distinguish pulmonary agenesis from the other lesions?

Is one lung more frequently affected?

What percent have associated anomalies?

- Unlike the other entities, affected lung is smaller and mediastinal structures displaced toward the involved side
- Both lungs equally affected
- Up to 50% have other anomalies; patent ductus arteriosus (PDA), tracheoesophageal fistula, hemivertebra, and other ipsilateral skeletal anomalies are common

FIGURE Caffey: 449

Diaphragmatic hernia

What is the most common type of hernia?

Which side is most frequently involved in diaphragmatic hernia?

What clues help in diagnosis?

- 95% are posterior Bochdalek hernia; only 5% are the anterior Morgagni type
- Left-sided hernia more common by a ratio of 9:1
- Clues include a gasless abdomen or clinical history of scaphoid abdomen; tip of endogastric tube may appear above the expected level of the diaphragm

FIGURE Kirks: 744

Neoplasms

What neoplasms may appear in the neonatal period?

- Congenital neuroblastoma and teratoma most common neonatal neoplasms; both may have calcifications, but neuroblastoma arises in posterior mediastinum, teratomas more common in anterior mediastinum
- Look for posterior mediastinal involvement, such as vertebral body changes or spreading of the posterior ribs

CYSTIC LUNG LESIONS

List causes of cystic lung lesions in children.

Congenital lobar emphysema
Congenital cystic adenomatoid malformation
Bronchopulmonary dysplasia
Congenital diaphragmatic hernia
Papillomatosis
Langerhans cell histiocytosis
Cystic fibrosis
Pneumatoceles
    Postinfectious
    Post hydrocarbon ingestion

Differential diagnosis

How is the differential diagnosis narrowed initially?

- Many of these lesions are congenital, appearing at or near birth, such as lobar emphysema, diaphragmatic hernia, bronchopulmonary dysplasia, and adenomatoid malformation
- Hydrocarbon ingestions most common in toddlers; pulmonary papillomatosis develops years after initial laryngeal infection
- Cystic bronchiectasis in cystic fibrosis also develops after years of recurrent infections

Bronchopulmonary dysplasia

What causes bronchopulmonary dysplasia?

What syndrome can appear identical radiographically?

- Caused by combined effect of oxygen toxicity and barotrauma in premature infants requiring ventilatory support
- Indistinguishable from Wilson-Mikity syndrome on radiographs

FIGURE Kirks: 608

10

Papillomatosis

Do papillomas have malignant potential?

What percent spread to the lungs?

- Papillomas are the most common laryngeal tumors in children
- Usually benign; rarely degenerate to squamous cell carcinoma
- Thought to spread to the lung after manipulation such as endoscopy or tracheostomy (in less than 1% of cases); average appearance in lungs occurs 10 years later

FIGURE Caffey: 624

Langerhans cell histiocytosis

What percent of cases of Langerhans cell histiocytosis have pulmonary involvement?

Are the changes more extensive in the upper or lower lobes?

Is it a common cause of cystic lung disease in childhood?

- Approximately 50% of cases have pulmonary involvement
- Upper lobes usually are more extensively involved than lower lobes
- Has been called the most common cause of cystic lung disease in children
- Spontaneous pneumothorax may occur in 10 to 25% of cases

FIGURE Caffey: 554

Cystic fibrosis

What organism colonizes children with cystic fibrosis?

Which lobe has the most extensive involvement with bronchiectasis?

- Children with cystic fibrosis (CF) eventually become colonized with *Pseudomonas aeruginosa* (rare mucoid type)
- Right upper lobe usually most severely involved
- Cystic bronchiectasis may become large and contain air-fluid levels
- Associated peribronchial thickening, hyperinflation, and mucus plugs distinguish CF from other causes of cystic lung disease

FIGURE Caffey: 499

Hydrocarbon ingestion

After how many hours does a normal chest film exclude the diagnosis of significant hydrocarbon ingestion?

What causes pneumatocele formation?

- Normal chest film 6 to 12 hours after hydrocarbon ingestion makes a significant ingestion unlikely
- Initial film finding: bibasilar airspace consolidation
- During healing phase, pneumatoceles may form as a result of bronchial necrosis with air trapping

FIGURE Kirks: 691

Postinfectious pneumatoceles

What infections are commonly associated with cavity or pneumatocele formation?

- Patients with coccidioidomycosis often develop thin-walled cavities
- Pneumatoceles are characteristic of staphylococcal pneumonias but also are described in bacterial pneumonias caused by other organisms, such as *Escherichia coli* or *Klebsiella* spp

FIGURES Caffey: 549; Kirks: 635

MILIARY INTERSTITIAL DISEASE

What is the differential diagnosis for miliary interstitial disease?

Tuberculosis and fungal infections
Sarcoid
Lymphocytic interstitial pneumonitis
Varicella pneumonia
Langerhans cell histiocytosis

Tuberculosis (TB)

What causes miliary pattern?

Does miliary TB heal with the formation of miliary calcifications?

Is adenopathy a common association?

- After primary infection, mycobacteria are hematogenously spread through lungs, inciting an inflammatory reaction
- It does not form calcifications when it heals
- Although adenopathy is more common in children than in adults, it is an uncommon finding

FIGURE   Caffey: 543

Sarcoid

What is the common age of presentation of childhood sarcoid?

How does it differ from the adult presentation?

- Uncommon in childhood; when it occurs, usually it presents between ages of 5 and 15 years
- More common in black children (80%)
- Thoracic adenopathy present in all children at diagnosis (versus present in 84% of adults)
- Classic 1-2-3 sign of adults (unilateral paratracheal adenopathy and bilateral hilar adenopathy) present in only 13% of children
- Usual pattern in children: bilateral paratracheal and hilar adenopathy

FIGURE   Kirks: 700

Lymphocytic interstitial pneumonitis (LIP)

What disease is LIP associated with?

What causes LIP?

Does LIP have prognostic implications?

- Associated with pediatric acquired immunodeficiency syndrome (AIDS)
- Children have an abundance of lymphoid tissue in the pulmonary interstitium
- Caused by immune response to an antigenic stimulus
- Positive prognostic indicator, because it implies that the child is still able to mount an immune response to a foreign antigen

FIGURES   Caffey: 538; Kirks: 695

Varicella pneumonia

Is varicella pneumonia common in the pediatric population?

- Only 15% of all patients with varicella develop pneumonia; varicella pneumonia is uncommon in the pediatric age group unless the child is immunocompromised
- Varicella and measles are infections common in children with lymphoma and leukemia
- History of skin lesions aids in diagnosis

FIGURE   Caffey: 568

10

Langerhans cell histiocytosis

What portion of the lungs is predominantly involved in Langerhans cell histiocytosis?

What feature can help distinguish it from the other processes in the differential?

Name a characteristic associated complication.

- Upper two thirds of lungs affected; costophrenic angles spared
- Presence of thin-walled cysts combined with fine nodules virtually diagnostic
- Recurrent pneumothoraces occur in 10 to 25%

FIGURES   Caffey: 629, 630

ANTERIOR MEDIASTINAL MASSES

What is the differential diagnosis for anterior mediastinal masses?

Teratoma (other germ cell tumors)
Lymphoma (Hodgkin's disease)
Thymoma
Thyroid lesions
Large normal thymus in young children

What percent of germ cell tumors in the anterior mediastinum are teratomas?

What CT findings suggest a malignant teratoma?

Teratoma

- Teratomas account for approximately 90% of germ cell tumors arising in anterior mediastinum; seminoma, embryonal cell carcinoma, endodermal sinus (yolk sac) tumor, and choriocarcinoma account for the other 10%
- Benign teratomas are well circumscribed with cystic spaces, fat, and calcific densities
- Malignant teratomas more solid, lack fat and calcifications, and can be seen infiltrating the surrounding fat

FIGURE Kirks: 663

What percent of mediastinal masses occur anteriorly?

What is the most common anterior mediastinal mass?

What type of lymphoma is most common in the anterior chest?

What is the most common type of Hodgkin's disease?

Are cystic changes common in the nodal masses before therapy?

What is the most common presentation?

Lymphoma

- Mediastinal masses divided fairly equally among compartments (30 to 40% anterior, 30% middle, 30 to 40% posterior)
- Most common anterior lesion is lymphoma (70%)
- Non-Hodgkin's lymphoma is more common overall, but Hodgkin's disease is the most common in chest
- Most common type is nodular sclerosing
- In 25% of cases, cystic-appearing nodes are seen at presentation; thought to be secondary to necrosis from rapid growth of tumor, do not appear to change prognosis
- Necrotic changes can also occur after therapy; if patient is stable, he or she can be monitored on serial examinations
- Most cases present with enlarged cervical nodes; thorax involved in 85%

FIGURE Kirks: 667

How common are thymomas?

At what age do they present?

Are they associated with myasthenia gravis?

What percent are malignant?

Thymoma

- Thymomas account for 2% of anterior mediastinal masses
- In children, usually present after age 10 years
- Unlike adults, children rarely have myasthenia gravis
- 10 to 15% considered malignant

FIGURE Kirks: 667

What is the differential for posterior mediastinal masses?

POSTERIOR MEDIASTINAL MASSES

Neurogenic tumors
Dural ectasia
Diaphragmatic hernia
   Extramedullary hematopoiesis
   Neurenteric cysts

What is the most common posterior mediastinal mass?

Are most masses benign?

A cervical or upper thoracic neuroblastoma can present with what syndrome?

What syndrome is associated with neurogenic tumors and dural ectasia?

Neurogenic tumors

- Neurogenic tumors account for 95% of posterior mediastinal masses
- Most are malignant neuroblastomas
- Approximately 10 to 15% of neuroblastomas appear in the posterior mediastinum
- They can present with Horner syndrome, which includes ptosis, miosis, and anhidrosis
- Nerve sheath tumors and dural ectasia are seen with neurofibromatosis; these lesions enlarge the neuroforamina and cause posterior vertebral body scalloping

FIGURES Kirks: 674–676

Neurenteric cysts

What spinal cord anomalies may be seen?

What vertebral anomalies may be seen?

- Associated cord anomalies include tethered cord, patent fistulous tract, or intradural cysts
- Associated vertebral anomalies include scoliosis, hemivertebra, butterfly vertebra, and dysraphism
- Vertebral anomalies at the same level or at a level higher than the cyst

Extramedullary hematopoiesis

What is an important cause of extramedullary hematopoiesis?

Where is it usually located?

What are some associated findings?

- Usually caused by hereditary anemias such as thalassemia or hereditary spherocytosis
- Most commonly seen in lower portion of posterior mediastinum bilaterally
- Look for splenomegaly and widened rib ends

AIRWAY

RETROPHARYNGEAL MASS

List five causes of retropharyngeal soft tissue thickening.

Retropharyngeal cellulitis/abscess
Cervical neuroblastoma
Cystic hygroma
Lymphoma
Hemorrhage

Retropharyngeal cellulitis/abscess

Retropharyngeal abscesses occur in what age group?

What plain film finding distinguishes cellulitis from abscess?

- Retropharyngeal abscess occurs most frequently in children aged less than 1 year
- Usual cause: previous oropharyngeal infection; occasionally secondary to penetrating trauma from a foreign body
- A definitive diagnosis of abscess requires the presence of air in the thickened tissues

FIGURE   Kirks: 565

Cervical neuroblastoma

What percent of neuroblastoma occurs in the neck?

Do cervical neuroblastomas have a better or worse prognosis than those arising in the adrenal gland?

What imaging is required?

- Primary cervical neuroblastoma occurs approximately 5% of the time
- Has better prognosis than neuroblastoma arising in adrenal gland given similar stage
- MRI usually recommended because many have intraspinal involvement; CT best for demonstrating calcifications

Cystic hygroma

What percent of cystic hygromas arise in the neck?

When are they usually detected?

- Developmental anomalies of the primitive lymphatic system
- Majority arise in the neck; some extend into mediastinum
- Approximately 90% discovered in first year of life

FIGURE   Caffey: 362

Lymphoma

What percent of neck masses are malignant?

What is the most common malignancy?

- Most neck masses either congenital or inflammatory; malignant lesions only 11% of the total
- Most common malignancy is lymphoma

10

ENLARGED EPIGLOTTIS

Epiglottitis
Angioneurotic edema
Omega epiglottis
Trauma/hemorrhage
Epiglottic cyst

Epiglottitis

What causes epiglottitis?

What percent of cases have associated subglottic edema?

- Most often caused by *Haemophilus influenzae*
- Approximately 25% of children also have subglottic edema; thus, lateral film of neck required to exclude the diagnosis, because frontal film could be misinterpreted as croup

FIGURE Kirks: 562

Angioneurotic edema

What causes angioneurotic edema?

How can it be distinguished from epiglottitis?

- Autosomal dominant condition caused by decrease in C1 esterase inhibitor, which activates complement system, causing transudation of fluid into extravascular spaces
- Involvement of other soft tissues of neck (e.g., retropharyngeal space) or swelling of extremities can help differentiate from epiglottitis

Omega epiglottis

What is an omega epiglottis?

- Normal variant caused by accentuated U shape of epiglottis
- On lateral view this results in enlarged appearance of epiglottis; however, aryepiglottic folds are normal, unlike those in epiglottitis

Trauma/hemorrhage

What entities can cause hemorrhagic enlargement of the epiglottis?

What other lesions can mimic epiglottitis?

- Trauma from foreign bodies or chemical ingestions can result in edema and hemorrhage of epiglottis in normal patients
- Hemophiliacs can experience increased complications from episodes of minor trauma, but more commonly experience episodes of recurrent bleeding into joints
- A benign cyst or papilloma can cause apparent enlargement of the epiglottis, but the clinical picture would be much different

GASTROINTESTINAL TRACT

GASLESS ABDOMEN

What is the differential diagnosis for a gasless abdomen?

Isolated esophageal atresia
Severe peritonitis
Diaphragmatic hernia, congenital
Central nervous system abnormalities
Vomiting
Paralysis

Esophageal atresia without distal fistula

What are the clinical symptoms of esophageal atresia?

What are the plain film findings?

- Children present with difficulty handling secretions and feeding intolerance
- May be history of failure to pass an orogastric (OG) tube
- Usually there is evidence of air-filled proximal blind-ended pouch in which OG tube may be coiled

- Incidence of esophageal atresia is increased in children with Down syndrome; plain film evidence of this should be sought
- Side of aortic arch should be noted so that surgeon may plan surgical approach
- Contrast study is not generally required for diagnosis; if requested, a few milliliters of barium may be administered, then removed at end of study

FIGURE   Kirks: 748

Diaphragmatic hernia, congenital

- Bochdalek hernia most common type (90%)
- Caused by patent communication between abdominal and pleural cavities and almost always on the left
- Clinical symptoms primarily are related to the degree of pulmonary hypoplasia; in addition, malrotation always occurs, increasing the risk of volvulus and obstruction

FIGURE   Kirks: 744

Central nervous system (CNS) abnormalities

- If associated intracranial hemorrhage exists, infant may have abnormalities of swallowing, which would decrease amount of bowel gas; in addition, infant may be paralyzed in order to be ventilated
- Patients at increased risk of peritonitis from necrotizing enterocolitis

DOUBLE BUBBLE

Duodenal atresia/stenosis
Malrotation with midgut volvulus or Ladd bands
Annular pancreas
Duodenal web
Preduodenal portal vein

Duodenal atresia/stenosis

- Duodenal atresia the most common cause of congenital duodenal obstruction
- Ratio of duodenal atresia to stenosis is 4:1
- Thought to be secondary to an intrauterine vascular insult
- Occasionally, a duodenal web can be seen as a circumferential filling defect on upper GI examination
- If web is distended, may give a "windsock" appearance

FIGURES   Kirks: 756, 757

Malrotation with midgut volvulus

- Double bubble sign can suggest midgut volvulus but is not specific
- Even if plain film is normal, bilious emesis is an emergency requiring further work-up to exclude malrotation and volvulus
- Upper GI series can confirm malrotation with or without volvulus; it may not be possible to differentiate the other entities
- Upper GI series shows characteristic corkscrew pattern to the second and third portions of the duodenum with abnormal fixation of the ligament of Treitz; if contrast passes into jejunum, loops are in the right abdomen

Is a study required for diagnosis?

What is the most common congenital diaphragmatic hernia?

Which side is most often involved?

What is the primary cause of morbidity and mortality?

Why is a gasless abdomen common in premature infants?

List five common causes of double bubble. Which is most common?

What is the most common cause of obstruction?

Which is more common, atresia or stenosis?

What is the cause of atresia and stenosis?

What would a duodenal web look like on upper GI examination?

Is there a characteristic plain film finding for midgut volvulus?

What study can distinguish among the causes of double bubble?

What are the characteristic upper GI findings of midgut volvulus?

- Ultrasound recently was described as a way to identify a volvulus: an abnormal inverted relationship between the superior mesenteric artery (SMA) and the superior mesenteric vein (SMV) is sought; normally, the vein is to the right of the artery; however, one third of patients with volvulus have normally related mesenteric vessels

What are Ladd bands? How do they cause obstruction?

- Abnormal peritoneal bands that extend from the cecum in the left upper quadrant to the liver in the right upper quadrant called *Ladd bands*; they cross anterior to duodenum causing obstruction

FIGURE   Kirks: 780

Annular pancreas

What causes annular pancreas?

- During fetal life, the ventral pancreatic anlage must rotate 180 degrees; if it passes behind the duodenum, it encircles it and narrows the second portion
- Annular pancreas is often associated with duodenal stenosis or atresia
- CT may identify the abnormal pancreatic tissue

DILATED BOWEL IN NEWBORN

Give the differential diagnosis for dilated bowel in infancy.

Intestinal atresia
Hirschsprung disease
Meconium ileus
Meconium plugs
Malrotation
Incarcerated inguinal hernia
Intussusception
Imperforate anus

Use the following mnemonic:
    A Atresia, aganglionosis (Hirschsprung)
    I Intussusception, imperforate anus, incarcerated inguinal
       hernia
    M Meconium, malrotation

Which causes of dilated bowel in a newborn are associated with a microcolon?

- Ileal atresia, total colonic aganglionosis, and meconium ileus are associated with microcolon; these entities do not allow succus entericus of small bowel to reach colon during development, which causes small, underdeveloped colon

FIGURES   Kirks: 772, 860

What is the association between meconium ileus and cystic fibrosis?

Which causes of dilated bowel in a newborn can be treated by the radiologist? How?

- Meconium ileus is a presenting symptom of cystic fibrosis in more than 95% of cases; however, only about 10% of patients with cystic fibrosis present with meconium ileus
- Meconium ileus, meconium plugs, and intussusception are amenable to therapeutic studies in radiology
- Enema with hyperosmolar water-contrast agents can draw fluid into bowel lumen and allow infant to evacuate meconium plugs or the thick tenacious meconium in terminal ileum in meconium ileus
- Intussusception can be reduced by either hydrostatic contrast enema or air reduction; the only contraindications to reduction are free air or peritoneal signs
- In neonates lead point is common, such as duplication, Meckel diverticulum, or meconium ileus; this makes reduction less successful

FIGURES   Kirks: 882, 886

10

What other plain film findings help distinguish among the various causes of dilated bowel in a newborn?

- Association exists between Hirschsprung disease and Down syndrome; 11 ribs or flattened acetabular angles should be sought
- Meconium ileus and atresias have an increased incidence of meconium peritonitis; flocculent abdominal calcifications should be sought
- Imperforate anus is in the VACTERL (vertebral, anal, cardiac, tracheal, esophageal, renal, and limb) associations; associated anomalies should be sought
- Inguinal hernias can cause thickening of inguinoscrotal fold

FIGURES Kirks: 859, 880

What does an obstructed appearance imply with malrotation and midgut volvulus?

- Obstructed appearance indicates complete venous obstruction because bowel gas is absorbed into venous system if the venous drainage system is patent

FIGURE Kirks: 781

ESOPHAGEAL STRICTURES

List the causes of esophageal strictures.

Caustic ingestion
Gastroesophageal reflux
Epidermolysis bullosa
Chronic granulomatous disease of childhood
After surgery for esophageal atresia

Caustic ingestion

What type of ingestion results in esophageal stricture?

What are the characteristics of the stricture?

What is a long-term complication?

- Alkaline ingestions (lye) commonly cause acute esophageal inflammation and necrosis, with the eventual formation of strictures (30%); acidic ingestions more often cause damage in the gastric antrum
- Strictures may be multiple and occur at any site, but long strictures involving middle and distal esophagus are most common
- Increased risk of carcinoma occurring years after the ingestion

FIGURE Kirks: 836

Gastroesophageal reflux

Why is gastroesophageal reflux more common in infants?

What are the clinical symptoms?

How is reflux diagnosed?

- Anatomy of gastroesophageal sphincter in children predisposes them to reflux: sphincter is narrower and less prominent, orientation of esophagus and stomach more direct, and intraabdominal length of esophagus shorter
- Most infants aged less than 1 year experience reflux, but it is usually asymptomatic; reflux is clinically significant if esophagitis, failure to thrive, aspiration, or weight loss occurs
- Upper GI series can diagnose only 25%, but can identify hiatal hernias, strictures, and gastric outlet obstructions
- More sensitive methods of detection include nuclear medicine study using Tc-labeled sulfur colloid or 24-hour pH probe monitoring, which do not provide anatomic detail
- Long-term reflux can lead to strictures in middle and distal esophagus

Epidermolysis bullosa

What are the clinical findings in epidermolysis bullosa?

Where do the strictures form?

- Rare congenital skin disorder that affects squamous epithelium, causing bullous skin lesions after mild trauma
- Esophageal strictures form at areas of minor trauma; are more common at level of carina or at proximal or distal end of esophagus
- Presence of skin lesions helps with diagnosis

FIGURE Caffey: 1012

10

Chronic granulomatous disease of childhood

What is the abnormality in chronic granulomatous disease?

How are the strictures formed?

- Hereditary disease characterized by abnormal phagocyte function: bacteria ingested but not killed by neutrophils; recurrent infections result in granuloma formation in the GI tract
- Strictures are thought to be secondary to inflammation from granulomatous process in esophagus
- Strictures usually are proximal and long

After surgery for esophageal atresia

What are the esophageal problems after surgical repair of esophageal atresia?

- Distal esophagus always demonstrates abnormal motility because of abnormal neural mechanisms distal to the site of atresia; this predisposes to increased risk of gastroesophageal reflux
- Stricture can form at the site of surgical repair; anastomotic leaks or recurrence of tracheoesophageal fistula can also occur

FIGURE   Caffey: 1003

RIGHT UPPER QUADRANT CYSTIC MASS

What are the causes of a cystic mass in the right upper quadrant?

Choledochal cyst
Hydropic gallbladder
Duodenal duplication
Pancreatic pseudocyst
Mesenteric or omental cyst
Ovarian cyst
Hepatic or renal cyst

Choledochal cyst

List the elements in the classic triad associated with choledochal cyst.

What are the complications of a choledochal cyst?

What is the treatment?

- Classic triad (20 to 50%) includes jaundice, right upper quadrant (RUQ) pain, and RUQ mass; jaundice is the most common presenting symptom (70%)
- Increased risk of cholangitis, choledocholithiasis, recurrent pancreatitis, and cholangiocarcinoma; risk of development of carcinoma increased twenty-fold
- Treatment of choice is complete surgical resection with enteric drainage

FIGURE   Kirks: 785

Hydropic gallbladder

Why do children with Kawasaki syndrome get a hydropic gallbladder?

What else causes a hydropic gallbladder?

- Kawasaki syndrome commonly is associated with hydropic gallbladder, which is thought to be a result of small vessel vasculitis
- Gallbladder wall thickness usually normal
- Usually resolves without sequelae
- Other reported causes include prolonged hyperalimentation, leptospirosis, and sepsis

FIGURE   Caffey: 952

Duodenal duplication

What is the most common location for an intestinal duplication?

Does duplication occur on the mesenteric or antimesenteric side of the bowel?

What percent contain ectopic gastric mucosa?

- Terminal ileum is the most common site of duplication (incidence approximately 35%); duodenal duplication is relatively uncommon (5% of total)
- Duodenal duplication is located on the mesenteric side of bowel
- 15 to 35% described as containing ectopic gastric mucosa, which may lead to bleeding and perforation

10

How can duplications be distinguished from other RUQ lesions?

- If echogenic lining consistent with bowel mucosa is identified, diagnosis is intestinal duplication

FIGURE   Kirks: 767

Pancreatic pseudocyst

What is the most common cause of pancreatitis in childhood?
List other common causes.

In what percent of cases does a pseudocyst develop?

How are pseudocysts treated?

- Trauma is the most common cause of pancreatitis in childhood; other causes are cystic fibrosis, medications (steroids), sepsis, hyperlipidemia
- Inflammatory pseudocyst occurs in approximately 5% of cases of pancreatitis
- Can be located anywhere in abdomen and less commonly in the pelvis or mediastinum
- May spontaneously decompress into bowel, but drainage (percutaneous or surgical) usually is required

FIGURE   Kirks: 841

Mesenteric or omental cyst

Which is more common, omental or mesenteric cyst?

How do patients usually present?

What is the most common complication?

- Mesenteric cyst is four to five times more common than omental cyst
- Several causes, including congenital, traumatic, infectious, and neoplastic
- Usually presents as asymptomatic abdominal mass
- Torsion is the most common complication (10%)
- May become infected

FIGURE   Kirks: 820

Ovarian cyst

Are ovarian cysts common in neonates?

What complications are associated with them?

How are they treated?

- Common in neonates
- Location commonly is abdominal
- Caused by follicular development secondary to maternal hormonal stimulation
- Presents as asymptomatic mass; may undergo hemorrhage or torsion
- Treated conservatively unless complicated or particularly large, in which case surgically removed

FIGURES   Kirks: 1030; Caffey: 1394

FOCAL HEPATIC LESIONS

What entities are in the differential diagnosis of a focal hepatic lesion?

Hemangioendothelioma
Hepatoblastoma
Hepatocellular carcinoma
Mesenchymal hamartoma

Hemangioendothelioma

What is the natural history of a hemangioendothelioma?

What are the findings on a contrast-enhanced CT?

- Natural course is to proliferate and grow for first several months of life, followed by regression with involution occurring by 1 to 1 1/2 years
- Usually solitary on CT and may have central fibrosis or cystic degeneration; calcifications common; after contrast administration intense enhancement seen from the periphery, spreading centrally; aorta may markedly diminish in size after take-off of celiac plexus

What is Kasabach-Merritt syndrome?

- Children may present with abdominal mass, congestive heart failure, or thrombocytopenia from consumptive coagulopathy (Kasabach-Merritt syndrome)

FIGURE Caffey: 956

Hepatoblastoma

At what age do hepatoblastomas present?

- Hepatoblastomas present in the first 3 years; most patients are less than 2 years old
- Distinguished from hemangioendothelioma by lack of centripetal contrast enhancement

What is the tumor marker?

- Serum alpha fetoprotein level is elevated in almost all patients

FIGURE Kirks: 814

Hepatocellular carcinoma

What are risk factors for the development of hepatocellular carcinoma?

- Usually occurs in children aged more than 3 years
- Chronic hepatitis, cirrhosis, glycogen storage disease, Wilson disease, and tyrosinemia are established risk factors

Which are more common malignant or benign tumors?

- Malignant tumors are twice as common as benign lesions

FIGURE Caffey: 961

Mesenchymal hamartoma

How does mesenchymal hamartoma present?

- Usually large; commonly presents as asymptomatic abdominal mass in children aged less than 2 years
- Benign lesion treated by surgical resection

Do they have malignant potential?

- Multiloculated cystic mass, no calcifications

FIGURE Kirks: 813

GENITOURINARY TRACT

ADRENAL MASSES

What are the causes of adrenal masses in children?

Adrenal hemorrhage
Pheochromocytoma
Adrenal carcinoma
Adenoma
Neuroblastoma
Teratomas and other germ cell tumors
Abscess

Adrenal hemorrhage

What clinical settings are associated with adrenal hemorrhage?

- Associated with birth trauma, maternal diabetes, hypoxemia, and hypovolemia

Is hemorrhage associated with adrenal insufficiency?

- Despite large bilateral hemorrhages, adrenal insufficiency rarely is present

How is hemorrhage differentiated from neuroblastoma?

- Initially may closely resemble congenital neuroblastoma, but is an avascular lesion and involutes over time; given the excellent prognosis of congenital neuroblastoma, it is safe to observe a neonatal adrenal lesion for several weeks to determine if it is resolving with time
- In utero adrenal mass most likely represents neuroblastoma because in utero hemorrhage is rare

FIGURE Kirks: 1026

Pheochromocytoma

What percent of pheochromocytomas present in childhood?

- Arise in neural crest cells; approximately two thirds arise in adrenal gland
- 5% develop in childhood

Describe the clinical presentation.

- Presents with symptoms of catecholamine production: hypertension, flushing, and tachycardia

What entities are associated?

- Associated with multiple endocrine neoplasia (MEN) syndromes, von Hippel-Lindau disease, and neurofibromatosis

FIGURE Kirks: 1029

Adrenal carcinoma

What syndrome predisposes to the development of adrenal carcinoma?

- Children with Beckwith-Wiedemann syndrome have an increased incidence of adrenal carcinoma

What paraneoplastic syndromes are associated with carcinoma?

- Usually hormonally active: androgen excess is the most common syndrome (seen in 33%); rarely, secretes estrogens
- In children aged less than 10 years, Cushing syndrome usually is caused by adrenal malignancy

Which is more common, carcinoma or adenoma?

- Carcinomas are far more common than adenomas in children

FIGURE Caffey: 1428

Neuroblastoma

Is neuroblastoma the most common childhood malignancy?

- Third most common malignancy in childhood after leukemia/lymphoma and CNS tumors
- Second most common abdominal malignancy after Wilms tumor

What is Verner-Morrison syndrome?

- Verner-Morrison syndrome occurs secondary to elevated vasoactive intestinal peptide, which causes hypokalemia and watery diarrhea

Is an adrenal primary a favorable prognostic factor?

- Extraabdominal location is a favorable prognostic factor; may be symptomatic and thus present earlier

HYDRONEPHROSIS

Give the differential diagnosis for hydronephrosis in childhood.

Primary megaureter
Prune-belly syndrome
Duplicated system with obstructed upper pole
Ureteropelvic obstruction
Vesicoureteral reflux
Posterior urethral valves

Imaging studies

What studies could help differentiate the entities?

- Initial study usually is ultrasound, which can usually identify an obstructed duplicated system; ultrasound is not as sensitive in detection of nonobstructed duplex kidney; most cases of prune-belly syndrome and posterior urethral valves result in bilateral hydronephrosis
- VCUG, the next examination, can exclude vesicoureteral reflux and presence of posterior urethral valves
- Excretory urogram can identify ureteropelvic junction obstruction or primary megaureter; fluoroscopic evaluation during study can show adynamic distal ureter of primary megaureter
- Nuclear medicine renal study can also show obstruction, but with less anatomical detail

Primary megaureter

What causes primary megaureter?

- A form of vesicoureteral obstruction caused by adynamic portion

10

Is it more common in males or females?

of distal ureter; incorrectly termed *ureteral achalasia* because the abnormality is caused by absence of longitudinal muscle, not the absence of ganglion cells
- Ratio of males to females affected is 4:1
- Associated anomalies include ureteropelvic junction obstruction and reflux
- Bilateral in 20%

FIGURE   Kirks: 1044

Prune-belly syndrome

What is the classic triad in prune-belly syndrome?

Are posterior urethral valves always present?

- Classic triad includes deficiency of anterior abdominal musculature, urinary tract anomalies, and undescended testicles
- Two groups of patients: those with obstruction of the urethra, such as valves, who die in the neonatal period and those with functional abnormality of bladder emptying but no urethral obstruction

FIGURE   Kirks: 981

Duplicated system

What percent of ectopic ureters is associated with a duplicated system?

Why are boys with an ectopic ureter always continent?

Is ectopic ureter more common in boys or girls?

- 90% of ectopic ureters are found with a duplicated system
- Insertion site of ectopic ureter in boys is above the external sphincter, so the patient always is continent; girls may present with constant wetting because the ureter may drain into the vestibule or vagina
- Ectopic ureter is up to four times more common in girls
- Ectopic ureterocele commonly leads to obstruction of upper pole moiety

FIGURE   Kirks: 965

Ureteropelvic junction obstruction

What is the most common cause of obstruction?

What is the mechanism?

- Most common cause of obstruction
- Secondary to intrinsic abnormalities (e.g., abnormal musculature or fibrosis) or extrinsic causes (e.g., crossing vessels or fibrotic bands)
- Bilateral in 10 to 30%

FIGURE   Caffey: 1258

BILATERAL ENLARGED KIDNEYS

List five causes of bilateral enlarged kidneys.

Nephroblastomatosis
Lymphoma
Autosomal recessive polycystic kidney disease
Bilateral Wilms tumors
Leukemia

Nephroblastomatosis

What is the definition of nephroblastomatosis?

Is it malignant?

- Caused by presence of fetal metanephric blastema after 36 weeks of gestation
- Histologically benign but believed to predispose to development of Wilms tumor
- Present in many unilateral and all bilateral Wilms tumors

FIGURE   Kirks: 1006

10

Lymphoma

Is renal involvement more common in Hodgkin's or non-Hodgkin's lymphoma?

What is the most common appearance in the kidneys?

- Renal involvement more common in non-Hodgkin's than in Hodgkin's lymphoma
- Most common pattern of involvement is multiple nodules (60 to 70%); diffuse involvement is less common

FIGURE Caffey: 1252

Autosomal recessive polycystic disease

Where are the cysts located in autosomal recessive polycystic disease?

How is the liver involved?

- Cysts in polycystic disease result from dilated collecting ducts
- Fibrosis of liver is associated; inverse relationship exists between degree of renal involvement and hepatic fibrosis

FIGURE Kirks: 952

Wilms tumor

What percent of Wilms' tumors are bilateral?

Does the prognosis change with bilateral involvement?

How are they treated?

- Approximately 5% are bilateral
- Prognosis the same in unilateral and bilateral involvement
- Kidney with dominant tumor excised and contralateral tumor resected; chemotherapy also instituted

FIGURE Caffey: 1245

MUSCULOSKELETAL SYSTEM

PERIOSTEAL REACTION

List causes of periosteal reaction.

Physiological
Metastatic disease
Caffey's disease
Syphilis
Prostaglandin therapy
Scurvy
Hypervitaminosis A
Trauma
Leukemia
Osteomyelitis

Physiologic

What is the most common cause of periosteal reaction?

- Periosteal reaction is physiologic in about 33% of cases; physiological periosteal reaction occurs during first 6 months of life
- Diaphysis of humerus, femur, and tibia are affected
- Patient is asymptomatic

Metastatic disease

What are the most common metastases to cause periosteal reaction?

- Neuroblastoma and retinoblastoma are the most common metastases to cause periosteal reaction
- Neuroblastoma is the most common solid extracranial malignancy of childhood
- Bone is the most common site of metastatic disease; children may present with bone pain
- Retinoblastoma is the most common ocular primary of childhood
- Hematogenous metastases to skeleton are common

FIGURES Kirks: 339; Caffey: 1908

Caffey's disease

What bone is most frequently affected in Caffey's disease?

What age group is most commonly affected?

- Affects mandible most frequently; other common sites include clavicles and ribs
- Most common in children aged less than 6 months
- Presence of fever, irritability, and elevated white blood cell count can distinguish from physiological periosteal reaction

FIGURE Kirks: 390

Syphilis

When do the characteristic bony changes of syphilis occur?

Describe other expected bony changes.

- Delay of 6 to 8 weeks between time of transplacental infection and development of bony abnormalities; changes may be present at birth or appear later, depending on time of infection
- Periosteal reaction involves diaphysis and metaphysis
- Presence of lucent metaphyseal bands and metaphyseal irregularities should be sought
- Wimberger sign is destruction of the medial aspect of proximal medial metaphysis

FIGURE Kirks: 332

Prostaglandin therapy

Why are children treated with prostaglandin therapy?

- Used to keep ductus arteriosus patent in children with ductus-dependent congenital heart lesion
- Periosteal reaction incorporated into developing bone

Scurvy

When do the bony changes of scurvy appear?

What are the white line of Frankel and Pelkan beaks?

Where do Wimberger rings appear?

- Secondary to deficiency of vitamin C
- Almost always occurs after 6 months
- Subperiosteal hemorrhage leads to extensive periosteal new bone formation
- White line of Frankel is preserved zone of provisional calcification.
- Scurvy (Trümmerfeld) zone is a lucent band proximal to the zone of provisional calcification
- Metaphyseal fractures may heal and form spurs at right angles to bone shaft (Pelkan beaks)
- Wimberger rings: fine white line of mineral deposition that occurs around epiphyses

FIGURES Caffey: 1757–1759

Hypervitaminosis A

When do the changes of hypervitaminosis A occur?

Which bones are affected?

- Caused by chronic overingestion of vitamin A
- Patients generally present at 1 to 3 years of age
- Bone changes typically occur 6 months after excessive intake begins
- Ulna and digits are most commonly involved; other tubular bones also are involved
- Metaphyses and epiphyses usually are normal
- Recovery usually complete when vitamin is stopped

FIGURE Caffey: 1761

Nonaccidental trauma

What skeletal findings should be sought in suspected nonaccidental trauma?

- Skeletal findings common in young children who have been abused
- Subperiosteal hemorrhage leads to periosteal reaction

- Fractures in various stages of healing or with an inappropriate history are suggestive
- Metaphyseal fractures in normal bones are virtually pathognomonic for abuse; other diseases may have metaphyseal irregularities, but bones generally are osteopenic
- Osteogenesis imperfecta with normal bone density may require collagen analysis

What other fractures have high specificity?
- Fractures of hands, feet, scapula, and spine are uncommon in accidental trauma

FIGURES Caffey: 1814–1817

Leukemia

What percentage of children with leukemia have skeletal changes?
- Most common childhood malignancy; acute lymphoblastic type (ALL) predominates
- More than 50% of patients have skeletal findings
- Periosteal reaction secondary to infiltration of leukemic cell into the subperiosteum

What are other skeletal manifestations?
- Generalized osteopenia usually is present; lucent bands seen around large joints are not caused by leukemic infiltration
- Multiple lytic lesions also are seen

VERTEBRA PLANA

List five causes of vertebra plana.

Langerhans cell histiocytosis
Leukemia/lymphoma
Idiopathic juvenile osteoporosis
Infection
Steroid effect
Cushing syndrome
Exogenous
Trauma

Langerhans cell histiocytosis

What is the most common cause of vertebra plana?
- Most common cause of vertebra plana
What causes the flattened vertebral body?
- Results from proliferation of histiocytes in bone with subsequent collapse; single vertebral body most frequently affected
- If contiguous vertebral bodies are involved, disc spaces are maintained

FIGURE Kirks: 205

Leukemia

What is the most common form of childhood leukemia?
- Acute lymphoblastic (ALL) type is the most common childhood leukemia

What percentage of patients have bony manifestations?
- Skeletal manifestations occur in 50% of patients and include lytic lesions, radiolucent metaphyseal bands, periosteal reaction, and diffuse osteopenia
- Multiple collapsed vertebral bodies are visible

What causes the associated osteopenia?
- Osteopenia is caused by change in mineral metabolism or leukemic infiltration

Idiopathic juvenile osteoporosis

What is idiopathic juvenile osteoporosis?
- Diagnosis is made by exclusion; results of laboratory studies usually are normal
- Uncommon, self-limited process caused by increased bone resorption

What are the findings in the spine?

- Generally occurs a few years before puberty
- Manifested by osteopenia of the spine, particularly in thoracic and lumbar regions
- Multiple compression fractures may occur
- Kyphosis has been described
- Fractures of long bones, especially in metaphyseal region
- Common entity in differential diagnosis: a tardive form of osteogenesis imperfecta

FIGURE Caffey: 1768

TIBIAL BOWING

List causes of tibial bowing in children.

Neurofibromatosis type I
Fibrous dysplasia
Congenital bowing
Osteofibrous dysplasia
Generalized dysplasias
Osteogenesis imperfecta
Hypophosphatasia

Neurofibromatosis (NF) type I

What percentage of patients with tibial bowing have NF type I?

Is it a late or early manifestation?

What is a common complication?

- Occurs in approximately 50% of patients with tibial bowing
- Tibial bowing may be earliest manifestation of NF type I
- Bowing may be complicated by development of pseudoarthrosis
- Tibial bowing in NF I has been classified by abnormality at site of bowing:
   Dysplastic with constriction at site
   Cystic with lucent expansile lesion at site
   Sclerotic with sclerotic focus at site

FIGURE Kirks: 377

Fibrous dysplasia

What percent of fibrous dysplasia involves the tibia?

What percent of these tibias have bowing?

- Tibia involved in approximately 20% of cases; of these, 24% have bowing
- Bowed tibias can be complicated by development of pseudoarthrosis

Congenital bowing

Which cause of tibial bowing is characterized by posterior bowing?

What is the origin of congenital bowing?

- Usually in a posteromedial direction, unlike other causes of bowing
- Benign condition is thought to be secondary to fetal positioning and intrauterine pressure

FIGURE Kirks: 377

Osteofibrous dysplasia

When does osteofibrous dysplasia usually present?

What bone is most commonly affected?

- Fibrous lesion that presents before age 10 years in 85% of cases
- Majority (>95%) present in tibia
- Lesions arise in diaphysis (middle third); anterior cortex is thinned, resulting in bowing that worsens with age

FIGURE Caffey: 1880

Osteogenesis imperfecta

What is underlying abnormality in osteogenesis imperfecta?

Which type is associated with bowing of the bones?

- Characterized by abnormality of collagen
- Commonly subdivided into four categories; type I is autosomal dominant and characterized by blue sclerae, presenile deafness, and bowing deformities of lower limbs
- Type I was previously described as tardive form because fractures increased in frequency with age

FIGURE   Kirks: 1678

Figure References

Kirks DE: *Practical Pediatric Radiology.* Boston: Little, Brown, 1991.
Silverman FN, Kuhn JP, eds: *Caffey's Pediatric X-ray Diagnosis.* St. Louis: CV Mosby, 1993.

PEDIATRIC IMAGING DISEASE ENTITIES

ADRENAL HEMORRHAGE

Clinical

- May present as abdominal mass, jaundice, or anemia
- Adrenal insufficiency is rare even in large bilateral bleeds
- Secondary to stress, asphyxia, birth trauma, or sepsis
- Right kidney only in 70%; bilateral in 10%

Imaging

- Abdominal film:
    May demonstrate calcifications in old hemorrhage; displacement of kidney
- Ultrasound:
    Echogenic suprarenal mass becomes anechoic as hemorrhage evolves; eventually, a focus of calcification can appear; differential includes neonatal neuroblastoma, which is usually more echoic; Doppler or color ultrasound can show vascularity; serial sonograms usually can distinguish from neuroblastoma, because hemorrhage should evolve with time
- CT:
    High-density suprarenal mass acutely; low-density center as hemorrhage resolves

ATRESIA, DUODENAL

Clinical

- Cause unknown: initially thought to be recanalization failure, but now thought to be caused by vascular insult
- Accounts for majority of duodenal obstructions
- Ratio of atresia to stenosis is 4:1
- Associated anomalies (50%): malrotation, congenital heart disease, other atresias of GI tract
- Down syndrome in 30% of cases; fewer than 5% of Down syndrome children have duodenal atresia
- Clinical presentation: vomiting in first days of life; may be bilious if distal to ampulla

Imaging

- Conventional films:
    "Double bubble" sign from distended stomach and duodenal bulb; amount of distal gas depends on degree of obstruction
- Contrast studies:
    Usually not indicated, but if diagnosis is in question, a small amount of contrast can be administered

ATRESIA, ESOPHAGEAL AND TRACHEOESOPHAGEAL FISTULA

Clinical

- Result of abnormal separation of primitive foregut
- May coexist with other anomalies occurring at same gestational age:
    Vertebral anomalies
    Anal atresia
    Cardiac anomalies
    Tracheoesophageal fistula
    Renal anomalies
    Limb anomalies
    These are associations, not a syndrome.
- Types:
    Isolated esophageal atresia   10%
    Atresia with proximal fistula   1%
    Atresia with distal fistula   81%
    Atresia with proximal and distal fistulas   2%
    Isolated fistula   6%
- Down syndrome is the most common abnormality associated with isolated atresia
- Right arch is associated in 5%, important for operative planning
- Tracheomalacia commonly is associated
- After repair, abnormal peristalsis of distal esophagus and reflux are common
- Complications: recurrent tracheoesophageal fistula, stricture, and leak

Imaging

- Conventional films:
    Air-distended proximal pouch
    Nasogastric tube coiled in pouch
    Distended stomach if distal fistula present
    Gasless abdomen if no distal fistula present
    May identify associated anomalies
- Contrast evaluation:
    Usually not necessary
    Air or small amount of contrast may be administered
    If contrast given, remove at end of study
    If isolated fistula suspected, 8-Fr feeding tube should be placed and contrast slowly administered throughout the length of the esophagus
    Postoperative esophagrams may identify leak or stricture

ATRESIA/STENOSIS OF SMALL INTESTINE

Clinical

- Result of in utero ischemic event
- More common than duodenal atresia
- Equal incidence in jejunum and ileum
- Atresia more common than stenosis
- Presents in first days of life with vomiting and abdominal distention; failure to pass meconium in ileal atresia; cystic fibrosis in 10%
- Treat with excision and reanastomosis

Imaging

- Abdominal film:
    Jejunal atresia
        Loops of small bowel indicating obstruction
        No other study usually indicated
    Ileal atresia
        Multiple loops of bowel with air-fluid levels
        Meconium peritonitis caused by in utero perforation in 12%
- Contrast enema:
    Usually required in ileal atresia to locate level of obstruction; microcolon occurs because small bowel secretions were not able to enter colon

AUTOSOMAL RECESSIVE POLYCYSTIC KIDNEY DISEASE

Clinical

- Inherited as autosomal recessive disorder
- Wide spectrum of clinical manifestations, depending on age
- *Perinatal form* most common: kidneys symmetrically enlarged, characterized by dilated collecting tubules (90%); most infants present at birth because of bilateral flank masses or respiratory distress resulting from lung hypoplasia; most affected infants die in newborn period from respiratory failure or renal failure
- *Intermediate forms* (neonatal and infantile): distinguished by renal ductal ectasia (25 to 50%) and mild to moderate hepatic periportal fibrosis; present after several months of life or in first few years; renal failure most common cause of death
- *Juvenile form*: characterized by diffuse progressive cystic dysplasia of bile duct accompanied by periportal fibrosis; usually presents at age 3 to 6 years with hepatosplenomegaly and portal hypertension; kidneys show tubular ectasia (10%) but renal function nearly or completely normal; death results from portal hypertension

Imaging

- Ultrasound:
    Demonstrate bilaterally enlarged kidneys with increased echogenicity because of multiple interfaces from dilated collecting tubules
    Loss of corticomedullary junction
    Small discrete macrocysts may be visualized
    Hypoechoic rim may be seen
    Hepatic fibrosis, portal hypertension, and varices may be seen in older patients
- Excretory urogram:
    Enlarged kidneys bilaterally, streaky nephrograms resulting from stasis of contrast in dilated tubules; poor function

BILIARY ATRESIA

Clinical

- Presents as obstructive jaundice in neonatal period
- Presentation similar to that of neonatal hepatitis, to which it may be related; atresia may be caused by an infectious process, but this has not been proved
- Jaundice results from focal or diffuse absence of extrahepatic bile ducts, causing obstruction
- Gallbladder usually absent or small, but reported as normal in 10%
- Treatment: surgery using direct anastomosis (12%) or Kasai procedure (portoenterostomy): anastomosis of porta hepatis to bowel loop
- Surgical correction must be performed in the first 3 months to be successful; after 90 days the success rate is 17%
- Long-term complications: development of cirrhosis; increased risk of neoplasms
- Eventually, patient may require liver transplant

Imaging

- Ultrasound:
    Initial imaging procedure; liver and intrahepatic ducts usually normal; gallbladder usually absent; 20 to 30% have identifiable gallbladder, usually less than 1 cm; periportal fibrosis may appear as increased echogenicity
- Hepatobiliary scintigraphy with ^{99m}Tc-IDA derivatives:
    Pretreatment with phenobarbital; delayed images may be required if excretion delayed; demonstrates normal uptake but no excretion into bowel; in older children, hepatic extraction may be abnormal because of advanced liver dysfunction; increased excretion through renal system

BRONCHOPULMONARY DYSPLASIA

Clinical

- Classic definition: chronic changes to lung requiring oxygen support at 28 days of life
- Secondary to mucosal damage, edema and fibrosis from oxygen therapy, and barotrauma from ventilator support
- Historically classified into four stages, which rarely are referred to today
- Treatment includes steroids and diuretics
- Chest radiograph may normalize in childhood; however, increased risk of respiratory tract infections exists, and pulmonary function is often abnormal

Imaging

- Chest film findings:
    Interstitial thickening with focal areas of atelectasis or air trapping, which may appear cystic
    Increased leakiness of lungs may result in episodes of superimposed edema

CAFFEY'S DISEASE

Clinical

- Infantile cortical hyperostosis
- Cause unknown, but viral process postulated
- Apparent in first few months of life
- Familial cases have been reported and may present at birth
- Clinical findings: fever, irritability, soft tissue swelling, and elevated white blood cell count
- Usually self-limited course

Imaging

- Conventional films:
    Periosteal thickening (epiphyses not involved); mandible (80%), ribs, clavicles affected most frequently; other sites include long bones, hands, feet, and skull

CAUSTIC INGESTION

Clinical

- Alkaline caustic ingestions produce penetrating burns of oropharynx and esophagus; agents include lye, household cleaners, and bleaches
- Early: intense inflammatory changes and sloughing of mucosa
- Later: formation of fibrotic tissue and long stricture formation
- Increased incidence of squamous cell carcinoma in injured area
- May treat with balloon dilation

Imaging

- Chest radiograph: widened mediastinum; pneumomediastinum indicates perforation
- Esophagram: may be difficult to evaluate esophagus acutely; late esophagrams show strictures (7 to 30%), which may be multiple and of variable length, involving mid and distal thirds of esophagus

CELLULITIS/ABSCESS, RETROPHARYNGEAL

Clinical

- Predisposing upper respiratory tract infection
- Usually occurs in children aged less than 1 year
- Most common organisms: staphylococci and streptococci, although mixed oral flora also are seen
- Acute onset of dysphagia and neck stiffness; fever and elevated white blood cell count
- Differential diagnosis includes hemorrhage, myxedema, cystic hygroma, neuroblastoma, hemangioma, and lymphadenopathy

Imaging

- Soft tissue lateral of neck: increased thickness of prevertebral soft tissues; loss of normal cervical lordosis; if gas is seen, diagnosis of abscess is made
- CT:
     Can confirm the presence of abscess; can demonstrate small amounts of air; shows extent of involvement

CHILD ABUSE

Clinical

- Also called *nonaccidental trauma, battered child syndrome*
- Common cause of morbidity and mortality in infancy and early childhood
- Often, delay in seeking medical treatment and provided history may not adequately account for child's injuries
- Mortality usually related to head injuries
- Fractures occur in up to 50% of cases; metaphyseal corner fractures are virtually pathognomonic of abuse
- Associated injuries include retinal hemorrhage or detachment; duodenal hematomas; liver, spleen lacerations; pancreatic pseudocysts; subdural hematomas; shear injuries of brain parenchyma

Imaging

Conventional films
- Complete skeletal survey includes:
     Two views of skull and spine
     Anteroposterior projections of all bones of body including hands and feet
     Additional images can be obtained of suspicious areas
- Spiral fractures of long bones are the most frequent fractures, but are nonspecific
- Most specific fractures are metaphyseal fractures; secondary to twisting injury; may appear as bucket handle or corner fracture, depending on film projection
- Other high-specificity fractures: scapula, spine, and small bones of hands and feet (rarely injured in accidental trauma)
- Rib fractures are caused by compressive forces on thorax; also uncommon in accidental trauma or secondary to CPR
- Multiple fractures at different stages of healing are highly suggestive

Nuclear medicine
- Bone scans may be performed for screening or to seek occult fractures if clinical suspicion is high and initial bone survey is negative; not as sensitive for skull

fractures as plain films; plain films of suspicious areas often are required for further evaluation because of lower specificity

Other modalities
- CT: usually performed for acute head injuries; shows subdural hematoma, contusion, hemorrhage, and edema
- MRI: evaluation of chronic parenchymal changes or dating of hemorrhage; more sensitive for detection of shear injuries

CHLAMYDIAL PNEUMONIA

Clinical

- Caused by infection with obligate intracellular parasite
- Infection occurs during delivery
- Patient has history of conjunctivitis (30%)
- Presents at average age of 6 weeks
- May have associated pulmonary hemorrhage

Imaging

- Chest radiograph:
    Similar to that seen in viral infection with perihilar interstitial prominence; effusions uncommon; improvement on film lags behind clinical improvement

CHOLEDOCHAL CYST

Clinical

- Focal dilatation of biliary ductal system
- Cause
    Infants: obstructive cholangiopathy leading to stenosis or atresia of common bile duct with proximal dilatation
    Children: ascribed to anomalous connection of pancreatic duct and bile duct, which allows reflux of pancreatic enzymes into the biliary system, resulting in inflammation with dilatation
- Classification:
    Type I   Fusiform dilatation of the common bile duct with or without associated dilatation of the intrahepatic ducts
    Type II   Saccular diverticulum off common bile duct
    Type III   Focal dilatation of common bile duct in duodenal wall (choledochocele)
    Type IV   Multiple dilations of intrahepatic ducts without obstruction (Caroli's disease); may be unrelated entity
- Ratio of females to males affected, 4:1; increased incidence in Asians
- 50% diagnosed in first decade
- Classic triad in 25%: pain (50%), jaundice (80%), palpable mass (50%); recurrent pancreatitis; cirrhosis
- Complications: stone formation, cholangitis, carcinoma (20-fold increase), cirrhosis, and recurrent pancreatitis
- Treatment: surgical excision with enteric drainage
- Differential diagnosis: hepatic, ovarian, mesenteric, and duplication cysts

Imaging

- Conventional films:
    Right upper quadrant soft tissue mass
- Urography:
    Displacement of the antrum anteriorly
- Ultrasound:
    Cystic mass connected to intrahepatic ducts, separate from gallbladder
- Nuclear medicine:

Biliary scans show collection of radiopharmaceutical in dilated bile duct, with or without drainage into duodenum

CHYLOTHORAX

Clinical

- Most common cause of large pleural effusion in neonate
- Becomes chylous after ingestion of fatty milk or formula
- Usually seen in term infant
- Ratio of males to females affected, 2:1
- Cause unknown; may be secondary to traumatic rupture of thoracic duct

Imaging

- Chest film findings:
  Large pleural effusion that is more common on right side; 10% may be bilateral
  May cause mass effect with shift of mediastinum to opposite side

CONGENITAL CYSTIC ADENOMATOID MALFORMATION (CCAM)

Clinical

- Hamartoma composed of cysts lined by proliferating terminal bronchiolar structures
- Maintains a connection to the bronchial tree, normal vascular supply
- Respiratory distress in first month of life (70%)
- Boys and girls affected equally; equal frequency in both lungs
- Classification
  Type I   At least one dominant cyst >2 cm (50%)
  Type II   Multiple cysts <2 cm (40%)
  Type III   Solid appearing with microscopic cysts (10%)
- Type II associated with other abnormalities (55%); has worst prognosis
- May be multiple
- Pregnancy may be complicated by polyhydramnios and fetal hydrops

Imaging

- Chest film:
  Solid or cystic lesion, depending on type and whether lesion contains air; mediastinal shift

CONGENITAL DIAPHRAGMATIC HERNIA

Clinical

Bochdalek hernia (90%)
- Secondary to patent pleuroperitoneal foramen of Bochdalek
- Organs herniated most often: small bowel (90%) and stomach (60%)
- Most frequently on the left (80%) posteriorly (Bochdalek = back)
- Ratio of males to females affected, 2:1
- Severe respiratory distress caused by lung hypoplasia
- Extracorporeal membrane oxygenation (ECMO) has improved mortality
- Associated anomalies:
  Central nervous system   30%
  Cardiovascular   20%
  Malrotation   95%
- Increased risk of volvulus with malrotation
- Delayed presentation of right-sided hernias in infants with streptococcal pneumonia

Morgagni hernia (3 to 5%)
- Most frequently on the right anteriorly
- Bilateral in 15 to 30% of cases
- Usually asymptomatic and present at older age; mnemonic: M = mature, mild

Imaging

Bochdalek hernia
- Conventional radiographs show the following:
    Opaque hemithorax, may see mass effect
    Bowel loops in the hemithorax after swallowing air
    Nasogastric tube in the hemithorax for diagnosis and bowel decompression
    Gasless abdomen
- Contrast studies generally not required
- Ultrasound can reveal defect in diaphragm

Morgagni hernia
- Chest film findings:
    Cystic lucency or opaque mass in the right cardiophrenic area
    May require contrast to identify
- Ultrasound can identify defect in diaphragm

CONGENITAL LOBAR EMPHYSEMA

Clinical

- Progressive overdistention of lobe or lobes
- Rarely contains increased number of alveoli
- Cause unknown in 50% of cases
- Known causes include cartilage deficiency, stenosis, external compression, endo-bronchial obstruction
- Ratio of males to females affected, 3:1
- Distribution
    Left upper lobe   45%
    Right middle lobe   30%
    Right upper lobe   20%
    Multiple   5%
- Respiratory distress for first 6 months
- Associated ventricular septal defect (VSD) or patent ductus arteriosus (PDA) in 15%

Imaging

- Chest film findings:
    Early films may show opaque mass caused by slow fluid clearance
    Late films show progressive distention of involved lung with air trapping
    Compression of adjacent lobes
    Mediastinal shift to opposite side

CROUP

Clinical

- Laryngotracheobronchitis
- Occurs at ages 6 months to 3 years
- "Barking" cough
- History of previous upper respiratory infection
- Usually viral in origin; parainfluenza most common
- Membranous croup: bacterial in origin; thick membrane in subglottic trachea

Imaging

- Frontal and lateral plain films of neck:
    Narrowing of subglottic trachea: "steeple" sign on frontal view, indistinctness and narrowing on lateral view
    Normal epiglottis and aryepiglottic folds
    Ballooning of hypopharynx
    Bacterial croup: membranes may be visualized by plain film

CYSTIC FIBROSIS

Clinical

- Autosomal recessive
- Incidence: 1 in 2000 births
- Whites more often affected than blacks or Asians
- Diagnosis by serum sweat test (in neonates, serum trypsinogen test)
- Characterized by exocrine gland dysfunction
- Most present with pulmonary manifestations: bronchitis, bronchiectasis (6 months), *Pseudomonas* (rare mucoid form) infection, and staphylococcal infection
- 5% present with gastrointestinal complaints: meconium ileus, distal intestinal obstruction syndrome (DIOS), malabsorption, steatorrhea, or rectal prolapse
- Complications: sinusitis, pneumothorax, infertility, cirrhosis, pancreatitis, hemoptysis, pulmonary hypertension, and cor pulmonale

Imaging

- Chest radiograph/CT:
    Increased interstitial markings, peribronchial cuffing, bronchiectasis with or without air-fluid levels; mucous plugging, enlarged pulmonary arteries, increasing heart size (indicates cor pulmonale), segmental or lobar collapse (usually right upper lobe), hilar adenopathy from recurrent infections
- Abdominal film: *infants:*
    Meconium ileus; *older children:* distended, stool-filled colon; calcific chronic pancreatitis; gallstones

CYSTIC HYGROMA

Clinical

- Caused by abnormal development of the primitive lymphatic system
- 75% in posterior neck, 20% in axilla; other locations: mediastinum, retroperitoneum, bone, and abdominal viscera
- Majority diagnosed at birth; 90% by the age of 2 years
- Associated syndromes: Turner, Noonan, fetal alcohol syndrome; trisomy 13, 18, 21
- May cause stridor or dysphagia
- Size increases rapidly if hemorrhage or infection is present
- Difficult to remove surgically because of infiltrative nature and high recurrence rates

Imaging

- Ultrasound:
    Good screening tool demonstrating multiple cysts
- Contrast CT:
    Enhancement if cyst infected
- MRI:
    Useful for delineating borders, which may be poorly circumscribed
    If lesion not infected, cysts usually low signal on T1 and high signal on T2
    Signal may be increased on T1 if lesion infected, hemorrhage present, or lipid content high

DEVELOPMENTAL DYSPLASIA OF THE HIP

Clinical

- Congenital hip dislocation
- Increased incidence in first-born infants, breech births (25%), oligohydramnionic pregnancy (related to uterine crowding), and children swaddled with legs in adduction
- Ratio of females to males affected, 8:1
- Whites affected more often than blacks
- Location:

  Left hip   70%
  Right hip   25%
  Bilateral   5%
- Ortolani-Barlow maneuvers performed clinically to assess hip stability
- If clinical instability is suspected, further radiographic work-up is required
- Treatment: double diapering, Pavlik harness, closed or open (surgical) reduction
- Complications of therapy: aseptic necrosis, development of coxa magna

Imaging

- Ultrasound:
    - Performed before extensive ossification of femoral head; involves combined static and dynamic study; standard views obtained in coronal and transverse planes with linear transducer and evaluated for morphology of femoral head, limbus, and acetabulum
    - Coronal images: normal for 50% of head to be covered; alpha angle may be measured between straight iliac edge and bony acetabular margin: mature is more than 60 degrees (in children less than 12 weeks, angle may be between 50 and 60 degrees, indicating physiological immaturity; such children are rescanned to ensure that normal angle is achieved by 12 weeks); angle less than 50 degrees indicates dysplasia
    - Transverse images: femoral head should be centered over triradiate cartilage; anterior transverse plane has been described for children in a harness
    - Dynamic scanning reproduces clinical examination and seeks evidence of subluxation or dislocation
    - Hips are classified as mature, subluxable or subluxed, or dislocated (reducible or irreducible)
- Plain film anteroposterior view of pelvis:
    - Not common except to seek associated anomalies or in older children after ossification of femoral head
    - Y-Y or line of Hilgenreiner: horizontal line drawn through superior aspect of triradiate cartilages
    - Perkins' line: line drawn perpendicular to Hilgenreiner's line at lateral aspect of acetabulum
    - Shenton's line: line formed by superior aspect of obturator foramen and medial femoral neck
    - Medial edge of proximal femoral metaphysis should lie in lower inner quadrant formed by intersection of Y-Y and Perkins' lines; if lateral or superior, dislocation is present
- Associated findings: increased acetabular angle (more than 30 degrees); formation of pseudoacetabulum; disruption of Shenton's line; delayed ossification of femoral head

EPIGLOTTITIS

Clinical

- Usual organism: *Haemophilus influenzae*
- Usual age range, 3 to 6 years
- Thickening of aryepiglottic folds is the predominant cause of airway obstruction
- Children appear toxic, with fever and elevated white blood cell counts
- Patients may have severe dysphagia

- Tripod position should be maintained to maintain airway
- Pediatric emergency: child should never be left unattended
- Classic presentation: no radiographic evaluation required until airway is secure

Imaging

- Plain film: soft tissue lateral view of the neck:
    Child should maintain position of comfort
    Child must be accompanied in radiology suite by someone familiar with pediatric airway
    Enlargement of epiglottis and thickened aryepiglottic folds
    Ballooning of hypopharynx
    Up to 25% of patients have associated subglottic narrowing
    Patient may have pneumonia or septic arthritis; thus, other imaging studies may be indicated

EXTRALOBAR SEQUESTRATION

Clinical

- Secondary to abnormal budding of the primitive foregut
- Most common location: left base posteriorly
- Contained in own pleural covering
- Systemic arterial and venous connections
- Initially may be thought to represent pneumonia
- No connection to bronchial tree unless infected
- Associated anomalies occur in 60%
    Types of anomalies include:
    Cystic adenomatoid malformation type II
    Lobar emphysema
    Diaphragmatic hernia

Imaging

- Chest film:
    Retrocardiac density; may or may not show air-fluid level
- Ultrasound:
    Doppler may show abnormal vascular connections; echogenic mass in lung base
- MRI or contrast-enhanced CT:
    Vascular connections should be sought

FOREIGN BODIES, IN AIRWAY

Clinical

- Common problem in childhood
- Aspirated foreign bodies usually not radiopaque (85% are vegetable matter)
- May or may not have positive history; symptoms coughing and wheezing; peak age, 1 to 2 years
- More common on right than left side because of more vertical position of right bronchus
- Complications include pneumomediastinum or pneumothorax
- Bronchoscopy necessary in all children if strong clinical suspicion exists, even if chest radiograph is normal

Imaging

- Chest radiograph:
    May be normal; areas of hyperinflation or atelectasis; expiratory films or decubitus films necessary to demonstrate air trapping
- Fluoroscopic evaluation:
    May demonstrate hyperinflation and mediastinal shift with expiration

FOREIGN BODY, ESOPHAGEAL

Clinical

- Coins are the most common objects ingested
- Location of lodging:

Thoracic inlet	75%
Aortic arch or left mainstem bronchus	20%
Gastroesophageal junction	5%

- If foreign body lodges elsewhere, underlying abnormalities must be excluded; most common is stricture
- Symptoms: gagging, dysphagia; airway symptoms may predominate
- Complications: perforation, stricture, and aspiration pneumonia

Imaging

- Conventional films:
    Include mouth to anus; foreign bodies larger than an American quarter may not pass ileocecal valve
- Esophagram:
    If nonradiopaque, barium esophagram may be required; contrast may obscure small foreign bodies
- Removal:
    Some centers use Foley catheter to pull object into mouth or push into stomach; attempt this only if object is blunt and has been in place a short time; endoscopic removal is the procedure of choice at other institutions

HEMANGIOENDOTHELIOMA

Clinical

- Benign vascular tumor
- Most common location is right hepatic lobe posteriorly
- Usually solitary, but occasionally lesion may be multicentric
- Natural history: proliferate for several months, then regress and involute by age 12 to 18 months; 90% are present by 6 months of age
- Female to male ratio, 2:1
- Clinical presentation: palpable abdominal mass, 50% have cutaneous hemangiomas; most present with high-output heart failure; occasionally infants present with Kasabach-Merritt syndrome characterized by consumptive coagulopathy or hemoperitoneum from rupture; serum alpha fetoprotein levels normal
- Treatment includes diuretics, digitalis, steroids, chemotherapy, radiation therapy, embolic therapy, or surgical ligation of feeding vessels

Imaging

- Ultrasound:
    Appearance varies from hypoechoic to hyperechoic, ± calcifications
- CT:
    Calcification (40%); *precontrast* images show single or multiple low-density lesions; *postcontrast* lesions enhance from periphery to center; lesions may fill in completely; if center is fibrotic or thrombosed, it may not fill completely
- MRI:
    T1 images show single or multiple low-signal intensity lesions
    T2 images reveal increased signal intensity
    Peripheral enhancement can be seen after contrast administration
- Angiography:
    Enlarged hepatic arteries; hypervascular tumor with abnormal vessels; pooling of contrast in sinusoidal lakes; arteriovenous shunting
- All imaging may reveal significant decrease in diameter of aorta after take-off of celiac plexus

HEMOLYTIC UREMIC SYNDROME

Clinical

- Immune-mediated disease caused by infection with verocytotoxin-producing and endotoxin-producing organism, usually *E. coli; Shigella, Salmonella, Yersinia,* and *Campylobacter* spp also reported
- Classic triad: microangiopathic hemolytic anemia, thrombocytopenia, renal failure
- Presents with diarrheal illness (90%) from hemorrhagic colitis of variable severity; soon after, child develops oliguria/anuria and anemia
- Leading cause of acute renal failure in childhood from thrombi in glomerular arterioles; 15 to 35% develop end-stage renal disease, reduced glomerular filtration rate, hypertension, and proteinuria
- CNS manifestations (40 to 50%): seizures, irritability, hemiparesis, coma, cortical blindness; secondary to metabolic abnormalities and intravascular microthrombi

Imaging

- Contrast studies of colon:
    Thumbprinting from edema and hemorrhage and mucosal abnormalities
- Ultrasound:
    Thickened bowel wall; increased echogenicity of kidneys; kidneys may be normal or increased in size; resistive index elevated, return to normal heralds clinical improvement
- MRI/CT of brain:
    May show large or small vessel infarcts, edema, hemorrhage, or cortical signal abnormalities

HEPATOBLASTOMA

Clinical

- Most common malignant hepatic neoplasm in children
- Third most common abdominal malignancy after Wilms tumor and neuroblastoma
- Increased incidence in Beckwith-Wiedemann syndrome; fetal alcohol syndrome; hemihypertrophy; and maternal exposure to metals, paint, oral contraceptives
- Usually single, with predilection for posterior segment of right hepatic lobe
- Male to female ratio, 2:1
- Usually presents before age 3 years; 50% < 1 year of age
- Clinical presentation: usually presents with abdominal mass; less common presentations include pain, weight loss, and precocious puberty; serum alpha fetoprotein levels are elevated in nearly all children
- Must be differentiated from hepatocellular carcinoma, which occurs in older children and those with predisposing factors such as chronic active hepatitis, glycogen storage disease, alpha-1 antitrypsin disease, and tyrosinemia
- Treatment: primary surgical resection or initial chemotherapy followed by surgical resection

Imaging

- Abdominal films:
    Large hepatic silhouette; calcifications may be seen
- Ultrasound:
    Lesions usually hyperechoic and heterogeneous, indicating hemorrhage or necrosis
- CT:
    Shows single or multiple low-density lesions; calcifications (in up to 50%); minimal enhancement after contrast administration; hepatocellular carcinoma is similar in appearance but calcifies less frequently (25%); evaluate for metastatic disease to lungs, which occurs in 10%
- MRI:
    As good as CT at demonstrating lesion; vascular invasion better delineated; lesion or lesions decreased in intensity on T1 images, increased in intensity on T2 images

10

HIRSCHSPRUNG DISEASE

Clinical

- Incidence: 1 in 4,500 term births
- Caused by absence of ganglion cells in the myenteric plexus
- Length:
  - 80% Short segment
  - 15% Intermediate length
  - 5% Total colon ± variable length of distal small bowel
  - Some texts report an ultrashort segment form, others question its existence
- Ratio of males to females affected, 4:1 in short and intermediate length involvement
- Equal gender incidence in total colonic aganglionosis
- Increased incidence in children with Down syndrome
- Clinically, failure to pass meconium in first 24 hours of life; if missed in perinatal period, most present in the first few months of life with constipation
- Risk of life-threatening colitis secondary to stasis and bacterial overgrowth
- Diagnosis by enema, rectal suction biopsy, or full-thickness rectal biopsy
- Treat with decompression colostomy followed by surgical anastomosis of normal colon to rectum:
  - Swenson pull-through: resection of aganglionic segment and reanastomosis
  - Soave procedure: pull the bowel through the anus and resect aganglionic portion
  - Duhamel procedure: leave the aganglionic segment intact, but bypass with an end-to-side anastomosis

Imaging

- Abdominal films:
  - May reveal distal obstruction
- Contrast enema (unprepped examination) findings:
  - Transition zone identified: normal bowel dilated above aganglionic segment
  - Rectosigmoid ratio <1.0 (normal >1)
  - Once transition zone is seen, no more contrast is administered
  - In infants, transition zone may not be seen
  - Delayed evacuation on 24-hour film is characteristic
  - Irregular contractions can be seen in aganglionic segments
  - In total aganglionosis, colon usually is normal (75%), but microcolon may be seen
  - Mucosal irregularity if colitis is present

HYDROCARBON ASPIRATION

Clinical

- Result of ingestion of substances such as furniture polish, gasoline, or kerosene
- Low viscosity and surface tension allow easy aspiration
- Chemical pneumonitis occurs in several hours, characterized by hyperemia, edema, bronchial necrosis, and small vessel thromboses

Imaging

- Chest film:
  - If normal after 12 hours, no significant aspiration has occurred
  - Findings usually located in lower lobes
  - Basilar consolidation with evidence of volume loss is typical appearance
  - Changes may persist after clinical resolution has occurred
  - Pneumatoceles present in healing stages as result of bronchial lumen obstruction with ball-valve effect

HYPERTROPHIC PYLORIC STENOSIS

Clinical

- Caused by hypertrophy of muscles of pyloric channel; cause of hypertrophy unknown

- Most common cause of gastric outlet obstruction
- Ratio of males to females affected, 4 to 5:1
- Questionable statistical increase in first-born males, but familial predisposition is known (5%)
- Usual age at presentation, 2 to 6 weeks
- Clinical presentation: nonbilious vomiting; weight loss, irritability, hypochloremic alkalosis, dehydration
- Experienced examiner may palpate an olive-shaped mass in the epigastric area
- Treatment is surgical pyloromyotomy after stabilization

Imaging

- Plain films:
    - Normal or suggestive of gastric outlet obstruction; stomach may show a caterpillar sign resulting from deep peristaltic waves
- Ultrasound:
    - Usually first diagnostic study; muscle width more than 4 mm is 100% specific for diagnosis; muscle width between 2 and 4 mm is suspect, and requires follow-up
- Associated findings: fluid-filled stomach (unless nasogastric tube has been placed or patient recently vomited); active peristaltic waves with little or no fluid passing through the pylorus
- Because of increased incidence of renal anomalies (ureteropelvic junction obstruction, reflux, agenesis, ectopia, nephroblastomatosis), kidneys should be examined
- Upper GI series: classic findings include:
    - String or track signs: lengthened, narrowed pyloric channel
    - Beak and mushroom signs: impression of pyloric muscle on antrum and duodenal bulb, respectively
    - Teat sign: mammiform projection along distal lesser curve
- Contrast should be removed after study

IMPERFORATE ANUS

Clinical

- Abnormal termination of hindgut; associated with abnormal separation of hindgut and genitourinary systems
- Cause unknown
- Categories

High lesion	Hindgut terminates above puborectalis sling
Intermediate lesion	Hindgut terminates at level of sling
Low lesion	Hindgut passes through sling

- Treatment: *high* and *intermediate* lesions are treated with abdominal surgery; *low* lesions can be treated by perineal approach
- Associated with vertebral, cardiac, GI, renal, and skeletal anomalies (VACTERL)
- Associated urinary tract abnormalities in 25% of infants with low lesions, 40% of infants with high lesions

Imaging

- Goal of imaging:
    - To identify level of lesion, associated malformations, and presence of any fistulas
- Conventional films:
    - Kidneys, ureter, bladder: bowel obstruction; associated skeletal anomalies
    - Prone lateral rectum: performed after 24 hours to allow for adequate gas distention; marker placed on anal dimple, level of sling determined (M line); meconium in distal rectum can mimic high lesion
- VCUG:
    - May identify reflux into hindgut

10

- Ultrasound:
    Transperineal imaging can detect level of hindgut; skin to hindgut distance of less than 1.5 cm indicates low lesion
- MRI:
    Can locate level of termination preoperatively and development of levator sling; complications should be sought after surgical repair

INGUINAL HERNIA

Clinical

- During fetal development, peritoneal cavity connects to scrotum via processus vaginalis
- Processus vaginalis patent in 80% of newborns; 20% are patent at 2 years
- 90% of patients are male; 80% of hernias occur on right side
- Persistent patency increases risk of developing hernia or communicating hydrocele (or both)
- Complication: incarcerated inguinal hernia
- Incarcerated inguinal hernia is the most common cause of obstruction in the first 4 months of life

Imaging

- Conventional films:
    Normal; evidence of bowel obstruction; if air in hernia, gas collection may be visualized below inguinal ligament; hemiscrotum may be enlarged or inguinoscrotal fold asymmetrical
- Ultrasound:
    May show hydrocele or loops of bowel in hemiscrotum
- Contrast study may be needed to visualize loops of bowel in hemiscrotum

INTESTINAL DUPLICATION

Clinical

- Spherical or tubular structures in continuity with normal bowel
- Location:

Ileal	35%
Esophageal	21%
Gastric	8%
Jejunal	8%
Duodenal	5%
Colonic	Rare

- Gastric mucosa present in 15 to 35%
- Duplications occur on mesenteric side of bowel lumen; gastric located on greater curve (65%)
- Colonic duplications occur along right colon or posterior to rectum
- Esophageal duplications in lower paraspinal location (60%)
- Unusual to communicate with bowel
- Clinical presentation: abdominal mass, distention, vomiting, bleeding, and perforation
- Treat by surgical excision of duplication and short segment of adjacent bowel

Imaging

- Conventional films:
    May demonstrate soft tissue mass; lesions near ileocecal valve may present as obstruction
- Ultrasound:
    Anechoic or mixed echogenic mass, depending on contents; echogenic lining consistent with mucosa should be sought (helps separate from omental, mesenteric, or ovarian cysts)

- Nuclear medicine:
    Pertechnetate scans can help localize duplications with gastric mucosa

INTUSSUSCEPTION

Clinical

- Caused by invagination of bowel into more distal segment: *intussusceptum*, herniated bowel; *intussuscipiens*, receiving bowel lumen
- Usual age ranges from 3 months to 2 years
- Male to female ratio, 2:1
- Clinical symptoms: pain (95%), palpable mass (65%), emesis (90%), and bloody (currant jelly) stools (65%)
- Usually idiopathic (95%); thought to be secondary to hypertrophied lymphoid tissue (Peyer patches) in terminal ileum from viral infection
- Majority (90%) are ileocecal
- In neonates and older children, a lead point should be sought: lymphoma, duplication, polyps, Meckel diverticulum

Imaging

- Plain films:
    May be normal (50%); mass in right upper or lower quadrant; small bowel obstruction
- Contrast enema:
    Filling defect in colon with coiled spring appearance; after reduction, valve and terminal ileum may be edematous
- Ultrasound:
    Pseudokidney sign on long images; target or bull's eye on transverse views

Reduction

- Contraindications: free air or signs of peritonitis; length of symptoms not a contraindication, but chance of successful reduction decreases after time
- Contrast or air may be used; effectiveness approximately the same
- Early studies suggest higher perforation rate with air, but fewer complications from perforation because peritoneal soiling is absent
- Contrast reduction: remember rule of threes:
    Bag 3 feet above table
    Three attempts
    3 minutes duration each
- Air reduction:
    120 mm Hg should not be exceeded (child's valsalva efforts may exceed this)
    Three attempts
    3 minutes duration each
- Reduction is successful when contrast or air is seen refluxing into small bowel
- Risk of recurrence: 10% after contrast reduction; 5% after surgical reduction

JUVENILE RHEUMATOID ARTHRITIS

Clinical

- Subset of juvenile chronic arthritis
- Classification
    Seropositive adult type (15%)
    Seronegative Still's disease (85%)
        Associated splenomegaly and adenopathy
        Variants: systemic, polyarticular, pauciarticular
- Presents with pain and swelling of joints; skin rash; fever
- Females affected more often than males
- Manifests at 3 to 5 years

10

- Locations

Knee	90%
Ankle/wrist	70%
Hand	55%
Hip	35%
Cervical spine	21%

Imaging

Conventional films:
- Similar to adult arthritis except in early involvement of large joints
- Early findings:
    Soft tissue swelling
    Accelerated bone maturity
    Juxtaarticular osteopenia
    Overgrown epiphyses
- Late findings:
    Premature physeal fusion
    Erosions
    Joint space narrowing
    Widening of intercondylar notch
    Ankylosis of spinal apophyseal joints
    Protrusio acetabuli

MRI:
- Shows joint effusions
- Synovial cysts well demonstrated
- Subtle changes in cartilage and soft tissues seen when conventional films are negative

LANGERHANS CELL HISTIOCYTOSIS

Clinical

- Histiocytosis X
- Result of proliferation of histiocytes of the Langerhans cell variety
- Cause unknown
- Varied clinical findings, with considerable overlap in presentation between historically described subgroups
    Letterer-Siwe disease (less than 10%): infantile form characterized by acute disseminated disease; hepatosplenomegaly, skin lesion, otitis media, and adenopathy; bone lesions uncommon; poor prognosis
    Hand-Schüller-Christian disease (15%): chronic disseminated form in older children of 3 to 6 years; classic triad (10%) includes diabetes insipidus, exophthalmos, and skull lesions; prognosis related to extent of visceral involvement
    Eosinophilic granuloma (75%): limited to bone, usually monostotic; seen in older children and young adults; 20% have lung involvement with possible development of pneumothorax (10 to 25%); best prognosis

Imaging

Conventional radiographs:
- Most common radiographic findings are skeletal lesions
- Most common order of involvement: skull, ribs, femur, pelvis, spine, mandible
- In disseminated disease, bones may appear osteopenic
- More commonly, well-defined lytic lesions seen
- In long bones, lesions usually are diaphyseal, often with associated periosteal reaction
- Margins may be sclerotic; pathologic fractures are common
- Skull lesions usually beveled because of uneven involvement of inner and outer tables

- Button sequestrum may be seen in skull lesions
- "Floating teeth" resulting from lytic lesions in mandible
- Vertebra plana and paravertebral soft tissue masses seen in spine

Other modalities:
- Nuclear medicine: bone scans may be falsely negative in 30%; extraskeletal lesions may be imaged, depending on presenting symptoms
- Chest radiograph and CT: can show interstitial disease; high-resolution CT is more sensitive to detection of mild disease
- MRI: best defines extent in CNS; better delineation of marrow involvement and soft tissue extension

LEGG-CALVÉ-PERTHES DISEASE

Clinical

- Idiopathic avascular necrosis of capital femoral epiphysis
- Symptoms: pain, limp
- Ratio of males to females affected, 4:1; rare in blacks
- Usually unilateral; if bilateral (less than 20%), usually at different stages
- Common age at presentation, 3 to 7 years
- Associated with delayed skeletal maturation
- Initial avascular insult usually is asymptomatic, so imaging abnormalities usually present at time of clinical presentation
- Prognosis depends on amount of femoral head involved

Imaging

- Conventional films:
    Anteroposterior and frog-leg views of the hip
    Early
      Reduced size of femoral head, which can mimic joint effusion
      Head may appear sclerotic
    Later
      Subchondral lucency or fracture can be seen (seen best on frog-leg view)
      Fragmented appearance to femoral head
      Cysts in metaphyseal region
      Head may be flattened and laterally uncovered
      Neck may be widened
    After healing
      Head may appear normal or demonstrate coxa magna
      Early degenerative joint disease
- Bone scan:
    Decreased uptake in the femoral epiphysis early during avascular stage; increased uptake during reparative stage
- MRI:
    Marrow edema evidenced by decreased signal intensity on T1 images and increased intensity on T2 images

KAWASAKI SYNDROME

Clinical

- Mucocutaneous lymph node syndrome
- Cause unknown
- Peak age, 1 to 3 years; 85% of patients less than 5 years of age
- Major criteria: fever, cervical adenopathy, skin rash, desquamation of palms and soles, strawberry mucosa, conjunctivitis
- Cardiac manifestations (25%): dysrhythmias, acute myocarditis, coronary artery aneurysms (20%), acute myocardial infarction caused by thrombus, and valvular dysfunction
- Aneurysms also described in aorta and renal, hepatic, and cerebral arteries

- Renal manifestations in fewer than 10% because of local vasculitis with elevated blood urea nitrogen (BUN) and creatinine levels
- Transient gallbladder hydrops caused by vasculitis
- Treatment: gamma globulin and aspirin therapy instituted during the febrile stage of illness decreases the frequency of coronary artery abnormalities

Imaging

- Conventional films:
    Cardiac enlargement; mass in right upper quadrant caused by enlarged gallbladder
- Ultrasound:
    Hydropic gallbladder; kidneys may be enlarged with increased echogenicity
- Angiography:
    Reserved for patients with echocardiographic evidence of aneurysms

MALROTATION/VOLVULUS, MIDGUT

Clinical

- Anomaly of intestinal rotation and fixation
- Duodenal obstruction caused by Ladd bands (abnormal peritoneal bands attempting to fix malrotated bowel) or volvulus
- Volvulus is a surgical emergency; may be life threatening
- Volvulus is secondary to an abnormally short mesenteric pedicle that allows bowel to twist clockwise, causing obstruction and constriction of the superior mesenteric artery (SMA) and vein, as well as impeding lymphatic return
- Associations: omphalocele, congenital diaphragmatic hernia, gastroschisis
- Clinical presentation:
    Infants: often present with bilious vomiting (any infant with bilious vomiting should be considered to have possible midgut volvulus and should receive appropriate work-up)
    Older children: present with intermittent pain, vomiting, and malabsorption
- Complications: bowel ischemia in distribution of SMA; may lead to surgical short gut
- Surgical correction with Ladd procedure: untwist bowel, lyse Ladd bands, small bowel fixed in right abdomen, colon fixed in left abdomen, and incidental appendectomy

Imaging

- Abdominal film:
    May be normal or demonstrate complete small bowel or duodenal obstruction (double bubble)
    Multiple loops of dilated small bowel could indicate bowel ischemia
    If evidence of complete obstruction seen, no further imaging is required
- Upper GI series: demonstrates malrotation with ligament of Treitz lower and to the right of normal position; volvulus has characteristic "corkscrew" appearance
- Contrast enema: may be misleading because cecum in young children may be high in right upper quadrant
- Ultrasound: shows inversion of normal position of superior mesenteric artery and vein; (unfortunately may be unreliable, so upper GI series remains the study of choice)
- CT: vessel inversion seen, as well as swirling appearance to bowel

MECKEL DIVERTICULUM

Clinical

- Omphalomesenteric duct remnant
- Occurs on antimesenteric side of small bowel
- Rule of twos:

2% of population
2 feet from ileocecal valve
2 cm in size
Complications usually before age of 2 years
- 20% contain ectopic gastric mucosa; more likely to be present in symptomatic patients
- Complications include GI bleeding, inflammation, intussusception, and volvulus

Imaging

- Abdominal film:
    Usually normal; may show obstruction
- Contrast studies:
    May occasionally show Meckel diverticulum with small bowel follow-through
- Nuclear medicine:
    Because most symptomatic diverticula contain gastric mucosa, Tc ^{99m} pertechnetate scan is a sensitive examination
    False negative: Very brisk bleeding, too little gastric mucosa
    False positive: Duplication cyst, vascular malformation, inflammatory process, dilated ureter

MECONIUM ASPIRATION

Clinical

- Increased incidence in postterm infants
- Infants defecate in utero secondary to perinatal stress
- History of meconium-stained amniotic fluid or meconium suctioned from airway
- Meconium staining seen in 10% of deliveries, but only 10% of these develop respiratory distress
- May lead to mechanical obstruction
- May cause chemical pneumonitis
- ECMO used to treat severe cases

Imaging

- Chest film:
    Patchy infiltrates with atelectasis or air trapping; airleaks such as pneumothorax or pneumomediastinum in 25%

MECONIUM ILEUS

Clinical

- Secondary to inspissated meconium in distal ileum
- Initial manifestation of cystic fibrosis
    >95% of patients have cystic fibrosis
    15% of patients with cystic fibrosis present with meconium ileus
- Small bowel obstruction in older children with cystic fibrosis referred to as *distal intestinal obstruction syndrome* (DIOS), secondary to dehydration or inadequate pancreatic enzyme replacement
- Increased incidence of volvulus, perforation, meconium peritonitis

Imaging

- Abdominal film findings:
    Multiple dilated bowel loops consistent with distal obstruction
    Bubbly appearance of bowel contents, particularly in right lower quadrant
    Paucity of air fluid levels
    If complicated, peritoneal calcifications or free air
- Contrast enema findings:
    Microcolon with filling defect in distal ileum

Treatment

- Hypertonic, water soluble contrast enema
- Hypertonicity may cause fluid shifts, so make sure child is well hydrated

MECONIUM PERITONITIS

Clinical

- Secondary to prenatal bowel perforation with spillage of meconium
- Caused by atresias, meconium ileus, or volvulus
- Causes chemical peritonitis
- May cause formation of a cystic mass

Imaging

- Abdominal film findings:
    Dystrophic calcifications scattered in abdomen
    Calcifications may be in rim of soft tissue mass
    Calcifications in scrotum are the result of patent processus vaginalis
    Bowel obstruction caused by primary problem may be seen

MECONIUM PLUG SYNDROME

Clinical

- Thick plugs of meconium in colon are the result, not cause, of functional obstruction
- Consequence of colonic hypotonia causing functional obstruction secondary to immaturity of myenteric plexus; child outgrows the problem
- Infants usually term, may have diabetic mothers
- Occasionally associated with small left colon syndrome
- History of failure to pass meconium
- Increased incidence in Hirschsprung disease

Imaging

- Abdominal film:
    Distal obstruction; meconium plug in rectum may look like mass "pseudo-tumor"
- Contrast enema with hypertonic, water soluble agents for diagnosis and therapy:
    Filling defects seen within colonic lumen; left colon usually normal caliber, may be small

MESENCHYMAL HAMARTOMA, HEPATIC

Clinical

- Benign developmental lesion composed of mesenchymal elements, hepatic parenchyma, and bile ducts
- Usually presents before age 2 years; asymptomatic mass; alpha-fetoprotein levels are normal
- Treated by surgical excision

Imaging

- All modalities demonstrate a predominantly cystic lesion
- More common in right lobe than left lobe, 6:1
- No calcifications

MESOBLASTIC NEPHROMA

Clinical

- Most common neonatal renal neoplasm
- Arises from metanephric blastema; usually histologically benign
- Mean age at diagnosis, 3 months
- Clinical presentation: large abdominal mass, hypertension rare
- Prenatal history may reveal polyhydramnios
- Male to femal ratio, 2:1
- Treatment is surgical excision; may recur locally

Imaging

- Ultrasound, CT:
    Usually reveals solid renal mass identical in appearance to Wilms tumor; calcification is rare; rarely may have cystic changes that resemble multilocular cystic nephroma

MULTICYSTIC DYSPLASTIC KIDNEY

Clinical

- Result of pyeloinfundibular atresia early in development
- Rare, hydronephrotic form retains some function; probably the result of atresia occurring late in fetal development
- Abnormalities of opposite kidney, present 10 to 30% of the time, include ureteropelvic junction obstruction most commonly; others are ureterovesical junction obstruction, renal malrotation, and reflux
- Benign lesion that tends to regress; thus, resection no longer routine; necessary only if mass is symptomatic or child has hypertension
- Clinical presentation: found on prenatal ultrasound or palpable abdominal mass

Imaging

- Ultrasound:
    Multiple cysts of varying sizes that do not communicate with each other; usually no demonstrable renal parenchyma; if there is a large central cyst, it may be difficult to distinguish from severe hydronephrosis
- Nuclear medicine renal scan:
    In classic case, no evidence of function in affected kidney; in rare, hydronephrotic form, may have slight function
- VCUG:
    May show reflux into atretic ureter or opposite kidney

MULTILOCULAR CYSTIC NEPHROMA

Clinical

- Benign lesion
- Usually present in childhood
- Biphasic sex distribution: boys more commonly affected in childhood, women more commonly affected in adulthood
- Clinical findings include mass or, less likely, pain
- Treated by nephrectomy
- Foci of nephroblastomatosis or Wilms tumor have been described

Imaging

- Ultrasound:
    Demonstrates cysts separated by thick septa
- CT:
    Calcification rare; shows cystic appearance; capsule, well-circumscribed mass

NECROTIZING ENTEROCOLITIS

Clinical

- Ischemic bowel disease
- Associated with prematurity (80%), hypoxemia, stress, and infection
- Uncommonly seen in term infants with Hirschsprung disease or congenital heart disease
- Results in mucosal damage with loss of normal bowel wall integrity
- Commonly involves terminal ileum and right colon
- Clinical findings: distention, bloody stools, feeding intolerance, sepsis
- Treatment usually includes bowel rest, antibiotic therapy, and supportive care
- Surgery reserved for bowel perforation or signs of peritonitis

Imaging

- Abdominal films:
    Loss of normal bowel mosaic pattern
    Focal or multiple loops of dilated bowel
    Persistent loop of abnormal bowel (adynamic focal ileus)
    Thickened bowel wall
    Most specific finding is pneumatosis intestinalis
    Air in portal venous system (does not affect outcome)
    Pneumoperitoneum indicating bowel perforation
- Ultrasound:
    Thickened bowel wall; ascites; may show air in portal venous system
- Contrast enemas:
    Usually contraindicated acutely unless necessary to exclude another cause of bowel distention; follow-up contrast studies may be required to assess for strictures, which occur in 20%

NEONATAL PNEUMONIA

Clinical

- Acquired in utero or in perinatal period
- Transplacental or ascending infection
- Group B β-hemolytic streptococcus most common organism
- 25% of mothers colonized with this organism
- Other organisms include *Enterobacter*, *Staphylococcus*, and *Klebsiella* spp

Imaging

- Chest film findings:
    Bilateral infiltrates; may be patchy or diffuse
    Pleural effusions in 66%
    May be identical in appearance to hyaline membrane disease or retained fetal lung fluid
    During healing stage pneumatoceles may form, particularly with staphylococcal or *Klebsiella* spp infections

NEPHROBLASTOMATOSIS

Clinical

- Persistent rests of fetal metanephric blastema after 36 weeks gestation
- May be intralobular or perilobular; if intralobular, age of presentation with Wilms tumor usually is younger
- Not malignant, but precursor of Wilms tumor
- Found in 100% of kidneys with bilateral Wilms tumor and in 30 to 40% of those with unilateral tumor
- Increased incidence in those conditions that predispose to Wilms tumor, including hemihypertrophy, Beckwith-Wiedemann syndrome, and Drash syndrome

- Diffuse form more common before age of 2 years; may present as flank masses
- Focal form can occur at all ages; detected incidentally or at surgery for Wilms tumor
- Treatment: chemotherapy and radiation therapy; usually responds well to treatment, but must be followed closely to assess for development of Wilms tumor

Imaging

- Ultrasound:
    - Isoechoic to hypoechoic rind surrounding normal parenchyma or hypoechoic nodules
- CT:
    - Better delineation than ultrasound; nonenhancing focal or confluent subcortical masses; usually asymmetric

NEUROBLASTOMA

Clinical

- Derived from primitive neuroblasts
- Arises within sympathetic neural system or adrenal medulla
- Second most common solid abdominal tumor of childhood (after Wilms tumor)
- Third most common malignancy of childhood after hematopoietic malignancy and CNS tumors
- Mean age at diagnosis, 2 years; 85% of patients < 4 years
- Unique in its ability to spontaneously regress or mature into ganglioneuroblastoma or ganglioneuroma
- 50% present with palpable abdominal mass
- Location:
    - Abdomen 65% (50% of patients present with abdominal mass)
        - (Adrenal gland 40%)
        - (Other abdominal 25%)
    - Chest 15%
    - Unknown primary 10%
    - Neck and pelvis 5% each
- Three staging systems:
    - Evans: based on imaging
    - Pediatric Oncology Group (POG)
    - International Staging System (ISS)
- Staging by Evans classification:
    - I   Tumor confined to structure of origin
    - II   Tumor in continuity with structure of origin, not crossing midline (ipsilateral lymph nodes may be involved)
    - III   Tumor extending in continuity beyond midline or bilateral extension of midline disease (bilateral lymph node involvement)
    - IV   Remote disease involving skeleton, organs, soft tissue, and distant nodes (70% of children aged more than 1 year have metastatic disease at presentation)
    - IVS   Stage I or II disease with remote disease limited to liver, skin, or bone marrow
- Midline tumors with penetration and extension to positive lymph nodes on ipsilateral side classified as stage II
- Bilateral extension classified as stage III
- Associated syndromes:
    - Verner-Morrison (7%): hypokalemia and watery diarrhea caused by elevated vasoactive intestinal peptide (VIP)
    - Myoclonal encephalopathy of infancy (MEI) (2%): opsoclonus ("dancing eyes"), myoclonus ("dancing feet"), and cerebellar ataxia (which may be autoimmune response), higher incidence with thoracic lesions, may persist after tumor resected, associated with better prognosis
    - "Blueberry muffin" syndrome: metastatic skin lesions (exclusively in stage IVS)
    - Hutchison syndrome: multiple bony metastases

10

Pepper syndrome: hepatomegaly from multiple metastases
- Increased urinary catecholamine excretion in 90%
- "Raccoon eyes" resulting from retrobulbar and orbital metastases

Treatment

- Surgery: for diagnosis and therapy
    May be curative in stages I and II
    Used after chemotherapy in stages III and IV
    Controversial whether primary surgery is indicated in stages III and IV
- Radiation therapy:
    Control of tumors that cannot be excised or do not respond to chemotherapy
    Palliation for unresectable masses
    For stage IVS if patient is symptomatic
    Total body irradiation prior to bone marrow transplantation
- Chemotherapy: mainstay of treatment
- Bone marrow transplant for patients at high risk for relapse

Prognosis

- Favorable factors:
    Patient <1 year of age
    Primary tumor in extraabdominal site
    Stage I, II, or IVS tumor
    Favorable Shimada classification
    Low concentration of neuron-specific enolase
    Low level of serum ferritin
    <10 copies of the N-myc oncogene in tumor cells

Imaging

- Conventional film findings:
    Abdominal films may show soft tissue mass or calcifications (50%)
    Skeletal metastases usually permeative or lytic and have periosteal new bone formation
    Widened cranial sutures indicate dural or epidural involvement
- Ultrasound findings:
    Inhomogeneous mass with echogenic foci of calcification
    Liver metastases
    Useful to identify that mass is distinct from kidney
- CT findings:
    Demonstrate mass and calcification (50 to 75%) and may show extension around celiac plexus or superior mesenteric artery
    Retrocrural adenopathy
    Metastatic disease; may not optimally show extension into spinal canal
- MRI:
    Equal to CT for imaging primary but superior for demonstration of marrow and vascular involvement as well as epidural extension
- Nuclear medicine:
    Tc^{99m} methylene diphosphonate (Tc-MDP) excellent for imaging bony metastatic disease; commonly taken up by primary
    I^{131} metaiodobenzylguanidine (MIBG) behaves like norepinephrine analog; detects 85% of primary lesions, 70% of metastases
    I^{123} MIBG more specific for neuroblastoma; used in higher doses for therapy in relapsed cases

PAPILLOMA, LARYNGEAL

Clinical

- Most common tumor of larynx in childhood
- Infected during delivery by human papillomavirus

- May spread through tracheobronchial tree from instrumentation, resulting in multiple pulmonary nodules or multiple cavitary lesions (1%)
- Symptoms: progressive hoarseness, stridor, cough, and hemoptysis
- Morbidity may be secondary to hemorrhage and restrictive lung disease
- Rarely undergoes malignant transformation into squamous cell carcinoma
- Location: uvula, soft palate, vocal cords and subglottic region, and tracheobronchial tree

Imaging

- Neck films:
    Irregular nodular soft tissue masses
- Chest radiograph:
    Multiple nodules or cavitary lesions

POSTERIOR URETHRAL VALVES

Clinical

- Most common cause of urethral obstruction in males
- Classification:
    I   Extend below verumontanum
    II   Above verumontanum to bladder neck
    III   Diaphragm with central opening below verumontanum
          Most are type I; existence of other types is controversial
- Usually present in first 3 months of life; abnormal stream, UTI, hydronephrosis, distended bladder
- Treatment: fulguration of valves
- Prognosis depends on renal function

Imaging

- Ultrasound:
    Shows dilated collecting systems, thickened bladder wall, and dilated posterior urethra; may have urinary ascites
- VCUG, procedure of choice:
    Shows dilated posterior urethra with abrupt narrowing reflux (30%), trabeculation of bladder wall, and large post-void residual

PRUNE-BELLY SYNDROME

Clinical

- Eagle-Barrett syndrome
- Classic triad: abdominal muscle hypoplasia, cryptorchidism, urinary tract dilation
- Occurs predominately in males (90%)
- Associated anomalies: scoliosis, foot abnormalities, lung hypoplasia, imperforate anus, and congenital heart disease
- Two subsets: *neonatal* form with urethral atresia or posterior urethral valves; second group has no obstruction but functional problems with bladder emptying

Imaging

- Ultrasound:
    Demonstrates presence of hydronephrosis; dilated ureters; large bladder
- VCUG:
    Hypertrophied bladder, urachal diverticulum, reflux, dilated posterior urethra, and large post-void residual

RESPIRATORY DISTRESS SYNDROME

Clinical

- Hyaline membrane disease; pink staining of membrane caused by protein leakage
- Primarily affects premature infants, although infants born by cesarean section and infants of diabetic mothers at increased risk
- Caused by immature levels of surfactant from type II pneumocytes
- Surfactant production begins at 24 to 28 weeks gestational age
- Maturity assessed by lecithin:sphingomyelin ratio
- Infants present with respiratory distress before 4 to 6 hours of life
- Treated by intratracheal delivery of exogenous surfactant
- Most patients on positive-pressure ventilation (PPV)
- Complications of PPV include pulmonary interstitial emphysema (PIE) (treated by selective intubation, decubitus positioning, or high-frequency ventilation), pneumothorax, pneumomediastinum, pneumopericardium, and pneumoperitoneum

Imaging

- Chest film findings:
    Classically, decreased lung volumes, but if patient received exogenous surfactant, lung volumes normal to increased
    Diffuse, symmetrical, finely granular appearance of lungs
    Air bronchograms usually visible
    Pleural effusions unlikely
    Exogenous surfactant therapy may result in patchy appearance of lungs
    Sudden diffuse opacity may be secondary to PDA, superimposed pneumonia, or hemorrhage
    PIE: air in interstitial space; linear lucencies from hilar areas to periphery of lungs; distinguished from air bronchograms by lack of peripheral tapering
    Pneumothorax: air may rupture into pleural space; usually collects anteriorly, adjacent to cardiac margins in supine infant
    Pneumomediastinum: extension of air into mediastinal compartment; air beneath thymic lobes results in "angel wing" appearance; air in inferior pulmonary ligament is beneath hilum on lateral film; may appear to be in heart on frontal film
    Pneumopericardium: air in pericardial sac; air completely surrounds heart and does not extend above level of great vessels
    Pneumoperitoneum: air in mediastinum dissects into peritoneal cavity

RHABDOMYOSARCOMA

Clinical

- Most common soft tissue neoplasm of childhood
- Cell types:
    Embryonal (most common)
        Sarcoma botryoides is type of embryonal cell that has characteristic grapelike appearance as it grows and invades hollow organs
    Pleomorphic (rare)
    Alveolar
- Locations: has been described in all parts of the body except the brain

Head and neck	31%
Genitourinary tract*	39%
Orbit	10%
Extremities	20%

    *Most common in bladder
- Malignant, with ability to invade locally or spread hematogenously or via lymphatic system
- Males and females affected equally; peak incidence, between 2 and 6 years; symptoms related to mass effect in head and neck; in genitourinary tract, may present with frequency, dysuria, hematuria
- Staging is based on anatomic site, size, and presence of nodes

- Stages are grouped based on whether complete surgical resection is performed, microscopic residual is present, and site of primary tumor

Imaging

- Head and neck:
    CT or MRI is the best method for visualizing extent of involvement and response to therapy
- Genitourinary tract:
    Ultrasound may demonstrate mass in bladder and obstructive hydronephrosis, if present
- CT:
    Findings similar to those of ultrasound
- VCUG or excretory urogram may show filling defects in the bladder
- No imaging modality may be able to tell if tumor originated in bladder or extended from adjacent prostate or vagina

ROUND PNEUMONIA

Clinical

- Secondary to acute bacterial pneumonia; primarily pneumococcal
- Found before age 8 years; unusual after this age, because collateral pathways (pores of Kohn and channels of Lambert) are fully developed
- If present at a later age, suggests immunocompromise or atypical organism
- Presents as acute febrile illness; white blood cell count is elevated
- Clinical presentation should distinguish from primary or metastatic lung lesions

Imaging

- Chest film:
    Initially, well-circumscribed round lesion; usually single but may be multifocal; air bronchograms may be seen in 20%; with antibiotic therapy, margins become less defined and lesion slowly clears

SACROCOCCYGEAL TERATOMA

Clinical

- Sacrococcygeal area is the most frequent location for teratoma
- Most common tumor of sacral region in childhood
- Ratio of females to males affected, 4 to 5:1
- Most are benign and identified at birth
- Increasing malignancy with age; 90% are malignant at 2 months
- Benign lesions predominantly are cystic; malignant lesions predominantly are solid
- Types:
    I   Primarily external
    II   Intrapelvic portion but predominantly external
    III   Predominantly intrapelvic with external component
    IV   Presacral
- Treatment: complete excision of tumor with coccyx

Imaging

- Conventional films:
    Soft tissue mass with calcifications in 60%
- Ultrasound:
    Shows cystic components
- CT or MRI:
    Shows extent of lesion and identifies presence of calcifications and fat

SLIPPED CAPITAL FEMORAL EPIPHYSIS

Clinical

- Fracture of proximal femoral physeal plate; neck moves in anterior and superolateral direction; epiphysis moves posterior and inferomedial
- Mechanical and endocrine factors probably play a role
- Males affected twice as often as females; increased incidence in obese children
- Usually occurs at age 10 to 15 years
- Associated with hypothyroidism, growth hormone therapy, and avascular necrosis
- Bilateral slippage in 10 to 15%
- Treatment: pinning of epiphysis; reduction increases risk of avascular necrosis

Imaging

- Conventional films:
    - Widened physeal plate; epiphysis may appear decreased in height on frontal view; loss of intersection of lateral femoral neck line with epiphysis; frog-leg view best demonstrates slippage
- Ultrasound:
    - May be used to screen for contralateral slip

SUBGLOTTIC HEMANGIOMA

Clinical

- Most common mass causing upper respiratory tract obstruction in infancy
- No malignant potential
- 50% have associated cutaneous hemangiomas
- Calcifications are rare
- Treatment includes steroids or endoscopic laser resection

Imaging

- Frontal film of neck reveals asymmetric narrowing of the subglottic trachea
- Small hemangiomas may require endoscopy for diagnosis

TODDLER'S FRACTURE

Clinical

- Nondisplaced spiral fracture of the mid to distal tibia
- Usual age less than 3 years
- Presents with limp or failure to bear weight
- Treated by casting

Imaging

- Conventional films:
    - May be negative initially; oblique images may be helpful; follow-up films in 10 to 14 days reveal periosteal reaction if fracture is not identified acutely
- Nuclear medicine:
    - If initial films are negative, bone scan may demonstrate increased uptake in area of suspected fracture

TRANSIENT TACHYPNEA OF NEWBORN

Clinical

- Retained fetal lung fluid, wet lung
- Fluid normally is expelled by compression during delivery or absorbed into capillary and lymphatic systems
- Increased incidence in cesarean section, precipitous delivery, sedated mother, diabetic mother
- Symptomatic in first 6 to 8 hours of life

Imaging

- Chest film:
    Interstitial prominence with fluid in fissures; pleural effusions
- Findings nonspecific; diagnosis made by rapid clearing (usually within 48 to 72 hours)

URETEROPELVIC JUNCTION OBSTRUCTION

Clinical

- Most common congenital obstruction
- Caused by narrowing from a variety of causes, including abnormal muscle, fibrous bands, extrinsic vascular compression, prominent mucosal folds
- May present as abdominal mass, infection, or intermittent flank pain; majority on left side; contralateral ureteropelvic junction obstruction in 20%; obstruction ranges from partial to complete
- If severe or progressive, treatment is surgical pyeloplasty

Imaging

- Conventional films:
    May show mass effect
- Ultrasound:
    Detects dilated collecting system; if severe may resemble cystic dysplasia
- VCUG:
    Excludes reflux or urethral obstruction as cause of dilated system
- Excretory urogram or nuclear medicine renal scan:
    Confirms site of obstruction and determines degree of renal function

VESICOURETERAL REFLUX

Clinical

- Uncommon in asymptomatic children
- Found in 29 to 50% of children who present with UTI
- Present in 8 to 26% of siblings of children with vesicoureteral reflux; siblings usually screened with VCUG
- Primary reflux: caused by incompetence of vesicoureteral junction
- Secondary reflux: caused by Hutch diverticulum, bladder-sphincter dyssynergy
- Incidence decreases with age; 95% resolve by age of 6 years
- Scarring increased with higher grades of reflux; usually requires presence of UTI to develop
- Scarring is most prevalent in polar regions where compound papillae allow intrarenal reflux of infected urine
- Incidence of scarring is highest in first year of life
- Scarring is the cause of end-stage renal failure in 20 to 40% of patients aged less than 40 years and increases risk of hypertension
- Grading
Grade I	Ureteral reflux only
Grade II	Reflux into nondilated collecting system
Grade III	Reflux into dilated collecting system with normal calyces
Grade IV	Reflux into dilated collecting system with blunted calyces
Grade V	Progressive dilatation of collecting system with tortuosity of ureters and intrarenal reflux
- Management: lower grades treated medically; children with higher grades or whose urine cannot be kept sterile may require surgical correction

Imaging

Children aged less than 5 years with initial UTI

- Undergo VCUG to exclude vesicoureteral reflux and ultrasound to evaluate kidneys

- Ultrasound alone cannot screen for vesicoureteral reflux, because it can be normal in cases with gross intermittent reflux; it is also insensitive in the detection of mild scarring
- Follow up with radionuclide VCUG and ultrasound at yearly intervals to monitor
- If further questions exist regarding scarring (such as unexplained hypertension and a normal ultrasound), DMSA renal cortical scan can be performed

Older children and adolescents with initial UTI
- Can be screened with ultrasound; if abnormality is detected, can be evaluated as indicated; if normal, no other imaging is required

WILMS TUMOR

Clinical

- Most common abdominal malignancy of childhood
- Usually sporadic, but may be familial (15 to 20%); familial forms usually present at earlier age and all have nephrogenic rests
- Clinical presentation: mean age, 3 years (90% less than 8 years); boys and girls affected equally; usually asymptomatic mass (90%); other symptoms: pain, hematuria, hypertension, anemia; those with associated syndromes present at earlier age
- Predisposing conditions: nephroblastomatosis, hemihypertrophy, Drash syndrome, Beckwith-Wiedemann syndrome, and sporadic aniridia (30% of patients with sporadic aniridia have Wilms tumor and 1% of children with Wilms tumor have sporadic aniridia)
- Staging
    - I   Limited to kidney and totally excised
    - II   Extends beyond kidney but totally excisable (includes venous extension)
    - III   Extends beyond kidney and not excisable*
    - IV   Hematogenous metatases
    - V   Bilateral disease at presentation (5%)
    - *Stage III recently changed to include patients with positive regional lymph nodes, even if they are resectable
- Favorable histology with blastemal, epithelial, and stromal elements (seen in 90%)
- Unfavorable histology includes Wilms tumor with anaplastic elements
- Also included under unfavorable histology are the following tumors:
    - Clear cell sarcoma: male to female ratio, 2:1; unilateral, bone metastases common
    - Rhabdoid tumor: present in infancy, brain metastases common or second primary brain tumor
- Surgery required for resection and staging; tumor in inferior vena cava (IVC) or right atrium changes surgical approach
- All stages require chemotherapy except stage I patients <24 months old with tumor <550 g
- Radiation reserved for stages III and IV and all tumors of unfavorable histology
- Currently, 90% of affected children are cured

Imaging

- All modalities show intrarenal origin of tumor
- Central necrosis and hemorrhage usually seen
- Ultrasound and MRI best demonstrate vascular involvement; 20% have extension into the renal vein and IVC; MRI with multiplanar capabilities may help differentiate between neuroblastoma invading the kidney and Wilms tumor
- CT:
    - Mixed enhancement seen in primary tumor after contrast administration
    - Calcifications seen in 15%
    - Contrast administration best reveals hepatic metastases
    - Best demonstrates lung metastases
    - Dispute exists as to whether CT should be performed to look for metastatic

disease; some screen with chest films, because the presence of occult metastatic lung disease does not seem to affect prognosis

WILSON-MIKITY SYNDROME

Clinical

- Occurs in premature infants breathing room air (no history of supplemental oxygen)
- Cause unknown; may result from insult from oxygen in room air
- Gradual onset of symptoms at 10 to 14 days of life
- Uncommonly encountered
- Some doubt the existence of this syndrome

Imaging

- Chest film:
    Indistinguishable from bronchopulmonary dysplasia; diagnosis made on clinical grounds

10

Ultrasound

■ **Maitray D. Patel,** M.D.

■ **Douglas Sides,** M.D.

OVERVIEW

It is difficult to discuss an overview of the approach one should use when evaluating a sonographic examination, because ultrasound is used throughout the body to evaluate vastly different organ systems. Other chapters of this textbook, like their corresponding sections in board examinations, outline an approach to evaluation of specific body systems or areas (such as the musculoskeletal system, gastrointestinal tract, genitourinary system, central nervous system, and so forth). In the context of these specific body systems and areas, ultrasound findings and their differential considerations have been discussed in the appropriate chapter. For example, echogenic hepatic masses are discussed in the chapter on gastrointestinal organs. This chapter focuses on the use of ultrasound in obstetrics and gynecology, in which ultrasound is the primary imaging modality used to evaluate disease. In addition, because ultrasound is the primary modality used to evaluate scrotal pathology, differential considerations regarding findings on a scrotal sonogram are included in the next section of this chapter.

OBSTETRIC ULTRASOUND

There are two types of obstetric ultrasound examinations: standard and targeted. The standard examination is performed in every patient regardless of the request, whereas the targeted examination is performed when a specific abnormality is sought as a result of patient risk or as a follow-up to an earlier examination. A set of guidelines created by the American College of Radiology, with modifications by the American Institute of Ultrasound, defines the minimum standard for a complete obstetric ultrasound examination. When reviewing an ultrasound examination, therefore, the radiologist should determine not only if abnormalities are identified on the submitted views, but also if all appropriate structures have been documented. Inability to adequately document one or several recommended views of uterine or fetal anatomy should raise the suspicion for abnormality, unless satisfactory technical explanations exist (early gestational age or large maternal body habitus).

First Trimester

In the first trimester, a complete obstetric ultrasound examination should evaluate the location of the gestational sac, the appropriate measurements of embryonic or fetal structures, the presence or absence of fetal heart motion, the number of fetuses, and uterine and adnexal anatomy. The gestational sac should not be positioned within the cervix or in the cornua of the uterus; these locations are considered forms of ectopic pregnancy. The presence of a gestational sac normally positioned within the uterus makes ectopic pregnancy quite unlikely, but not impossible, especially in women who have undergone assisted fertilization. In such women, the risk of heterotopic gestation can be as high as 1 in 100. Without such history, the risk of heterotopic gestation has been recorded as approximately 1 in 7,000. If only "close-up" endovaginal images of the gestational sac are provided, it may be difficult to clearly identify the gestational location. By identifying the relationship of the gestational sac to the endometrial stripe and the endocervical canal, one can be assured that ectopic gestation is not overlooked.

Not all intrauterine fluid collections in pregnant women represent gestational sacs. The presence of embryonic structures within a sac is unequivocal proof that the sac is a gestational sac. The presence of a double decidual sac sign is strong evidence that the sac is a gestational sac, but unfortunately, this sign is not foolproof, because endometrial fluid surrounded by decidualized endometrium (which can occur in ectopic pregnancy) can mimic the double decidual sac sign to inexperienced observers.

If an embryo or yolk sac is not identified in an intrauterine fluid collection suspected of representing an intrauterine pregnancy, analysis of mean sac diameter (MSD) can be helpful. In early pregnancy, the size of the gestational sac, as expressed by the MSD, directly corresponds to the age of the developing gestation (menstrual age in days equals MSD plus 30). Different centers use different size thresholds for determining when an intrauterine fluid collection should always demonstrate embryonic structures if it truly represents a normally developing gestational sac. Evidence suggests that with most (but not all) gestational sacs, a yolk sac is evident sonographically by endovaginal scanning before the MSD exceeds 8 mm; by the time the MSD equals 13 mm, all normally developing gestational sacs exhibit a yolk sac on endovaginal sonography. Similarly, an embryo is sonographically visible by endovaginal scanning by the time the MSD exceeds 16 mm within most (but perhaps not all) normally developing gestational sacs, and definitely within all normally developing gestational sacs with an MSD equaling or exceeding 18 mm. Thus, when an intrauterine fluid collection is identified, determination of the mean sac diameter suggests what embryonic structures should be identified if the fluid collection represents a normally developing gestational sac.

If a technically satisfactory endovaginal sonogram of an intrauterine fluid collection fails to identify the embryonic structures that are expected given the size of the collection, a normally developing gestation can be excluded from the diagnostic possibilities. The intrauterine fluid collection can then be removed and examined pathologically to determine if it contains chorionic villi diagnostic of an abnormal intrauterine pregnancy. If it does not, the suspicion for ectopic pregnancy is greatly heightened.

Once an embryo is identified, measurement of the embryonic crown-rump length (CRL) is used to date the gestation. Measurements of the biparietal diameter (BPD), head circumference (HC), abdominal circumference (AC), and femur length (FL) are combined with the CRL once these additional structures are clearly defined. The CRL usually is not used at all after all four fetal measurements are clearly obtainable, usually after 13 weeks menstrual age.

Fetal heart motion is unmistakable when present. It can be identified as pulsating echoes adjacent to the yolk sac even before the embryo itself is clearly resolved. If an embryo can be clearly resolved and accurately measured and the CRL exceeds 5 mm, heart motion should always be present. The absence of heart motion in a fetus of this size signals embryonic demise. If there is a question about whether the CRL obtained is accurate and it is conceivable that the CRL has been overestimated and does not truly exceed 5 mm, a short interval follow-up study should be performed to confirm fetal demise. In early pregnancy, the gestational sac and the embryo grow at a rate of approximately 1 mm per day. Absence of expected growth indicates an abnormally developing gestation.

In the first trimester, the chorionicity of multiple gestations is usually easily defined. With twins, dichorionic gestations show clearly separate gestational sacs. Monochorionic gestations have one gestational sac with two separate yolk sacs. Identification of separate amniotic cavities proves diamniotic gestation. If both twins are present within a single amnion, monoamniotic pregnancy is proved. Recognition of each embryo and heartbeat can be difficult before 8 weeks menstrual age, with the major pitfall being the inability to identify a second embryo within a single gestational sac.

Uterine and adnexal structures generally are well assessed in the first trimester, particularly by endovaginal scanning. Commonly, an adnexal cyst is identified corresponding to the corpus luteum. It is important to identify any adnexal mass that might be present, because such identification may necessitate clinical or sonographic follow-up, or both. During pregnancy, adnexal surgery is best performed at approximately 18 to 20 weeks gestation, a relatively quiescent period for the gravid uterus.

Second and Third Trimesters

Complete obstetric ultrasound in the second and third trimesters includes evaluation of the following:

(1) Fetal life, number, and presentation
(2) Amniotic fluid volume
(3) Placental location and appearance
(4) Assessment of gestational age
(5) Uterus and adnexa
(6) Certain aspects of fetal anatomy: cerebral ventricles, posterior fossa, four-chamber view of the heart (including position in thorax), spine, stomach, urinary bladder, umbilical cord and its insertion site on anterior abdominal wall, and renal region

A complete discussion of the abnormalities that might be found in each aspect of the complete obstetric ultrasound examination is well beyond the scope of this chapter. The following discussion is a general overview of the subject, with emphasis on specific common queries that often arise on board examinations.

With regard to fetal number, determination of the chorionicity and amnionicity in twin gestations can be difficult with advanced gestation. One logical sequence for determining the chorionicity and amnionicity of a twin gestation is to first determine the gender of the twins. If the twins are of opposite gender, they are necessarily dizygotic, and therefore also dichorionic and diamniotic. If twins are the same gender, determine the number of placentas. Two separate placentas indicates dichorionicity and, perforce, diamnionicity. A single placental site can be a manifestation of two abutting separate placentas or a single placenta. If a single placental site is present, search for a chorionic peak, which is a projecting zone of placental tissue extending into the intertwin membrane that indicates dichorionic gestation. Absence of this finding does not exclude dichorionicity, however, because not all dichorionic gestations demonstrate the chorionic peak sign.

If a chorionic peak sign is not identified, evaluate the presence and thickness of the intertwin membrane. This is a subjective criterion for determining chorionicity. If no intertwin membrane is seen, the possibilities include monochorionic monoamniotic pregnancy, diamniotic pregnancy with one twin demonstrating complete oligohydramnios (stuck twin, usually a result of twin-twin transfusion in a monochorionic gestation), and finally diamniotic pregnancy with nonvisualization of the intertwin membrane because of thinness and position.

Amniotic fluid volume often is assessed subjectively by experienced observers. The single largest pocket of amniotic fluid not containing fetal parts or umbilical cord should not exceed 8 cm in the anteroposterior (AP) dimension. The amniotic fluid index (AFI) has more specificity in identifying polyhydramnios (fewer false-positive results). This index is the sum of the largest AP pocket of fluid identified in each of four quadrants, with normal dimensions varying between 5 and 24 cm. Oligohydramnios is suggested when the AFI is less than 5, when the single greatest pocket is less than 2 cm, or when the fluid appears abnormally low to an experienced observer. Differential diagnostic considerations for the finding of polyhydramnios and oligohydramnios are important to know (see section 2 in this chapter).

11

Placenta that covers the internal os of the cervix is classified as complete placenta previa. If the central portion of the placenta covers the os, the previa is sometimes called a *central* or *symmetric previa*. If the margin of the placenta covers the os, the previa is designated *asymmetric*. This is not the same as marginal previa, which means that the placental edge covers one lip of the cervix but not the internal os. *Partial previa* is a term that arose from digital examination of a dilated cervix at term, in which the edge of the placenta could be felt covering part but not all of the dilated internal os. As expected, it can be difficult to determine if a previa is marginal, partial, or asymmetrically complete before cervical dilatation. Usually it does not matter at term, however, because all three forms of previa are managed with cesarean section. Care should be exercised to avoid mistaking a lower uterine segment contraction as evidence of placenta previa. Furthermore, marginal subchorionic hematomas may cover the internal os; in the acute phase, these hematomas can simulate placental tissue, mimicking previa.

The placenta is usually homogeneous in echotexture. Occasionally, lucencies are seen in the placenta, representing venous lakes, subchorionic fibrin deposition, small placental hematomas, cystic degeneration, or intervillous thrombi. These entities are generally not clinically significant and can be lumped together conceptually because it can be impossible to differentiate between them sonographically. If the placenta appears abnormally large or heterogeneous, or if focal masses are present, the appropriate differential diagnostic considerations should be considered (see section 2 in this chapter). A rule of thumb regarding placental size is that the thickness of the midportion of the placenta (in millimeters) usually equals the gestational age (in weeks); the placenta is definitely abnormal if it exceeds the gestational age in weeks plus 10 (i.e., placenta measuring 3.5 cm in thickness at 25 weeks gestation is definitely abnormal).

The sonographic assessment of gestational age relies on composite measurements of the BPD, HC, AC, and FL. For the best results, measurements should be made with strict attention to detail. The BPD should be perpendicular to the orientation of the third ventricle, at the level of the thalami. The plane of section for the HC should include the occipital horns of the lateral ventricles and the thalami, without visualization of the cerebellar hemispheres. The AC image should be round and show both the left portal vein and the fetal stomach. The FL should not include measurement of the distal femoral point, a reflection of the edge of the cartilaginous epiphysis. Measurements are generally fairly concordant with each other in normally developing fetuses. An abnormally small AC raises the possibility of intrauterine growth retardation. Short FL is usually a normal variant but can be a manifestation of skeletal dysplasia or chromosomal abnormality.

Uterine and adnexal evaluation becomes increasingly difficult with advancing gestational age. One especially important aspect of uterine anatomy that should be evaluated is the appearance and length of the cervix. Images of the cervix may require transperineal scanning. The cervix is normally more than 2.8 cm in length. Shorter measurements before 35 weeks gestation should be viewed with suspicion for premature cervical change (either premature labor or cervical incompetence).

Recognition of fetal anatomic abnormalities relies on a thorough understanding of the normal appearance of fetal anatomy. Fetal observations requiring analysis of differential considerations include fetal cerebral ventriculomegaly, fluid-filled fetal skull, supratentorial lesions, posterior fossa abnormalities, nuchal thickening or abnormality, chest mass, abdominal wall defects, intraabdominal cysts, and hydronephrosis. These differential diagnoses are considered in section 2 of this chapter.

GYNECOLOGIC ULTRASOUND

Ultrasound is the primary imaging modality used to evaluate the uterus and adnexa. An examination is complete when the uterus and ovaries are identified in sufficient detail to answer the clinical question at hand. This can often be done via transabdominal scanning using a distended urinary bladder as an acoustic window. Endovaginal scanning is added when a complete study cannot be performed transabdominally. Although some practitioners forgo the transabdominal study, we cannot recommend this practice.

The uterus is evaluated for size, contour, endometrial thickness, and content. The size of the normal uterus varies with age, parity, and menstrual status. Sonographically, the premenopausal uterus is usually less than or equal to 10 cm in length, 5 to 6 cm in width, and 4 to 5 cm in AP dimension, with allowance for 1 or 2 cm more in each dimension with parity. The most common abnormality of the uterus is the presence of one or several leiomyomas. A large uterus can be a manifestation of congenital malformation, leiomyomas, adenomyosis, or a normal variant. These uterine abnormalities are further discussed in the genitourinary chapter of this textbook.

The endometrial thickness, measured as the combined width of the anterior and posterior endometrial lining measured on sagittal images of the uterus, varies considerably in menstruating women. The endometrium can be roughly divided into a superficial or functional layer and a thin, deeper basal layer. The opposed surfaces of the anterior and posterior layers of the endometrium create an echogenic line. During menstruation, only the echogenic thin basal layer remains, resulting in a thin echogenic stripe. During the proliferative phase, a "triple-line" appearance results, because the basal layer is echogenic and the functional layer is relatively hypoechoic. The endometrial stripe, measured from basalis layer to basalis layer, measures 4 to 8 mm during this phase. During the secretory phase, the endometrial functional layer becomes more echogenic and can match the echogenicity of the deeper basal layer, resulting in loss of, or a less conspicuous, triple-stripe appearance. Usually, the endometrium measures between 7 and 14 mm during the secretory phase.

After menopause, the normal endometrium is usually 8 mm or less in thickness. The incidental discovery of an endometrial stripe exceeding 8 mm in thickness in a postmenopausal woman should raise consideration of endometrial biopsy. If a postmenopausal woman has symptoms of vaginal bleeding, endometrial biopsy routinely is performed without sonographic evaluation. When the results of endometrial biopsy show atrophic cells or insufficient material for pathologic diagnosis, ultrasound is performed to measure the endometrial thickness. In this scenario, if the endometrial thickness exceeds 4 to 5 mm, a dilatation and curettage is indicated to obtain more material for pathologic evaluation. If dilatation and curettage results are negative but the patient continues to bleed, sonohysterography or hysteroscopic evaluation (or both) is indicated.

The sonographic approach to evaluation of the adnexa relies on identification of normal ovaries. When normal ovaries are visualized and no other masses are detected, many gynecologic pathologic processes that require intervention can be reasonably excluded. Of course, not all pathologic processes can be eliminated from consideration, including ectopic pregnancy, endometriosis, and pelvic inflammatory disease (PID). When an adnexal mass is identified, it can be difficult to distinguish a solid mass from a cystic mass with internal echoes because of blood, pus, or mucin. Color Doppler sonography can identify blood vessels within the mass, confirming its solid nature. Identification of increased sound transmission through a mass highly suggests that the mass is cystic. Differential considerations for solid-appearing and cystic adnexal masses are analyzed in section 2 of this chapter.

SCROTAL ULTRASOUND

Abnormalities of the testes found on scrotal sonography can be subdivided into three categories: (1) identification of a testicular mass; (2) identification of an abnormal area of echotexture in the testis, possibly but not definitely a mass; and (3) identification of diffusely abnormal-appearing testicular parenchyma without a focal mass. These three differential considerations are analyzed in section 2 of this chapter. Because the specific disease entities are properly considered in the body of knowledge reviewed in the genitourinary chapter, they are discussed in section 3 of the genitourinary chapter. The differential diagnosis of extratesticular abnormalities is discussed in the genitourinary chapter.

11

ULTRASOUND DIFFERENTIAL DIAGNOSES

First trimester bleeding
Third trimester bleeding
Elevated maternal serum alpha fetoprotein (AFP)
Decreased maternal serum AFP
Oligohydramnios

Polyhydramnios
Abnormal placental echotexture
Lower uterine segment abnormality
Fetal ventriculomegaly
Fluid-filled fetal skull
Fetal supratentorial lesion/mass
Fetal posterior fossa abnormality
Nuchal abnormality/thickening
Fetal chest masses
Fetal abdominal wall abnormality
Cyst in fetal abdomen
Fetal hydronephrosis
"Frozen uterus"
Thickened endometrium
Cystic adnexal mass
Solid-appearing adnexal mass
Testicular mass
Abnormal area within testis, not definitely a mass
Diffusely abnormal testicular parenchyma
Hepatic visceral echogenic foci

FIRST TRIMESTER BLEEDING

What is the differential diagnosis of first trimester bleeding?

Normal intrauterine pregnancy (IUP)
Abortion
Early pregnancy failure
Ectopic pregnancy
Hydatidiform mole

Normal IUP

- Most patients with first trimester bleeding have normal intrauterine gestations
- Subchorionic hematoma may be seen
- Increased chance of losing pregnancy with larger extent of subchorionic hematoma, but as long as fetal heart motion is identified, no threshold quantity exists for subchorionic hemorrhage beyond which one can reliably predict poor outcome

True or false: If a subchorionic hematoma extends over 50% of the surface of the gestational sac, the pregnancy almost always is subsequently lost.

Abortion

What features of an IUP suggest abortion in progress?

- Often, no residual evidence of IUP; uterus appears empty or contains blood
- If sac is visualized, often it is deformed and located in lower uterine segment or cervix
- Sonographic evidence of an embryo without a heartbeat is a specific sign of embryonic demise (must be larger than 5 mm CRL by endovaginal sonography)

FIGURE   Callen: 72

Early pregnancy failure

- Refers to abnormal development of an early gestation, in which embryonic structures do not develop normally
- Formerly called *blighted ovum*
- At our institution, a gestational sac 13 mm or more without a yolk sac or 18 mm or more without an embryo is considered an early pregnancy failure
- Sac margins tend to be irregular, with poorly echogenic, surrounding decidual reaction

At what size should all normal gestational sacs contain a sonographically visible yolk sac? At what size should they contain an embryo?

Ectopic pregnancy

Describe intrauterine findings seen with ectopic gestation.

- Possible findings within uterus:
  - ¶ "Normal" trilaminar appearance of decidualized endometrium
  - ¶ Decidual cyst: represents breakdown of decidualized endometrium
  - ¶ Endometrial fluid/blood
  - ¶ "Pseudogestational sac": represents focal collection of blood within endometrial cavity, surrounded by decidualized endometrium

What is the spectrum of adnexal findings seen with ectopic gestation?

- Possible findings seen in adnexa:
  - ¶ Normal ovaries and no free fluid ("normal" sonogram)
  - ¶ Direct visualization of embryonic products (yolk sac or embryo)
  - ¶ Adnexal "ring": represents extrauterine gestational sac surrounded by rim of trophoblastic tissue
  - ¶ Hematoma
  - ¶ Hematosalpinx
- Presence of more than physiologic free fluid, especially if echoes are present within the fluid is a worrisome finding that greatly raises the chance that there is an ectopic gestation
- Some endovaginal sonographic evidence of IUP expected when serum β-human chorionic gonadotropin (hCG) level exceeds 2,000 mIU/mL (IRP); absence of any evidence of IUP when β-hCG exceeds 2,000 mIU/mL raises the chance of ectopic gestation

FIGURES Callen: 653, 657

Hydatidiform mole

True or false: The presence of a yolk sac excludes all forms of molar pregnancy from the differential.

- No embryonic structures are seen with classic mole; thus, no yolk sac or embryo is visible
- In first trimester, the classic mole appears as echogenic material representing developing chorionic villi with occasional lucencies; the gestational sac itself is small and irregular
- Because partial moles have fetal components, it may not be possible to make this diagnosis in the first trimester; lucencies might be seen in the developing chorion

What adnexal findings suggest the presence of hydatidiform mole?

- May see enlarged ovaries with theca lutein cysts because of elevated hCG

FIGURES Callen: 616–618

THIRD TRIMESTER BLEEDING

What is the differential diagnosis for third trimester bleeding?

Placental abruption
Placenta previa
Premature rupture of membranes

Placental abruption

What are the two types of placental abruptions?

- Retroplacental hematoma (separation of basal plate of placenta from uterine wall) or marginal (subchorionic) hematoma may be seen
- Hematoma appearance varies from echogenic (acutely) to hypoechoic; not all placental abruptions are sonographically apparent

11

What might a retroplacental hematoma be confused with sonographically?

- Acutely, retroplacental hematoma may appear as thickening of placenta, and appearance may be mimicked by retroplacental fibroid or uterine contraction
- Marginal abruption, which has a much better prognosis than retroplacental hematoma, is visualized as elevation of the edge of the placenta

FIGURES   Callen 455, 456

Placenta previa

What is the significance of placenta previa?

What mechanisms may result in a false-positive diagnosis of placenta previa?

What finding my be a tip-off that one of these false-positive mechanisms is at work?

- Placental tissue is visualized overlying the internal cervical os
- Beware of causes of false-positive diagnosis: overly distended urinary bladder, alteration of lower uterine anatomy secondary to a contraction
- If it appears that the cervix measures more than 5 cm in the presence of previa, a lower uterine segment contraction or an overly distended maternal urinary bladder that is causing a false-positive diagnosis is likely
- The diagnosis mandates cesarean section

FIGURES   Callen 447–450

Premature rupture of membranes

- Patients do not always give classic history of fluid "gush"
- Amniotic fluid usually appears decreased, near oligohydramnios
- Fluid may be visualized within the vagina
- Endovaginal imaging is relatively contraindicated if suspected (risk of infection)

What finding supports the occurrence of premature rupture of membranes?

- Diagnosis made clinically by evaluation of vagina for evidence of amniotic fluid (fern test)

ELEVATED MATERNAL SERUM ALPHA FETOPROTEIN (AFP)

What is the differential diagnosis of elevated maternal serum AFP?

Incorrect dates
Twins
Fetal demise
Fetal abnormality
Normal variant

General comments

What is AFP?

- AFP is a glycoprotein, synthesized by the fetal liver, which peaks in fetal serum by week 14
- Maternal serum (MS) levels of AFP increase from weeks 7 through 32 of gestation

What defines an elevated MS-AFP?

- MS-AFP more than 2.5 times the median is considered elevated

Incorrect dates

Is the pregnancy less developed or further developed than expected when incorrect dating accounts for an elevated AFP level?

- If pregnancy is misdated and actual age of the fetus is older than stated age, maternal serum AFP appears falsely elevated

Twins

- Account for approximately 10% of cases of elevated MS-AFP

Fetal demise

- Accounts for approximately 5% of cases of elevated MS-AFP
- Breakdown of fetal tissues releases AFP

Fetal abnormality

What are some fetal abnormalities leading to increased MS-AFP?

- Any defect in fetus that allows spillage of fetal fluid into amniotic sac elevates MS-AFP
- Included are open neural tube defects, abdominal wall defects, teratomas
- Closed defects that elevate MS-AFP include cystic hygroma, closed neural axis abnormalities (including hydrocephalus and Dandy-Walker), esophageal atresia, renal abnormalities, and duodenal obstruction

Normal variant

- Diagnosis of exclusion

DECREASED MATERNAL SERUM AFP

What is the differential diagnosis for decreased MS-AFP?

Incorrect dates
Fetal demise
Chromosomal abnormality
Hydatidiform mole
Normal variant

Incorrect dates

Is the pregnancy less developed or further developed than expected when incorrect dating accounts for a decreased MS-AFP level?

- Maternal serum levels of AFP increase from weeks 7 through 32 of gestation
- If actual age of the fetus is younger than stated age, MS-AFP is falsely lowered

Fetal demise

- Before fetal tissue breakdown, demise results in a fetus that is not synthesizing new AFP and that is smaller than it should be (smaller fetus results in lower AFP)

Chromosomal abnormality

- Increased incidence of fetal trisomies, particularly trisomy 21, associated with a low MS-AFP
- 20% of fetuses with trisomy 21 found in women with low MS-AFP
- Improved detection of trisomy 21 with measurement of hCG and serum estriol (triple marker)

What fetal features suggest the presence of a chromosomal abnormality?

- Look for nuchal thickening, pyelectasis, shortened long bones, among other manifestations of trisomy 21; however, even if no abnormalities are identified, most experts recommend karyotype analysis if an alternative explanation of decreased AFP is not identified

Hydatidiform mole

- Molar pregnancy, because of the absence of fetal tissues, has a low MS-AFP

Normal variant

- Diagnosis of exclusion

OLIGOHYDRAMNIOS

What is the differential diagnosis of oligohydramnios?

Demise (fetal death)

Renal/genitourinary abnormalities
    Posterior urethral valves
    Bilateral renal agenesis
    Infantile polycystic kidney disease
    Bilateral multicystic dysplastic kidney
    Unilateral multicystic dysplastic kidney with contralateral
       agenesis or ureteropelvic junction obstruction
Intrauterine growth retardation (IUGR)
Post-dates pregnancy
Premature rupture of membranes
Syndromes and chromosomal abnormalities

General comments

- A simple mnemonic to remember the differential: DRIPPS

FIGURE Callen: 478

Demise

- Look for fetal heart motion

Renal/genitourinary abnormalities

What genitourinary abnormalities lead to oligohydramnios?

Does agenesis have to be bilateral to cause oligohydramnios?

- A normal-appearing urinary bladder is strong evidence that the cause of oligohydramnios is not renal
- Urinary bladder is absent or persistently appears small with all of the renal causes except bladder outlet obstruction, in which case the bladder is dilated
- Dilated proximal urethra seen in cases of posterior urethral valves resembles a keyhole extending from the bladder
- With agenesis, the ipsilateral adrenal gland assumes a long, thin shape in expected renal fossa, termed the "laying-down adrenal"
- Any combination of severe unilateral anomalies such as multicystic dysplastic kidney agenesis or severe ureteropelvic junction causes oligohydramnios

FIGURES Callen: 401 (urethral valves), 395, 396 (agenesis), 409–410 (multicystic dysplastic kidney)

Intrauterine growth retardation (IUGR)

What sonographic features suggest IUGR as the cause of oligohydramnios?

- Significant placental insufficiency causes a redistribution of flow from fetal kidneys to brain, resulting in decreased fetal urine production, which causes oligohydramnios
- One or more of the following features suggests IUGR as the cause of oligohydramnios
    ¶ Interval growth less than expected compared with previous ultrasound
    ¶ Size less than dates and fetal weight less than 10%
    ¶ Significantly smaller fetal abdomen size compared with other measurements

Post-dates pregnancy

- Compare size of fetus with age based on last menstrual period

Premature rupture of membranes

- Diagnosis established clinically, with appropriate history in combination with supporting findings from physical examination (i.e., presence of amniotic fluid in upper vagina)

- If suspected clinically, do not perform endovaginal or translabial imaging without sterile precautions because of risk of infection

Syndromes and chromosomal abnormalities

- Chromosomally abnormal fetuses and those with bizarre syndromes can demonstrate oligohydramnios, usually mediated through renal mechanisms outlined above or through IUGR that is not caused by placental insufficiency

POLYHYDRAMNIOS

What is the differential diagnosis for polyhydramnios?

Idiopathic
Maternal causes
    Diabetes
    Rh incompatibility
Fetal causes
  Unable to swallow fluid
    CNS abnormalities
    Cleft lip/palate
    Facial tumors
  Swallowed fluid meets obstruction
    Gastrointestinal (GI) obstruction (esophageal atresia, duodenal atresia, small bowel obstruction)
    Intrathoracic masses
    Short-limbed skeletal dysplasia
    Nonimmune hydrops
Twin pregnancy

Fetal inability to swallow

- Any severe central nervous system (CNS) anomaly leads to polyhydramnios, probably because of an inability to swallow
- Facial clefts and facial masses may lead to an inability to swallow and subsequent polyhydramnios
- Small stomach

Esophageal atresia

Does esophageal atresia usually occur in isolation?

What is the most common type of esophageal atresia?

- Small or absent stomach
- Proximal esophageal pouch is difficult to see sonographically
- Look for associated anomalies, which are common (VACTERL: vertebral, anorectal, cardiac, tracheoesophageal, renal, and limb)

Duodenal atresia

What chromosomal abnormality is often seen with duodenal atresia?

- Double bubble representing the dilated stomach and duodenal bulb
- 30% have trisomy 21

FIGURE Callen: 359

Small bowel obstruction

- Atresias of the jejunum and ileum, midgut volvulus, and meconium ileus may lead to polyhydramnios
- Appearance differs from duodenal atresia in that more than one loop of bowel not filled with stomach fluid is identified

FIGURES Callen: 359–360

11

Intrathoracic masses

How does an intrathoracic mass lead to polyhydramnios?

- Any intrathoracic mass that is large enough to compress the esophagus may lead to polyhydramnios
- More common possibilities include diaphragmatic hernia and congenital cystic adenomatoid malformation, although almost any fetal chest mass can be a cause

Nonimmune hydrops

What are the findings of a hydropic pregnancy?

- Any severe fetal anomaly may lead to hydrops, but an important one to recognize is arrhythmia because it is treatable
- Look for skin thickening, placental enlargement, and serous effusions (peritoneal, pleural, and pericardial spaces)
- Polyhydramnios

FIGURES   Callen: 433–437

Twin pregnancy

What type of placentation must be present for twin transfusion to occur?

- Look for two fetuses
- If one fetus is smaller than the other, consider twin transfusion syndrome, which can occur in monochorionic pregnancies

FIGURES   Rumack: 749–750

ABNORMAL PLACENTAL ECHOTEXTURE

What entities should one consider as a framework for evaluating the possible causes of abnormal placental echogenicity?

Clinically insignificant sonolucency
Infarct
Hematoma
Chorioangioma
Infection
Molar pregnancy
Hydrops
Placental maturation
Mimics of placental pathology

Clinically insignificant sonolucency

True or false: Most sonolucencies of the placenta are clinically insignificant.

- Several causes: venous lake, subchorionic fibrin deposition, cystic degeneration, intervillous thrombosis
- This is the favored diagnosis in the vast majority of cases, especially when only one or a few small areas of sonolucency are identified in the third trimester

FIGURES   Callen: 457, 458

Infarct

What clue may be present to suggest placental infarction as a cause of a focal placental abnormality?

True or false: Ultrasound should be able to detect a large placental infarct, if one exists.

- Can appear as focal lucency but usually heterogeneous in appearance
- No mass effect
- If large, can result in IUGR; thus, when considering this diagnosis, examine fetal biometry and amniotic fluid volume for evidence of IUGR
- Generally, placental infarctions are not detected sonographically, no matter what the size

FIGURE   Callen: 458

Hematoma

- Retroplacental
    - ¶ Hypoechoic maternal separating placenta from myometrium
    - ¶ If more than 30 to 40% of the maternal surface is involved, significant fetal hypoxia is likely
- Marginal/subchorionic
    - ¶ Seen at placental margin
    - ¶ Hypoechoic, lifts up the more echogenic edge of the placenta
- Preplacental (Breus mole)
    - ¶ Seen at placental surface
    - ¶ Appears as hypoechoic mass lying on surface of placenta, may show mass effect by bulging into the amniotic cavity

FIGURES Callen: 454–457

Chorioangioma

Where are chorioangiomas typically found when sonographically identified?

- Appears as heterogeneous echotexture associated with a mass
- Usually found near the insertion of the umbilical cord on the placenta
- Highly vascular, with blood flow easily demonstrable by color Doppler
- Look for associated findings: fetal hydrops, polyhydramnios

Why should frequent sonograms of the fetus be performed when a chorioangioma is identified?

- Frequent follow-up examinations of the fetus are indicated to evaluate for development of hydrops

FIGURE Callen: 459

Infection

- More likely to result in globally thickened placenta rather than a focal abnormality
- Diagnosis made on evaluation of amniotic fluid and maternal serum
- Look for manifestations of fetal hydrops

Molar pregnancy

In what types of molar pregnancy are fetal parts visualized?

- Multiple small, clustered sonolucencies can be an indication of partial molar pregnancy
- The fetus in a partial molar pregnancy has sonographically identifiable morphologic abnormalities in most, but not necessarily all, cases
- Consider also the possibility of twin pregnancy, in which one is normal and the other is a classic molar pregnancy; in this case, normal placenta is seen separate from the abnormal placental tissue
- Placenta usually enlarged

FIGURES Callen: 49, 619, 620

Hydrops

Does hydrops manifest as a focal placental abnormality?

- May manifest as a global placental abnormality, usually with enlargement, sometimes with a characteristic "ground-glass" appearance
- Look for other features of hydrops: serous effusions, polyhydramnios
- Consider both immune and nonimmune causes (including chromosomal abnormality)

FIGURE Callen: 426

11

Placental maturation

- Appears as areas of increased echogenicity, representing calcification of cotyledons
- More than 50% of placentas show some sonographic evidence of calcification after 33 weeks
- Accelerated maturation can occur in conditions that affect maternal placental vascularization, such as maternal smoking and hypertension

True or false: Areas of increased placental echogenicity seen in the third trimester are usually of clinical concern.

FIGURE Callen: 443

Mimics of placental pathology

- Myometrial contraction
- Prominent basal myometrial vascularity

LOWER UTERINE SEGMENT ABNORMALITY

Previa
Myometrial contraction
Placenta accreta
Myoma
Cervical change

If the lower uterine segment appears unusual, what entities should one consider?

Previa

- Consider strongly when amniotic fluid is not visualized abutting the internal os of the cervix
- In placenta previa, placental tissue covers the internal os (complete) or some part of one cervical lip (marginal); if present at the time of delivery, either necessitates cesarean section, but marginal previa may "resolve" before delivery
- In vasa previa, blood vessels leading to the placenta cover the internal os
- Be sure that the cervix does not appear abnormally long; if so, consider the possibility of a lower uterine contraction simulating previa

What is the difference between a complete placenta previa and a marginal placenta previa? Is there a difference in clinical consequence if either is present at the time of delivery?

FIGURE Callen: 447

Myometrial contraction

- May see a hypoechoic "line" extending from the amniotic fluid to the internal cervical os, representing the opposed layers of the myometrium; to the uninitiated, this hypoechoic line can appear as part of the endocervical canal, resulting in what appears to be a very long cervix
- Suspect contraction if the cervix appears too long (i.e., more than 5 cm)

What clue regarding the cervix can indicate that a lower uterine segment contraction exists?

FIGURES Callen: 450, 611

Placenta accreta

- When identified sonographically, it is almost always associated with an anterior placenta previa
- The hypoechoic zone normally seen beneath the placenta, representing the uterine myometrium, is absent

When should one suggest the diagnosis of placenta accreta?

FIGURE Callen: 453

Myoma

What features help distinguish a myoma from a contraction?

- Hypoechoic with attenuation of sound
- Round shape
- Symmetrically bulges the outer and inner myometrial contour, unless exophytic (contractions result in disproportionate inner myometrial contour bulging)

FIGURES   Callen: 611, 613

Cervical change

- Evaluation of the cervix is part of the recommended mimimum guidelines for obstetric sonography at any gestational age
- Cervical shortening/dilatation that occurs before 36 weeks gestational age is considered premature cervical change; can be caused by premature labor or cervical "incompetence"

At what length cervix should one consider the diagnosis of cervical change? What other features should be sought?

- Consider when cervix is less than 2.8 cm in length (transperineal scanning is useful to better evaluate cervical length)
- When cervix is less than 2.8 cm in length, features that favor cervical change rather than constitutionally short cervix include a funneled appearance of the internal cervical os and demonstration of progressive shortening on serial examination; the latter two findings are worrisome for cervical change even if the cervix is more than 2.8 cm in length

FIGURE   Callen: 612

FETAL VENTRICULOMEGALY

List the differential diagnosis of fetal ventriculomegaly.

Obstruction (hydrocephalus)
   Communicating: infection, hemorrhage
   Noncommunicating: Chiari II, Dandy-Walker malformation, aqueductal stenosis, space-occupying lesion
Destruction: porencephaly, hydranencephaly
Malformation: holoprosencephaly, megalencephaly, white matter dysgenesis, agenesis of corpus callosum, migrational abnormality
Normal variant

General comments

- Measure ventricular size at the level of the ventricular atrium, where the choroid plexus should fill or nearly fill the ventricle
- The down-side ventricular atrium should be less than 10 mm transversely throughout gestation

11

Communicating hydrocephalus

Name two causes of communicating hydrocephalus.

- Caused by extraventricular obstruction of cerebrospinal fluid (CSF) at level of arachnoid granulation (resulting from failure of absorption)
- Uncommon cause of ventriculomegaly in fetuses, secondary to intracranial hemorrhage or infection
- Intracranial hemorrhage can occur with immune thrombocytopenia and with severe maternal stress (severe illness, fetal surgery)
- Posterior fossa is normal, intracranial structural abnormality is not found
- If infection is suspected, next step is to evaluate maternal serum and amniotic fluid for relevant antibodies

Chiari II malformation

What sonographic features are seen with Chiari malformation?

If you suspect the Chiari malformation based on examination of the fetal brain, where else should you look?

- Most common single cause of fetal ventriculomegaly, accounting for approximately one third of all cases
- Normal-appearing cisterna magna not seen; conversely, normal-appearing posterior fossa excludes the diagnosis
- Signs:
    - ¶ Lemon sign: inward scalloping of frontal bones, mild forms more common in normal fetuses (1% of normal fetuses have mild lemon sign appearance of cranium)
    - ¶ Banana sign: cerebellum wrapping around the brain stem in a C-shaped configuration as it is crammed into a small posterior fossa
    - ¶ Beaked tectum: pointed appearance of the midbrain posteriorly
- If cisterna magna effaced, look carefully at fetal spine to identify the level of the associated myelomeningocele
- Identification of the level of the myelomeningocele is important in assessing fetal prognosis

FIGURES   Callen: 227, 229

Dandy-Walker malformation

What structure is absent in the Dandy-Walker malformation?

What is the usual sonographic appearance?

- Large cyst seen in posterior fossa; cerebellar vermis absent
- In structurally milder forms, only inferior vermis is absent, with clear communication demonstrable between the cisterna magna and the fourth ventricle
- These structurally milder forms are **not** associated with a better prognosis
- Often, several other fetal anomalies are detected
- Amniocentesis is indicated for karyotype analysis

FIGURES   Callen: 193, 194

Aqueductal stenosis

When should one consider the diagnosis of aqueductal stenosis?

- Fetal third ventricle should be dilated (more than 3 mm in width)
- This diagnosis is considered when other possibilities are excluded

Space-occupying lesion

Name three space-occupying lesions that can occur in the fetal brain.

- Unusual cause
- Intracranial anatomy appears abnormal and normal structures may be difficult to recognize
- Possibilities include arteriovenous malformation (vein of Galen), congenital neoplasm (rare, usually teratoma), and arachnoid cyst
- Hydrocephalus often asymmetrical

FIGURE   Callen: 217

Hydranencephaly

What feature distinguishes hydranencephaly from hydrocephalus?

- Severe destruction of brain parenchyma, thought to be caused by bilateral internal carotid obstruction
- No cerebral tissue overlying the ventricle, distinguishing this from severe hydrocephalus
- Falx is present to a variable degree
- Third ventricle generally not enlarged (unlike findings in hydrocephalus)
- Concomitant hydrocephalus often present, leading to a large head (in a purely destructive process without obstruction, a small head would be expected)

- Thalamus, basal ganglia, and brain stem are intact

FIGURE Callen: 205

Porencephaly

- Secondary to parenchymal hemorrhage or infarction
- Cystic lesion that communicates with the ventricular system
- Ex vacuo enlargement of the ipsilateral ventricle (no mass effect from the porencephalic cyst)

FIGURE Callen: 206

Holoprosencephaly

What sonographic features distinguish holoprosencephaly from hydrocephalus and hydranencephaly?

- Cortical mantle
- Large, monoventricular cavity that communicates with a dorsal cyst
- Cavum septi pellucidi absent
- Hippocampal ridge is the tissue that separates the monoventricular cavity from the dorsal cyst, which is an important point in differentiating this lesion from hydranencephaly and hydrocephalus
- Midline facial anomalies, when present, are always associated with holoprosencephaly; however, facial anomalies are not always seen with holoprosencephaly

FIGURES Rumack: 887; Callen: 202, 203

Agenesis of corpus callosum

What causes the interhemispheric cyst seen in agenesis of the corpus callosum?

What are the sonographic features of agenesis of the corpus callosum?

- Indentation of the medial walls of the lateral ventricles by Probst bundles causes "steer horn" appearance of the frontal horns
- Probst bundles also result in lateral displacement of the anterior portion of the lateral ventricles, making the ventricles appear parallel
- High-riding third ventricle can appear as an interhemispheric cyst; in addition, an associated extraventricular interhemispheric arachnoid cyst may be present
- Colpocephaly is caused by maldevelopment of the white matter surrounding the atria and occipital horns
- Absent cavum septi pellucidi

FIGURES Callen: 197–199

Normal variant

- Consider in a fetus with mild form of ventriculomegaly (less than 15 mm atrial width, usually less than 12 mm) when no other sonographic abnormality is seen after evaluation by an experienced sonologist (a situation known as isolated mild ventriculomegaly)
- Unfortunately, there is no way at this time to differentiate these normal fetuses from other causes of isolated mild ventriculomegaly (white matter dysgenesis, migrational abnormality, and aqueductal stenosis)

True or false: Fetuses with ventriculomegaly are always abnormal, even if the specific abnormality is not identified sonographically.

FLUID-FILLED FETAL SKULL

What three entities can lead to the appearance of a fluid-filled fetal skull?

Massive hydrocephalus
Hydranencephaly
Holoprosencephaly

What sonographic features suggest the diagnosis of massive hydrocephalus as the cause of a fluid-filled fetal skull?

Massive hydrocephalus

· Cortical mantle present
· Falx may be seen but can be fenestrated or be so thin as to be not visible sonographically

FIGURE Callen: 209

What sonographic features suggest the diagnosis of hydranencephaly as the cause of a fluid-filled fetal skull?

Hydranencephaly

· Absence of cerebral tissue overlying the ventricle distinguishes hydranencephaly from massive hydrocephalus
· Third ventricle generally not enlarged (unlike most forms of hydrocephalus)
· Thalamus is not fused; basal ganglia and brain stem are intact

FIGURE Callen: 205

What sonographic features suggest the diagnosis of holoprosencephaly as the cause of a fluid-filled fetal skull?

Holoprosencephaly

· In alobar forms, can appear as a fluid-filled skull
· In such cases, there is a monoventricular cavity that communicates with a dorsal cyst; thus, a cortical mantle of tissue is present anteriorly, with a hippocampal ridge marking the point of transition from the monoventricular cavity to the dorsal cyst
· Thalami fused
· Associated midline facial abnormalities may be present

FIGURE Callen: 202

FETAL SUPRATENTORIAL LESION/MASS

List entities to consider when the supratentorial region of the fetal brain has an abnormality.

Tumor
Hemorrhage
Arachnoid cyst
Vein of Galen malformation
High-riding third ventricle (agenesis of corpus callosum)
Choroid plexus cyst

Tumor

· Mass effect
· Generally heterogeneously isoechoic to hyperechoic compared with brain parenchyma
· Rare
· Types of lesions: teratoma, primitive neuroectodermal tumor (PNET), glioma

FIGURE Callen: 215

Hemorrhage

· Echogenic
· Often located in region of caudothalamic notch or periventricular white matter
· When present, occurs in setting of fetal stress (for example, maternal surgery, burn, acute illness) or with immune thrombocytopenia

In what clinical settings does fetal intracranial hemorrhage occur?

Arachnoid cyst

· Extraaxial location
· No solid elements

- Septations may be present
- The interhemispheric cyst seen with agenesis of the corpus callosum is a type of arachnoid cyst

FIGURES   Callen: 195, 206

Vein of Galen malformation

Where are vein of Galen malformations identified prenatally? What other fetal findings should be sought when the diagnosis has been established?

- Cystic
- Located adjacent to tectum of the midbrain
- Doppler interrogation makes the diagnosis
- Look for associated fetal hydrops, which may be present

FIGURE   Callen: 217

High-riding third ventricle

What sonographic features are associated with a high-riding third ventricle?

- Cyst between the hemispheres
- Look for other features of agenesis of the corpus callosum: absent cavum septi pellucidi, parallel orientation of the lateral ventricles, steer-horn appearance of the frontal horns

FIGURES   Callen: 197–199

Choroid plexus cyst

Which chromosomal abnormality is most often associated with choroid plexus cysts?

Name some sonographically identifiable fetal malformations associated with this karyotype abnormality.

- Obvious location of cyst within the choroid of lateral ventricle
- Look for other signs of trisomy 18, the most frequently associated chromosomal abnormality (occurs in about 1 of 50 cases of choroid plexus cyst): cardiac abnormalities, diaphragmatic hernia, omphalocele, esophageal atresia (manifests as small stomach and polyhydramnios), hydronephrosis, limb malformations (especially clenched hands), craniofacial abnormalities

FIGURES   Callen: 47, 48, 215, 216

FETAL POSTERIOR FOSSA ABNORMALITY

What entity leads to an effaced cisterna magna? What entities lead to the sonographic appearance of an enlarged cisterna magna?

Effaced cisterna magna
    Chiari malformation
Large cisterna magna
    Dandy-Walker malformation
    Arachnoid cyst
    Cerebellar hypoplasia
    Mega cisterna magna

Chiari malformation

What sonographic signs other than an effaced cisterna magna can be seen with Chiari malformations?

- Other sonographic signs include:
    ¶ Lemon sign: inward scalloping of frontal bones
    ¶ Banana sign: cerebellum wrapping around the brain stem in a C-shaped configuration as it is crammed into a small posterior fossa
    ¶ Beaked tectum: pointed appearance of the midbrain posteriorly
- Look carefully at the fetal spine to identify the presence and level of the associated myelomeningocele

FIGURES   Callen: 227, 229

True or false: Although inferior vermian agenesis has a poor prognosis, fetuses with this diagnosis tend to have a slightly better outcome than those with complete vermian agenesis.

Dandy-Walker malformation

- Cerebellar hemispheres appear splayed apart
- Cerebellar vermis is absent; sometimes only the inferior aspect of the vermis is missing and the superior aspect is intact (inferior vermian agenesis)
- Inferior vermian agenesis is **not** associated with a better prognosis

FIGURE Callen: 193

Arachnoid cyst

- Should show mass effect on the cerebellum, with flattening of the cerebellar contour where it abuts the arachnoid cyst
- If large, can result in obstructive hydrocephalus

FIGURE Callen: 195

What rule of thumb regarding the transverse measurement of the cerebellar hemispheres helps to exclude cerebellar hypoplasia as a cause of a large cisterna magna?

Cerebellar hypoplasia

- Vermis appears normal
- Normally, the transverse measurement of the cerebellar hemispheres (in millimeters) is approximately equal to the fetal gestational age (in weeks) up to about 24 weeks gestational age after which it slightly exceeds the gestational age; thus, if the transverse measurement of the cerebellar hemispheres equals the gestational age, cerebellar hypoplasia can be excluded

Mega cisterna magna

- Diagnosis of exclusion, made when vermis appears normal, no mass effect on the cerebellum exists to suggest the presence of an arachnoid cyst, and cerebellar dimensions are within normal limits

FIGURE Callen: 196

NUCHAL ABNORMALITY/THICKENING

What is the differential diagnosis of an abnormality in the nuchal region?

Normal variant
Chromosomal abnormality
Cystic hygroma
Encephalocele
Soft tissue mass
Teratoma
Hemangioma

What chromosomal abnormalities are associated with nuchal thickening?

What is considered abnormal nuchal thickness?

Chromosomal abnormality

- Nuchal thickening is defined by some as a measurement exceeding 6 mm
- To avoid false-positive results, must be imaged in suboccipital-bregmatic plane, in which both the cavum septi pellucidi and the cisterna magna are visualized
- The smallest measurement that one can obtain using the landmarks described above is the measurement to use
- Chromosomal abnormalities include trisomies (particularly 21) and 45,X
- Many cases result from involuted hygromas

FIGURE Rumack: 876

Cystic hygroma

What is the most common chromosomal abnormality associated with cystic hygroma?

- Appearance as large, septated fluid collection; the "septation" is usually oriented perpendicular to the skin surface, representing the nuchal ligament
- No associated cranial defect
- Adjacent skin and subcutaneous tissues are abnormal
- Associated hydrops (usually fatal)
- Most common associated karyotype abnormality is 45,X

FIGURE Callen: 223

Encephalocele

What is the most common site for encephalocele?

What alternative diagnosis should you think of when the defect in the calvarium is not midline?

- Fluid-filled sac that may contain meninges only or meninges and brain tissue
- Associated calvarial defect
- CNS anomalies are commonly associated
- May occur in the occiput (most common), frontal bone, or parietal bone
- Usually midline (if not midline, think of amniotic band syndrome)

FIGURE Rumack: 885

Soft tissue mass

- Masses such as hemangioma, teratoma, and thyroid goiter must be considered when a neck mass is encountered

FETAL CHEST MASSES

What is the differential diagnosis when a mass in the fetal chest is encountered?

Congenital cystic adenomatoid malformation
Congenital diaphragmatic hernia
Bronchopulmonary sequestration
Bronchial atresia
Teratoma
Neuroblastoma

Congenital cystic adenomatoid malformation

Does the diagnosis of congenital cystic adenomatoid malformation mandate fetal surgery?

What associated features are important to identify, if present?

How can ultrasound reliably distinguish between congenital cystic adenomatoid malformation and sequestration in some cases?

- Echogenic
- Cysts always evident pathologically but occasionally not evident sonographically (microcystic variety)
- May cause mass effect and mediastinal shift
- Features of associated hydrops are important to identify because they indicate poor prognosis
- May regress without intervention; thus, observation is initial management strategy
- Arterial supply arises from pulmonary system (as opposed to the systemic arterial supply of sequestration), which sometimes can be visualized sonograpically

Congenital diaphragmatic hernia

Which hernia location is more common, left side or right side?

What are some sonographic features that distinguish diaphragmatic hernia from other possibilities in this differential diagnosis?

- Left side is more common than right
- Heart is shifted to unaffected side
- Stomach is not seen in its usual location
- Stomach often seen as cystic structure in the chest, located next to or behind the heart
- False-positive finding may be caused by oblique imaging showing the fetal heart and stomach at the same level

11

- Complications include polyhydramnios, hydrops, and pulmonary hypoplasia
- Increased incidence of associated anomalies, particularly CNS

FIGURES   Callen: 338, 339

Bronchopulmonary sequestration

Where is sequestration most commonly located?

How can sequestration be distinguished from congenital cystic adenomatoid malformation and CDH?

Which is more commonly detected in utero, extralobar or intralobar sequestration?

- Well-circumscribed, echogenic mass
- Lower lobe location, left side more common than right side
- Can cause mass effect with resultant polyhydramnios and hydrops
- Color Doppler may detect the feeding systemic artery (which distinguishes sequestration from congenital cystic adenomatoid malformation and congenital diaphragmatic hernia [CDH])
- Because intralobar sequestration is thought to develop as a result of infection postnatally, all sequestrations detected in utero are extralobar

FIGURES   Callen: 341, 342

Bronchial atresia

What is the most common location of bronchial atresia?

- Focal obliteration of a segment of bronchial lumen
- Appears as an echogenic mass lesion
- Upper lobe location most common, left side affected more often than right side
- Rare in the lower lobes

Teratoma

- Solid mass with cystic areas
- May have areas of calcification
- In the chest, usually arises from pericardial sac

Neuroblastoma

- Posterior mediastinal mass
- Echogenic
- Rarely seen prenatally

FETAL ABDOMINAL WALL ABNORMALITY

11

What is the differential diagnosis for an abdominal wall abnormality in the fetus?

Omphalocele
Gastroschisis
Amniotic band syndrome
Limb-body wall complex

Omphalocele

What is more commonly associated with other anomalies, gastroschisis or omphalocele?

- Defect is midline and shows a smooth edge (resulting from covering membrane)
- Expect to find umbilical vein within the mass (umbilical cord inserts on the apex of the mass)
- Look for associated anomalies: cardiac, gastrointestinal, renal, and genitourinary
- Elevated MS-AFP (although typically lower than in gastroschisis)
- Recommend that patient get karyotype analysis because of risk of chromosomal abnormalities

FIGURE   Callen: 378

Gastroschisis

Where does the defect in gastroschisis typically occur?

What usually herniates through the defect?

- Multiple loops of bowel are seen to float freely within the amniotic cavity
- Defect is not covered by a membrane, and thus has an irregular edge
- Defect usually is to the right of the umbilical cord insertion
- MS-AFP is elevated
- Low incidence of associated anomalies

FIGURES   Callen: 375–377

Amniotic band syndrome

What features of an abdominal wall defect should suggest amniotic band syndrome?

- Consider if you see what appears to be gastroschisis with externalized liver (the liver does not extrude in straightforward gastroschisis)
- Defect usually asymmetric
- Look for other findings: constriction rings of the distal extremities, asymmetrical amputations, kyphosis

FIGURE   Callen: 384

Limb-body wall complex

What is limb-body wall complex and what are some of the abnormalities that are seen with it?

- Short umbilical cord
- Lateral thoracic and abdominal defect, usually left-sided
- Other anomalies are common, including limb, facial, and neural tube defects, as well as scoliosis

FIGURE   Callen: 386

CYST IN FETAL ABDOMEN

Posterior midabdomen (touches spine)
    Hydronephrosis
    Urinoma
    Multicystic dysplastic kidney
Anterior abdomen (not touching spine)
    Choledochal cyst
    Gut duplication
    Meconium pseudocyst
    Dilated bowel
    Urachal cyst
    Fluid within omental or mesenteric leaves
Pelvis/lower abdomen
    Ovarian cyst
    Hydrometrocolpos
    Sacrococcygeal teratoma

General comments

What feature in regard to the location of a fetal intraabdominal cyst makes a renal origin most likely?

- Cysts discovered in the fetal abdomen are almost always benign
- Origin can be difficult to determine; one rule is that if the cyst touches the fetal spine, it is most likely renal in origin
- List of entities above is not a complete list of all possible diagnoses

Hydronephrosis

- Renal cortex seen as rim of tissue around one margin of the fluid collection

- Calyces present as focal bulges extending off the dilated renal pelvis
- If the obstruction is not at the ureteropelvic junction, then a dilated ureter can often be seen extending off the hydronephrotic kidney

FIGURES   Callen: 405, 407

Urinoma

- Calyces not seen extending off the collection
- Large urinomas typically displace the kidney anteriomedially

FIGURE   Callen: 408

Multicystic dysplastic kidney

- Often one dominant cyst is present, with adjacent noncommunicating smaller cysts
- Closely evaluate the contralateral kidney and the amount of amniotic fluid, because the amniotic fluid volume and fetal prognosis depend entirely on normal function of the contralateral kidney

FIGURES   Callen: 409, 410

Choledochal cyst

- Typically in right upper quadrant, but can be large and extend out of this quadrant
- For this diagnosis to be considered, one margin of the cyst should touch the porta hepatis

FIGURE   Callen: 353

Gut duplication

What helpful feature may be seen that indicates that a cyst is a gut duplication?

- Can have internal echoes
- Wall of cyst usually shows hypoechoic muscle layer typical of bowel, but this can be difficult to appreciate prenatally

Meconium pseudocyst

How do meconium pseudocysts occur?

- Echogenic rim, often with acoustic impedance
- Associated with ascites (because meconium pseudocyst is a consequence of bowel perforation)

FIGURE   Callen: 361

Dilated bowel

- With duodenal or jejunal atresia, dilated duodenum and jejunum can appear as one or two "cysts" adjacent to the fetal stomach
- In meconium ileus, small bowel can become dilated
- In third trimester, normal fetal colon can appear dilated
- Tubular appearance, may show peristalsis

FIGURES   Callen: 356, 359, 360

Urachal cyst

- Located at dome of bladder
- Umbilical arteries may course around the cyst

FIGURE   Callen: 398

Fluid within omental or mesenteric leaves

- Can be seen in the presence of fetal ascites
- Mesenteric cyst rarely occurs without ascites

FIGURE   Callen: 364

Ovarian cyst

- Most likely diagnosis if fetus is female and cyst does not touch fetal spine
- Round, may have septations and internal echoes
- Because fetal pelvis is relatively small, these can appear to arise in the abdomen

FIGURES   Callen: 366, 417

Hydrometrocolpos

- Tubular shape, low in pelvis

Sacrococcygeal teratoma

- Large, heterogeneous in appearance, with cystic and solid elements
- Exophytic component seen in most sacrococcygeal teratoma

FETAL HYDRONEPHROSIS

Name six causes of fetal hydronephrosis.

Ureteropelvic junction obstruction
Apparent obstruction at the ureterovesical junction
      Ectopic ureterocele
      Megaureter
      Reflux
Apparent obstruction at the urethra
      Posterior urethral valves
      Caudal regression anomaly
      Urethral atresia
      Megacystis microcolon intestinal hypoperistalsis syndrome
      Persistent cloaca

General comments

- Measurement of the AP diameter of the renal pelvis has been used to determine which fetuses might have renal obstruction; experts differ as to the exact numbers that require follow-up and what type of follow-up is indicated

Define fetal pelviectasis. Which fetuses need sonographic follow-up? At what intervals?

- The most conservative measurement guidelines indicate that the renal pelvis should not exceed 4 mm before 33 weeks of gestation, or 7 mm after 33 weeks of gestation
- Other authors define pelviectasis as a renal pelvis exceeding 4 mm at 15 to 20 weeks, 5 mm at 20 to 30 weeks, and 7 mm at 30 to 40 weeks
- One approach to follow-up is to adopt the policy that any fetus exceeding threshold measurements needs a follow-up sonogram in 3 to 4 weeks; if the pelviectasis persists on the follow-up sonogram, a postnatal evaluation is indicated; another approach is to obtain a third-trimester follow-up for pelviectasis found in the second trimester, and a postnatal follow-up for pelviectasis found in the third trimester

FIGURE   Callen: 398

11

Ureteropelvic junction obstruction

Describe expected findings with mild ureteropelvic junction obstruction, moderate ureteropelvic junction obstruction, and ureteropelvic junction severe obstruction.

- In mild cases, ureteropelvic junction obstruction may manifest only as pelviectasis
- In moderate cases, clearly defined dilated renal pelvis, infundibula, and calyces are visualized
- In severe cases, only a single fluid-filled structure representing the dilated renal pelvis is seen, with a thin parenchymal rim; in such cases, careful evaluation of the margin of the renal pelvis demonstrates small lobulations that represent the flattened dilated calyces
- Urinary bladder and amniotic fluid volume are normal, unless the contralateral kidney also is abnormal

FIGURE Callen: 407

Ectopic ureterocele

What constellation of features can be found with ectopic ureterocele? What findings are characteristic of the diagnosis?

- Hydronephrosis can be asymmetric, with more dilatation usually seen in upper pole of affected kidney
- Hydronephrosis can be bilateral with unilateral ectopic ureterocele because the ureterocele in the bladder can obstruct the contralateral ureterovesical junction
- Cyst-within-a-cyst appearance of the urinary bladder is characteristic, when visualized

FIGURES Callen: 404, 405

Megaureter

What is the typical appearance of the urinary tract when a unilateral megaureter exists?

- Degree of ureteral enlargement is more pronounced than degree of hydronephrosis
- Diagnosis confirmed postnatally

FIGURE Callen: 406

Reflux

Are there any prenatal features that distinguish vesicoureteral reflux from megaureter?

- Generally indistinguishable from megaureter prenatally, unless one happens to see hydronephrosis develop after urinary bladder emptying
- Diagnosis established after birth

Posterior urethral valves

Describe expected findings with posterior urethral valves. Does the absence of oligohydramnios make the diagnosis unlikely?

- Bilateral hydronephrosis; often, dilated ureters are clearly identified
- Male fetus
- Urinary bladder has a characteristic keyhole appearance, unless it has ruptured, in which case fetal urinary ascites is present
- Oligohydramnios is seen in about 50% of cases

FIGURES Callen: 402, 403

Caudal regression anomaly

Why does hydronephrosis develop with caudal regression?

- Distal spine does not appear normal
- Urinary tract dilatation is caused by reflux

Urethral atresia

- Looks like posterior urethral valves but can occur in male or female fetus

11

Does the absence of oligohydramnios exclude the diagnosis of urethral atresia?

- Absence of oligohydramnios excludes this diagnosis, practically speaking

Megacystis microcolon intestinal hypoperistalsis syndrome

Describe the typical findings of the fetus with megacystis intestinal hypoperistalsis syndrome.

In what trimester is oligohydramnios an expected finding in this syndrome?

- Much more common in female fetus
- Sonographic appearance of urinary tract similar to that of posterior urethral valves
- Small bowel dilatation occurs but is not apparent sonographically until late in the third trimester
- Because bladder is not obstructed, no association with oligohydramnios exists, in fact, these pregnancies usually demonstrate polyhydramnios in the third trimester

Persistent cloaca

Describe findings suggestive of persistent cloaca.

- Female fetus
- Urinary tract dilatation caused by reflux
- Spinal anomalies common: tethered spinal cord, sacral agenesis, spina bifida, segmentation anomalies
- Septated/bilobed pelvis cystic mass is often observed, representing dilated vagina, uterus, or rectum (or all three)

FIGURE   Callen: 363

"FROZEN UTERUS" (UTERUS SURROUNDED BY ILL-DEFINED MATERIAL IN CUL-DE-SAC OR ALONG ADNEXA)

What entities should be considered when the uterus appears surrounded by ill-defined material?

Pelvic abscess
Endometriosis
Ectopic pregnancy
Ovarian cancer
Exophytic myomas

General comments

- Except for exophytic myomas, no distinguishing sonographic features exist that allow differentiation among the possibilities

Pelvic abscess

- May be a sequela of pelvic inflammatory disease or of a nongynecological process
- Clinical features suggest infection

Endometriosis

- Subacute presentation
- Patient not pregnant

Ectopic pregnancy

- Positive pregnancy test
- IUP not seen

Ovarian cancer

- Usually in older women

Exophytic myomas

- Only entity in this differential diagnosis in which a "normal" uterus is not identified
- Contours of the uterus are obscured, and endometrial stripe is difficult or impossible to identify with confidence
- Marked sound attenuation usually occurs

THICKENED ENDOMETRIUM

What is the differential diagnosis when a thickened endometrial stripe is found?

Secretory phase of menstrual cycle
Pregnancy related
      Intrauterine pregnancy
      Ectopic pregnancy
      Molar pregnancy
      Retained products of conception
Hyperplasia
Polyp
Carcinoma
Endometritis

Secretory phase of menstrual cycle

- Endometrium gradually thickens throughout the menstrual cycle
- Superficial layer is hypoechoic to the deeper layer in the proliferative phase and becomes isoechoic to the deeper layer in the secretory phase

FIGURE Callen: 576

Intrauterine pregnancy

By what gestational age is the gestational sac first visible?

- A gestational sac imbedded in the decidua usually becomes sonographically evident as a 2- to 3-mm sac by 4.5 weeks after last menstrual period
- Until this time, the endometrial stripe of a pregnant woman is identical to that of any woman in the proliferative phase

Ectopic pregnancy

True or false: The endometrial stripe in ectopic pregnancy is different from that seen early (less than 4.5 weeks in pregnancy).

- Unlikely to coexist if intrauterine gestation is present (but risk can be as high as 1 in 100 in cases of assisted fertilization)
- Pseudogestational sac is an endometrial fluid collection surrounded by decidualized endometrium; this is distinguished from an IUP, which is embedded within the decidualized endometrium
- Most often a pseudogestational sac is not seen, and the endometrial stripe appears similar to that seen during the proliferative phase of menstrual cycle

FIGURE Rumack: 712

Molar pregnancy

- Classic appearance of an echogenic mass with cystic spaces describes a second trimester mole
- First trimester moles may not show cystic spaces

FIGURE Callen: 616

Retained products of conception

- Thick, echogenic endometrium, usually asymmetrical or focal in appearance
- Definitive diagnosis can be made if recognizable fetal or placental structures can be identified
- May show increased color flow in the suspicious area in acute stage
- Chronic retained products can appear as focal area of calcification or ossification

Hyperplasia

What are some causes of endometrial hyperplasia?

- Nonspecific finding of a thickened endometrial stripe
- Can demonstrate cystic spaces but usually does not

FIGURE   Rumack: 393

Polyp

What procedure reliably distinguishes between endometrial hyperplasia and endometrial polyp?

- May appear as a discrete mass or as nonspecific endometrial thickening
- Often but not always has cystic spaces
- Can escape detection on blind endometrial biopsy; in such cases, sonohysterography can be useful to further characterize location and presence, if suspected

FIGURE   Callen: 601

Carcinoma

What is the normal endometrial thickness for an asymptomatic postmenopausal woman?

What feature of endometrial thickening is especially worrisome for the presence of cancer?

- Thickening of endometrium that may be heterogeneous or echogenic
- Thickness of 8 mm or less is considered normal for postmenopausal women without bleeding
- Look for extension of echogenic endometrial tissue into myometrium, which would make carcinoma very likely

FIGURE   Callen: 609

Endometritis

- May see fluid, gas, or echogenic material within the endometrium
- Diagnosis made clinically

11

CYSTIC ADNEXAL MASS

List considerations for a cystic adnexal mass.

Physiological ovarian cyst
Benign neoplasm
Malignant neoplasm
Endometrioma
Hydrosalpinx
Paraovarian cyst
Peritoneal inclusion cyst
Ectopic pregnancy
Abscess

General comments

True or false: When an adnexal cystic mass is encountered sonographically, unless there are features that indicate that the mass is clearly benign, the mass should be surgically removed as soon as possible.

- Because most adnexal cysts are benign and self-limiting (resolve spontaneously), unless compelling clinical or sonographic findings suggest a specific diagnosis that needs immediate attention (e.g., malignancy, ectopic pregnancy, or abscess), it is reasonable to obtain a follow-up sonogram in a few weeks to determine if the cystic mass is self-limiting or not; if the mass is not self-limiting, it is usually removed surgically, even if it has benign features, in order to make a specific diagnosis and because of the risk of torsion
- The presence of a retracting clot within a cystic mass argues for a benign process, usually hemorrhagic cyst; retracting clots are characterized by scalloped, concave margins, as opposed to mural nodules, which have convex margins
- Some experts argue that evaluation of resistive indices can be helpful in distinguishing benign processes from malignant processes, but this is not our experience at the University of California, San Francisco, and we do not advocate resistive index evaluation

FIGURES Callen: 634–637

Physiological ovarian cyst

When is the diagnosis of nonneoplastic ovarian cyst most likely? What types of cyst are included in this category?

- Includes follicular, corpus luteum, and theca lutein cysts
- Most likely diagnosis when the mass is unilocular, thin-walled, smoothly contoured, and less than 5 cm in diameter
- Presence of wispy strands of linear echoes within cyst are highly suggestive of hemorrhage
- Should resolve or decrease in size on follow-up sonogram
- Although postmenopausal women do not develop physiological cysts, these cysts can persist into the postmenopausal period

FIGURE Callen: 628

Benign neoplasm

What features suggest that a cystic adnexal mass is a benign neoplasm?

- May be unilocular or septated
- Presence of solid nodules (either septal or wall based) suggests malignancy
- May or may not have internal echoes
- Unchanged in appearance on short-interval follow-up sonogram
- Presence of echogenic sound-attenuating region indicates dermoid; other features of dermoids include echogenic lines and dots (hair) within the cyst and fluid-fluid level (which is not specific for dermoid)

FIGURE Callen: 632

Malignant neoplasm

What features suggest that a cystic adnexal mass is malignant?

- For practical purposes, these never appear sonographically as a unilocular cyst
- Look for mural or septal nodules
- Avoid mistaking a retracting clot for a mural nodule; mural nodules should not have concave margins

FIGURES Callen: 634, 635, 638

Endometrioma

Describe the classic appearance of an endometrioma.

- Classic appearance: cystic mass with diffuse, low-level internal echoes, without retracting clot, occasionally with punctate hyper-

echoic foci on the inner wall of the cystic mass that are thought to represent cholesterol deposition
- Often does not have the classic appearance
- Not self-limiting
- Absence of endometrioma does not exclude endometriosis; endometriosis is a laparoscopic diagnosis

FIGURES Callen: 629, 630

Hydrosalpinx

Describe features suggesting hydrosalpinx as the cause of a cystic adnexal mass.

- Tubular shape, often with "incomplete septations" that represent folds
- Sonographic diagnosis much more certain when an adjacent, normal-appearing ovary is identified

Paraovarian cyst

When should one consider paraovarian cyst as one of the most likely diagnoses?

- Adjacent to normal-appearing ovary
- Can be mistaken for an exophytic cyst

Peritoneal inclusion cyst

- Adjacent to normal-appearing ovary
- Often with history of previous surgery

Ectopic pregnancy

- Consider in any woman of child-bearing age
- For practical purposes, does not appear as a unilocular "simple" cyst
- Consider strongly in appropriate clinical setting if cyst has echogenic rim ("adnexal ring" sign) and is located adjacent to ovary
- Look for coexisting hemoperitoneum

FIGURES Callen: 655, 657

Abscess

- Usually heterogeneous in appearance
- Ovary on affected side usually is not discretely identified separate from the abscess
- Clinical features are generally characteristic

SOLID-APPEARING ADNEXAL MASS

List considerations for a solid-appearing adnexal mass.

Exophytic leiomyoma
Ovarian torsion
Hemorrhagic cyst
Endometrioma
Abscess
Ectopic pregnancy
Dermoid
Solid ovarian tumor (primary and metastatic)

Exophytic leiomyoma

- Poor sound transmission
- Hypoechoic, heterogeneous
- Try to identify attachment to uterus

• Presence of other uterine myomas makes this diagnosis more likely
• Clearly identified separate ovary makes diagnosis more certain (ovarian fibromas have the same sonographic characteristics as leiomyomas, but in these lesions a separate, normal-appearing ovary is not identified)

Ovarian torsion

• Classically has multiple enlarged follicles, which may not be seen

Hemorrhagic cyst

• Diffuse internal echoes can make this appear solid, but increased through-sound transmission helps to characterize the hemorrhagic cyst as a cystic mass with internal echoes

Endometrioma

• Diffuse internal echoes can make this appear solid, but increased through-sound transmission helps to characterize the endometrioma as a cystic mass with internal echoes

Abscess

• Heterogeneous in appearance

Ectopic pregnancy

• Pelvic hematoma can appear solid, with echogenic and heterogeneous areas
• Consider in appropriate clinical setting, especially if IUP not identified

Dermoid

• Can appear solid; in such cases, it is characterized by poor acoustic transmission and the leading edge of the mass is echogenic, without a clearly defined back edge

Solid ovarian tumor (primary and metastatic)

• Fibromas, adenofibromas, thecomas, Brenner tumors
• Krukenberg's tumor (metastatic gastric adenocarcinoma)

TESTICULAR MASS

What is the differential diagnosis when an intratesticular mass is discovered?

Tumor
Cyst
Abscess
Hematoma
Adrenal rest

Tumor

• Unless sonographic observation or clinical history strongly suggests another entity, intratesticular masses are presumed to represent malignant tumor until the pathologist states otherwise

What sonographic features reliably distinguish between benign and malignant tumors?

What is the typical appearance of seminoma?

Of nonseminomatous germ cell tumor?

How can one reliably distinguish between malignant and benign intratesticular tumors using ultrasound?

- Both benign and malignant tumors occur, but orchiectomy is usually performed because they cannot be reliably differentiated by imaging
- Most common primary malignancy is seminoma, which typically appears as a fairly well-circumscribed, uniformly hypoechoic mass
- Cystic areas and calcification are more suggestive of a nonseminomatous germ cell tumor
- Epidermoid cyst is a benign germ cell tumor that is generally well-circumscribed and hypoechoic, often demonstrating hyperechoic rim

FIGURES   Rumack: 571–575

Cyst

- Common, can be multiple
- Well-defined, anechoic, smooth-walled mass, with increased sound-through transmission
- Often located near mediastinum
- Must distinguish from cystic necrosis of neoplasm (not difficult because the necrotic areas of tumors are irregular, with clearly abnormal solid areas)

FIGURE   Rumack: 576

Abscess

- Testis usually enlarged
- Epididymis typically abnormal and hyperemic, unless infection has been partially treated
- Intratesticular abscess appears as a heterogeneous, mass-like area; do not expect an intratesticular abscess to be easily recognizable as a fluid collection
- Clinical history important in considering diagnosis

FIGURE   Rumack: 577

ABNORMAL AREA WITHIN TESTIS, NOT DEFINITELY A MASS

What are the possibilities when an abnormal focus without a discrete mass is discovered in the testis?

Tumor
Infarct
Abscess
Tubular ectasia of rete testis

Tumor

- Unless there is compelling clinical or sonographic evidence to suggest an alternative diagnosis, the abnormal area should be regarded as suggestive of neoplasm

Infarct

What are some distinguishing features of infarct compared with testicular mass?

If one suspects infarct as the cause of an abnormal area in the testis, what other test may be helpful?

- Think of infarct when the abnormal area is band-like or zone-like, extending out to the periphery of the testis in a wedge shape
- Masses have convex margins, whereas infarcts tend to have concave margins
- Involved testis often significantly smaller than contralateral testis (if contralateral testis is normal)
- Testicular MR examination may help confirm infarct if suggested by lack of vascularity on sonogram

FIGURE   Rumack: 578

Abscess

- Testis usually enlarged
- Epididymis typically abnormal and hyperemic, unless infection has been partially treated
- Intratesticular abscess may appear as an ill-defined heterogeneous area without definite mass effect; do not expect an intratesticular abscess to be easily recognizable as a fluid collection
- Clinical history important in considering diagnosis

FIGURE Rumack: 577

Tubular ectasia of rete testis

Describe the sonographic appearance of tubular ectasia. What other abnormality is usually present?

- Dilatation of efferent tubules, thought to be caused by obstruction
- Often bilateral
- Subtle striated linear pattern that follows the mediastinum
- Associated spermatocele almost always seen

DIFFUSELY ABNORMAL TESTICULAR PARENCHYMA

What is the differential diagnosis when a diffusely abnormal appearing testicle is encountered?

Atrophy
Torsion
Orchitis
Infiltrating tumor
Testicular microlithiasis

Atrophy

- Atrophic testicle typically small and hypoechoic relative to the contralateral testis
- Search for history of previous torsion or inflammation

Torsion

- In the later stages of torsion, the testis becomes hypoechoic and heterogeneous in echotexture
- Absence or significant relative decrease of blood flow on color Doppler imaging makes the diagnosis

Orchitis

Where does the infection/inflammation of the scrotum generally begin?

- Inflammation generally begins in the epididymis and may subsequently involve the testis
- Color Doppler abnormalities with hyperemia of epididymis and testicle seen earlier than gray-scale abnormalities
- As inflammation progresses, epididymis and testicle become enlarged and hypoechoic
- Must be distinguished clinically and sonographically from torsion

FIGURE Rumack: 585

Infiltrating tumor

What neoplasms can result in testicular enlargement but maintain homogeneous echotexture?

- Consider if testis is markedly enlarged and heterogeneous
- If enlarged and homogeneous, consider possibility of lymphoma or leukemia

Testicular microlithiasis

- Multiple intratesticular echogenic foci, usually without acoustic shadowing
- Usually diffuse but may be clustered
- Usually bilaterally symmetrical
- Associated with cryptorchidism

What is the recommended course of action when testicular microlithiasis is discovered, and why?

- Tumor seen in up to 40% of cases, so surveillance ultrasound is recommended

HEPATIC VISCERAL ECHOGENIC FOCI

What is the differential diagnosis for echogenic foci within the abdominal viscera?

Prior infection
Intrahepatic ductal stones
Pneumobilia
Portal venous gas
Hepatitis

Prior infection

- TB and histoplasmosis may demonstrate 2- to 3-mm echogenic foci, seen within the spleen and liver

What infectious agents are responsible for echogenic foci in the spleen in patients with AIDS?

- Tiny echogenic foci may be seen in the spleen, liver, and kidneys in patients with acquired immunodeficiency syndrome (AIDS), secondary to disseminated pneumocystis, mycobacteria, or cytomegalovirus (CMV).

FIGURES Rumack: 61 (*Pneumocystis carinii* pneumonia [PCP]), 95 (granulomatous disease), 101 (*Mycobacterium avium–intracellulare* [MAI])

Intrahepatic ductal stones

What is the usual cause of intrahepatic ductal stones?

- Usually secondary to recurrent pyogenic cholangitis
- Shadowing, medium-echogenicity foci are seen within the intrahepatic and extrahepatic ducts

FIGURE Rumack: 128

Pneumobilia

- Can be secondary to incompetent sphincter of Oddi, surgery, or erosion into the common bile duct of a stone or ulcer

What features of hepatic echogenic foci suggest pneumobilia?

- Echogenic foci are linear, and more are seen in the left lobe of the liver in supine patient (nondependent)

FIGURE Rumack: 129

Portal venous gas

- Usually secondary to pneumatosis intestinalis

What characteristic finding is seen on pulse-wave Doppler examination of the portal venous system in cases of portal venous gas?

- Look for evidence of bowel ischemia (thick-walled bowel, echogenic foci within bowel wall), and echogenic foci within the liver
- Unlike pneumobilia, no left-sided preference
- May see high-amplitude spikes on Doppler examination of the portal venous system

11

True or False: The liver is normally slightly echogenic relative to renal cortex.

Diffuse gallbladder wall thickening is fairly specific for an intrahepatic process, such as hepatitis.

Hepatitis

- Liver parenchyma may have decreased echogenicity, accentuating the portal triads, which appear bright
- The liver is hypoechoic relative to renal cortex (usually isoechoic to slightly hyperechoic)
- Gallbladder wall thickening is a nonspecific finding that is often associated

FIGURE   Rumack: 55

Figure References

Callen PW: *Ultrasonography in Obstetrics and Gynecology,* 3rd ed. Philadelphia: WB Saunders, 1994.
Rumack CM, Wilson SR, Charboneau JW: *Diagnostic Ultrasound.* St. Louis: Mosby–Year Book, 1991.

ULTRASOUND DISEASE ENTITIES

OBSTETRICS

Abruptio Placenta

Clinical
- Defined as premature separation of a normally implanted placenta
- 1% of all pregnancies
- Associated with pain and vaginal bleeding
- Can be retroplacental or marginal
- Retroplacental abruption, usually result of rupture of spiral arteries, is associated with hypertension and vascular disease and has a worse prognosis
- Marginal abruption results from tearing of marginal veins and is associated with cigarette smoking
- Accounts for up to 25% of all perinatal deaths

Imaging
- Appearance varies with the age of the hematoma
- Acutely, the hematoma may be isoechoic with the placenta, detectable only as thickening of the placenta
- Becomes hypoechoic by 1 to 2 weeks
- Leiomyoma or contraction may mimic hematoma
- Retroplacental hematoma may be detected as hypoechoic material separating the placenta from the myometrium
- Marginal abruption is associated with subchorionic hemorrhage

Agenesis of Corpus Callosum

Clinical
- May be a developmental disorder or may be acquired
- Insult occurs early in gestation
- Other anomalies found in 80% include holoprosencephaly, Dandy-Walker cysts, intracranial lipomas, heterotopias, encephaloceles, and microcephaly
- Also associated with trisomies
- Defect can be asymptomatic, but low intelligence found in 70% and seizures in 60%

Imaging
- Poorly developed white matter around the atria and lateral horns leads to culpocephaly
- Steer horn configuration of the frontal horns of the lateral ventricles is the result of lateral displacement from bundles of Probst
- Third ventricle extends superiorly, the "interhemispheric cyst"

11

- Presence of a cavum septi pellucidi excludes the diagnosis of complete agenesis; partial agenesis may not be detectable sonographically

Amniotic Band Syndrome

Clinical
- A set of congenital malformations attributed to entanglement of the fetus by bands of amnion
- Cause unknown
- Incidence: approximately 8 in 10,000 live births
- Males and females affected equally
- Prognosis depends on the associated anomalies

Imaging
- Calvarial involvement includes off-midline encephaloceles, asymmetrical anencephaly and facial clefts
- Asymmetrical amputations and constriction of limbs, distal lymphedema, and clubfoot deformity
- Spinal deformities include scoliosis, kyphosis, lordosis, and marked angulation deformities
- Truncal defects include rib clefting, gastroschisis, omphalocele, and bladder extrophy
- Other band-like structures that may be seen without fetal deformity include the amnion itself and uterine synechiae, both of which have no untoward consequence for the fetus

Anencephaly

Clinical
- Most common open neural tube defect
- Ratio of females to males affected, 4:1
- Increased familial incidence
- Results from failure of neural tube to close at cephalic end; occurs between second and third weeks of gestation
- Discovered during prenatal ultrasound performed to investigate elevated maternal serum AFP
- Universally fatal

Imaging
- Bony calvarium absent
- May be diagnosed before 14 weeks but may not be readily apparent by transabdominal ultrasound before 14 weeks gestation
- Angiomatous stroma is tissue that can look like brain and is located over the fetal orbits
- Symmetry of the defect distinguishes it from amniotic band syndrome

Aqueductal Stenosis

Clinical
- Narrowing at the aqueduct of Sylvius
- Several causes
- When isolated, patients have a good chance of normal development, both functionally and mentally
- Associated anomalies occur in approximately 75% of cases and are associated with a poor outcome

Imaging
- Dilatation of the lateral and third ventricles with a normal-sized fourth ventricle
- Posterior fossa structures appear normal

Autosomal Dominant Polycystic Kidney Disease

Clinical
- Potter type III
- Rarely manifests antenatally; mean age at diagnosis is 43 years

11

- Associated with cysts in the liver, spleen, pancreas, and seminal vesicles and with CNS aneurysms ("berry")

Imaging
- Disease suspected when cystic and echogenic kidneys are seen with normal amniotic fluid when a known family history exists
- If prenatal sonogram suggestive of autosomal dominant polycystic kidney disease, sonographic examination of the parents should help to confirm or lower the suspicion

Autosomal Recessive Polycystic Kidney Disease

Clinical
- Potter type I
- Medullary ectasia with innumerable small (1- to 2-mm) cysts
- 25% risk of recurrence
- Associated with fibrotic hepatic disease (severity of hepatic disease correlates inversely with severity of renal disease)
- High mortality rate when renal disease is severe as a result of oligohydramnios and pulmonary hypoplasia

Imaging
- Bilaterally enlarged kidneys
- Reniform shape is maintained
- Early on, cortical echogenicity is increased
- Late in gestation, the cortex becomes hypoechoic relative to the echogenic medulla
- Normal sonogram in a fetus at risk for the disease does not ensure disease absence because of biological variability

Bronchopulmonary Sequestration

Clinical
- Represents a bronchopulmonary foregut malformation
- Divided into extralobar (enveloped by its own pleura) and intralobar
- Extralobar accounts for 25%, but is usually the type detected prenatally; some authors think that intralobar sequestrations are acquired lesions
- Most common location of both types is the left lower lobe
- Both types receive systemic arterial supply from the abdominal aorta
- Extralobar type has systemic venous drainage, whereas venous drainage for intralobar sequestrations is pulmonary
- Extralobar sequestrations commonly associated with other abnormalities, particularly congenital diaphragmatic hernia and foregut anomalies

Imaging
- Well-circumscribed mass that is echogenic, often with "triangular" shape reflecting the cross-sectional appearance of a pulmonary lobe
- Color Doppler may show the feeding arterial supply, which differentiates sequestration from congenital diaphragmatic hernia or congenital cystic adenomatoid malformation
- May see results of mass effect on the mediastinum, including polyhydramnios and hydrops

Chorioangioma

Clinical
- Benign vascular malformation of the placenta that acts as an arteriovenous shunt
- Small chorioangiomas are pathologically detectable in 1% of placentas
- Symptomatic chorioangiomas occur in 1 in 3,500 to 1 in 20,000 pregnancies
- Can be a source of elevated MS-AFP
- Can result in polyhydramnios, hydrops, hemorrhage, preterm labor, growth retardation, and fetal death

Imaging
- Well circumscribed
- Solid or heterogeneous on ultrasound imaging
- Most commonly located on fetal surface of placenta near umbilical artery insertion
- Color Doppler shows hypervascularity

Choroid Plexus Cyst

Clinical
- Common lesion, seen in about 1% of normal fetuses
- Associated with chromosomal abnormalities, particularly trisomies 18 and 21
- Controversy over whether a detailed sonographic evaluation of the fetus can select out a subgroup of fetuses with choroid plexus cysts that do not require karyotype analysis

Imaging
- May be unilateral or bilateral
- May be as large as 2 cm
- May be multilocular
- Most regress by 25 to 26 weeks

Cleft Lip and Palate

Clinical
- Second most common congenital malformation
- Caused by lack of fusion of the facial grooves
- Isolated cleft lip occurs in 25% and has a 2:1 female predominance
- Cleft palate in isolation occurs in 25%
- Cleft lip and palate occur in 50%
- Clubfoot most common associated anomaly with both isolated cleft lip and palate
- Polydactyly most common associated anomaly of combined cleft lip and palate
- Karyotyping should be performed when these anomalies are identified

Imaging
- Cleft lip more often identified than palatal clefting
- Polyhydramnios and a small stomach alerts the sonographer to the possible diagnosis
- Median cleft lip is associated with holoprosencephaly

Cystic Adenomatoid Malformation

Clinical
- Hamartoma of the lung
- Stocker classification divides them into three types: macrocystic, medium-sized cystic, and solid (histologically, the solid lesions contain tiny cysts)
- May displace mediastinal structures and compress the heart and inferior vena cava (IVC)
- May be associated with hydrops, pulmonary hypoplasia (mass effect), and polyhydramnios
- Prognosis related to the size of lesion and degree of mass effect
- Some have been noted to regress in utero

Imaging
- Bulky mass
- May range in appearance from multiple large cysts to solid appearance (tiny cysts cause multiple interfaces; thus, mass appears echogenic)
- Mass effect with mediastinal shift and development of complications such as hydrops or polyhydramnios
- Differential diagnosis includes sequestration, diaphragmatic hernia, bronchogenic cyst, neurenteric cyst, bronchial atresia

Cystic Hygroma

Clinical
- Pathologically defined as a multilocular lymphatic malformation lined by lymphatic endothelium
- Occurs in 1 in 6,000 pregnancies
- Thought to represent dilated obstructed jugular lymph sacs
- Often seen with generalized lymphedema, which is invariably fatal
- 75% have chromosomal abnormalities, most commonly Turner syndrome
- Associations include Turner syndrome, trisomy 21, Noonan syndrome, fetal alcohol syndrome

Imaging
- Multiseptate cystic mass that is often bilateral and located posterolaterally along the neck, occasionally extending into the upper thorax
- Differential diagnosis of a cystic neck mass includes encephalocele, brachial cleft cyst, thyroglossal duct cyst, teratoma, cervical meningocele, and nuchal edema
- Locations other than nuchal include mediastinum, axilla, chest wall, face, retroperitoneum, abdominal viscera, scrotum, and bones

Dandy-Walker Syndrome

Clinical
- Result of abnormal development of the cerebellar vermis and fourth ventricle
- Caused by several factors
- Commonly associated with agenesis of the corpus callosum and hydrocephalus
- Poor prognosis with high mortality and high likelihood of intellectual impairment
- Dandy-Walker variant, which is more common, has a smaller degree of vermian agenesis and less hydrocephalus

Imaging
- Can be detected before 20 weeks
- Posterior fossa cyst (Dandy-Walker cyst) that communicates with the fourth ventricle through a defect in the vermis
- Cerebellar hemispheres are splayed apart, differentiating the condition from retrocerebellar arachnoid cyst (which causes mass effect and anterior displacement of the cerebellum)
- Main differential diagnosis is arachnoid cyst, but other entities in differential diagnosis include mega cisterna magna, communicating hydrocephalus, and cerebellar hypoplasia

Diaphragmatic Hernia (Congenital)

Clinical
- Occurs about 1 in 2,000 to 1 in 5,000 live births
- Usually occurs on the left
- Results from failure of fusion of a portion of the primitive diaphragm
- Associated malformations occur in up to 50% of fetuses and include cardiac defects, neural tube defects, spinal defects, and trisomies (particularly 18 and 21)
- Extremely high mortality because of pulmonary hypoplasia and persistent fetal circulation

Imaging
- Findings that raise suspicion for congenital diaphragmatic hernia include polyhydramnios, absence of a normally placed stomach, and mediastinal shift
- Finding bowel on a transverse image at the level of the four-chamber view of the heart makes the diagnosis
- Coronal views of the fetal thorax can be useful to identify the presence of liver in the thorax, a poor prognostic sign
- Differential diagnosis includes cystic adenomatoid malformation, bronchogenic cysts, and extralobar sequestration

Encephalocele

Clinical
- Mesodermal defect with herniation of meninges (meningocele) or brain and meninges (encephalocele)
- Least common open neural tube defect
- Midline defect that occurs in the frontal, parietal, or occipital bones
- Off-midline defect suggests amniotic band syndrome
- MS-AFP generally is not elevated because the defect usually is skin covered
- Brain tissue within the sac implies a worse prognosis
- Associated with agenesis of the corpus callosum, Meckel-Gruber syndrome, Dandy-Walker syndrome, and Chiari III malformation (high cervical encephalo-meningocele containing medulla, fourth ventricle, and most of cerebellum)

Imaging
- Fluid-filled sac extending from calvarium
- Associated with a bony defect that is often difficult to detect
- Main differential diagnosis is cystic hygroma, which does not show a skull defect

Esophageal Atresia

Clinical
- Occurs in 1 in 2,500 live births
- Cause unknown
- Five types; esophageal atresia with distal tracheal fistula is the most common (90%)
- Part of VACTERL (vertebral, anal, cardiac, tracheoesophageal, renal, and limb) spectrum of associated anomalies
- If diagnosis is suspected, fetal morphologic survey and karyotyping are indicated

Imaging
- Absent stomach (although this is insensitive because most fetuses have a connection to the stomach via the tracheal tree)
- Small amount of fluid in stomach
- Esophageal pouch
- Polyhydramnios
- Differential diagnosis for an absent stomach includes obstruction of esophagus, oligohydramnios, facial clefting, CNS abnormalities, and congenital diaphragmatic hernia

Gastroschisis

Clinical
- Occurs in 1 in 4,000 live births
- Elevated MS-AFP
- Believed to occur secondary to abnormal involution of the right umbilical vein or disruption of the omphalomesenteric artery
- Occurs sporadically without recurrence risk or genetic association (thus, if diagnosis is certain by sonography, amniocentesis is not indicated)
- Complications include prematurity, sepsis, and bowel ischemia; mortality less than 10%
- Associated bowel-related abnormalities occur in up to 30% of fetuses, but other anomalies are rare
- Main differential diagnosis is omphalocele

Imaging
- Abdominal defect almost always located to the right of the umbilicus
- Usually small defect
- Extraabdominal organs always include the small bowel but can be accompanied by other organs, including large bowel, stomach, and genitourinary system
- Defect is not membrane covered
- Bowel loops may be mildly dilated

11

Holoprosencephaly

Clinical
- Group of disorders arising from failure of normal forebrain development
- Occurs in approximately 6 in 10,000 live births
- Spectrum of severity from alobar to semilobar to lobar
- Most affected fetuses die in utero or shortly after birth
- Survivors usually have severe mental retardation
- Karyotype abnormalities are common, particularly trisomy 13

Imaging
- Septum pellucidum is absent in all three subtypes
- Alobar subtype shows a monoventricular cavity that communicates posteriorly with a dorsal sac, fused thalami, absence of the falx, and cephalically displaced cortical tissue
- Semilobar is less severe and shows fused thalami, separated ventricles posteriorly, and a frontal cortical mantle
- Lobar subtype is least severe and displays fusion of only the rostral-most portion of the cerebral hemispheres with separation posteriorly, as well as separate ventricles that communicate as a result of the absence of the septum pellucidum

Hydranencephaly

Clinical
- Complete or near complete destruction of cerebral cortex and basal ganglia that had been normally formed
- Thought to represent bilateral internal carotid artery occlusion
- Poor prognosis, although it may initially evade clinical detection

Imaging
- Calvarial contents are almost totally fluid without rim of cortex
- Falx is present
- Main differential diagnosis includes alobar holoprosencephaly and severe hydrocephalus

Hydrops Fetalis

Clinical
Immune Hydrops
- Refers to maternal antibodies to fetal red blood cells with consequent development of fetal anemia
- Secondary to maternal sensitization to fetal antigens from prior pregnancy; antigens cross the placenta during the next pregnancy, resulting in fetal hemolysis
- Liver responds to this anemia by replacement of parenchyma with erythropoietic and fibroblastic tissues, which then leads to portal hypertension and eventual decreased placental perfusion and edema
- Before Rh_o (D) immune globulin (RhoGAM), the most common cause was Rh incompatibility
- Currently, other fetal antibodies are more common causes

Nonimmune Hydrops
- Now accounts for 90% of cases of hydrops
- Several causes; in general, hydrops is a manifestation of heart failure or plethora, so any fetal anomaly that can lead to heart failure or cause plethora can cause hydrops
- Maternal causes include hypoalbuminemia, hypertension, and anemia
- Prognosis of nonimmune hydrops, particularly that associated with a structural defect, is poor

Imaging
- Diagnosis based on finding either serous effusions in two body cavities or a serous effusion in addition to anasarca
- Skin thickening more than 5 mm
- Placental enlargement more than 4 cm

Intrauterine Growth Retardation (IUGR)

Clinical
- Defined as fetal weight less than tenth percentile of normal for the population being examined
- Most fetuses with weight less than tenth percentile are normal
- If oligohydramnios is present, probability of IUGR is high
- Uteroplacental insufficiency accounts for approximately 80%
- Fetal causes account for the remaining 20% (congenital heart disease, genitourinary anomalies, CNS anomalies, viral infection, and chromosomal abnormalities)

Imaging
- Comparison of the estimated fetal weight based on sonographic biometry with the fetal age based on last menstrual period or early sonogram identifies those fetuses who are smaller than expected (less than 10%)
- Doppler evaluation has been used to further evaluate, but its usefulness is controversial
    > High resistance in the umbilical artery or low resistance in the fetal cranial circuit are worrisome findings
    > Reversed diastolic flow in the umbilical artery is an ominous finding
- Fetal abdominal measurements may be relatively small compared with other measurements when IUGR is caused by uteroplacental insufficiency; this is termed *asymmetrical IUGR*
- IUGR is considered "symmetrical" when it exists with no discrepancy between fetal abdominal circumference and other fetal measurements; this type of IUGR is often caused by early insults, such as infection or chromosomal abnormalities

Limb–Body-Wall Complex

Clinical
- Fetal malformation characterized by neural tube defects, lateral body-wall defects, limb defects, and scoliosis
- Occurs sporadically, without known predilection or recurrence rates
- Approximately 1 in 4,000 births
- Invariably fatal

Imaging
- Truncal defects involving the thorax, abdomen, or both, with herniation of viscera through the defect
- Spinal anomalies in nearly all cases
- Cranial defects (anencephaly, encephalocele) are common
- Limb defects include clubfoot, absent extremities, and syndactyly

Meckel-Gruber Syndrome

Clinical
- Autosomal recessive
- Diagnosis established sonographically with at least two of the following: bilateral multicystic dysplastic kidneys, occipital encephalocele, postaxial polydactyly
- Fatal
- Accounts for up to 5% of neural tube defects

Imaging
- Look for other features of the syndrome if bilateral renal cysts or occipital encephalocele are seen because of the 25% recurrence risk

Meconium Ileus

Clinical
- Small bowel obstruction from impaction of viscous meconium in the distal ileum
- Nearly always associated with cystic fibrosis

11

Imaging
- Microcolon
- Dilated, distended ileum, which may be confused with colon
- Difficult diagnosis to make in utero

Meconium Peritonitis

Clinical
- Occurs secondary to in utero bowel perforation
- Extraluminal meconium incites a chemical peritonitis that then calcifies
- May be associated with obstructive bowel lesions and malformations (atresias, volvulus, malrotation), as well as cystic fibrosis

Imaging
- Abdominal calcifications may extend into the scrotal sac in males (patent processus vaginalis)
- Calcifications often seen on the surface of the liver
- Meconium can encyst, becoming meconium pseudocyst
- Commonly accompanied by fetal ascites and polyhydramnios

Mesoblastic Nephroma

Clinical
- Also known as *fetal renal hamartoma*
- Most common neonatal renal neoplasm; may be detected during fetal life
- Benign tumor but may invade locally
- Nephrectomy is curative

Imaging
- Solid mass within the kidney
- Looks like Wilms' tumor, but neonatal Wilms' is rare

Multicystic Dysplastic Kidney

Clinical
- Potter type II
- Result of ureteral atresia causing failure of induction of the metanephric blastema
- Collecting tubules become cystically enlarged
- Kidney is functionless
- Contralateral renal abnormalities in about 40%, most commonly obstruction of ureteropelvic junction
- Survival of fetus depends on viability of contralateral kidney

Imaging
- Paraspinous flank mass characterized by numerous cysts
- Cysts do not communicate with the renal pelvis (distinguishes this abnormality from the main differential diagnosis of ureteropelvic junction obstruction)

Myelomeningocele

Clinical
- Second most common open neural tube defect; thus causes elevated MS-AFP
- Most occur in lumbosacral area, although can occur anywhere
- Results from failure of closure of the neural tube
- Prognosis relates to size of lesion and location, with higher lesions having a worse prognosis
- Deficits range from mild sensory impairment to death
- Associated anomalies are common, particularly Chiari II malformation, which has a high association with meningomyelocele

Imaging
- Most common cause of hydrocephalus in fetus (because of Chiari II malformation)
- Because not all meningomyeloceles are readily detected, a small posterior fossa mandates a careful search for meningomyelocele

11

- "Lemon" and "banana" signs are two cranial abnormalities that may be seen in fetuses with meningomyelocele/Chiari II
- Frontal bones may be scalloped, giving the calvarium the appearance of a lemon (seen at 16 to 24 weeks), although this may be seen in normals and in cephaloceles
- "Banana" sign refers to the appearance of the cerebellum when wrapped around the posterior brain stem (because of the small posterior fossa)
- Meningomyelocele may be detected directly if large or if the sac contacts the amniotic fluid
- Abnormal morphology of the posterior ossification centers of the spine (spina bifida) must be used if the sac cannot be visualized directly
- Normally, the posterior ossification centers are parallel or converge toward each other, whereas in spina bifida the centers diverge and are farther apart than the adjacent levels

Oligohydramnios

Clinical
- Amniotic fluid below the normal range
- Causes include fetal demise, renal abnormalities, IUGR, post-dates pregnancy, premature rupture of membranes (mnemonic: DRIPP)
- Prolonged oligohydramnios may have severe effects on the fetus, including Potter facies, flexion contractures, pulmonary hypoplasia, and umbilical cord compression

Imaging
- Measurements include single deepest pocket less than 1 to 2 cm and four-quadrant amniotic fluid index less than 5
- Finding oligohydramnios at 30 to 32 weeks is more sensitive than trying to find it at term

Omphalocele

Clinical
- Occurs with approximately the same frequency as gastroschisis, 1 in 4,000 live births
- Increased incidence with advanced maternal age
- Can be isolated but is often associated with other abnormalities (up to 66% of cases)
- Associated syndromes include pentalogy of Cantrell (omphalocele, anterior diaphragmatic defect, sternal cleft, ectopia cordis, and cardiovascular malformations); cloacal extrophy; Beckwith-Wiedemann syndrome; and trisomies, particularly 13 and 18
- Mortality rate depends on the presence of other anomalies

Imaging
- Membrane covered
- Umbilical cord inserts centrally on the membrane
- Because of the limiting membrane, MS-AFP is lower than with gastroschisis
- Presence of liver in the defect distinguishes it from gastroschisis
- Bowel-only omphaloceles have a higher association with chromosomal abnormalities than those containing liver

11

Placenta Previa

Clinical
- Occurs in 1 in 200 pregnancies
- Manifests as painless vaginal bleeding
- 3 to 5% of pregnancies complicated by third-trimester bleeding, but only 7 to 11% of these are caused by placenta previa
- Factors predisposing to previa include prior surgery, older age, and multiparity
- Diagnosis mandates cesarean section

Imaging
- Divided into marginal, partial, and complete by location relative to the internal os
- Because the radius of the cervix does not exceed 2 cm, all forms of placenta previa are excluded when the placenta edge is more than 2 cm from the internal os

- When placental tissue covers one lip of the cervix without covering the os, it is termed *marginal*
- Placental tissue only partially covering the os is termed *partial previa*
- *Complete previa* is defined by placental tissue completely covering the internal os
- Many early diagnoses of placenta previa "resolve" by term because of involution of marginal, low-lying placental tissue (presumably because of poor blood supply) in combination with growth of the lower uterine segment
- Overly distended urinary bladder or uterine contraction can also result in a false-positive diagnosis because of apposition of lower uterine walls with incorrect localization of the internal os
- Transperineal (translabial) scanning may be helpful in difficult cases

Polyhydramnios

Clinical
- Defined as amniotic fluid above the normal amount
- Several causes: 20% maternal, 20% fetal, 60% idiopathic
- Severe polyhydramnios is associated with fetal abnormalities 75% of the time
- Maternal causes include diabetes, immune hydrops, placental tumor, and twins
- Fetal causes include nonimmune hydrops, gastrointestinal malformations, CNS abnormalities
- Complications include preterm labor, lower extremity edema from IVC compression, and pain
- Treatment for severe polyhydramnios includes early delivery and therapeutic amniocentesis

Imaging
- Measurements for diagnosis include single largest pocket of fluid larger than 8 cm, as well as four-quadrant amniotic fluid index more than 25
- Subjective visual inspection also used by some
- Full maternal bladder can push fluid out of the lower uterus, causing the appearance of polyhydramnios in the fundus

Porencephaly

Clinical
- Milder form of hydranencephaly
- Develops from cerebral hemorrhage or infarction with necrosis and cyst formation
- Prognosis depends on the amount and location of destroyed brain

Imaging
- Cystic spaces that communicate either with the ventricular system or the CSF spaces at the brain surface
- Enlargement of ipsilateral ventricle
- No mass effect (it represents an ex vacuo event)

Posterior Urethral Valves

Clinical
- Refers to obstruction of the posterior urethra by redundant epithelium
- Common cause of urinary obstruction
- Three types described, but they are not sonographically distinct

Imaging
- Dilated, thick-walled urinary bladder
- Dilatation of proximal urethra, which in combination with the distended urinary bladder results in a "keyhole" appearance
- May not see oligohydramnios or pelvocaliectasis (the bladder may decompress or the kidneys may cease urine production from dysplasia)
- Poor prognostic signs include oligohydramnios, lack of caliectasis, large amount of urinary ascites, and dystrophic bladder wall calcification

Renal Agenesis

Clinical
- Occurs in approximately 1 in 4,000 births
- Result of absent ureteral bud formation
- If bilateral, leads to severe oligohydramnios with subsequent pulmonary hypoplasia and is uniformly fatal
- Associated with cardiac and musculoskeletal abnormalities

Imaging
- Adrenal glands may assume a reniform shape and occupy the renal fossa
- Identification of the bladder excludes bilateral agenesis
- Normal amniotic fluid at up to 14 weeks of gestation does not exclude the diagnosis, because the fetal kidneys are not the major source of amniotic fluid until after weeks 14 to 16

Sacrococcygeal Teratoma

Clinical
- Occurs in approximately 1 in 35,000 births
- Usually an isolated abnormality
- Arises from the coccyx and can extend internally or externally
- Most are benign
- Prognosis is good if polyhydramnios is not present
- Fetus is delivered by cesarean section to avoid rupture and hemorrhage

Imaging
- Cystic, with or without solid components
- Can have arteriovenous shunting with subsequent polyhydramnios and hydrops
- Differential diagnosis mainly includes meningomyelocele, ovarian cysts, and duplication cysts

Schizencephaly

Clinical
- Bilateral clefts in the cerebral cortex thought to be secondary to bilateral middle cerebral artery (MCA) infarction
- Lined by gray matter
- Extend from ventricular lumen to cerebral surface
- Similar to porencephaly, prognosis depends on extent and location of brain injury

Imaging
- Lesions are bilateral, but the reverberation artifact in the near field may lead the sonographer to believe that the lesion is unilateral and therefore a porencephalic cyst

Subependymal Hemorrhage

Clinical
- Common among premature infants (less than 32 weeks)
- Greatest risk with gestational age less than 32 weeks or weight less than 1,500 g
- Generally originates in germinal matrix of subependyma, a fine network of vessels that is susceptible to metabolic and blood pressure changes
- Four grades:

I	Limited to subependyma
II	Intraventricular extension without hydrocephalus
III	Intraventricular extension with hydrocephalus
IV	Intraparenchymal hemorrhage (although not all intraparenchymal hemorrhage develops from subependymal hemorrhage)

- Most hemorrhages occur within the first week of life
- Prognosis depends on location and size of hemorrhage, as well as degree of hydrocephalus; in general, grades I and II do well, with few neurologic sequelae

11

- Complications include hydrocephalus and porencephalic cysts

Imaging
- Hemorrhage appears homogeneous and echogenic acutely
- May see focal enlargement of the choroid at the caudothalamic notch as a result of clot (germinal matrix regresses toward term, and caudothalamic notch is the last place to regress)
- Clot becomes less echogenic with time, and the center becomes hypoechoic
- May completely resolve or subependymal cyst may be seen
- Porencephalic cyst develops from intraparenchymal hemorrhage

Trisomy 13

Clinical
- Occurs in 1 in 5,000 births
- Severe mental retardation
- Other associated problems include seizures, apneic episodes, and failure to thrive
- Early death (50% die within first month)

Imaging
- Early IUGR
- Polyhydramnios
- Congenital heart disease, particularly septal defects
- CNS abnormalities, including holoprosencephaly and agenesis of the corpus callosum
- Facial abnormalities including micrognathia, microphthalmia, and cleft lip or palate (or both)
- Omphalocele
- Renal malformations
- Limb abnormalities include polydactyly and overlapping digits

Trisomy 18

Clinical
- Edward syndrome
- Occurs in 1 in 3,000 births
- Severe retardation
- Failure to thrive, apneic episodes
- 90% die within first year

Imaging
- Early IUGR
- Polyhydramnios
- Omphalocele
- Congenital diaphragmatic hernia
- Renal malformations
- Cardiac malformations, particularly septal defects
- Limb deformities include clubfoot and arthrogryposis
- Choroid plexus cysts are common, but isolated choroid plexus cyst without other recognizable malformation is rare
- Large cisterna magna
- Facial abnormalities include micrognathia and sloped occiput

Trisomy 21

Clinical
- Down syndrome
- Occurs in approximately 1 in 700 live births
- 15 to 20% die within the first year of life, and mortality rates exceed those of normals at any age
- Increased incidence with increased maternal age
- Maternal age older than 35 years and low MS-AFP are indications for amniocentesis
- 30% of patients with duodenal atresia have trisomy 21
- 40% of patients have congenital heart disease

Imaging
- Nuchal fold thickening (measured on a transverse axial image from a suboccipital-bregmatic plane) of more than 6 mm suggests the diagnosis
- Double bubble from distention of the stomach and duodenal bulb seen in duodenal atresia
- Nonimmune hydrops
- Renal pyelectasis seen in up to 25%
- Other findings include clinodactyly of the fifth digits, short femurs and humeri, widely spaced first and second toes (sandal gap), cystic hygroma, esophageal atresia, and diaphragmatic hernia

Turner syndrome

Clinical
- Usually XO karyotype
- Majority result in fetal demise
- Occurs in 1 in 2,500 liveborn females
- Phenotype includes short stature, webbed neck, shield chest with wide-spaced nipples, and cubitus valgus
- Also associated with renal malformations (especially horseshoe kidney), deafness, and cardiac disease (especially aortic coarctation)
- Affected females are infertile

Imaging
- Cystic hygroma
- Lymphangiectasia (universally fatal)
- Hydrops
- Renal and cardiac anomalies

Twin-Twin Transfusion Syndrome

Clinical
- Occurs in monochorionic placentas
- Caused by arteriovenous shunting in the placenta from one fetus to the other
- Spectrum of severity ranging from mild chronic shunting to death of both fetuses

Imaging
- One fetus is growth retarded and anemic (donor twin), whereas the other is plethoric and occasionally hydropic (recipient twin)
- Discordant amniotic fluid
- Poor prognostic indicators include hydrops, oligohydramnios with "stuck" twin (twin in oligohydramniotic sac that is stuck against the wall of the endometrial cavity), and early diagnosis (less than 28 weeks)
- Serial, large volume amniocentesis improves the dismal survival rate in stuck twins

Ureteropelvic Junction Obstruction

Clinical
- Most common cause of neonatal hydronephrosis
- Bilateral in 10 to 30%, although usually asymmetric
- Associated with contralateral multicystic dysplastic kidney
- Neonate may appear normal on examination, so prenatal detection is important

Imaging
- Hydronephrosis
- Normal amniotic fluid if contralateral kidney is normal or only mildly affected
- Polyhydramnios is paradoxically seen in 25%

Vein of Galen Aneurysm

Clinical
- Really an arteriovenous malformation with dilatation of the vein of Galen
- Frequently leads to cardiac failure or hydrops

11

- Associated CNS abnormalities
- Treated by embolization postnatally
- High morbidity and mortality

Imaging
- Aneurysmal dilatation of the vein of Galen seen sonographically, located near tentorial hiatus
- Turbulent Doppler flow within the vein
- Features of hydrops may be seen, as well as cardiac enlargement
- Brain infarction from "steal" may develop; leukomalacia may be seen

GYNECOLOGY

Adenomyosis

Clinical
- Defined as the presence of endometrial tissue within the myometrium
- Common; found in about 25% of hysterectomy specimens
- Increased incidence with multiparity
- Varied symptoms, often mimicking leiomyomas

Imaging
- Difficult diagnosis with sonography
- Diffuse uterine enlargement with a normal contour
- Myometrium may appear heterogeneous or normal
- Focal adenomyosis may be difficult to differentiate from leiomyomas
- MRI is the imaging modality of choice

Choriocarcinoma

Clinical
- 1 in 40,000 pregnancies
- 50% are preceded by molar pregnancies, 25% occur after an abortion, 22% after a normal pregnancy, and 3% after an ectopic pregnancy
- Only about 5% of molar pregnancies result in choriocarcinoma
- Widespread metastases, particularly to lung and brain

Imaging
- In a patient with elevated β-hCG, ultrasound is used to detect intrauterine pregnancy
- Ultrasound can also detect liver metastases (typically hyperechoic), which dictate a different chemotherapy protocol
- Theca lutein cysts may be seen in ovaries

Ectopic Pregnancy

Clinical
- 1 in 100 to 1 in 400 pregnancies
- Accounts for 15% of maternal deaths
- Incidence has increased over last few decades, only recently stabilizing
- Risk factors include previous ectopic pregnancy (25% recurrence risk), pelvic inflammatory disease, previous tubal surgery, endometriosis, and ovulation induction
- Classic clinical triad of pain, adnexal mass, and bleeding (complete triad seen only in 45% of patients with ectopic pregnancy)
- Differential diagnosis for positive β-hCG includes IUP, molar pregnancy, recent spontaneous abortion, and ectopic pregnancy
- In 48 hours, should see doubling of the hCG with IUP, decreasing hCG with abortion, subnormal increase with ectopic pregnancy (although may be normal)

Imaging
- Finding IUP makes the diagnosis highly unlikely in naturally conceiving women (risk decreases to 1 in 4,000 to 1 in 8,000)

- With endovaginal sonography, should see evidence of IUP in 20% with hCG less than 1,000 mIU/mL (IRP), 80% with hCG between 1,000 and 2,000 mIU/mL, and 100% with hCG more than 2,000 mIU/mL; thus, if a woman has no sonographic evidence of IUP and her serum β-hCG exceeds 2,000 mIU/mL, ectopic pregnancy is likely
- May see pseudogestational sac, which represents decidual reaction and hypoechoic fluid from bleeding
- May directly visualize living extrauterine gestation
- Adnexa should be scrutinized for the presence of any mass that is not a simple cyst and for the presence of intraperitoneal fluid
- If a cystic mass is identified in the ovary, it is more likely a corpus luteum cyst, because intraovarian ectopic pregnancy is rare

Endometrial Carcinoma

See *Genitourinary Imaging Disease Entities*

Endometrial Hyperplasia

Clinical
- Result of unopposed estrogen
- Most common cause of abnormal uterine bleeding
- Causes include exogenous estrogen, estrogen-producing tumors, polycystic ovarian disease, obesity, and estrogen receptor binders (tamoxifen)
- Categorized histologically as cystic, adenomatous, and atypical adenomatous (risk of progression to endometrial cancer with atypia)

Imaging
- Nonspecific finding of a thickened endometrial stripe
- Can show cystic spaces

Endometrial Polyp

See *Genitourinary Imaging Disease Entities*

Endometriosis

Clinical
- Endometrial tissue in ectopic locations (termed *adenomyosis* when it occurs in the uterus)
- Affects 5 to 15% of women
- May be caused by retrograde menstruation
- Symptoms include pain and dyspareunia
- Common cause of female infertility
- Common sites include pouch of Douglas, ovary, broad ligament, and rectovaginal septum
- May occur as implants, nodules, or endometriomas
- Endometrioma is a cystic structure lined with endometrial endothelium

Imaging
- Sonography can identify endometrioma but cannot visualize endometrial implants; therefore, laparoscopy is the "imaging" modality of choice when endometriosis is suspected
- Endometriomas can have a variety of appearances sonographically; classic appearance consists of a cystic mass with fairly uniform, diffuse low-level echoes
- Barium studies may show submucosal lesions of endometriosis
- Endometriomas appear cystic on CT with rim enhancement

Hydatidiform Mole

Clinical
- Incidence varies around the world; 1 in 2,000 in the United States
- Increased risk toward the end of reproductive years

11

- 20 to 40 times higher risk if patient had prior mole
- Clinical features include abnormal vaginal bleeding, uterus large for dates, pre-eclampsia, hyperemesis gravidorum
- *Classic* mole refers to fertilization of an empty egg by haploid sperm; 80% have benign course, 15% develop invasive mole, 5% develop choriocarcinoma
- *Partial* mole is usually result of polyploidy (often triploidy); generally, no malignant potential
- *Invasive* mole refers to local recurrence after uterine evacuation, with penetration of adjacent vascular structures

Imaging
- *Classic* mole appears sonographically in one of two ways, based on trimester discovered
    First trimester: mass of tissue that looks like placenta fills the endometrial cavity
    Second trimester: villous hypertrophy is evident with numerous small cystic structures scattered throughout an echogenic mass that fills the uterine cavity
- *Partial* mole shows combination of villous hypertrophy and abnormal fetal tissue
- In *invasive* mole, ultrasound may detect villous extension into the myometrium; however, the role of ultrasound is to rule out pregnancy when β-hCG is elevated in a patient with previous mole
- Associated feature is theca lutein cyst, which occurs in 20 to 50% of cases (caused by elevated β-hCG)

Hydrometrocolpos

Clinical
- Enlargement of obstructed uterus and vagina from uterine secretions
- Obstruction may be secondary to imperforate hymen, vaginal membranes, atresia of the vagina or cervix, uterine duplication anomalies, and anorectal malformations

Imaging
- Hypoechoic mass posterior to the bladder that extends into the abdomen
- May compress the urinary tract, causing hydronephrosis or hydroureter

Leiomyoma

Clinical
- Most common neoplasm of uterus
- Occurs in approximately 40% of women over 35 years of age
- Secondary changes include calcification, hemorrhage, fatty degeneration, and necrosis
- Increases in size during pregnancy

Imaging
- Usually hypoechoic with decreased sound-through transmission, although appearance may vary because of secondary changes
- MRI is better at differentiating leiomyoma from adenomyosis

Ovarian Hyperstimulation Syndrome

Clinical
- Occurs as a complication of drugs used in ovulation induction and is the most serious complication of these drugs
- Multiple follicles are induced, and multiple corpus luteum cysts develop after ovulation
- Symptoms occur 5 to 7 days after ovulation
- Divided into mild, moderate, and severe clinically
- With severe hyperstimulation, ovaries are at risk for torsion
- Pleural effusions and ascites may develop from fluid exuded by the ovaries
- May result in death
- If patient does not become pregnant, syndrome generally resolves within 1 week

11

Imaging
- Enlarged ovary
- Multiple, peripheral, thin-walled cysts

Ovarian Torsion

Clinical
- Acute abdominal condition in which ovarian pedicle rotates on its axis, compromising vascular supply and drainage, and eventually infarcting if untreated
- Most patients present with pain, nausea, and vomiting
- Mass may be palpable
- Occasionally, may escape clinical detection, then be discovered as a pelvic calcification
- More generally occurs in childhood or adolescence
- Ovary may be involved with mass or cyst or may be normal
- Unusual for an ovary that is involved by malignancy to undergo torsion because of the adhesive effects of malignancy

Imaging
- Enlarged ovary
- Multiple cortical follicles
- Doppler may demonstrate absent flow, but the presence of flow signal does not exclude torsion

Pelvic Inflammatory Disease (PID)

Clinical
- Most commonly caused by sexually transmitted diseases, especially gonorrhea and chlamydia
- Less common causes include adjacent inflammation, intrauterine device (IUD) with actinomycosis infection, systemic tuberculosis, and recent surgery or abortion
- Patient presents with pain, fever, and vaginal discharge
- Pyosalpinx develops from occlusion of fallopian tube
- Fitz-Hugh-Curtis syndrome refers to pelvic inflammatory disease from gonorrhea with perihepatitis

Imaging
- Endometrial thickening or fluid indicating endometritis
- Echogenic pus in cul-de-sac
- Fluid-filled tubes containing low-level echoes from pus
- Tuboovarian abscess may occur; appears as a multiloculated mass

Polycystic Ovary Disease

Clinical
- Also known as *Stein-Leventhal syndrome*
- Deficient aromatase (needed for conversion of androgen to estrogen) results in excess androgen
- Exaggerated pulsatile follicle-stimulating hormone (FSH) secretion stimulates ovarian androgen production at the expense of estradiol; reduction of local estrogen impairs FSH activity; this results in accumulation of multiple small or medium-sized atretic follicles that cannot mature into graffian follicle
- Occurs late in second decade
- Presents with symptoms of excess androgen: amenorrhea, reduced fertility/sterility, obesity, acne, hirsutism, and baldness
- Can result in endometrial cancer at young age because of unopposed estrogen

Imaging
- Increased ovarian size
- Multiple cysts
- Hypoechoic ovary with irregular contour has been described
- Ultrasound often performed at midcycle to document ovulation in patients treated with clomiphene

11

Nuclear Medicine

- **Stanley J. Goldsmith,** M.D.

- **Barbara Binkert,** M.D.

- **James Hurley,** M.D.

Central nervous system	Skeletal system
Cardiology	Oncology
Pulmonary system	Inflammation
Gastrointestinal system	Genitourinary system
Endocrinology	Basic science

Nuclear medicine as a functional imaging modality differs from the other mainly anatomical divisions of radiology. This chapter reflects the differences. The chapter is divided into ten sections, with the last being a brief review of the basic science of nuclear medicine. The other nine are a mixture of anatomical regions and pathological processes. Each section contains the elements of radiopharmaceuticals, normal distribution of the administered radionuclides, and clinical applications. Thus, the chapter provides a concise overview of many aspects of nuclear medicine in a format that is uniform and easily learned.

CENTRAL NERVOUS SYSTEM

RADIOPHARMACEUTICALS

Regional Cerebral Perfusion (rCBF: Regional Cerebral Blood Flow); SPECT Imaging

Tc-99m hexamethyl-propyleneamineoxime (HMPAO) is lipophilic, crosses the blood-brain barrier, has limited stability, and must be prepared fresh (10–20 minutes prior to use). Stabilized kit containing methylene blue (oxygen scavenger) is now available; 20 mCi; approximately 60% extraction—first pass; inject under basal conditions of sensory-motor activation for diagnostic applications. Image 20 minutes after tracer injection.

Tc-99m ECD is lipophilic, crosses the blood-brain barrier, 20 mCi. In general, more rapidly extracted than Tc-99m HMPAO with less washout. It can be imaged as early as 5–10 minutes after tracer injection.

Intervention test of Diamox (acetazolamide) challenge is 1 gram IV (2 minutes). Diamox is a carbonic anhydrase inhibitor that increases pCO_2 promoting cerebral vasculature dilatation. It increases sensitivity for the detection of cerebral vascular stenoses.

Blood-brain barrier disruption is demonstrated with Tl–201, 3–4 mCi; SPECT imaging.

Vascular anatomy is demonstrated with Tc-99m diethylenetriamine-penta-acetic acid (DTPA), 20 mCi; bolus injection technique, planar imaging technique, anterior projection, and vertex projection.

Cerebrospinal fluid (CSF) flow is demonstrated with In-111 DTPA (special preparation for cisternography and subdural space injection); 0.5 mCi and planar imaging.

NORMAL DISTRIBUTION

Regional Cerebral Perfusion: SPECT Imaging

Transverse sections are most valuable; 3D volume also useful. Activity is taken up proportional to regional blood flow, reflecting underlying neurological activity. Radionuclide uptake is seen in the "cortical stripe" representing an increased flow to the gray matter. Basal ganglia are seen in the midbrain transverse slices. There is considerable variation ($\pm$ 10%) in the blood flow to various portions of the cortical stripe. The pattern is dependent upon sensory-motor activity at the time of injection.

Transverse SPECT slices should be combined to 2–3 pixel thickness since pixel (or voxel) thickness is less than the resolution of the SPECT imaging technique. The cortical stripe should be evaluated and compared with the opposite side. If possible, surface weighted, 3D volume displays should also be examined. In rCBF imaging, the basal ganglia should be identified and compared. The cerebellar activity should be noted. The possibility of head tilt to the left or right side should be considered as this factor will produce asymmetrical patterns. This possibility may be inferred from transverse images, but it is most clear in coronal sections and 3D volume projections.

Radionuclide Angiography

On sequential anterior planar imaging every 1–3 seconds, following bolus injection of a nondiffusable tracer like Tc-99m DTPA (approximately 20 mCi), activity is seen in the carotid arteries bilaterally. The two columns join in the midline at the circle of Willis at the base of the brain. A midline stream of activity, representing the anterior cerebral arteries, is seen next at the same time that flow is seen to the right and left hemispheres—initially representing the corresponding middle cerebral arteries. In order to image the posterior circulation, a vertex view can be obtained with the patient on his/her back and the head tilted back so that the activity in the body does not obscure the cerebral data. Within several seconds, the activity is seen as a "blush." This is called the "watershed phase" and represents the capillary phase of cerebral perfusion. It is followed by the venous phase, which is characterized by the visualization of the superior sagittal sinus—prominent focal activity in the midline at the most cephalad portion of the brain.

Tumor Identification (Differentiation from Abscess)

Tl-201 is excluded from the normal brain. SPECT images (usually transverse slices) demonstrate activity only in the skull, representing the marrow and vascular component. Vascular perfusion of a tumor is seen as an active focus (corresponding to the lesion on CT/MRI), whereas foci due to inflammatory processes, such as toxoplasmosis, do not take up the tracer.

12

Cisternography

In-111 DTPA is injected into the subdural space in the lumbar spine via lumbar puncture. Imaging is performed in the anterior and lateral projections at 4 and 24 hours and at 24-hour intervals thereafter until the study is terminated. Within hours, the tracer moves cephalad. Although normally excluded from the lateral ventricles, some regurgitant activity may be seen briefly at 4 hours, particularly in younger patients. The tracer is identified in the spaces (cisterns) between the brain and the bony structure. The cisterna magnum and lateral cisterns should be seen at 4–6 hours. At 24–48 hours, the activity has moved up over the cerebral hemispheres and pools in this area. Activity persisting in the lateral ventricles is abnormal. There is delay in the usual transit pattern with age.

CLINICAL APPLICATIONS

Regional Cerebral Perfusion SPECT Scintigraphy

1. Cerebral vascular accident (CVA); cortical stroke, subcortical stroke
2. Dementia; multistroke dementia vs. Alzheimer's disease
3. Transient ischemic attack (TIA); perform Diamox challenge
4. Seizure disorder, medical refractory for the location of seizure focus
5. Psychological provocation tests

Thallium Cerebral SPECT

1. Brain tumor (lymphoma) vs. infection/abscess

Tc-99m DTPA Vascular Imaging

1. Brain death
2. Subdural hematoma
3. Carotid occlusion
4. Middle cerebral artery occlusion

Cisternography and CSF Dynamics

1. Normal pressure hydrocephalus
2. Cerebral spinal fluid rhinorrhea/otorrhea
3. Recurrent meningitis
4. Evaluation of ventriculo-peritoneal (VP) shunt

Cerebral Vascular Accident (CVA)

This is the principal indication and the basis for the FDA approval of rCBF imaging. In CVAs involving the cerebral cortex, there is interruption of the cortical stripe, typically involving the gray matter cephalad to the basal ganglia. This finding is accompanied by a decrease in activity in the contralateral cerebellum (crossed cerebellar diaschisis) due to interruption of cortical-cerebellar communication. The rCBF SPECT scan becomes abnormal shortly after the onset of "stroke," prior to changes in the computed tomography (CT) scan or magnetic resonance imaging (MRI). The defect reflects the infarcted area (or area destined to become infarcted) as well as the ischemic penumbra. On later imaging, the defect may be smaller than seen on earlier images. Considerable differences may exist between the size of the area seen on CT or MRI and that of the rCBF. The defects in rCBF images may be greater than those of the CT/MRI because of the penumbra. In small strokes, however, the rCBF may not resolve the defect. Likewise in subcortical strokes affecting the white matter, the cerebral cortex may be intact. The cerebellum, however, demonstrates crossed cerebellar diaschisis. Based on asymmetry in the cerebellar uptake, a subcortical stroke should be suspected in patients with a suitable clinical history and a normal cortical pattern.

Dementia: Multi-infarct vs. Alzheimer's Disease

This is probably the most frequently requested indication for rCBF imaging. Utilization of rCBF imaging to differentiate between multi-infarct dementia and Alzheimer's disease is justified based on approval of these agents for the diagnosis of acute and/or chronic stroke. In multi-infarct dementia, there is a series of defects in the cerebral cortical stripe of activity. By contrast, in Alzheimer's disease, there is classically a bilateral decrease in the parietal or parietal-occipital lobes with so-called frontalization of brain activity. Occasionally, the defect is asymmetric.

Transient Ischemic Attack

Under basal conditions, the images (rCBF SPECT transverse slices) may be normal or may reflect previous cerebral infarcts. However, reimaging after a Diamox challenge (1.0 gram IV, 2–3 minutes prior to injection of the diagnostic tracer Tc-99m HMPAO or Tc-99m ECD) should be performed. In subcritical stenosis of the carotid or cerebral arteries, a defect is seen in the affected area, which may be normal under basal conditions.

Evaluation of Potential Surgical Sacrifice of an Internal Carotid Artery

Patients are injected and imaged before and after balloon occlusion of the artery at risk. If performed on one day, rest imaging is performed first, following a 5–8 mCi injection of tracer. Subsequently, during the trial occlusion, 20 mCi of the tracer is injected.

Seizure Disorders, Medical Refractory

Imaging during the interictal period reveals a small area of decreased uptake in the involved area, usually the temporal lobe in spontaneous onset seizure disorders. If the patient is injected during a seizure episode, a focal area of increased uptake is visualized.

Psychological Provocation Tests

These are investigational only at this time but of great interest in the psychology and psychiatry communities. Patients are injected via an indwelling catheter while they perform psychological tasks, such as the Wisconsin Card Sort Test. Images obtained following this injection are compared with those obtained following injection during a controlled situation.

Brain Death

Radionuclide (Tc-99m DTPA) is excluded from the brain. Sequential planar images demonstrate a remarkably clear image with activity confined to the vascular structures of the skull. If dynamic imaging is performed, no activity is seen in the intracerebral arterial phase.

Normal Pressure Hydrocephalus

A condition in which the normal CSF dynamics are altered. With In-111 DTPA, activity is seen to persist in the lateral ventricles. An intermediate pattern, in which there is some reflux into the ventricles and a slow clearing pattern over the cerebral hemispheres, can be found and probably represents significant cerebral atrophy that will not respond to shunting.

Shunt Evaluation

Only In-111 DTPA prepared for CSF dynamics should be introduced into CSF shunts or pumps. Imaging sequences vary with the clinical indications.

12 CARDIOLOGY

Nuclear cardiology is a term that describes a number of procedures to evaluate the heart. The two most common procedures are (1) myocardial perfusion scintigraphy that evaluates the blood supply to the myocardial tissue and (2) gated blood pool imaging that evaluates the ventricular function and wall motion of the cardiac chambers.

Other procedures performed less frequently are as follows:

1. Infarct-avid imaging in which areas of recent infarction are identified with radiopharmaceutical uptake.
2. First pass scintigraphy as an alternate to gated blood pool imaging or to evaluation of shunts.

3. Receptor imaging in which the adrenergic receptors of the myocardium are imaged.
4. Metabolic imaging to evaluate energy substrate (glucose, fatty acids) utilization.

RADIOPHARMACEUTICALS

Myocardial Perfusion Scintigraphy

	Thallium (Tl)-201	Tc-99m MIBI	Tc-99m Tetrofosmin
Dose	2–4 mCi	20–30 mCi	20–30 mCi
Energy	60–80 keV	140 keV	140 keV
	Hg X-rays	Gamma rays	Gamma rays
Decay	Electron capture	Isomeric transition	Isomeric transition
Half-life	73 hours (3 days)	6 hours	6 hours
Extraction			
Normal	80%	65%	70%
High Flow	Decreased	Decreased	Decreased
Clearance	Relatively fast (Depends on flow)	Slow	Slow

Myocardial perfusion scintigraphy is a technique that produces images of the myocardial tissue (ventricles) following injection of a tracer, which is taken up in proportion to blood flow and tissue perfusion. The images depict tissue perfusion at the time of tracer delivery. Images obtained when the tracer is injected near peak exercise or pharmacological intervention are called *stress images*. Images obtained when the patient receives the tracer under basal conditions are known as *rest images*.

Since Tl-201 washes out of tissue relatively quickly, images reflecting "stress" conditions should be obtained within 10–15 minutes after injection. Images obtained 3–4 hours after injection reflect *redistribution* of the radionuclide under basal conditions. These are termed *redistribution* or *rest* images. Some laboratories inject a second smaller dose (1.0 mCi at rest 20–30 minutes prior to reimaging) after a period of redistribution to enhance ischemia detection.

Tc-99m MIBI rapidly penetrates cell membranes and irreversibly binds to intracellular (mitochondrial) proteins; thus, it does not redistribute. Separate injections are necessary for *stress* and *rest* imaging. A variety of protocols may be used.

1. *Rest* injection *first* (8 mCi); followed by *stress* (25 mCi). This is the most common same day protocol.
2. *Stress* injection (25 mCi); *rest* imaging only is performed after analysis of the *stress* images, if there is a need to compare with the *rest* images. In these cases, the *rest* injection is usually performed 24 hours later.

Dual isotope imaging may also be performed using Tl-201 at rest, allowing an assessment of myocardial viability, followed by stress imaging with a Tc-99m–labeled perfusion compound (MIBI or Tetrofosmin).

Since myocardial perfusion imaging is a noninvasive technique, the procedure is often used to identify patients at risk of having coronary artery disease for appropriate angiography. Alternately, it may be utilized to assess the functional significance of known coronary artery lesions and to follow the effect of therapy or the evolution of these lesions.

The technique is based upon the rapid intracellular transfer of radioactive tracers. Thallium-201 behaves biochemically like potassium, entering the cell via the Na–K ATPase pump. Thallium-201 enters the cell rapidly with an extraction efficiency of approximately 80%. It slowly exchanges with plasma K^+ ions and is taken up again by tissues until it has been completely excreted or has undergone decay. Several Tc-99m–labeled compounds (Tc-99m MIBI, Tc-99m Teboroxime, Tc-99m Tetrofosmin) have become available that are rapidly taken up by viable tissue in proportion to blood flow. These compounds provide radiolabeled alternatives to Tl-201 with the advantages of the physical characteristics of Tc-99m, but do not precisely follow Tl-201 kinetics in their rate of uptake or washout. Nevertheless, images can be obtained as either planar images or SPECT images.

12

Planar images; minimally three views
- Anterior (or RAO)
  - LAO (usually 45 degrees)
  - Left lateral (alternately a 30- and 60-degree LAO are obtained)
- SPECT images
  - Uniform display pattern is recommended by the Society of Nuclear Medicine, American College of Cardiology, and American Society of Nuclear Cardiology.
    - Short axis slices ("O")
    - Horizontal long axis ("Inverted U")
    - Vertical long axis ("Reverse C")

CLINICAL APPLICATIONS

In each pattern, attenuation artifacts must be considered. Most common in women are breast artifact and decreased septal activity. In men diaphragm and abdominal organs and decreased inferior wall activity are most common.

Indication and Type of Myocardial Perfusion Scintigraphy Protocol

Indication	Protocol
Detect coronary artery disease	stress, rest
Determine myocardial viability	rest, rest
Measure area at risk/infarct size	rest
Provide prognostic information	stress, rest
Revascularization vs. medical therapy	stress, rest

Stress Protocols

In stress protocols, exercise is the most commonly used or standard technique. Treadmill exercise involves the upright walking on a treadmill; the standard is the modified Bruce Protocol in which pace and inclination increase every 2–3 minutes. Patient's heart rate, blood pressure, and ECG are monitored throughout the test. The goal is 85% of predicted age determined maximum heart rate (i.e., 220 − age = beats per minute). As this rate is approached, administer tracer through previously established IV line. The patient continues walking even if it is necessary to slow the treadmill rate somewhat. The procedure is terminated based on the patient's fatigue, dyspnea, symptoms of chest pain, arrhythmia, or ischemic changes on ECG. Tracer is usually administered prior to terminating exercise regardless of rate achieved to determine perfusion pattern when procedure is symptom- or stress-limited. Other forms of exercise include the bicycle and hand grips. The forms of exercise demonstrate many defects, but are less stressful (usually lower, double product = product of heart rate (HR) × systolic blood pressure (BP), also known as rate-pressure product).

Limitations of Exercise Imaging

1. Sensitivity decreases with suboptimal exercise.
2. Beta-adrenergic drugs interfere with achieving rate-pressure product.
3. Orthopedic and/or neurological problems interfere with treadmill use.

Pharmacological "stress" tests, with adenosine or dipyridamole, produce pharmacological vasodilatation of coronary arteries resulting in increased myocardial perfusion. This effect provides contrast with areas of coronary stenosis, which do not respond in an equivalent fashion. Imaging defects indicate areas of "limited coronary reserve."

Agents used are dipyridamole (Persantine) IV infusion of 0.15 mL/kg/min for 4 minutes and adenosine 0.14 gm/kg/min for 6 minutes. Adverse reactions are rare; occasional A-V conduction defects, heart block, and bronchoconstriction are noted. Undesirable effects, such as headache, breathlessness, chest fullness, epigastric discomfort, nausea and/or flushing, dissipate rapidly when the adenosine infusion is stopped (effective half-life is 15 sec). Dipyridamole effective half-life is longer and may require treatment with aminophylline IV.

12

Comparison of Dipyridamole and Adenosine

	Dipyridamole	Adenosine
Mechanism	Blocks adenosine uptake	Direct blood vessel dilatation
Blood flow	Increases $\times$ 3 (15% may not obtain maximal vasodilatation)	Increases $\times$ 4–5
Duration	15–30 seconds	2 seconds
Side effects	Sometimes	Almost always (80%)

Pharmacological stress tests with the β-antagonist dobutamine produces an increase in the chronotropy and inotropy (rate and force of myocardial muscle contraction), as well as in the vasodilatation of the peripheral, and to a lesser extent, coronary arteries, producing an increase in heart rate and contractile function. Dobutamine is infused initially at 5 mcg/kg/min for 3 minutes, increasing by 5–10 mcg/kg/min every 3 minutes, attempting to achieve 85% of the maximum predicted heart rate. The maximum infusion rate is 40 mcg/kg/min. Adverse reactions are palpitations, shortness of breath, headache, atrial ectopy or fibrillation, ventricular ectopy, or nonsustained ventricular tachycardia.

Comparison of "Stress Protocol" Effect on Coronary Blood Flow

	Ischemia	NI	Difference
Exercise	$\times$ 2	$\times$ 5	60%
Pharmaceutical			
Dobutamine	?	$\times$ 2	?
Dipyridamole	$\times$ 2	$\times$ 3	33%
Adenosine	$\times$ 2	$\times$ 5	60%

Interpretation

Images are examined for the degree and uniformity of tracer uptake. Uptake may be graded as normal, mild, moderate, severe, or completely absent. A 0 to 4 grading system is used for semiquantitative assessment: normal (4+) or completely absent (0) with degrees of partial uptake between these two extremes. Quantitative profiles provide a more objective measure. Tracer uptake reflects myocardial perfusion that usually indicates coronary blood flow under the physiological conditions at the time of tracer administration. Images obtained following tracer administration during stress reflect the coronary artery reserve, the ability of the coronary circulation to increase blood flow in response to physiological demand (myocardial oxygen consumption), or the pharmacological effect. If an area of decreased perfusion is seen, the segment involved should be identified.

Rest images indicate perfusion at rest; defects indicate infarction or chronic ischemia (so-called hibernating myocardium). Attenuation artifacts from breast tissue must also be considered. Differential diagnosis depends upon the demonstration of viability in a chronically ischemic myocardium by Tl-201 uptake or by greater uniformity of the perfusion pattern as late as 24 hours after injection following exercise, a separate rest injection, or following nitroglycerin. (See PET Imaging.)

Myocardial areas that are normal under stress conditions and develop "defects" on delayed imaging indicate rapid washout of tracer or reverse redistribution. This finding may be seen in healthy patients as well as in those with mild disease or cardiomyopathy.

	Pattern	Interpretation
Stress	*Rest*	
Normal	Normal	Normal myocardial perfusion scintigraphy; very low likelihood of coronary artery disease
Defect	Normal	Abnormal myocardial perfusion scintigraphy; mild, moderate, severe ischemia involving the (name of segment)

12

	Pattern		Interpretation
Stress	*Rest*		
Defect	Defect		Abnormal myocardial perfusion scintigraphy compatible with myocardial infarction involving the (name of segment) or chronic ischemia

Gated Blood Pool Imaging

Red blood cells (RBCs) labeled with Tc-99m are preferred over labeled albumin because the latter diffuses into the extracellular fluid and provides poorer contrast. RBC labeling with Tc-99m is based on stannous ion (Sn^{+2}) diffusing into the RBC and chelating Tc with the -globin portion of the hemoglobin molecule.

There are three methods to label RBCs as follows:

In vivo. "Cold" pyrophosphate or medronate methylene diphosphonate (MDP) in saline is injected IV. After 10–20 minutes, 10–30 mCi Tc-99m pertechnetate is injected.

Advantage: This is the *simplest* method and good-to-excellent labeling is frequently achieved. No blood is removed.

Disadvantage: If the Sn^{+2} dose is unsatisfactory or the Tc-99m/Tc-99 ratio is not high enough, pertechnetate is seen in the thyroid and gastric mucosae. Gastric activity interferes with the quantity of LV function.

In vivtro. "Cold" pyrophosphate or MDP in saline is injected IV. After 10–20 minutes, a 10–20-mL aliquot of blood is withdrawn into a syringe containing Tc-99m pertechnetate and an anticoagulant (acid-citrate-dextrose). Heparin should not be used as the anticoagulant because it may label. The Tc-99m and whole blood aliquot incubate, with occasional inversion, for 10–20 minutes. The labeled aliquot is reinjected.

Advantage: More opportunity for Tc-99m to label the RBCs before reinjection into the circulation; some but minimal blood handling.

Disadvantages: Two to 3 injections are needed unless a line is kept open. Blood handling is involved. Potential unbound Tc-99m is injected.

In vitro: A 10–20-mL aliquot of blood is withdrawn into a tube containing Sn^{+2} ion. After incubation, 10–30 mCi (or more) Tc-99m is added, inverted, and incubated. After 10–30 minutes, the tube is gently centrifuged, the supernatant is removed, and the cells are resuspended in saline. These steps are repeated two or three times or until Tc-99m no longer appears in the supernatant.

Advantages: Best label, only labeled RBCs are injected and least free pertechnetate.

Disadvantages: Increased blood aliquot handling; more time, labor, and expense; sample removed from patient and transported to laboratory; potential for misadministration.

Gated blood pool imaging provides cine imaging of the cardiac chambers and great vessels and is useful to assess regional wall motion and overall left ventricular function. Images are typically obtained in one or more planar projections although it is possible to perform SPECT imaging. The two most common views are the *anterior projection,* which provides the best view of the anterior wall motion, and the LAO (45 degrees) projection, which distinguishes the right ventricle blood pool from the left ventricle blood pool. The LAO view is best for selection of a region of interest (ROI) necessary for determination of the left ventricular ejection fraction (LVEF). The inferior wall is best seen in a left lateral or left posterior oblique projection.

A second ROI is needed for background correction. Currently, many software programs automatically select an area. The nuclear medicine physician should evalu-

12

ate images for excess activity in the lung or gastric region that might result in a background that is too high, causing artefactual lowering of the LVEF.

Time-activity curves provide additional measures of ventricular function, such as LV systolic emptying time and rate and diastolic filling times. LVEF measurements from gated blood pool imaging are reproducible within 5%.

Images should be evaluated qualitatively for the degree of wall motion of the major segments, ventricular chamber size, myocardial wall thickness, and coordinated contractility. Anterior, lateral, and posterior wall exhibit more dynamic motion than the septum and inferior wall. Septal thickening and movement toward the left ventricle are observed during systole in the LAO projection. Following coronary artery by-pass surgery, paradoxical septal wall motion is seen. Wall motion is reported as normal or variable degrees of decreased motion, mild or moderate hypokinesis, no wall motion, akinesis, paradoxical motion, or dyskinesis (i.e., sign of ventricular aneurysm or pseudoaneurysm).

Gated blood pool imaging is performed at rest. Stress imaging can be obtained most commonly with a bicycle ergometer with the patient in the supine position. LVEF normally increases greater than 5% with exercise.

Decreases in LVEF as well as single or multiple segmental decreases in qualitative wall motion are seen in coronary artery disease. Decreased LVEF and LV enlargement are early findings in LV decompensation in patients with aortic or mitral valve disease. Decreased LVEF and global hypokinesis are seen in cardiomyopathy, either idiopathic or secondary to hypertension, cardiotoxic chemotherapy, or other metabolic abnormalities.

First Pass Scintigraphy

Ventricular function and imaging can also be obtained during first-pass recording of a 20–30 mCi Tc-99m (pertechnetate, DTPA, or other tracer) bolus, passing through the cardiac chambers. On cine review, a left ventricle ROI is identified. The subsequent time-activity curve allows identification of beat-to-beat LV function during passage of the bolus. These frames can be "summed" and images viewed to evaluate LV wall motion.

Infarct-Avid Imaging

Infarct-avid imaging is infrequently performed in the United States. It is based upon the uptake of a radiolabeled tracer by infarcted myocardium. Tc-99m pyrophosphate binds to calcium exposed or released from the actin-myosin complex during severe (irreversible) ischemic injury. Tc-99m pyrophosphate accumulates readily in recent infarcts (>12 hour old), and the uptake gradually diminishes with time so that most patients have negative images after 4 weeks. Occasionally, positive images are seen many years later. Late positive images are seen with calcified ventricular aneurysms. In-111–labeled antimyosin antibody is also available to obtain images of infarcts. This antibody is more specific for recent injury since it recognizes the exposed myosin.

PET Imaging

PET imaging is based upon the use of radiopharmaceuticals that decay by positron emission.

Tracer	Application
N-13 NH$_3$	Myocardial perfusion
Rb-82	Myocardial perfusion
F-18 FDG	Glucose metabolism

Ischemic myocardium preferentially metabolizes glucose (traced by F-18 FDG) instead of the high energy substrate—free fatty acids—the usual energy source for well-perfused myocardium with adequate oxygen.

PET Perfusion/Metabolism Patterns

Perfusion Image	F-18 FDG Image	Clinical Significance
Normal	Uniform; uptake depends on plasma glucose	Normal myocardium
Perfusion defect	No FDG accumulation in hypoperfused area	Infarcted, fibrotic myocardium
Perfusion defect	Relative increased FDG accumulation in hypoperfused area	Ischemic myocardium

Receptor Imaging

I-123 MIBG provides images of the myocardial distribution of adrenergic nerve endings that normally are abundant and uniform. These nerve endings are very sensitive to ischemic injury. The technique is also of interest in evaluating certain congenital arrhythmias. It is not a routine clinical procedure, however.

PULMONARY SYSTEM

Ventilation:perfusion scintigraphy is a useful, noninvasive screening test for pulmonary embolism (PE). The classic appearance of PE is a ventilation: perfusion mismatch in which perfusion defects are present that conform to segmental anatomy and correspond to areas of normal ventilation without chest radiograph opacities or cystic air spaces.

RADIOPHARMACEUTICALS

To evaluate the perfusion pattern of the lungs, 200,000 to 400,000 particles (upper limit of 1 million) of macroaggregated albumin (MAA), with a range of particle size from 10 to 90 microns, radiolabeled with 3.0–5.0 mCi of Tc-99m (4+ or 5+ valance), are administered intravenously. These particles temporarily occlude about 0.1% of the precapillary arterioles in the normal lung. They break down with a half-life of 4–6 hours, followed by renal clearance. Patients are injected while in the supine position to more equally distribute the particles throughout the lungs. Some differential perfusion, however, is still present in the supine position with activity diminishing from posterior to anterior, secondary to the posterior dependent lung being the more perfused.

Tc-99m-MAA is prepared by reconstitution with normal saline and addition of Tc-99m-pertechnetate followed by silica gel–thin layer chromotography (SG–TLC) (>90% purity). The vial contained within a lead pig is refrigerated and removed for dose preparation until the expiration time (6 hours). Prior to injection, each Tc-99m-MAA syringe within its lead shield should be gently agitated to prevent clumping of aggregates. In addition, if blood is in contact with Tc-99m-MAA during an attempted injection, a new dose, syringe, and needle should be obtained as blood mixed with macroaggregated albumin for even a short period of time promotes clumping or aggregation of particles. Injected, these aggregates produce the characteristic pattern of well-defined focal areas of intense increased uptake distributed in a random, typically peripheral pattern in both lung fields. As segmental perfusion defects may be seen distal to these aggregates, repeat perfusion imaging may be required. While the Tc-99m-MAA is injected, the patient is instructed to take several deep breaths to ensure a more homogeneous distribution of radiopharmaceutical. (Microspheres, which are particles more uniform in size than macroaggregated albumin, are no longer manufactured.)

Perfusion lung imaging is a safe test and rarely causes an allergic reaction (typically hives), which can be treated with diphenhydramine (Benadryl). With neonates and with patients with severe pulmonary hypertension and right-to-left shunts, it is not a contraindication to obtain perfusion lung imaging, but it is prudent to be conservative in terms of the number of particles injected (i.e., 200,000). Statistically, a certain number of particles are necessary in order to obtain good count statistics and good scan quality.

Less than 60,000 particles may produce inhomogeneous distribution of MAA, and less than 15,000 may produce a pattern of segmental defects. Breakdown of MAA occurs with a half-life of 4–6 hours after which clearance is seen in the kidneys. When a vial of MAA is initially prepared, the specific activity is high. As time passes, a larger volume and, therefore, more particles will have to be injected to achieve an equivalent dose.

Dosimetry for a perfusion dose of 3.0 mCi is 3.5 rads to the lungs, which for perfusion imaging are both the critical and the target organ.

To improve specificity, the ventilation pattern of the lungs is typically assessed and compared with the perfusion pattern to determine whether they are the same (matched) or mismatched. Four FDA-approved agents are available: Xenon-133,

Xenon-127, aerosolized Tc-99m-DTPA, and Krypton-81m—all of which have advantages and disadvantages. Experimental agents currently include Technegas and Pertechnegas.

Xenon-133 imaging has three phases. Initially, via a closed system, the patient takes a deep breath of Xenon-133 and holds his/her breath for the initial single breath image that is acquired for 30 seconds. The distribution of this single breath ventilation image shows regional distribution similar to those of the Krypton-81m and aerosolized Tc-99m-DTPA ventilation images. The second phase is the equilibrium phase during which the patient breathes Xenon-133 for approximately 4–5 minutes in a closed system to fill the ventilatory volume of the lung. An extended breathing period is necessary in patients with airway diseases to fill the entire ventilatory volume via the pores of Kohn and the canals of Lambert. This step defines "air trapping" during the washout or third phase when the patient breathes oxygen only. A normal Xenon-133 scan shows homogeneous distribution during the single breath phase. The single breath image is obtained in the posterior projection with a second image possible if the patient maximally exhales and re-inhales pure Xenon. Xenon-133 imaging should occur prior to perfusion imaging, as the gamma emission of Xenon-133 (81 keV) is lower than that of Tc-99m (140 keV), which can cause downscatter and degradation of the xenon images. The advantages of Xenon-133 are that it is inexpensive and able to show areas of air trapping during the washout phase.

NORMAL DISTRIBUTION

For evaluation of a lung scan, the perfusion pattern of both lungs should be carefully assessed. It is important to determine whether perfusion is normal, homogeneous in distribution, or abnormal. If abnormal, is there inhomogeneity or are there discrete defects and, if so, do the defects conform to segmental anatomy or are they nonsegmental or regional? If the VQ scan is abnormal, a frontal and lateral chest radiograph should be obtained as close as possible in time to the VQ scan.

CLINICAL APPLICATIONS

The interpretation of the VQ lung scan is based upon well-recognized criteria obtained more recently, confirmed, and/or modified with data from the prospective investigation of pulmonary embolism diagnosis (PIOPED) study. The scan pattern should be assessed as to whether it meets the criteria for high or low probability for PE. All others belong in the indeterminate/non-diagnostic/intermediate probability for PE for which further testing should be obtained whether it be a Doppler study for deep vein thrombosis (DVT), a helical CT for PE, or an MRA. The minimum criterion for high probability for PE is two segmental or subsegmental equivalents that are mismatched and are not in the region of any opacities on the chest radiograph. In the PIOPED study, all patients with two segmental mismatches or subsegmental equivalents had PE, whereas only 79% of those with two mismatches had PE. The more mismatches, the higher the essential probability. A normal perfusion lung scan excludes the possibility of PE. The criteria for a low probability scan are inhomogeneous perfusion, small matched or mismatched defects, matched segmental or subsegmental defects without opacities on the chest radiographs, and nonsegmental matched defects. The incidence of PE with a low probability scan is about 10%. All others are in the indeterminate category, including single segmental or subsegmental mismatched defects without an opacity on chest radiographs. In the PIOPED study, 33% of patients with a single subsegmental mismatched defect had PE.

A segmental defect, according to Biello's original criteria, is more than 75% of an anatomical segment; a subsegment is 25–75% of a segment; and a smaller defect (<25% of a segment) is not recognized as an anatomical defect.

Pulmonary embolism is a difficult clinical diagnosis to make. Algorithms for the workup of patients for PE are continually changing. VQ imaging remains a good noninvasive, well-tried initial screen for PE, especially in cases of low clinical suspicion for PE and no clinical evidence for DVT.

GASTROINTESTINAL SYSTEM

The scintigraphy evaluation of gastrointestinal (GI) hemorrhage with either Tc-99m–sulfur colloid or Tc-99m-pertechnetate–labeled RBCs provides a useful, noninvasive method for the accurate localization of an active bleeding site. The classic appearance of an active bleeding site in the GI tract is a focus of activity representing extravasation of blood into the bowel lumen, which becomes visible during image acquisition and increases in intensity. It then moves with time in an antegrade and/or a retrograde fashion in bowel. Accurate assessment of the site of an active bleed helps to focus the medical management and the surgical approach.

RADIOPHARMACEUTICALS

Two methods are currently utilized for detection of bleeding site, one using RBCs radiolabeled with Tc-99m-pertechnetate and the other using Tc-99m–sulfur colloid. Although not as widely utilized, the advantage of Tc-99m–sulfur colloid (0.1–1.0 microns in size) is that, after IV administration, it is rapidly cleared from the intravascular space by the reticuloendothelial system with a half-life of 2–3 minutes, allowing adequate visualization of an abdominal bleeding site without interference from background activity. If the patient is not actively bleeding at the time of Tc-99m–sulfur colloid administration and bleeding recurs, even within several hours after the initial scan, a second dose of Tc-99m–sulfur colloid can be administered followed by additional imaging, because no interfering background activity is present in the mid and lower abdomen.

The disadvantage of Tc-99m–sulfur colloid is the difficulty in evaluating the upper abdomen for an upper GI bleed because of scatter from radiopharmaceutical in the liver and spleen. In addition, as clearance from the intravascular space is so fast, limiting the time radiopharmaceutical is available to extravasate at a bleeding site, the patient must be actively bleeding at the time of Tc-99m–sulfur colloid administration for a site to be accurately localized. This method, therefore, may be useful for late night emergency evaluation of a bleeding site which, if negative, may be repeated the following day with Tc-99m–RBCs.

The advantages of Tc-99m–RBC imaging, currently the method of choice, are that acquisitions with adequate count statistics can be obtained continually up to 24 hours—limited only by the decay characteristics of Tc-99m. With frequent imaging, therefore, the site can be localized if bleeding occurs any time over this 24-hour period, particularly for the evaluation of intermittent bleeding. This method can help to adequately evaluate the presence of an active bleeding site in the upper as well as the lower GI tract.

The major disadvantage of the Tc-99m–RBC study is that, although it has the potential of identifying a bleeding site over an extended period, the patient must be actively bleeding during the time of actual imaging to accurately localize the site. If bleeding occurs when the patient is not being imaged, radiolabeled RBCs will be present in the GI tract on delayed images, but the actual site of bleeding cannot be identified. A minor disadvantage is the presence of minimal background activity.

Compared with angiography, the Tc-99m–RBC study can detect a bleeding site with a slower rate of bleed (0.1–0.3 mL/minute) than can angiography (0.5–1.0 mL/minute), and it can be repeated at frequent intervals, limited only by the decay characteristics of Tc-99m-pertechnetate (half life = 6 hours). The low absorbed radiation dose from this study allows safe repetition at frequent intervals. In addition, as contrast material is not administered, renal compromise and adverse reactions are not anticipated.

Dosimetry for all organs and the whole body for both radiopharmaceuticals is available in the package inserts. The target organ and the critical organ for Tc-99m–sulfur colloid are the same—the liver, which receives a dose of 3.4–3.6 rads/10 mCi. For a 20-mCi dose of Tc-99m-pertechnetate, labeled to RBCs, the target organ is the heart wall, which receives a dose of 2.2 rads. The critical organs are blood, spleen, and bladder wall with doses of 2 rads.

Preparation of Radiopharmaceuticals

Red blood cell labeling can be done using the in vivo, in vivtro, or in vitro methods. In all methods, a reducing agent, 10 µg/kg of stannous ion (stannous pyrophosphate), is administered IV by direct venous access because this ion tends to adhere to the surface of plastic tubing. Stannous ion is injected IV in both the in vivo and in vivtro methods. In the in vitro method, it is mixed with the removed blood. In all methods, a waiting period of 20 minutes takes place, after which the RBCs are mixed with 20 mCi of Tc-99m-pertechnetate by either IV injection (in vivo) or mixing with withdrawn blood (in vivtro or in vitro).

The labeling (tagging) efficiency is variable for in vivo labeling (60–90%), very good for in vivtro (90–95%), and optimal for in vitro (95–100%) with use of the Brookhaven kit. With the in vivo method, many factors may modify tagging efficiency.

NORMAL DISTRIBUTION

It is essential to know the normal distribution of radiolabeled RBCs as well as the potential causes of false-positive and false-negative or inaccurate findings for the most accurate interpretation of bleeding studies. The normal whole body distribution of radiolabeled RBCs includes visualization of activity in the heart, liver, spleen, aorta, vena cava, and other vascular structures including collateral vessels, kidneys, bladder, and male genitalia. It is imperative, when evaluating the pelvic region, therefore, to obtain a lateral view of the pelvis. On a lateral view, the anterior position of male genitalia, the posterior position of a bleeding site in the rectum, and the position of the bladder can be appreciated.

CLINICAL APPLICATIONS

For Tc-99m–sulfur colloid studies, images are obtained in the dynamic mode, at 1 minute per frame for 30 minutes, or as static acquisitions, every 5 minutes for 30 minutes. Formatting must include images of high intensity so that the bony structures of the pelvis are seen in order to adequately localize a bleeding site. Normal distribution of sulfur colloid is to the reticuloendothelial system, liver, spleen, and bone marrow.

Imaging should begin immediately after the readministration of radiolabeled RBCs with anterior static imaging, every 5 minutes, or dynamic imaging, at 1 minute per frame for 1 hour, followed by dynamic and/or static images, every 5 minutes or every 15 minutes, until active bleeding occurs. At this time, dynamic or static imaging at more frequent intervals should begin again.

It is important, when an active bleeding site is identified, that the imaging continues until the interpreter is able to accurately localize the finding to the small bowel or colon. An active bleeding site that can be localized accurately appears while the patient is being imaged. It is initially a discrete focus of increased activity that moves on sequential images in an antegrade and/or retrograde fashion. When active bleeding occurs, the bowel is irritable and often responds with increased motility and peristalsis. The extravasated radiolabeled RBCs, therefore, tend to move rapidly throughout the bowel. It is imperative that patients be imaged at frequent intervals in order to accurately identify the site of active bleeding.

Inaccurate localization of a site may occur if a significant time has elapsed between images, so much so that bleeding has occurred when the patient is not being imaged. Radiolabeled RBCs are then seen on subsequent images throughout the bowel and the bleeding site cannot be accurately determined.

For accurate interpretation of bleeding scans, it is important that a reliable patient history be obtained to include recent and prior surgical interventions, particularly with regard to resection of bowel, polypectomy, anastomotic sites, or previous arteriovenous malformation (AVM). To aid in the localization of a bleeding site, it may be helpful to correlate scintigraphic images with abdominal radiographs or recent barium study findings to confirm bowel patterns.

Patterns that are variants of the normal biodistribution include the appearance of a linear pattern of gastric activity along the borders of the stomach, which can be from free pertechnetate or from hemorrhagic and nonhemorrhagic gastritis. Typically, if an upper GI bleed is suspected, endoscopic evaluation and assessment of the gastric aspirate adequately determines whether the source is related to gastric or duodenal pathology. If free pertechnetate is present, activity is usually present in the thyroid gland, which is visualized with an image of the anterior neck region.

Occasionally, more than 12 hours after RBCs have been tagged and readministered, activity appears in the gallbladder. Although hemobilia can occur secondary to hepatic artery pseudoaneurysm, it is rare. The delayed appearance of activity in the gallbladder has been associated with chronic renal failure and/or multiple transfusions. The mechanism for biliary excretion has been postulated to be the breakdown of blood products into heme and globin and the appearance of heme—a precursor of bilirubin in the biliary system. Other potential causes for false-positive results in radiolabeled RBC studies include renal activity, bladder activity, collaterals, and vascular tumors.

For Tc-99m–sulfur colloid studies, false-positive results may be secondary to activity in renal transplant or splenosis. In addition, if marrow replacement (e.g., secondary to radiation therapy, tumor, and fibrosis) has occurred in the bony structures of a hemipelvis, activity in the opposite hemipelvis may mimic a focus of activity and a bleeding site.

Several studies have determined the sensitivity and specificity for the two tests. In one study, each of 100 patients had a Tc-99m–sulfur colloid scan with imaging for 20 minutes followed by a Tc-99m–RBC scan. The sensitivity for the Tc-99m–RBC study was 93% and the specificity was 95%.

Scintigraphic methods and Tc-99m–RBC studies that detect and localize an active bleeding site in the GI tract are noninvasive and safe and yield high sensitivities with specificities and low radiation doses, when bleeding occurs during the imaging process.

ENDOCRINOLOGY

THYROID

Radiopharmaceuticals

Since the thyroid concentrates iodine, radioactive iodine is used as a tracer to measure function and to image the gland, as well as to ablate remnants of normal thyroid tissue and to treat hyperthyroidism and thyroid carcinoma.

Tc-99m, as the pertechnetate ion, mimics the size and ionic charge of the iodide ion. Consequently, it can be used also to image the thyroid gland.

	Iodine-131	Iodine-123	Tc-99m
Mode of decay	Beta minus	Electron capture	Isomeric transition
Physical half-life	8.1 days	13.2 hours	6 hours
Photon energy	364 keV	159 keV	140 keV
Abundance	81%	83.4%	89%
Time after administration to image	24 hour	4–6 hour and/or 24 hour	20 minutes

A significant radiation dose is delivered to the thyroid with Iodine-131. Consequently, although convenient and inexpensive, other radionuclides, most commonly Tc-99m-pertechnetate, are selected for diagnostic imaging purposes of the thyroid gland. I-131 images thyroid carcinoma metastases since delayed visualization is usually necessary to achieve satisfactory contrast between the lesions and background.

Organ IV	Dosimetry (for Typical Adult Imaging Dose)		
	Iodine-131 (rads/100 uCi PO)	Iodine-123 (rads/400 uCi PO)	Tc-99m-pertechnetate (rads/5 mCi IV)
Thyroid (15% uptake)	78	7.7	0.65
Bladder wall	0.27	0.16	0.425
Stomach	0.15	0.089	0.25
Intestine	0.11 (small)	0.065 (small)	0.55 (large)
Red marrow	0.021	0.012	0.10
Testes	0.018	0.007	0.05
Ovaries	0.012	0.017	0.15
Total body	0.047	0.014	0.05

12

Clinical Procedures

A 24-hour thyroidal iodine uptake, normal range, depends upon dietary iodine content. Uptake is inversely proportional to dietary iodine content, and decreases with high dietary iodine (e.g., kelp, dietary supplements).

Thyroid Function
- "Normal": 10–25%
- Hyperthyroid: 25–95%
- Subacute thyroiditis: 0–5%
- Nonthyroidal causes

Increased Uptake
- Iodine deficiency
- Pregnancy
- Rebound after thyroid suppressive drugs (antithyroid drugs, thyroid hormone)
- Following subacute thyroiditis
- Choriocarcinoma, hydatidiform mole (ectopic TSH–like activity)

Decreased Uptake
- Thyroid hormone treatment
- Expanded iodine pool

Excessive Iodine Intake
- Medications
- Mineral supplements
- Dietary supplements
- High iodine foods (shellfish, kelp, seafood, red food dyes as in herbal teas, prepared sauces, Chinese food)
- Iodinated contrast material

Decreased Iodine Excretion
- Renal failure

Imaging

Thyroid Gland
- Pinhole collimator
  - Energy independent (use with all three radionuclides)
  - Magnifies thyroid gland
  - Good resolution
  - Permits oblique views (LAO, RAO, and anterior)
  - Concern about pinhole distortion, parallax distortion
  - Difficult to "mark" nodules
- Parallel hole collimator (use electronic zoom)
  - Collimator chosen depends on gamma energy
  - Image Tc-99m-pertechnetate at 20 minutes after injection; thereafter, radionuclide washes out (not bound).
  - Image Iodine-131 at 24 hours
  - Image Iodine-123 at 3–4 hours or at 24 hours (combine with 24-hour uptake)

Whole Body
- Iodine-131, 2–5 mCi oral dose
- High energy collimator
- ROI views for 10 minutes/view or
- Whole body imaging
- Optimal imaging: 72 hours (3 days)
- Detection may improve further with more delay.
- If dosimetry is performed, it may image at 24, 48, 72, or more hours.
- Concern at high tracer dose
  - "Star" artifact due to septal penetration.

Clinical Applications

Euthyroid Patient

Evaluate Function of Palpable Nodule.

Cold Nodule (Decreased to Absent Function or Activity). About 20–35% of solitary cold nodules are malignant, most commonly well-differentiated thyroid carcinoma: papillary carcinoma, mixed papillary-follicular, or follicular carcinoma. Cold nodules should be biopsied or removed. A cold nodule may coexist with other conditions but a multinodular goiter may contain areas of decreased function, which are usually not malignant. Most frequently, these are an expression of a chronic thyroid dysfunction, such as Hashimoto's thyroiditis—a chronic low-grade inflammatory process, usually without acute symptoms. Symptoms develop related to decreased thyroid function or to thyroid enlargement as the thyroid-stimulating hormone (TSH) rises to stimulate compensatory thyroid activity. The patient may be euthyroid or hypothyroid.

Other Causes. Other causes of a cold nodule are thyroid cyst, nonfunctioning or hypofunctioning adenoma, focal Hashimoto's thyroiditis, hemorrhage (usually painful with rapid onset), nonthyroid malignancies (rare), and granuloma.

Uniform or Normal Activity. This is usually benign and most commonly a functioning adenoma. It may be treated with thyroid hormone to suppress TSH. Reevaluate and/or perform surgical removal if the size continues to increase. Adenomas may be "autonomous," i.e., nonsuppressible. In patients who have had subtotal thyroidectomies, the remainder of the thyroid gland enlarges. It may become palpable or visible if the patient has not received thyroid hormone supplements.

Increased Activity or "Hot" Nodule. This is usually a functioning adenoma; if the remainder of the gland is absent or decreased in activity, the nodule is likely suppressing endogenous TSH. The patient may be euthyroid or hyperthyroid (thyrotoxic). In this circumstance, the nodule is called a "toxic" nodule.

Multinodular Thyroid. Multiple areas of increased and decreased activity are seen in multinodular goiter and Hashimoto's thyroiditis. Both conditions may be associated with normal, increased, or decreased thyroid function. Functional diagnosis is based upon clinical and laboratory assessment. Imaging evaluates thyroid functional anatomy; characterizes palpable findings; provides a baseline to monitor clinical management; evaluates size; and identifies areas for biopsy, surgical removal, or observation.

Patient With A Goiter (An Enlarged Thyroid). Evaluate the pattern of thyroid gland function (functional anatomy). A scan may reveal focal areas of altered function—palpable or nonpalpable. Subsequent management is similar to that for the thyroid gland with palpable nodules. Evaluate size as an index (baseline) for future management.

Hyperthyroid Patient

Confirms clinical impression of enlargement or diffuse activity or establishes whether clinical and laboratory findings of increased function are of thyroid origin (usual) or not (rare). Nonthyroidal causes of clinical hyperthyroidism include overmedication (may be surreptitious, Münchausen syndrome) and ectopic thyroid (rare). Hyperthyroidism is most commonly due to Graves' disease (diffuse gland activity), toxic multinodular goiter (may be Graves' superimposed on a multinodular thyroid gland or an independent disease), or toxic nodule (remainder of the thyroid gland is suppressed). Rarely, thyrotoxicosis may be due to Graves' disease in a congenital or postsurgical remnant. Scans are also useful in hyperthyroid patients to assist in assessment of thyroid size in selecting radioactive iodine (I-131) therapy doses.

Other Applications of Thyroid Scans

Palpable masses in the neck region may be ectopic thyroid or metastatic thyroid carcinoma. In the presence of the intact thyroid gland, carcinoma of the thyroid usually appears as an area of decreased function. Occasionally, metastases take up radioactive iodine even in the presence of the normal thyroid.

A mass at the base of the tongue, so-called lingual thyroid, is most commonly identified in the neonatal period in association with neonatal hypothyroidism. Routine screening of thyroid function is performed on cord blood. It does not require surgical removal and responds (decrease in size) to suppression with thyroid hormone replacement therapy.

Follow-up thyroid cancer requires that Iodine-131 should be used in increased doses

(1.0–5.0 mCi) following discontinuation of thyroid replacement until the patient is clinically hypothyroid. Plasma TSH assay is greater than 35 ulU/mL. Delayed imaging is required (48–72 hours or longer). Whole body scans to identify functioning metastases are obtained with a high energy (364 keV) collimator.

Radioiodine Therapy with Iodine-131. Hyperthyroidism: fixed dose may vary with rough estimate of size. Dose is based upon mCi retained per gram. It requires 24-hour uptake and size (weight) estimate. Dosimetry to deliver predetermined rad dose (7000–14,000) is needed.

Dose for hyperthyroidism determined and based upon
  Clinical goal (control, ablation)
  Gland weight
  Percent uptake
  Turnover rate (half-life effective)
Thyroid cancer
  Ablate remnant
    29 mCi (maximal outpatient dose)
    75 mCi (requires hospital admission in United States until retained dose <30 mCi)
  Treat metastases
    Fixed dose (Beierwaltes): 100 mCi for local disease only
    150 mCi for distant metastases
    Dosimetric Method
    Regional lymph nodes: 8000 rads (Maxon)
    Distant Metastases
      Maximal recommended dose based upon rad dose to blood, which is more readily measured than marrow dose (Memorial Sloan-Kettering Cancer Center).
        Marrow dose does not exceed blood dose.
        No bone marrow toxicity at <200 rads to blood per year.
        Requires blood sampling daily for 3–5 days; whole body counting (use gamma camera).

ADRENAL GLANDS

Radiopharmaceuticals

Adrenal cortex: I-131 NP-59; I-131 norcholesterol—Dose, 1.0 mCi, inject slowly (tracer dissolved in alcohol). Premedication, 15 drops Lugol's solution or soluble solution of potassium iodide (SSKI) tid for 3–5 days prior to tracer and throughout duration of imaging (3–5 days). Additional premedication (dexamethasone) depends upon indication. Image: high energy (364 keV) collimator—organ (region of interest) views × 10 minutes, anterior and posterior abdomen. Lateral views are optional to assess depth of adrenals.

Normal Distribution

Liver uptake and hepatobiliary excretion into bowel are seen. Gallbladder may be visualized in right upper quadrant (region of right adrenal). In nondexamethasone suppressed patients, both normal adrenals are seen. Failure to identify adrenal cortex is abnormal—compatible with replacement by tumor. In dexamethasone-suppressed patients neither adrenal is seen. Identification of activity indicates autonomous function—adrenal cortical adenoma or macroadenoma. Bilateral activity indicates bilateral function—hyperplasia secondary to nonsuppressible ACTH stimulation or bilateral macroadenoma. Preoperative differential diagnosis is based upon ACTH measurement. The source of the ACTH may be a pituitary adenoma or an ectopic ACTH-producing tumor (bronchial, intestinal, or pancreatic carcinoid).

Clinical Applications

Dexamethasone Suppression Not Required
"Incidentaloma" (i.e., mass found on CT) identifies functioning adrenal cortical adenoma vs. nonfunctioning "tumor."

Cushingoid patient has a unilateral or bilateral source of adrenal cortical function. It is particularly useful if ACTH is suppressed. More sensitive than CT to identify focus of "functioning" adrenal cortical tissue. The finding of adrenal cortical carcinoma frequently is negative on imaging as the degree of iodocholesterol incorporation is low.

Dexamethasone Suppression Required
Suspected hyperaldosteronism: Functioning aldosterone-producing adenoma will not suppress.

ADRENAL MEDULLA

Radiopharmaceuticals

I-131 MIBG (metaiodobenzylguanidine): Adult dose, 500 uCi; pediatric dose is based upon 1000 uCi/m^2; maximum dose 500 uCi; image at 72 hours (day 3) or later.

I-123 MIBG (not yet commercially available) up to 10 mCi: Image not later than (NLT) 24 hours. Uptake and contrast (lesion to background) increase with time, but after 24 hours physical decay is a more important factor.

MIBG is a pharmacologically inert analogue of guanethidine and epinephrine, which is concentrated in the presynaptic adrenergic nerve terminals via the secretory granule reuptake mechanism.

Premedicate with Lugol's solution or SSKI 3 days prior to study and throughout the imaging procedure. Premedication blocks the thyroid uptake of radioactive iodine that is released from the radiopharmaceutical. Image the thorax, abdomen, and pelvis at 72 hours or later. With I-123, earlier images can be obtained.

Normal Distribution

With I-131 MIBG, low level activity is seen in the liver and bone marrow. Cardiac (myocardial) activity is seen with I-123 MIBG imaged at 24 hours.

Clinical Applications

Adrenal medulla imaging is used to identify suspected, known, or recurrent pheochromocytoma. It can also be used to identify neuroblastoma and the extent of involvement.

Pheochromocytomas usually arise in the adrenal medulla but may arise in ectopic locations in chromaffin tissue throughout the abdomen and pelvis and even the thorax and neck.

PARATHYROID SCINTIGRAPHY

Radiopharmaceuticals

Tc-99m-MIBI, 20 mCi adult dose. See Cardiology for details.
Multiple protocols exist
    Dual phase protocol (most common): Early (20–30 minutes) imaging and delayed (2 hours) imaging
    Planar imaging (parallel hole collimator with zoom)
    SPECT (optional)
Dual tracer protocol (alternate)
    (1) Tc-99m-pertechnetate (4.0–5.0 mCi)
    Image 500,000 cts at 10–20 minutes
    Parallel hole collimator (HiRes) with zoom and markers followed by
    (2) Tc-99m-MIBI, 20–30 mCi, 500,000 cts at 10–20 minutes
                OR
    (1) I-123, as NaI, 300–400 uCi, image after 2 to 4 hours, 5 minutes acquisition
    (2) Tc-99m-MIBI, 20–30 mCi, 500,000 cts at 10–20 minutes.
Each image must undergo background subtraction image normalization.

Normal Distribution

Thyroid and parathyroid tissue are identified on early images with Tc-99m-MIBI, but thyroid tissue usually "washes out" on the delayed images, whereas parathyroid adenoma tissue retains its activity. Frequently, parathyroid adenomas are better identified (i.e., have greater uptake) even on early image. Iodine-123 and Tc-99m-pertechnetate are taken up by the iodine trap of thyroid tissue. The thyroid image is subtracted from the Tc-99m-MIBI image of the thyroid and parathyroid, leaving the residual parathyroid tissue.

Clinical Applications

Thyroid carcinoma and adenoma may have differential washout characteristics from the remainder of the thyroid gland and thus retain Tc-99m-MIBI on the delayed phase image. Significant differences in the trapping of the Tc-99m-pertechnetate or I-123 images are less likely. Subtraction imaging is based on the following:

Tc-99m-MIBI images = parathyroid + thyroid
I-123 images = thyroid
Subtracted image = parathyroid

Accuracy depends upon the size of the adenoma. Sensitivity usually is greater than 90%. Limit of detection is 0.5 gram (500 mg); SPECT may improve detection to 300 mg tissue.

For identification and localization of parathyroid adenoma in primary hyperthyroidism (1) Detect and localize the recurrent parathyroid adenoma; (2) evaluate the mediastinum for ectopic localization of parathyroid adenoma; and, rarely, (3) parathyroid hyperplasia is active enough to be identified.

SOMATOSTATIN RECEPTORS

Radiopharmaceuticals

In-111-DTPA-pentetreotide (OctreoScan)
   An 8 amino acid somatostatin analogue
   The amino acid portion is similar to octreotide, an agent used therapeutically to inhibit secretion of metabolically active substances by neuroendocrine tumors. Use a 6.0 mCi dose.

Acquisition Parameters

Image at 4 and 24 hours
Because of 10–15% GI excretion, bowel preparation is after administration
ROI or planar views, 10-minute acquisition
SPECT required to evaluate liver, abdomen, and thorax for suspected involvement
Medium energy collimator

Clinical Application

Pituitary tumors, functional or nonfunctional
Medullary cancer of the thyroid
Carcinoid, bronchial
Carcinoid, bowel
Islet cell tumors
Pheochromocytomas
See Oncology.

SKELETAL SYSTEM

RADIOPHARMACEUTICALS

Tc-99m-MDP (methylene diphosphonate) is the most common tracer for diagnostic imaging of the skeleton. It rapidly exchanges with the outer active regions of the hydroxyapatite crystal and is a marker of bone (mineral) turnover. Tc-99m-pertechnetate is added to a vial of desiccated stannous ion and MDP. A stannous chelate is formed with the Tc and MDP.

Pharmacokinetics is as follows: 50% to bone, 50% excreted by kidneys (critical organ, bladder), and the image quality is affected by decreased renal function. Typical Tc-99m-MDP imaging dose is 20–30 mCi, Tc-99m-MDP. Imaging may occur concurrently with injection of the diagnostic dose (i.e., 3-phase imaging) or after a suitable delay (usually 2 hours) to allow for skeletal uptake and clearance of the body background activity. Rarely, delayed imaging at 24 hours is performed (so-called 4-phase imaging).

Imaging at 2 hours after injection, so-called static imaging, can be performed with the static images of each region of the skeleton with a single or dual head gamma camera or with a scanning camera to provide whole body images. Alternately, SPECT acquisition is done over a body part or region of interest (ROI).

The 3-phase imaging consists of the sequential (1–3 sec/frame) images of the arrival of the radionuclide *(vascular phase)*, the immediate postvascular images *(equilibrium or tissue phase)*, and the delayed images *(osseous phase)*. SPECT has increased sensitivity for the detection of vertebral lesions, such as from trauma and metastases.

NORMAL DISTRIBUTION

Visualization of active skeleton can be done as follows:

Activity in the extremities decreases with age, but normal or increased activity may be seen in individuals with the exercise effect. Increased activity is normally seen in the sacroiliac joints and thyroid cartilage. The kidneys retain activity for 2–4 hours following injection. Decreased activity is seen in renal disease (decreased renal function) and in images obtained greater than 2 hours after injection.

CLINICAL APPLICATIONS

Bone pain, differential diagnosis
Infectious or noninfectious inflammation
Tumor, benign
     Osteoid osteomas
     Dermoid cysts
Tumor, malignant
     Primary or secondary (metastatic)
     Osteogenic sarcoma (may also see uptake in soft tissue metastases)
     Ewing's sarcoma
     Osteoblastic metastases
          Breast, prostate, colon, gastric, melanoma, lymphoma
     Mixed osteoblastic-osteolytic
          Nonsmall cell lung cancer
     Predominantly osteolytic (may have minor blastic component)
     Osteolytic metastases (photogenic)
          Myeloma, hypernephroma, thyroid cancer
          Most soft tissue sarcomas involving bone are photogenic.
Trauma
     Radiographically occult fractures appear as focal areas of increased uptake.
     Onset of increased uptake may be delayed in the elderly. Reimage at second
         injection at 72 hours if negative results are seen early.
     Less common, *metabolic bone disease* is characterized by increased uptake:
         hyperthyroidism, hyperparathyroidism, and myelofibrosis. Evaluation of
         the extent of disease, such as Paget's disease and fibrous dysplasia
         neuroblastoma, is possible.
Metastatic disease
     Most common, prostate, breast, lung cancer
     Most common sites, ribs 35%; vertebrae 25%; pelvis or extremities 15%; skull
         5% (as a memory aid, think −10% decrease per location)
Soft tissue uptake
     Liver: metastatic colorectal and breast cancer

Abdomen: Neuroblastoma in children

Lungs: Osteogenic sarcoma

Brain: Cerebral infarct

Myocardium: Myocardial infarction (activity appears in pleural and peritoneal effusions)

Lungs, stomach, kidneys: hypercalcemia—kidney uptake is normal at 2 hours.

Osteomyelitis

Both active osteomyelitis and fracture are positive findings on all three phases. Differential diagnosis depends upon the clinical setting and/or history.

Bone scintigraphy is useful to differentiate between cellulitis alone and osteomyelitis (with or without cellulitis). Cellulitis has increased uptake (positive scan) in the flow and blood pool phases (1 and 2). The delayed image appears negative without associated osteomyelitis. The pattern is also different from that of cellulitis. The area of increased uptake does not correspond to the position of the bones. *Caution:* The patient may have focal osteomyelitis and surrounding cellulitis. Diabetic foot ulcers may overlie bone and appear as focal areas of increased uptake. A labeled white blood cell (WBC) scan may be needed to differentiate.

Osteitis Neoformans. Bony growth following trauma is probably caused by the interruption of periosteum. Increased tracer indicates proliferating active bone.

Reflex sympathetic dystrophy. This follows osseous or soft tissue trauma, e.g., mastectomy, fractures:

Increase in phases 1 and 2 during the acute process is followed by a gradual decrease. After 1 year, the process is arrested. Decreased activity is noted during flow and on delayed images.

ONCOLOGY

RADIOPHARMACEUTICALS

Gallium-67 Citrate

8–10 mCi, medium energy collimator

Image 48–72 hours after injection to allow blood pool clearing

Delayed imaging with bowel preparation (laxatives and/or enema) to clear GI tract

Whole body imaging and/or 10-minute planar images (approximately 500–750 K counts).

SPECT is $64 \times 64 \times 16$ matrix, 40 sec/frame, 360° orbit.

Ga-67 binds to the plasma iron–binding protein transferrin.

Gallium-transferrin receptor: lymphoma, malignant

Melanoma, hepatoma

Dissociation from the Ga-transferring complex at lower pH:

Adenocarcinoma

Tl-201

3–4 mCi, 20–30 minutes after injection, low energy collimator

10-minute planar images (500–750 K counts)

SPECT of relevant area

Biochemical analogue of K^+ enters cell NA/K ATPase pump. Blood flow, tumor type, and vascular permeability influence TI-201 uptake.

Tc-99m-MIBI

15–20 mCi, 20–30 minutes after injection, low energy collimator

Planar (500,000–1 million counts)

SPECT of relevant area

Introduced as myocardial perfusion imaging agent

Marker of tumor perfusion

Binds to mitochondrial protein

Eliminated from tumor cells by multiple drug resistance mechanism (p-glycoprotein)

In-111-DTPA pentetreotide (OctreoScan)
    6.0 mCi, image at 24 hours
        Additional earlier imaging at 4 hours helpful
        Medium energy collimator
        Planar images of ROI (may be whole body)
    500,000–800,000 counts or 10-minute views
    Whole body imaging
    10 cm/min at 4 hours; 8 cm/min at 24 hours
    SPECT of ROI (even if planar result is negative).
Monoclonal Antibodies
    Satumomab pendetide (OncoScint): First antibody approved by FDA
    6.0 mCi In-111-labeled intact murine immunoglobulin (IgG)
    Medium energy collimator
    Planar and SPECT of ROI at 72–96 hours
Arcitumomab carcinoembryonic antigen (CEA) scan
    20–30 mCi Tc-99m-labeled murine Fab fragment (IgG)
    Image at 4–6 hours
    Planar and SPECT of ROI
    General purpose or high resolution collimator
Capromab pendetide (ProstaScint)
    6.0 mCi In-111-labeled intact murine monoclonal antibody (IgG)
    Medium energy collimator
    Image at 1 hour (vascular phase) and 72–96 hours (specific uptake phase)
    SPECT imaging for interpretation:
        Transverse sections, also coronal, sagittal
FDG
    5–10 mCi F-18 fluorodeoxyglucose (2-hour half-life)
    Cyclotron-produced product
    Image at 45 minutes, preferably after overnight fast
    Coincident imaging
        Ring detector or modified dual-headed camera
        Imaging with 511 keV collimator is *not* appropriate for tumor detection.

NORMAL DISTRIBUTION

Ga-67 Citrate
    Liver (most prominent), bone, and bone marrow
    Lactating women
    Variable uptake: spleen, salivary glands, lacrimal glands, nasal mucosa,
        genitalia, female breasts, kidneys (usually only seen faintly)
    Large bowel excretion (10–15%)
    Bladder activity usually not seen at 24 hours or later
Tl-201
    Myocardium, kidneys, liver, spleen, splanchnic areas, muscles (variable with
        activity), lacrimal glands, salivary glands, thyroid
Tc-99m-MIBI
    Myocardium, liver, gallbladder (secretion into small bowel), spleen, kidneys
        and urinary bladder, salivary and parotid glands, thyroid
In-111 Pentetreotide
    Liver, spleen, kidneys
    Variable minimal activity, thyroid, pituitary
    Bladder activity at 4 hours
    Bowel activity at 24 hours (approximately 10% excretion)
Monoclonal Antibodies
    Early imaging: vascular pool
    Delayed imaging: liver, spleen, bone marrow, genitalia, body background
F-18 FDG (fluorodeoxyglucose)
    Liver, spleen, brain
    Myocardium varies with blood glucose level
    Muscles, skin

12

CLINICAL APPLICATIONS

Nonspecific organ imaging

Cold spots (space-occupying defects): liver, lung, brain, bone, thyroid
Malignant tumors vs. benign tumors
    Adenoma, cysts (clinical history, ultrasound)
    Hemangioma (labeled RBC scan)
    Abscess, inflammation (labeled WBC scan)
    Necrosis (perfusion imaging: Tl-201, Tc-99m-MIBI)
Hot spots (foci of increased radiopharmaceutical uptake)
    Bone
        Malignant (usually osteoblastic tumor)
        Infection (osteomyelitis)
        Trauma (even with negative X-ray findings)
        Degenerative process (osteoarthritis)
        Paget's disease
        Vascular lesions
        Benign bone tumors (osteoid osteoma)
    Gallium: Increased uptake
        Inflammation and infectious processes, abscesses
        Osteomyelitis, septic arthritis, sinusitis
        Occult infections (postoperative, antibiotic therapy, perforated viscera)
        Salivary glands (following radiotherapy)
        Active sarcoid
        Bone marrow (rebound following chemotherapy)
        Thymus (rebound following chemotherapy)
        Kidneys (interstitial nephritis, pyelonephritis, glomerulonephritis, transfusions)
        Lungs (inflammation, following chemotherapy, e.g., bleomycin, contrast lymphangiography)
        Recent surgical wounds
        Delayed bowel clearance
        Trauma, fractures, hematomas
        Paget's disease of bone
    Although not used for clinical management, Ga-67 uptake is seen in the following:
Melanoma
Lung cancer
Hepatoma
Bone and soft tissue sarcoma
Gastric cancer
Colon cancer
Pancreatic cancer
Seminoma
Embryonal cell cancer
Teratoma
Mesothelioma
Head and neck tumors
Uptake is poor in the following:
Gynecological tumors
Chondrosarcoma
Thallium increased uptake is a nonspecific indicator of perfusion/viability. Very active inflammatory lesions may mimic tumor uptake.
Tc-99m-MIBI uptake depends on perfusion/viability/metabolic activity. Very active inflammatory lesions may mimic tumor uptake. Absent uptake may indicate multiple drug resistance (MDR) mechanism.
In-111-DTPA pentetreotide (OctreoScan)
    Inflammatory lymphoid tissue
        Sarcoid, tuberculosis
    Viral infections
    Radiation pleuritis
Radiolabeled antibodies
    Difficult to distinguish lymph node activity from vascular structures early.

12

Bladder activity, bowel activity
F-18 FDG
Inflammatory activity
Bladder, ureters (urine)
Increased muscle metabolism (swallowing, vomiting)
Sweating

Screening for Tumor Presence

Staging

Localize primary tumor
Determine local extent and metastases

Evaluation of Therapy

Response to therapy
Tumor recurrence
Gallium-67
Hodgkin's disease and non-Hodgkin's lymphoma
Hodgkin's disease: sensitivity: 85–97%; specificity: 90–100%
Non-Hodgkin's lymphoma: sensitivity > 85%
Except low-grade non-Hodgkin's lymphoma
Evaluate response to therapy (persistent CT mass)
Predict response to therapy (absent activity following chemotherapy)
Detect recurrent activity
Limited application in staging of Hodgkin's disease
Soft Tissue Sarcoma
Response to therapy
Detection of recurrence
Not currently used clinically for management of lung cancer, head and neck cancer, colorectal cancer, breast cancer, or melanoma.
Thallium [Tl-201]
Differentiate benign from malignant diseases
Determine the grade of malignancy
Evaluate response to therapy
Differentiate changes following therapy from recurrent/residual tumor.
Brain Tumors
Tl-201 uptake not dependent on breakdown of blood-brain barrier (BBB)
Greater uptake, more malignant
Recurrence vs. necrosis
Soft Tissue Sarcoma
Evaluate before and after therapy to determine tumor viability

Immunocompromised Patients

	Tl-201	Ga-67
Pulmonary Kaposi's sarcoma	+	−
Lymphoma	−	−
Opportunistic infections	−	+
Tuberculosis and chronic inflammatory lesions	+	+
Pneumocystis carinii pneumonia	±	+

Tc-99m MIBI
Similar to Tl-201
Absent activity may indicate MDR; predicts poor response.
Monoclonal Antibody Imaging
Detection of recurrence sites in patients with rising tumor markers
Prostate cancer—PSA (prostate-specific antigen)
Colon cancer—CEA (carcinoembryonic antigen)
Confirmation of tumor sites demonstrated on other imaging techniques
Identification of occult tumors

In-111 Pentetreotide
    Neuroendocrine tumors
        Detect
            Extent of disease
            Somatosatin receptor positive (i.e., therapeutic potential)
            Progression of disease
            Effect of therapy
            Recurrence
        Pituitary tumors, functioning or nonfunctioning
        Medullary cancer thyroid
        Bronchial carcinoid (may secrete ACTH)
        Islet cell tumors, functioning or nonfunctioning
            Insulinoma, gastrinoma, glucagonoma
        Small bowel carcinoid (may secrete serotonin)
        Pheochromocytoma
        Paraganglioma, ganglioma, carotid body tumors
        Lymphoma (variable) and Hodgkin's disease
F-18 FDG
    Characterization of known or indeterminate lesions
    Staging extent of disease
    Monitoring response to treatment
    Detect recurrence
Lung Tumors
    Solitary pulmonary nodule: Malignant vs. benign: sensitivity, 95%; specificity, 80%
    False-positive findings include granulomatous disease and inflammatory lesions.

Staging of mediastinal lymph node involvement (NSCLC):

	FDG	CT
Sensitivity	>76%	65%
Specificity	98%	87%
Accuracy	93%	82%

Recurrent tumor vs. scar: sensitivity, 90%; specificity, 62%. False-positive findings include acute inflammation and reactive mesothelial cells.
Head and neck tumors
    Recurrence vs. fibrosis

	FDG	CT
Sensitivity	88%	25%
Specificity	100%	75%

Colorectal cancer

	FDG	CT
Local disease recurrence	95%	65%
Liver metastasis	98%	93%
Unsuspected extrahepatic malignant	32%	0%

Pancreatic cancer

	FDG	CT
Sensitivity	95%	80%
Specificity	93%	74%

False-positive findings include chronic active pancreatitis, cystadenomas, mass forming pancreatitis, and retroperitoneal fibrosis.
Brain tumors
    Tumor grade directly proportional to FDG uptake

Patients prognosis inversely proportional
Detect recurrence
Recurrence vs. radiation necrosis
Lymphoma
    Staging concordant with conventional imaging: 82%
    Better than conventional imaging: 18%
Breast cancer
    Recurrent disease vs. fibrosis: sensitivity, 93%; specificity, 79%
    False-positive findings include muscle uptake, inflammation, blood pool, and
        bowel uptake.
    False-negative findings include bone lesions.
Melanoma
    Sensitivity, 100%.
    Potential false-negative findings: small pulmonary lesions (<1 cm) due to
        respiratory motion or recent therapy.
Prostate cancer
    Sensitivity, 65%
    Detection of bone lesions, 20%
Ovarian cancer
    Recurrence vs. fibrosis

	FDG	CT
Sensitivity	93%	87%
Specificity	80%	50%

INFLAMMATION

RADIOPHARMACEUTICALS

Gallium-67 citrate
    See Oncology.
    Localization is based upon increased delivery due to hyperemia and exudation.
Decreased pH in inflamed area promotes dissociation of transferrin bound Ga.
Greater binding to lactoferrin found in inflamed area (from necrotic polys and from
binding to some bacterial siderophores). Ga-67 uptake occurs in acute and chronic
infections. With chronicity, it is frequently more sensitive than labeled WBC imaging
(i.e., primarily polys).
In-111 oxine WBCs
    Adult: 45-ml aliquot of patient's blood
    Currently the standard imaging agent for inflammation.
    Caution: Careful identification of patient and sample required. Confirm identity with
witness prior to reinjection.
    Separate WBCs by sedimentation
    Remove WBCs
    Separate from plasma
    Wash
    Incubate with In-111 oxine, 5.0 mCi
    Wash and resuspend in saline
Tc-99m HMPAO
    Separate as just described.
    Incubate with Tc-99m HMPAO, 30 mCi; wash and resuspend.

ACQUISITION PARAMETERS

	Ga-67	In-111 WBCs	Tc-99m WBCs
Dose	10 mCi	5 mCi	20 mCi
Collimator	Medium	Medium	Low energy
Time after	48 hours	24 hours	1 hour
injection	(4–48 hours)	(4–24 hours)	(1–4 hour)

Whole body imaging is recommended to rule out unsuspected areas; follow with ROI images. In-111 and Ga-67, 10 minute views; Tc-99m: 500 K cts vs. 10-minute view.

NORMAL DISTRIBUTION

Gallium-67
See Oncology.
In-111 WBCs and Tc-99m WBCs: Liver, spleen, active bone marrow
Ga-67
> Although in most instances an infectious etiology is suspected, Ga-67 localizes in many situations such as noninfectious inflammation: e.g., sarcoid (characteristic pattern, panda-lambda sign); parotid, lacrimal, and submandibular glands (panda); mediastinal and subhilar lymph nodes (lambda).
>> Acute trauma
>> Increased bone remodeling: inactive osteomyelitis
>> Iron injection sites
>> Other intramuscular/subcutaneous injection sites: insulin, heparin
>> Tumors (see Oncology)
>> Recent fractures
>> Noninfectious inflammation (sarcoid, rheumatoid arthritis)
>> Paget's disease
>> Hemochromatosis, hemosiderosis

Gallium is excreted into the bowel (large intestines). Diffuse or focal Ga-67 may persist for days. Consider bowel preparation: enema and/or laxative
In-111 WBCs
> The causes of false-positive scan findings are *most commonly a problem in the abdomen.*

> Swallowed WBCs: Nasal secretions are usually associated with sinusitis, oral pharyngeal infection, pneumonia, or esophagitis.
>> Bleeding
>> Ostomies
>> Accessory spleen
>> Transplanted kidney (even without clinical rejection)
>> Surgical wound, recent, uninfected
>> Heterotopic bone
>> Tumors, infarcted
>>> Tc-99m WBC *only:* Appearance of label in bowel increases after 1 hour; regularly seen at 4 hours.
False-negative WBC scan findings
> Leukemia
> Chronic infection
> Antibiotic treatment

CLINICAL APPLICATION

In general, In-111 WBCs are the standard for identification of acute pyogenic infection and certain fungal or viral infections in which there is a prominent polymorphonuclear leukocyte (PMN) response (e.g., *Candida* esophagitis, cytomegalovirus colitis).
In-111 WBC imaging
> Differentiate contrast-enhancing CNS ring lesions
> Head and neck abscesses, interstitial infections
> Bacterial pneumonia
> Valve infections
> Infected aneurysms
> Infected vascular grafts
> Osteomyelitis, extremities
> Osteomyelitis, vertebral
>> Focal increase—diagnostic
>> Focal decrease—consider chronic infection (Ga-67)
>> Normal (uniform) activity (Compare with Tc-99m sulfur-colloid marrow scan).

12

Periprosthesis osteomyelitis (may need Tc-99m sulfur-colloid to differentiate from active marrow).

Diabetic ulcer with or without osteomyelitis

Colitis

Bowel fistula

Acute cholecystitis

Postsurgical intraabdominal abscess (may be remote in time or location).

Inflamed bowel, appendicitis

Tuboovarian abscess

Septic abortion

Fever of undetermined origin (FUO)

Gallium-67 imaging is positive in all of the aforementioned. Uptake is generally less intense than that of In-111 WBCs. For Ga-67 image lesion, the background contrast is usually 2 to 3:1 when compared with In-111 WBC in which the contrast may be 15:1. Gallium-67 imaging is more sensitive than labeled WBCs.

Fungal infections

Opportunistic infections (*Pneumocystis carinii* pneumonia)

Granulomatous infections (tuberculosis, *Mycobacterium avium-intracellular*, histoplasmosis, coccidioidomycosis)

Chronic osteomyelitis

Chronic infection

Chronic or partially treated FUO

Diagnosis of osteomyelitis depends on visualizing increased activity *greater in area or intensity than expected* from corresponding bone scan.

Pulmonary Uptake of Ga-67 Grading

0	No uptake
1+	Equivocal uptake
2+	Definite uptake (> cardiac blood pool; = ribs)
3+	Uptake > ribs; = liver
4+	Uptake > liver

GENITOURINARY SYSTEM

RADIOPHARMACEUTICALS

1. Tc-99m-DTPA. A chelate that is filtered at the glomerulus and not reabsorbed. In a patient with normal glomerular filtration, it is rapidly cleared from the blood and excreted into the urine. The clearance of Tc-99m-labeled DTPA can be used to determined the glomerular filtration rate.
2. Tc-99m-MAG 3. A triamide monomercaptide that is tightly bound to protein in the blood. Virtually none is filtered by the glomeruli, but it is quantitatively extracted by the tubular cells and is present in high concentration in the urine. Tc-99m-MAG 3 is cleared more rapidly than DTPA because its clearance approximates effective renal plasma flow (ERPF), which is about 500 mL/min as opposed to glomerular filtration (GFR), which is about 120 mL/min. This agent reaches high concentrations in the urine. Tc-99m-MAG 3 can be used to estimate the ERPF.
3. Tc-99m-DMSA (2,3-diMercaptosuccinic acid). This is taken up and retained by the renal tubular cells with little urinary excretion. It is used as a cortical imaging agent.
4. Tc-99m-glucoheptonate. About 80 to 90% is excreted by glomerular filtration (like Tc-99m-labeled DTPA). However, the remainder is fixed in the renal cortex and is used for its imaging.

In individuals with normal renal function and excretion, Tc-99m-DTPA and Tc-99m-MAG 3 deliver very little radiation to the kidney. The bladder receives the

12

largest radiation dose. The cortical imaging agents, Tc-99m-DMSA and Tc-99m-glucoheptonate, deliver a larger dose to the kidney and a smaller dose to the bladder.

IMAGING PARAMETERS

Tc-99m-DTPA or Tc-99m-MAG 3 dynamic renal blood flow and function; 3-5–mCi
  Patient supine, camera beneath table
  IV bolus; record every 3 seconds × 20 (1 minute)
  Record 1 min/frame for 30 minutes
  If excretion is complete by that time, study is terminated. Patients with stasis or obstructions require longer imaging times.
  Draw ROI around kidney, collecting system, or both.
  Generate activity vs. time curves.
  Split function is equal to the area under the renogram curve 1.5–2.5 minutes after injection.
Tc-99m-DMSA, 2–3 mCi. Image at 2 hours; slow cortical uptake
  Anterior, posterior, and both posterior oblique views for 500,000 counts or 5 minutes. Pinhole images may also be obtained.
  Split function: ROI, posterior images at 2 hours; subtract background; express each kidney as a percent of the summed counts.
Tc-99m-glucoheptonate. Renogram is performed in a fashion similar to that for patient studies with Tc-99m-DTPA or Tc-99m-MAG 3, followed by cortical imaging 2 hours later.

NORMAL DISTRIBUTION

On the initial blood flow images activity should be observed in both kidneys either simultaneously with visualization of the aorta or on the next image. Flow should be symmetrical. On a summed image of the first minute after injection, the kidneys should be sharply defined and should contain more radionuclide than other structures in the abdomen.

On the renogram images there should be rapid uptake of radiotracer with activity first seen in the collecting system by 3 to 4 minutes. This is the cortical transit time. Activity should be seen in the bladder, if in the field of view, by 4 to 5 minutes. Normal patients who are not adequately hydrated may have delay in both cortical transit and appearance of activity in the bladder. The most intense activity should be in the renal cortex at 3 to 5 minutes, with subsequent rapid clearance of activity from the kidney and accumulation in the bladder. Virtually all activity should have left the kidneys by 30 minutes. Not uncommonly there is intense activity in the urine within the collecting system on the early images, but essentially all of this activity should have left the collecting system by 20 to 30 minutes.

The renogram curve shows an initial rapid upstroke as the first bolus of radiotracer is delivered to the kidney. This is followed by a continual rapid rise as the kidney continues to accumulate radionuclide. The peak of the curve occurs at approximately 3 to 5 minutes, followed by a rapid downstroke during the excretory phase. The excretory phase slows as more activity is excreted. By 30 minutes, this tail of the curve should be virtually flat. When split function is calculated, each kidney should contribute between 45 and 55% to the total.

Pharmaceutical Intervention

1. Furosemide (Lasix) is a potent loop diuretic that may be given IV to cause a sudden increase in urine production by the kidneys. Furosemide is given in cases of possible obstruction to flush residual activity from the collecting system.
2. An ACE inhibitor, most commonly captopril 25 mg by mouth, may be given 1 hour prior to injection of Tc-99m-labeled MAG 3 or DTPA for a renogram. This blocks formation of angiotensin II resulting in decreased perfusion to a kidney with hemodynamically significant renal artery stenosis.

CLINICAL APPLICATIONS

Obstructive Uropathy

Patients with dilated renal collecting systems may have significant obstruction or simply urine stasis in a dilated but not obstructed collecting system. This type of renogram can be used to differentiate between obstruction that requires surgical correction and stasis that does not.

The renogram is performed in the usual manner with either Tc-99m-labeled DTPA or MAG 3. Twenty minutes after injection of the radiopharmaceutical, furosemide is given IV in a dose of 0.5 mg/kg (adult dose, 40 mg). However, if the dilated collecting system is not filled with radioactive urine at 20 minutes, the injection of furosemide should be delayed until filling is achieved. Imaging is continued for an additional 20 minutes after injection of furosemide.

In a dilated but nonobstructed collecting system, subsequent images show a rapid clearance of radioactive urine into the bladder. The renogram curves show a precipitous drop. In severe obstruction, there is no change in the appearance of the collecting system on the images. The renogram curve continues to rise or comes to a plateau. Some patients manifest an intermediate response with a gradual but incomplete clearance or radioactive urine.

Patients in the first category (dilated, nonobstructed) do not need surgery, patients in the second category (severe obstruction) do, and patients in the third category (intermediate response) need repeat renograms. Sequential determination of split function may also help to detect obstruction that is sufficient to cause renal damage. The test is of particular value in following patients after they have undergone surgery for significant obstruction.

There are several instances in which these renograms may be inaccurate or misleading. In premature infants and for the first month or so after delivery in normal infants, the kidneys are less responsive to furosemide and the result may show a false-positive finding. Very poorly functioning kidneys may be unresponsive to furosemide and result in a false-positive test finding.

Renovascular Hypertension

In a patient with hemodynamically significant renal artery stenosis, there is a decrease in perfusion pressure in the kidney. The juxtaglomerular apparatus is stimulated to release renin leading to an increase in angiotensin II and an increase in systemic blood pressure, which normalizes perfusion pressure in the kidney and maintains glomerular filtration and urine output at normal levels.

Radionuclide renography in such a patient may be normal in the early stages. However, the stenosis increases and the compensatory mechanisms are no longer adequate. Glomerular filtration and urine output gradually decrease. Renography in such a patient shows prolonged cortical transit time, delayed visualization of the bladder, delayed renogram peak, and prolonged cortical retention in the radionuclide kidney. If renal artery stenosis is severe enough the affected kidney may be significantly smaller. Eventually there may be no excretion from the affected kidney, and the renogram curve may rise progressively and continuously throughout the study.

In very severe end-stage renal artery stenosis, the kidney may be extremely small and may have virtually no function. Patients with hemodynamically significant renal artery stenosis—who are restudied after the administration of an angiotensin-converting enzyme inhibitor (ACEI)—show deterioration in the renogram of the affected kidney. The standard test is to perform a renogram without an ACEI and one with an ACEI to document deterioration. Since most patients with suspected renal artery stenosis are actually healthy, it makes sense to perform the first renogram following administration of an ACEI. If it is normal, no further renograms need to be performed.

Renal Failure

Radionuclide renography may be helpful in the differential diagnosis of patients with renal failure. A standard renogram with Tc-99m-labeled DTPA or MAG 3 is performed. Patients with chronic renal failure have small kidneys, usually with markedly diminished but symmetrical renal blood flow. Renogram curves are usually normal in shape but very low in amplitude. If the patient has superimposed renal artery stenosis the affected kidney may be smaller and may demonstrate an abnormal renogram. Captopril testing can be performed in such a case.

In acute renal failure the kidneys are normal in size or enlarged. Renal blood flow is usually relatively well preserved. The renogram curve is variable. In patients with complete renal failure it rises continually. In those patients with partial renal failure it may have either a plateau or a delayed peak, with gradual excretion and prolonged cortical retention. Cortical defects may be seen in patients with pyelonephritis and those with renal emboli. These defects are best detected by delayed imaging after injection of Tc-99m-labeled DTPA or glucoheptonate.

Renal Transplantation

Radionuclide renograms are a standard for following patients after renal transplantations. The renograms are performed with the patient supine and the camera positioned above the transplanted kidney, which is usually in the iliac fossa. The imaging parameters are the same as those used for renograms in patients with native kidneys.

Normal Transplant. In patients with living related donor transplants, normal renal function is seen within the kidney immediately after visualization of activity in the external iliac vessel to which the renal artery is anastamosed. Subsequent images show rapid uptake, cortical transit, and excretion into the bladder, which is usually detected by the 5-minute image. The renogram curve appears normal with a sharp peak and rapid washout.

Rejection. The first change is usually a slight delay in the appearance of radiotracer in the bladder and a slight delay in the peak of the renogram. Progressive rejection involves gradual decrease in blood flow and gradual prolongation of the excretory phase with increasing delay in excretion. Eventually excretion ceases. The renogram curve gradually deteriorates to a delayed peak, then to a plateau, and finally to a continually rising curve.

Acute Tubular Necrosis. Cadaver kidneys often manifest renal tubular necrosis at the time of transplantation. If severe, renal blood flow is delayed and diminished. Images show poor uptake and no bladder activity. The renogram curve is very low and rises continuously. In the absence of rejection, there is usually gradual improvement in the renogram results with progressive increase in renal blood flow, renal uptake, and excretion. Patients with cadaver transplants are usually studied every 3 to 5 days. The curve improves slowly over weeks. If there is a delayed appearance of radionuclide in the urine, and/or a lower renogram curve and/or a revision of the curve shaped to a more pathological form, superimposed rejection can be diagnosed. In some cases of acute tubular necrosis, superimposed ejection and cyclosporine toxicity may be identical. Clinical information is required to differentiate between these two possible etiologies.

Rejection, Hyperacute. Patients with preformed antibodies to transplanted kidneys develop hyperacute rejection. There is sudden loss of all blood flow to the kidney. This appears as a photon-deficient image on the flow phase.

Urine Leaks [Urinomas]. These usually occur at the anastomosis of the ureter to the bladder. Radionuclide is seen outside the kidney and bladder. Often, a photogenic halo is seen in the early part of the study that "fills in."

Testicular Torsion

The testicle twists on its axis and remains fixed in that position producing ischemia. The condition is markedly painful. If testicular torsion is not relieved within a few hours, necrosis may occur. The condition usually occurs in young males, ages 5 to 12 years, but also occurs in fetuses (in utero), infants, and adults.

The condition must be differentiated from the other causes of acute pain in the testicle:

Orchitis
Epididymitis
Torsion of the testicular appendix
Tumor, abscess

RADIOPHARMACEUTICAL

Tc-99m DTPA is preferred but pertechnetate or any other soluble Tc-99m radiopharmaceutical can be used; 10–20 mCi adult dose (70 kg). Adjust the pediatric dose based on weight.

ACQUISITION

Separate thighs
Support scrotal contents with towel or tape sling
Tape penile shaft to lower abdomen
Mark (optional) scrotal midline with lead strip
Flow sequence of 2–3 second/frame × 20–30 frames (= 1 minute)
300,000–500,000 counts, ROI images

PATTERNS

Correlate image findings with clinical history (side with pain).
Normal Pattern
    Uniform flow and redistribution pattern
Torsion
    Ischemic flow phase
    Decreased perfusion of tissue phase
Missed Torsion
    Ischemic or markedly reduced flow
    Photogenic testes with increased rim of activity (halo) (represents late
        imaging; torsion and testicular infarct occurred more than 12–24 hours
        previously).
    Testicle cannot be salvaged.
    Orchipexy performed on opposite side.
Orchitis
    Increased flow and tissue perfusion involving most of scrotal contents.
Epididymitis
    Small focus of increased activity near upper pole of testicle.
Abscess
    Increased flow and tissue phase.
Tumor
    Variable; patient may present with tissue hemorrhage, necrosis, and
    diminished flow associated with pain. Usually distinguished by examination.

12   BASIC SCIENCE

RADIOPHARMACEUTICALS

Modes of Decay of Radionuclides

Mode	Example
Beta (minus) decay (pure beta minus)	Iodine-131 ($\beta-$ and γ); strontium-89
Positron (beta plus) decay	Fluorine-18; rubidium-82 ($\beta+ - 2[511\text{ keV}]$)
Electron capture	Thallium-201 (γ and x-rays); gallium-67, Indium-111 (γ)
Isomeric transition	Tc-99m (γ)

The most commonly used radionuclide is technetium-99m. Technetium-99m decays by isomeric transition to technetium-99. Technetium-99m as eluted from a generated aqueous solution is in the form of the pertechnetate ion (TcO$_4-$). Tc-99m-pertechnetate is used to prepare various Tc-99m-labeled compounds with the so-called technetium kits. Most commonly this procedure is accomplished by using stannous ion to chelate the Tc and the carrier molecule.

Technetium Kits

Principal Component	Chemistry	Application
DTPA	Sn^{+2} ion chelation	Renal flow, function, imaging (glomerular filtration); short-lived vascular pool agent
MDP	Sn^{+2} ion	Bone imaging
MAG-3	Sn^{+2} ion	Renal flow, function, imaging (tubular excretion)
HMPAO*	Sn^{+2} ion	Cerebral perfusion SPECT imaging
ECD	Sn^{+2} ion	Cerebral perfusion SPECT imaging
Sulfur colloid	Coprecipitation	Liver, spleen, bone marrow imaging Reticuloendothelial imaging Lymphoscintigraphy
MAA	Sn^{+2} ion	Pulmonary perfusion imaging Intraarterial perfusion imaging Shunt detection
RBCs	Sn^{+2} ion	Gated blood pool scintigraphy Vascular imaging
DTPA†		Cisternography

*Tc-99m-Sn-HMPAO is also used to label isolated WBCs.
†DTPA provides a tight bound that ensures insolubility.

Other Techniques

WBCs (Indium-111 oxine)	Infection/inflammation imaging
Platelets (Indium-111 oxine)	Thrombus Detection/imaging
Monoclonal antibodies	Tumor specific imaging (using DTPA or other links)
Peptides (DTPA link)	Somatostatin receptor imaging

Other radionuclides used in Nuclear Medicine include the following:

Radionuclide (Source)	Mode of Decay
Gallium-67 (accelerator produced)	Electron capture
Indium-111 (accelerator produced)	Electron capture
Iodine-123 (accelerator produced)	Electron capture
Krypton-81m (generator produced from rubidium-81)	Isomeric transition
Xenon-133 (reactor fusion product)	Beta-minus decay
Iodine-131 (reactor fusion or bombarded target product)	Beta-minus decay

12

Index

Note: Page numbers followed by the letter t refer to tables.

Histiocytoma *(Continued)*
    lesion with sequestrum in, 218
Histiocytosis, Langerhans cell, in children, 620, 621, 635
    clinical and imaging signs of, 654–655
Histiocytosis X, clinical and imaging signs of, 78–79
    mediastinal lymphadenopathy in, 34
Histoplasmosis, clinical and imaging signs of, 83
    mediastinal lymphadenopathy in, 33
HIV. See *Human immunodeficiency virus (HIV).*
Hodgkin's lymphoma, 89–90
Holoprosencephaly, 687, 688
    clinical and imaging signs of, 196–197, 712
Honeycomb lung, 47
Honeycombing, radiographic definition of, 23
Human immunodeficiency virus (HIV). See also *Acquired immunodeficiency syndrome (AIDS).*
    encephalitis due to, 180
    esophageal ulceration associated with, 301
    esophagitis due to, 360
Hydatid cyst, lung cavity due to, 43
Hydatid disease, 83–84
Hydatidiform mole, 677, 679
    clinical and imaging signs of, 721–722
Hydranencephaly, 686, 688
    clinical and imaging signs of, 712
Hydrocarbon aspiration, 650
Hydrocarbon ingestion, by children, 620
Hydrocele, 463
    clinical and imaging signs of, 474
Hydrocephalus, 134–135, 260
    communicating, 135–136, 685
    congenital, 135
    massive, 688
    normal pressure, 728
Hydrometrocolpos, 722
Hydronephrosis, 438–439
    fetal, 693–694
        differential diagnosis of, 695–697
    in children, 631–632
Hydrops, 683
Hydrops fetalis, 712
Hydrosalpinx, 701
Hydroxyapatite deposition, 252
    clinical and imaging signs of, 272
Hygroma, cystic, fetal, 691
    clinical and imaging signs of, 710
    in children, 623
Hyperlucent lung, unilateral, 48
    clinical and imaging signs of, 104–105
Hyperostosis, cortical, 219–220
Hyperparathyroidism, 230, 238, 253
    clinical and imaging signs of, 272–273
Hyperplasia, adrenal, 457
    adrenocortical, 467
    breast, 527
        clinical and imaging signs of, 539
    Brunner's gland, 319, 324, 351
    endometrial, 721
    hepatic, focal nodular, 399
        clinical and imaging signs of, 422
    lymphoid, angiofollicular, 28, 29
        clinical and imaging signs of, 71
        benign, 350–351
        duodenal, 319
Hypersensitivity, T1, 137
Hypersensitivity pneumonitis, 84
Hypertension, portal, 400–401, 589

Hypertension *(Continued)*
    clinical and imaging signs of, 598–599
    film of, questions and answers about, 610–611
    intervention for, 599
    pulmonary, 563
        clinical and imaging signs of, 99
        radiographic definition of, 23
    renal artery, 599–600
    renovascular, 490
        nuclear imaging of, 754
Hypertensive heart disease, 569
Hyperthyroid patient, nuclear imaging of, 740–741
Hypervitaminosis A, 222
    in children, 634
Hypervitaminosis D, 228
Hypogenetic lung syndrome, 84–85
Hyposensitivity, T2, 137
Hypotension, intracranial, 134
Hypothyroidism, 229

I

Idiopathic juvenile osteoporosis, 635–636
Ileum, terminal, narrowed with abnormal cecum, 332
Ileus, 326, 345
    meconium, clinical and imaging signs of, 657–658, 713–714
Iliac artery aneurysm, 452
Iliac artery occlusion, film of, questions and answers about, 607
Iliac lymphadenopathy, 452
Immotile cilia syndromes, 85
Immunocompromised patient, nuclear imaging of, 748–749
    clinical applications of, 747–750
    distribution of, 746
    radiopharmaceuticals in, 745–746
Implants, breast, 539–540
    fibrous capsule adjacent to, 514
In-111-DTPA pentetreotide imaging, in oncologic nuclear medicine, 746
Inclusion cyst, peritoneal, 701
Infarct, bone, immature, 217
    mature, 216
    cerebral, 115
        clinical and imaging signs of, 190–191
        in young adult, 127–128
        venous, 130–131
    hepatic, 399, 402
    intramedullary, 138
    pulmonary, radiographic definition of, 23
    renal, 438, 439, 440
        clinical and imaging signs of, 486–487
    splenic, 408
    testicular, 703
    thromboembolic, 130
Infarct-avid imaging, in nuclear cardiology, 733
Infection(s). See also specific infection, e.g., *Pneumonia*; specific type, e.g., *Tuberculosis.*
    acromioclavicular joint, 226
    causing gastric fold thickening, 310
    epiphyseal, 215
    esophageal, 297
    opportunistic, 56
    placental, 683
    pulmonary, 17–21
    renal, focal, 446
    small bowel, in immunocompromised patients, 330

Infection(s) *(Continued)*
    TORCH, 227, 228, 229
Infectious aneurysm, 586
Infectious gastritis, 362
Inferior vena cava (IVC) filters, complications of, 581
    film of, questions and answers about, 603–604
    indications for, 581
    types of, 582
Infiltrate, radiographic definition of, 23
Inflammatory disorders, nuclear imaging of, 750–752
    acquisition parameters in, 750–751
    clinical applications in, 751–752
    distribution in, 751
    radiopharmaceuticals in, 750
Inflammatory polyp(s), in trachea, 35
Infrahyoid neck, 157
Infundibular mass, in adults, 123
    in children, 123
Ingested agents, causing gastric fold thickening, 310
Inguinal hernia, 652
Innominate artery, aneurysmal dilatation of, 27
Insulinoma, 406, 421
Interlobular septal thickening, CT definition of, 25
Interstitial lung disease. See *Lung disease, interstitial.*
Interstitium, radiographic definition of, 23
Interventricular septum, rupture of, 567
Intestinal duplication, 652–653
Intraaxial brain hemorrhage, 129–131
    in elderly patient, 131
    in young adult, 131
    multifocal, 132
Intraaxial brain lesions, 158–161
    ring-enhancing, differential diagnoses of, 115–116
Intraconal mass, 149–150
Intracranial hypotension, 134
Intrahepatic ductal stones, 404, 705
Intralobular interstitial thickening, CT definition of, 25
Intramammary lymph node(s), 517
    clinical and imaging signs of, 540
Intramedullary spinal lesions, clinical and imaging signs of, 168–169
    differential diagnoses of, 137–139
Intrathoracic mass(es), fetal, 682
Intrauterine growth retardation, 680
    clinical and imaging signs of, 713
Intrauterine pregnancy, 698
Intraventricular mass, cerebral, 125–126
    clinical and imaging signs of, 165–167
Intussusception, clinical and imaging signs of, 364–365
    colonic, 341, 344
    in children, 653
    jejunogastric, 306
    small bowel, 334
Invasive ductal carcinoma, of breast, 513, 518
    clinical and imaging signs of, 540–541
Invasive lobular carcinoma, of breast, 520–521
    clinical and imaging signs of, 541
Iodine-131, radioiodine therapy with, 741
Ischemia, colonic, 339, 343, 345
    clinical and imaging signs of, 365
    gastric, 312
    intramedullary, 138
    mesenteric, 587
    small bowel, 328